Ellis'
Clinical Anatomy
For Medical Students

To my wife, Wendy, and my late parents

H. E.

To my wife, Neila, and my late parents

V. M.

To my wife, Manorama, and my late parents

V. S.

Ellis'
Clinical Anatomy

For Medical Students

Harold Ellis

CBE, MA, DM, MCh, FRCS, FRCP, FRCOG, FACS (Hon)
Clinical Anatomist, Guy's, King's and St Thomas' School of Biomedical Sciences
Emeritus Professor of Surgery, Charing Cross
and Westminster Medical School, London
Formerly Examiner in Anatomy, Primary FRCS (Eng)

Vishy Mahadevan

MBBS, PhD, FRCSEd, FDSRCSEng (Hon), FRCS
Barbers' Company Professor of Anatomy & Professor of Surgical Anatomy
The Royal College of Surgeons of England
Lincoln's Inn Fields
London
Member of the Court of Examiners, RCS England

Vishram Singh

MBBS, MS, PhD (hc), FASI, MICPS
Professor and Head
Department of Anatomy
Santosh Medical College, Member of the Academic Council and Core Committee PhD Course
Santosh University
Ghaziabad, NCR Delhi
Editor-in-Chief, Journal of the Anatomical Society of India

First Indian Adaptation

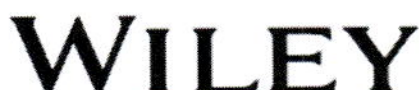

Clinical Anatomy
For Medical Students

Harold Ellis, Vishy Mahadevan and Vishram Singh

Authorised reprint by Wiley India Pvt. Ltd., 4435-36/7, Ansari Road, Daryaganj, New Delhi-110002.

First Indian Adaptation: 2015

ISBN: 978-81-265-5263-4

www.wileyindia.com

Printed at: Sanat Printers, Kundli

Contents

Preface to the First Indian Adaptation

Anatomy is the foundation for all branches of medicine, especially for the surgical branch. Unfortunately, there is a big gap between the anatomy taught to preclinical students and that they come across in wards and operation theatres of clinical specialities, viz. surgery, orthopaedic, ENT, gynaecology, paediatric, etc. Ellis' textbook on Clinical Anatomy was written to fill this gap. Anatomy is a vast subject, and Professor Harold Ellis and Professor Vishy Mahadevan performed a rigorous selection of the material to meet the needs of clinical students. This is one of the most interesting and readable resources in anatomy with frequent common clinical applications, enabling students to remember various important details. The text is well complemented by clear illustrations and imaging.

The First Indian Adaptation is prepared keeping in mind the needs of students, especially those of Indian subcontinent. A careful revision and modification of the text and illustrations has been carried out. A number of new figures and relevant text have been added wherever required. Moreover, the text has been made simple and student friendly. All the four-colour illustrations have followed the standard colour code of anatomical illustrations. While revising this edition, it has been ensured to preserve the essence of the original book compiled by Professor Ellis and Professor Mahadevan. I sincerely hope that this book will be of immense help not only to students of the Indian subcontinent but also to students across the globe.

Vishram Singh
February 2015

Preface to the Thirteenth Edition

As a teacher of medical students and surgical trainees, I know that much of clinical examination and diagnosis depends on an adequate knowledge of anatomy. No matter how good the doctors are at communication skills and patient empathy, unless they know what lies beneath their examining fingers or under the bell of their stethoscopes, they will have great difficulty in the interpretation of clinical signs. Understanding the exquisite details of modern radiological imaging also requires a good knowledge of the structure of the human body.

This was true over 50 years ago when I wrote the first edition of this book, and is perhaps even more so today, when anatomy in the medical student's curriculum has been greatly reduced.

Over these many years, during which time I have taught students and postgraduates in five medical schools, and examined them in eight countries and sixteen universities, my belief in the importance of an adequate knowledge of anatomy as an adjunct to clinical training has been strongly reinforced.

In the preparation of the 12th edition and this edition, I have been fortunate indeed in having been able to recruit Professor Vishy Mahadevan, the Barbers' Company Professor of Anatomy at the Royal College of Surgeons of England, as co-author. He is a renowned and revered teacher of surgical trainees as well as being a current examiner in the MRCS and in overseas medical schools. Together, in this new edition, we have carried out a careful revision and updating of the text and diagrams, as well as adding new figures and images.

We hope that this book will continue to help our students and postgraduate trainees throughout the English-speaking world.

Harold Ellis
July 2013

Preface to the First Edition

Experience of teaching clinical students at three medical schools has convinced me that there is still an unfortunate hiatus between the anatomy which the student learns in his pre-clinical years and that which he later encounters in the wards and operating theatres.

This book attempts to bridge this gap. It does so by high-lighting those features of anatomy which are of clinical importance, in medicine and midwifery as well as in surgery. It presents the facts which a student might reasonably be expected to carry with him during his years on the wards, through final examinations and into his post-graduate years; it is designed for the clinical student.

Anatomy is a vast subject and therefore, in order to achieve this goal, I have deliberately carried out a rigorous selection of material so as to cover only those of its thousands of facts which I consider form the necessary anatomical scaffolding for the clinician. Wherever possible practical applications are indicated throughout the text – they cannot, within the limitations of a book of this size, be exhaustive, but I hope that they will act as signposts to the student and indicate how many clinical phenomena can be understood and remembered on simple anatomical grounds.

Harold Ellis
Oxford, 1960

Acknowledgements to the First Indian Adaptation

We are delighted to see the publication of the First Indian Adaptation of Clinical Anatomy, a book which originally appeared in England more than 50 years ago! We wish to thank the many students, both undergraduates and postgraduates in the UK and overseas, who have taken the trouble to send us many helpful and constructive suggestions. Several of these have been incorporated in this edition. CT and MRI scans used in this edition were provided by Dr Sheila Rankin and Dr Jeremy Rabouhans of the Department of Radiology at Guy's Hospital, London, and Professor Adrian Dixon of the Department of Radiology at Addenbrooke's Hospital, Cambridge. Our thanks to all three. We extend our gratitude to Jane Fallowes for some of the artworks in this edition.

We wish to thank Dr Vallika Devi for initiating work on the Indian Adaptation. We would like to express our sincere thanks to Dr Deepa Singh of the Department of Anatomy at Himalayan Institute of Medical Sciences, Jolly Grant Dehradun, Uttarakhand, for going through the entire text and making valuable comments. We are highly indebted to Mr Krishna Chaitanya Reddy, PhD scholar in the Department of Anatomy at Santosh Medical College, Ghaziabad, NCR Delhi, for going through proofs sincerely and making corrections wherever necessary. Finally, we wish to express our debt to Dr Bushra Rashid and her colleagues at Wiley India for their invaluable help, support and guidance.

Harold Ellis
Vishy Mahadevan
Vishram Singh
(February 2015)

About the Companion Website

Clinical Anatomy has its own resources website:
www.ellisclinicalanatomy.co.uk/13edition
with digital flashcards of the images from the book for easy revision.

Part I

The thorax

Introduction

The clinical anatomy of the thorax is in daily use in clinical practice. The routine examination of the patient's chest is nothing more than an exercise in relating the deep structures of the thorax to the chest wall. Moreover, so many common procedures – chest aspiration, insertion of a chest drain or of a subclavian line, placement of a cardiac pacemaker, for example – have their basis, and their safe performance, in sound anatomical knowledge.

Surface anatomy and surface markings

A good clinician should be able to relate the surface anatomy of his patients to their deep structures (Fig. 1.1; *see also* Figs 1.12 and 1.27).

The following bony prominences can usually be palpated in the living subject (corresponding vertebral levels are given in brackets):

- Superior angle of the scapula (T2)
- Upper border of the manubrium sterni, the suprasternal notch (T2/3)
- Spine of the scapula (T3)
- Sternal angle (of Louis) – the transverse ridge at the manubriosternal junction (T4/5)
- Inferior angle of the scapula (T8); it also overlies the 7th rib
- Xiphisternal joint (T9)
- Lowest part of the costal margin – 10th rib (the subcostal line passes through L3)

Note from Fig. 1.1 that the manubrium sterni corresponds to the 3rd and 4th thoracic vertebrae and overlies the aortic arch, and that the body of the sternum corresponds to the 5th–8th vertebrae and neatly overlies the heart.

Since the 1st and 12th ribs are difficult to feel, the ribs should be counted from the 2nd costal cartilage, which articulates with the sternum at the angle of Louis.

The spinous processes of all the thoracic vertebrae can be palpated in the midline posteriorly, but it should be remembered that the first spinous process that can be felt is that of C7 (the **vertebra prominens**).

The position of the *nipple* varies considerably in the female, but in the male it usually overlies the 4th intercostal space approximately 4 in. (10 cm) from the midline. The *apex beat*, which marks the lowest and outermost point at which the cardiac impulse can be palpated, is normally in the 5th intercostal space 3.5 in. (9 cm) from the midline and within the midclavicular line. (This corresponds to just below and medial to the nipple in the male, but it is always better to use bony rather than soft-tissue points of reference.)

The *trachea* is palpable in the suprasternal notch midway between the heads of the two clavicles.

Trachea (Figs 1.1 and 1.2)

The trachea commences in the neck at the level of the lower border of the cricoid cartilage (C6) and runs vertically downwards to end at the level of the sternal angle of Louis (T4/5), just to the right of the midline, by dividing to form the

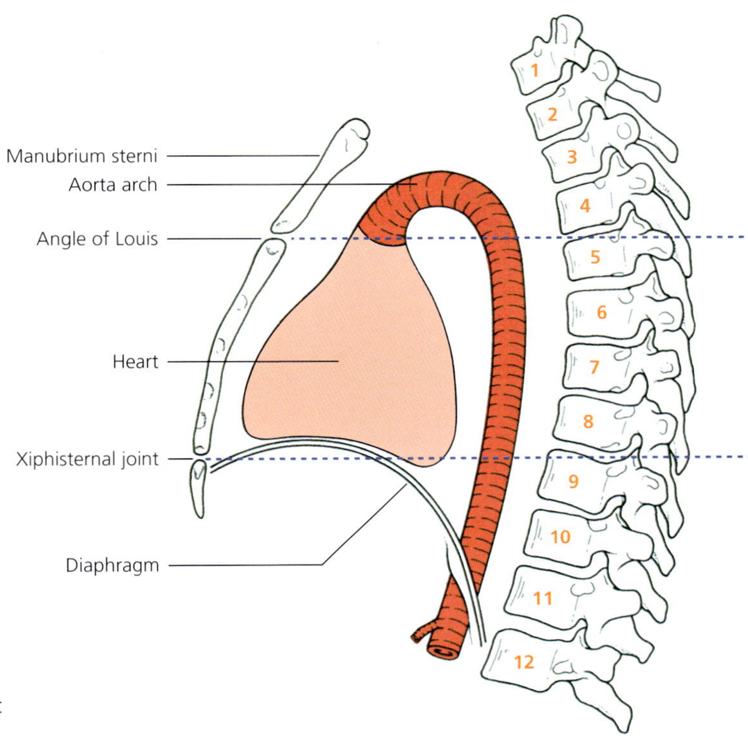

Figure 1.1 Lateral view of the thorax – its surface markings and vertebral levels. (Note that the angle of Louis (T4/5) demarcates the superior mediastinum, the upper margin of the heart and the beginning and end of the aortic arch.)

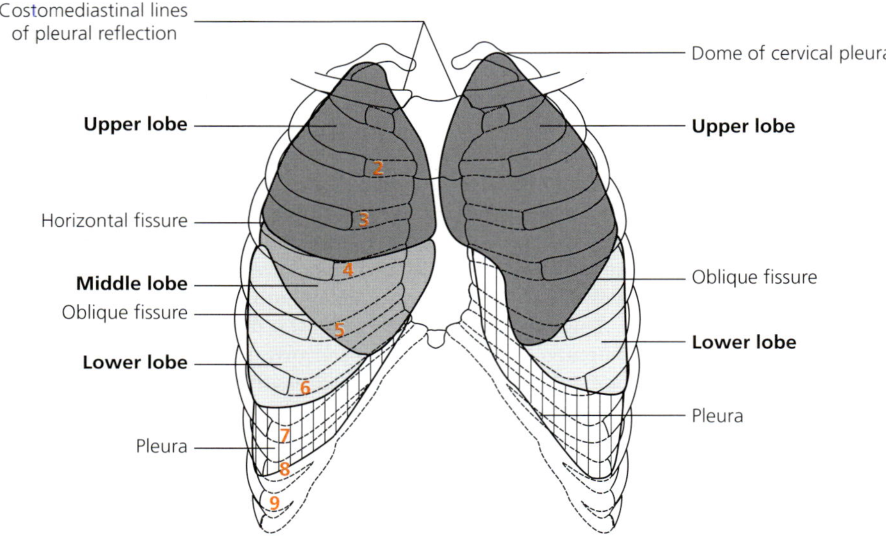

Figure 1.2 The surface markings of the lungs and pleura – anterior view.

right and left principal/main bronchi. In the erect posture and in full inspiration, the level of tracheal bifurcation lies at the level of lower border of T6.

Pleura (Figs 1.2 and 1.3)

The *cervical pleura* can be marked out on the surface by a curved convex line drawn from the sternoclavicular joint to the junction of the medial and middle thirds of the clavicle; the apex of the pleura is approximately 1 in. (2.5 cm) above the clavicle. This fact is easily explained by the oblique slope of the 1st rib. It is important because the pleura can be wounded (with consequent pneumothorax) by a stab wound – and this includes the surgeon's knife and the anaesthetist's needle – above the clavicle, or, in an attempted subclavian vein catheterization, below the clavicle. The *costomediastinal lines* of pleural reflexion pass from behind the sternoclavicular joint on each side to meet in the midline at the 2nd costal cartilage (the angle of Louis). The right pleural edge then passes vertically downwards to the 6th costal cartilage and then crosses the following:

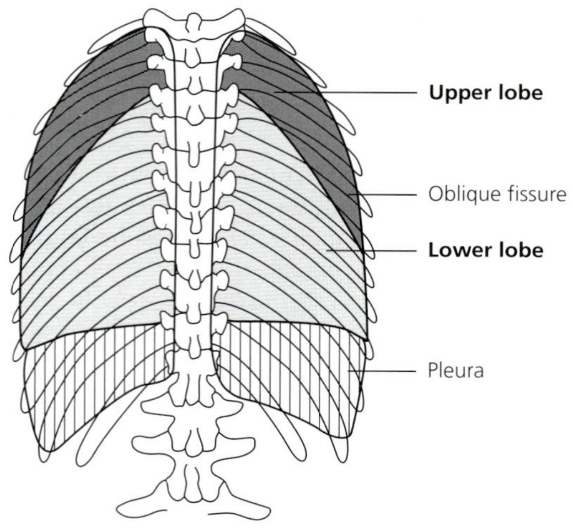

Figure 1.3 The surface markings of the lungs and pleura – posterior view.

- The 8th rib in the midclavicular line
- The 10th rib in the midaxillary line
- The 12th rib at the lateral border of the erector spinae

On the left side the pleural edge arches laterally at the 4th costal cartilage and descends lateral to the border of the sternum, up to the 6th costal cartilage, owing, of course, to its lateral displacement by the heart; apart from this, its relationships are those of the right side.

The inferior margin/costodiaphragmatic line of pleural reflection passes laterally from the lower end of costomediastinal line of pleural reflection. In this event, it crosses 8th rib in the midclavicular line, 10th rib in the midaxillary line and 12th rib at the lateral border of sacrospinalis muscle. Further, it continues below the 12th rib to the lower border T12 vertebra 2 cm lateral to the upper border of T12 spine.

As the pleura descends just below the 12th rib margin at its medial extremity – or even below the edge of the 11th rib if the 12th is unusually short; obviously, in this situation, the pleura may be opened accidentally in making a loin incision to expose the kidney, perform an adrenalectomy or drain a subphrenic abscess.

Lungs (Figs 1.2 and 1.3)

The surface projection of the lung is somewhat less extensive than that of the parietal pleura as outlined above, and in addition it varies quite considerably with the phase of respiration.

The *apex* of the lung closely corresponds to the line of the cervical pleura. The surface marking of the *anterior border of the right lung* corresponds to that of the right mediastinal pleura. On the left side, however, the *anterior border* has a distinct notch (the ***cardiac notch***) that passes behind the 5th and 6th costal cartilages. The *lower border* of the lung has an excursion of as much as 2–3 in. (5–8 cm) in the extremes of respiration, but in the neutral position (midway between inspiration and expiration) it lies along a line which crosses the 6th rib in the midclavicular line, the 8th rib in the midaxillary line and the 10th rib at the lateral border of sacrospinalis and ends 2 cm lateral to the T10 spine posteriorly.

The *oblique fissure*, which divides the lung into upper and lower lobes, is indicated on the surface by a line drawn obliquely downwards and outwards from 1 in. (2.5 cm) lateral to the spine of the 3rd thoracic vertebra (T3) along the 5th intercostal space to the 6th costal cartilage approximately 1.5 in. (4 cm) from the midline. This can be represented approximately by abducting the shoulder to its full extent; the line of the oblique fissure then corresponds to the position of the medial border of the scapula.

The surface markings of the horizontal *transverse fissure* (separating the middle and upper lobes of the right lung) is a line drawn horizontally along the 4th costal cartilage and meeting the oblique fissure where the latter crosses the 5th rib in the midaxillary line.

Heart (Fig. 1.4)

The outline of the heart can be represented on the surface by an irregular quadrangle bounded by the following four points (Fig. 1.4):

1. Point on the 2nd *left* costal cartilage 0.5 in. (1.25 cm) from the edge of the sternum
2. Point on the 3rd *right* costal cartilage 0.5 in. (1.25 cm) from the sternal edge
3. Point on the 6th *right* costal cartilage 0.5 in. (1.25 cm) from the sternum
4. Point on the 5th *left* intercostal space 3.5 in. (9 cm) from the midline (corresponding to the apex beat)

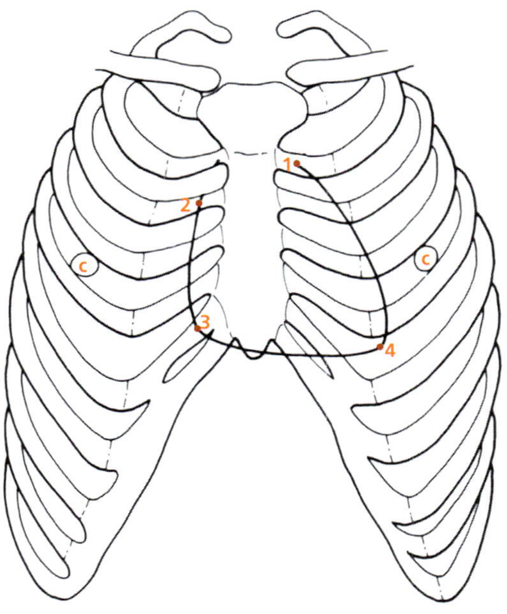

Figure 1.4 The surface markings of the heart.

The *left border* of the heart (indicated by the curved line fairly convex to the left joining points 1 and 4) is formed almost entirely by the left ventricle (the auricular appendage of the left atrium peeping around this border superiorly); the *right border* (marked by the line joining points 2 and 3) is formed by the right atrium (*see* Fig. 1.29(a)); the *lower border* (the horizontal line joining points 3 and 4) corresponds to the right ventricle and the apical part of the left ventricle.

A good guide to the size and position of your own heart is given by placing your clenched right fist palmar surface down immediately inferior to the manubriosternal junction. Note that the heart is approximately the size of the subject's fist, lies behind the body of the sternum (therefore anterior to thoracic vertebrae 5–8) and bulges over to the left side.

The surface markings of the vessels of the thoracic wall are of importance if these structures are to be avoided in performing aspiration of the chest. The *internal thoracic* (*internal mammary*) *vessels* run vertically downwards behind the costal cartilages 0.5 in. (1.25 cm) from the lateral border of the sternum. The intercostal vessels lie immediately below their corresponding ribs (the vein above the artery) so that it is safe to pass a needle immediately *above* a rib, but dangerous to pass it immediately *below* (*see* Fig. 1.8).

Thoracic cage

The thoracic cage is formed by the vertebral column behind, the ribs on either side and the sternum and costal cartilages in front. Above, it communicates through the 'thoracic inlet' with the root of the neck; below, it is separated from the abdominal cavity by the diaphragm (Fig. 1.1).

Thoracic vertebrae

See 'Vertebral column', page 197. Fig. 5.48.

Ribs

The greater part of the thoracic cage is formed by the 12 pairs of ribs. Of these, the first seven ('**true ribs**') are connected anteriorly by way of their costal cartilages to the sternum, the cartilages of the 8th, 9th and 10th articulate each with the cartilage of the rib above ('**false ribs**') and the last two ribs are free anteriorly ('**floating ribs**').

Each typical rib (Fig. 1.5(a)) has a *head* bearing two articular facets, for articulation with the upper demifacet on the side of the body of the numerically corresponding thoracic vertebra and the lower demifacet of the vertebra above (*see* Fig. 5.48). Thus, the head of the 3rd rib articulates with its own third vertebral body and the one above. The head continues as a stout *neck*, which gives attachment to the costotransverse ligaments, a *tubercle* with a rough non-articular portion and a smooth facet, for articulation with the transverse process of the corresponding vertebra, long shaft is flattened from side to side and twisted at an 'angle' of the rib. The angle of rib lies 2 in. (5 cm) lateral to tubercle. The angle demarcates the lateral limit of attachment of the erector spinae muscle.

The features of the first two and last three ribs differ from that of a typical rib; hence, they are termed as atypical ribs.

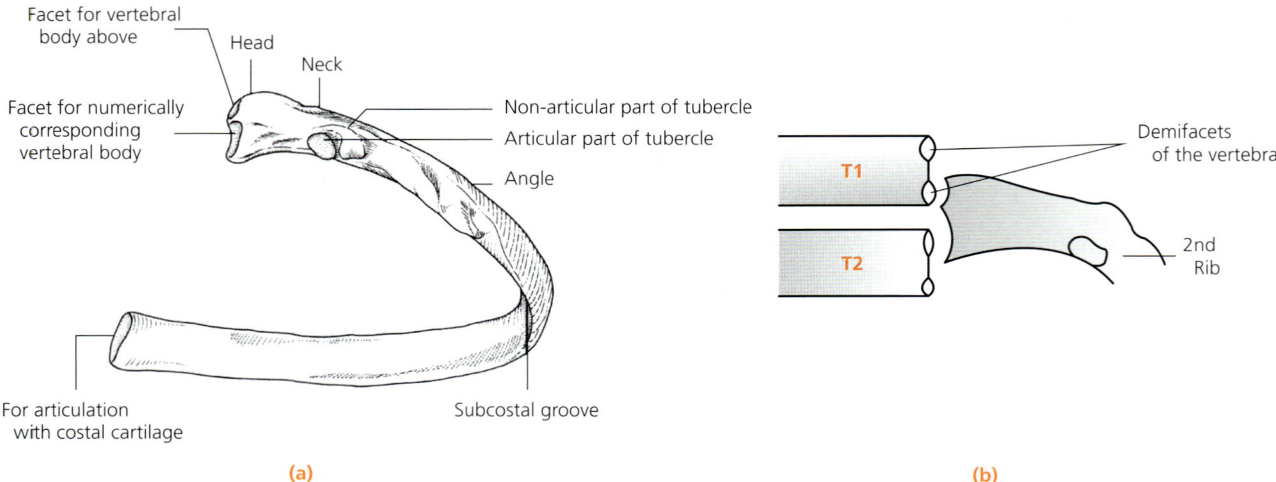

Figure 1.5 (a) A typical rib. (b) Costovertebral joint.

The following are the significant features of the 'atypical' ribs.

The *1st rib* (Fig. 1.6) is flattened from above downwards. It is not only the flattest but also the shortest and most highly curved of all the ribs. It has a prominent *tubercle* on the inner border of its upper surface for the insertion of scalenus anterior. In front of this tubercle, the subclavian vein crosses the rib; behind the tubercle is the *subclavian groove*, where the subclavian artery and lowest trunk of the brachial plexus lie in relation to the bone. This is one of the sites where the anaesthetist can infiltrate the plexus with local anaesthetic.

Crossing the front of the neck of the 1st rib from the medial to the lateral side are the sympathetic trunk, the 1st posterior intercostal vein, the superior intercostal artery (from the costocervical trunk) and the large branch of the ventral ramus of the 1st thoracic nerve to the brachial plexus.

The *2nd rib* is much less curved than the 1st, and its length is approximately twice that of the 1st rib.

The *10th rib* has only one articular facet on the head.

The *11th* and *12th ribs* (*the* ***'floating ribs'***) are short, have no tubercles and only a single facet on the head. The 11th rib has a slight angle and a shallow subcostal groove; the 12th has neither of these features.

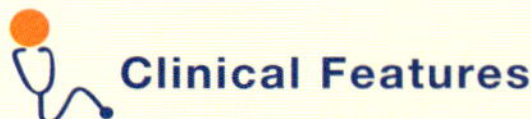

Clinical Features

Rib fractures

The chest wall of the child is highly elastic and therefore fractures of the rib in children are rare. In adults, the ribs may be fractured by direct violence or indirectly by crushing injuries; in the latter, the rib tends to give way at its weakest part in the region of its angle. Not unnaturally, the upper two ribs, which are protected by the clavicle, and the lower two ribs, which are unattached anteriorly, and therefore swing freely, are the least commonly injured.

In a severe crush injury to the chest several ribs may fracture in front and behind so that a whole segment of the thoracic cage becomes torn free ('stove-in chest'). With each inspiration, this loose flap sucks in; with each expiration, it blows out; thus undergoing paradoxical respiratory movement. The associated swinging movements of the mediastinum produce severe shock, and this injury calls for urgent treatment by insertion of a chest drain with underwater seal, followed by endotracheal

(Continued ...)

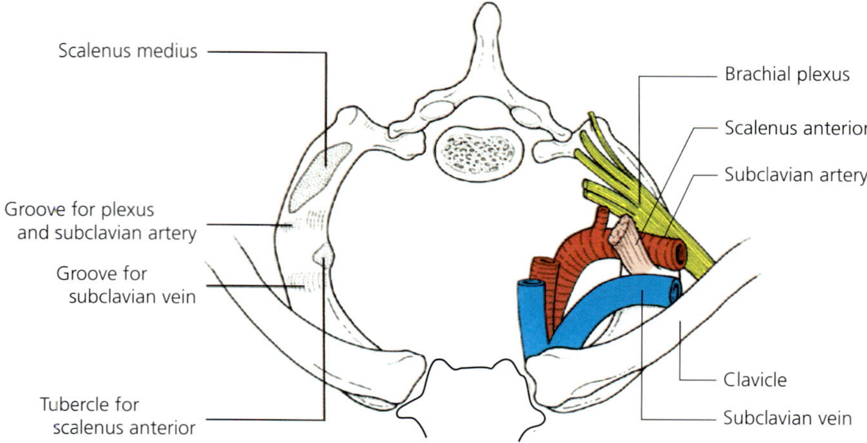

Figure 1.6 Structures crossing the 1st rib.

(... *continued*)

intubation, or tracheostomy, combined with positive pressure respiration.

Coarctation of the aorta (*see* Fig. 1.40(b) and page 27)

In coarctation of the aorta, the intercostal arteries derived from the aorta receive blood from the superior intercostals (from the costocervical trunk of the subclavian artery), from the anterior intercostal branches of the internal thoracic artery (arising from the subclavian artery) and from the arteries anastomosing around the scapula. Together with the communication between the internal thoracic and inferior epigastric arteries, they provide the principal collaterals between the aorta above and below the block. In consequence, the intercostal arteries undergo dilatation and tortuosity and erode the lower borders of the corresponding ribs to give the characteristic irregular *notching of the ribs*, which is very useful in the radiographic confirmation of this lesion.

Cervical rib

A cervical rib (Fig. 1.7) occurs in 0.5% of subjects and is bilateral in half of these. It is attached to the transverse process of the 7th cervical vertebra and articulates with the 1st (thoracic) rib or, if short, has a free distal extremity which usually attaches by a fibrous strand to the (normal) 1st rib. Pressure of such a rib on the lowest trunk of the brachial plexus arching over it may produce paraesthesiae along the ulnar border of the forearm and wasting of the small muscles of the hand (T1). Less commonly, vascular changes, even gangrene, may be caused by pressure of the rib on the overlying subclavian artery.

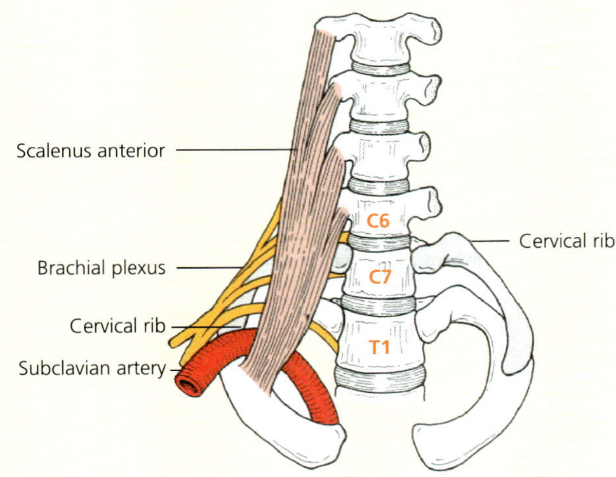

Figure 1.7 Bilateral cervical ribs. On the right side the brachial plexus is shown arching over the rib and stretching its lowest trunk.

Costal cartilages

These bars of hyaline cartilage serve to connect the upper seven ribs directly to the side of the sternum and the 8th, 9th and 10th ribs to the cartilage immediately above. The cartilages of the 11th and 12th ribs merely join the tapered extremities of these ribs and end in the abdominal musculature.

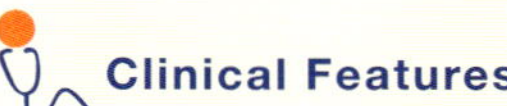

1. The cartilage adds considerable resilience to the thoracic cage and protects the sternum and ribs from more frequent fracture.
2. In old age (and sometimes also in young adults), the costal cartilages undergo progressive ossification; they then become radio-opaque and may give rise to some confusion when examining a chest radiograph of an elderly patient.

Sternum

This dagger-shaped bone, which forms the anterior median part of the thoracic cage, consists of three parts. The *manubrium* is roughly triangular in outline and provides articulation for the clavicles and for the first and upper part of the 2nd costal cartilages on either side. It is situated opposite the 3rd and 4th thoracic vertebrae. Opposite the disc between T4 and T5 it articulates at an oblique angle at the manubriosternal joint (the **angle of Louis**) with the *body of the sternum* (placed opposite T5–T8). This is composed of four parts or '**sternebrae**', which fuse between puberty and 25 years of age. Its lateral border is notched to receive part of the 2nd and the 3rd to the 7th costal cartilages. The *xiphoid process* is the smallest part of the sternum and usually remains cartilaginous well into adult life. The cartilaginous manubriosternal joint and that between the xiphoid and the body of the sternum may also become ossified after the age of 30.

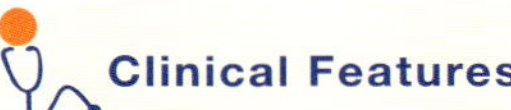

1. The attachment of the elastic costal cartilages largely protects the sternum from injury, but indirect violence accompanying fracture dislocation of the thoracic spine may be associated with a sternal fracture. Direct violence to the sternum may lead to displacement of the relatively mobile body of the sternum backwards from the relatively fixed manubrium.
2. In a *sternal puncture*, a wide-bore needle is pushed through the thin layer of cortical bone covering the sternum into the highly vascular spongy bone beneath, and a specimen of bone marrow aspirated with a syringe.
3. In operations on the thymus gland, and occasionally for a retrosternal goitre, it is necessary to split the manubrium in the midline in order to gain access to the superior mediastinum. A complete vertical split of the whole sternum is one of the standard approaches to the heart and great vessels used in modern open cardiac surgery.

Intercostal spaces

There are slight variations between the different intercostal spaces, but typically each space contains *three muscles*, comparable to those of the abdominal wall, and an associated *neurovascular bundle* (Fig. 1.8).

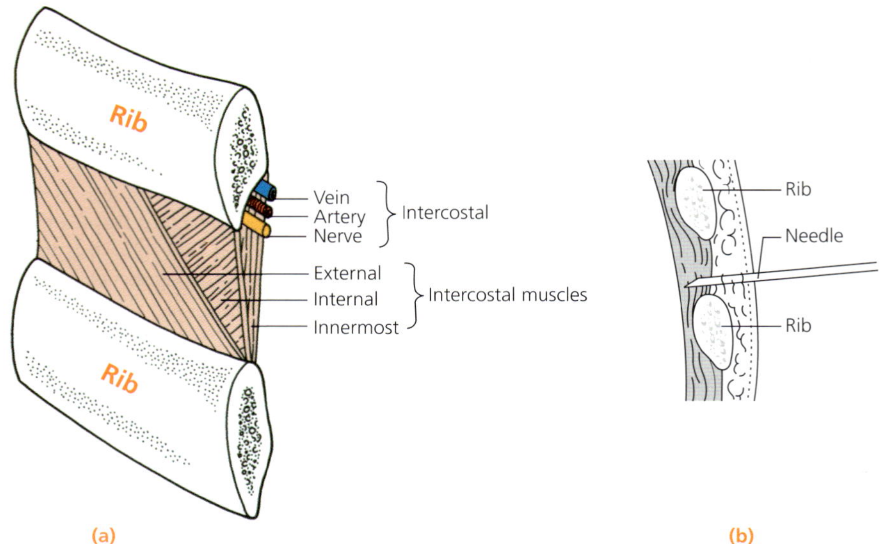

Figure 1.8 The intercostal space. **(a)** The relationship of structures in an intercostal space. **(b)** A needle passed through intercostal space into the chest immediately *above* a rib will avoid the neurovascular bundle.

Muscles

The muscles are as follows:

1. **External intercostal:** Its fibres pass downwards and forwards from the rib above to the rib below and reach from the vertebrae behind to the costochondral junction in front, where muscle is replaced by the *anterior intercostal membrane.*
2. **Internal intercostal:** It runs downwards and backwards from the sternum to the angles of the ribs where it becomes the *posterior intercostal membrane*.
3. **Innermost intercostal:** It is only incompletely separated from the internal intercostal muscle by the neurovascular bundle. The fibres of this sheet cross more than one intercostal space and it may be incomplete. Anteriorly, it has a more distinct portion that is fan-like in shape, termed the ***transversus thoracis*** (or ***sternocostalis***), which spreads upwards from the posterior aspect of the lower sternum to insert onto the inner surfaces of the 2nd to the 6th costal cartilages.

Neurovascular bundles

Just as in the abdomen, the nerves and vessels of the thoracic wall lie between the middle and innermost layers of muscles. This neurovascular bundle consists, from above downwards, of vein, artery and nerve, the vein lying in a groove on the undersurface of the corresponding rib (remember: v,a,n).

Intercostal arteries

They comprise the posterior and anterior intercostals.

The *posterior intercostal arteries* of the lower nine spaces are branches of the thoracic aorta, while the first two are derived from the superior intercostal branch of the costocervical trunk, the only branch of the second part of the subclavian artery. Each runs forward in the subcostal groove to anastomose with the anterior intercostal artery. Each has a number of branches to adjacent muscles, to the skin and to the spinal cord. The corresponding veins are mostly tributaries of the azygos and hemiazygos veins. The 1st posterior intercostal vein drains into the brachiocephalic or vertebral vein. On the left, the 2nd and 3rd veins often join to form a superior intercostal vein, which crosses the aortic arch to drain into the left brachiocephalic vein.

The *anterior intercostal arteries* are branches of the internal thoracic artery (1st–6th space) or of its musculophrenic branch (7th–9th spaces). The lowest two spaces have only posterior arteries. Perforating branches pierce the upper five or six intercostal spaces; those of the 2nd–4th spaces are large in the female and supply the breast.

Intercostal nerves

They are the anterior primary rami of the thoracic nerves, each of which gives off a collateral muscular branch and lateral and anterior cutaneous branches for the innervation of the thoracic and abdominal walls (Fig. 1.9).

Internal thoracic artery (Fig. 1.10)

The internal thoracic artery arises from the first part of the subclavian artery opposite the thyrocervical trunk. It runs downwards and medially, in front of cervical pleura up to the 1st costal cartilage. Thereafter, it runs vertically downwards behind the thoracic cage up to the 6th intercostal space where it terminates by dividing into superior epigastric and musculophrenic arteries.

Branches

The internal thoracic artery gives off six sets of branches as follows:

1. **Pericardiophrenic artery:** This arises in the root of the neck.
2. **Mediastinal arteries:** They supply mediastinal structures.

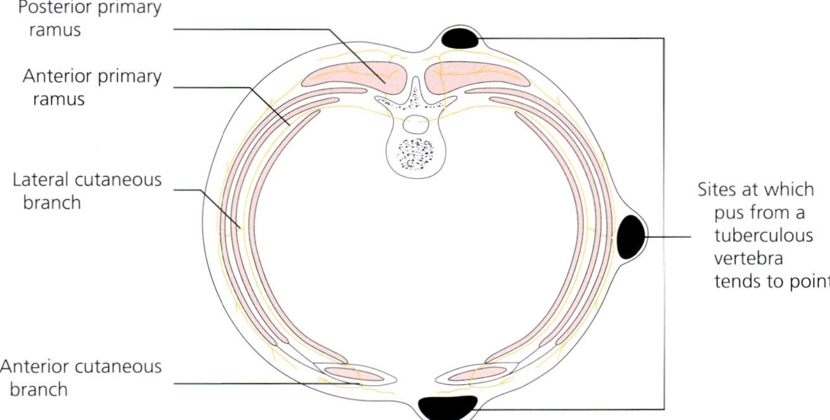

Figure 1.9 Diagram of a typical spinal nerve and its body–wall relationships. On the left side, the sites of eruption of a tuberculous cold abscess tracking forwards from a diseased vertebra are shown – these occur at the points of emergence of the cutaneous branches.

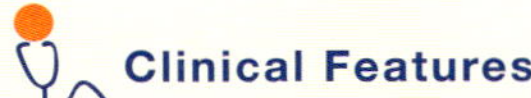

Clinical Features

1 Local irritation of the intercostal nerves by such conditions as Pott's disease of the thoracic vertebrae (tuberculosis) may give rise to pain that is referred to the front of the chest or abdomen in the region of the peripheral termination of the nerves.
2 Local anaesthesia of an intercostal space is easily produced by infiltration around the intercostal nerve trunk and its collateral branch – a procedure known as *intercostal nerve block*.
3 Insertion of an emergency chest drain, for example for a traumatic haemo-pneumothorax, is performed through the 5th intercostal space in the midaxillary line. Under local anaesthetic, an incision is made through the skin and subcutaneous tissue. The rest of the procedure is carried out by blunt dissection over the upper edge of the lower rib. In this way, injury to the intercostal bundle in the subcostal groove is avoided. A finger is passed into the pleural space to ensure that there are no lung adhesions in the vicinity and to confirm that the pleural cavity is entered. A chest tube is then placed into the pleural space, connected to an underwater drain and firmly sutured in place.
4 In a conventional posterolateral thoracotomy (e.g. for a pulmonary lobectomy) an incision is made along the line of the 5th or 6th rib; the periosteum over a segment of the rib is elevated, thus protecting the neurovascular bundle, and the rib is excised. Access to the lung or mediastinum is then gained though the intercostal space, which can be opened out considerably owing to the elasticity of the thoracic cage.
5 Pus from the region of the vertebral column tends to track around the thorax along the course of the neurovascular bundle and to 'point' to the three sites of exit of the cutaneous branches of the intercostal nerves, which are lateral to erector spinae (sacrospinalis), in the midaxillary line and just lateral to the sternum (Fig. 1.9).
6 The internal thoracic artery, especially, that of the left side (due to its easy access) is often used for coronary graft. It is observed that the internal thoracic artery is less prone to develop atherosclerosis due to its histological peculiarity.

3. **Aterior intercostal arteries:** They are two for each of the upper six intercostal spaces.
4. **Perforating branches**: These branches accompany anterior cutaneous nerves. In females, branches to 2nd, 3rd and 4th intercostal spaces are large and supply the breast.
5. **Superior epigastric artery:** It runs downward to enter the rectus sheath.
6. **Musculophrenic artery:** It runs downwards and laterally and gives off arterial intercostal arteries to 7th, 8th and 9th spaces.

Diaphragm

The diaphragm is the dome-shaped septum dividing the thoracic from the abdominal cavity. It comprises two portions: a peripheral muscular part that arises from the margins of the thoracic outlet and a centrally placed aponeurosis (Fig. 1.11).

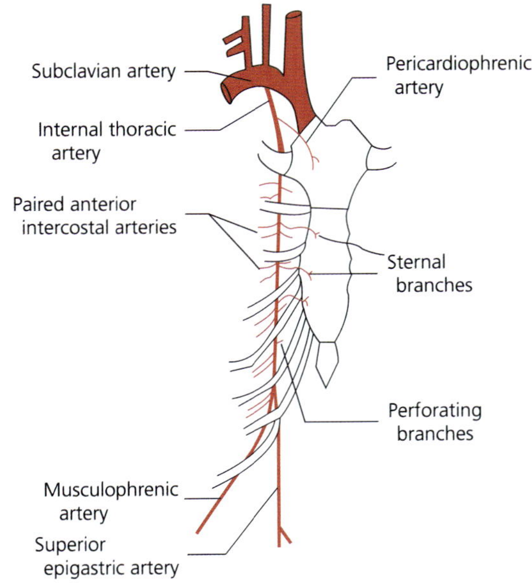

Figure 1.10 Origin, course, termination and branches of internal thoracic artery.

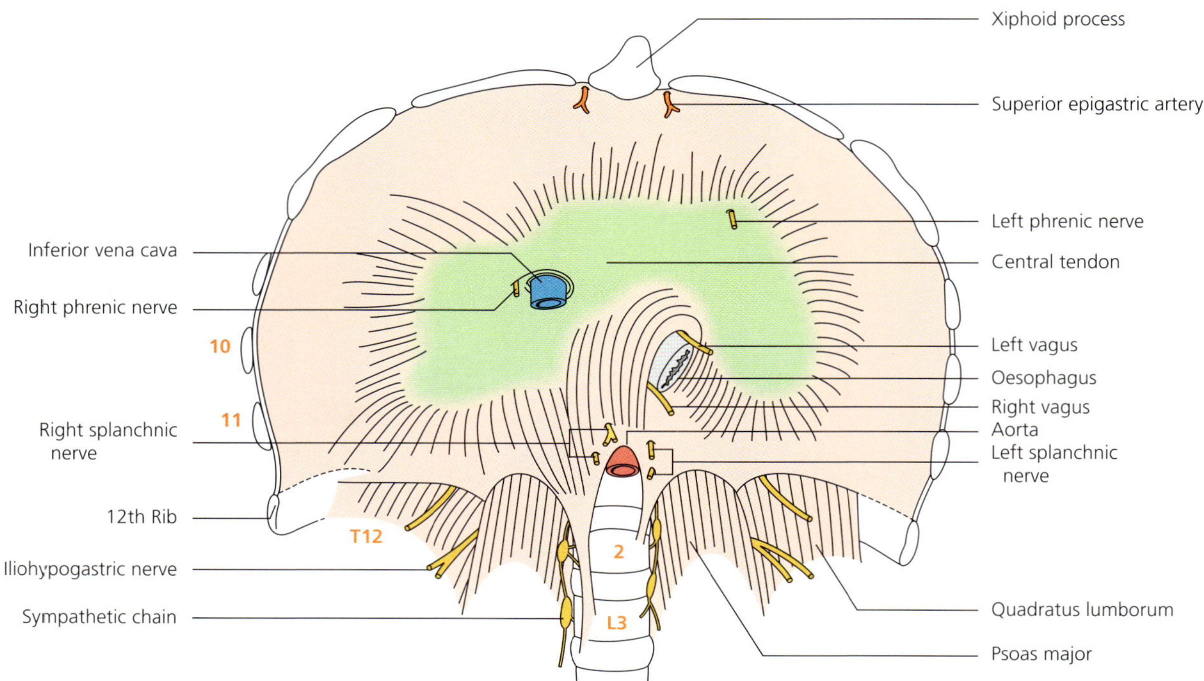

Figure 1.11 The diaphragm – inferior aspect. The three major orifices, from above downwards, transmit the inferior vena cava, oesophagus and aorta.

The muscular fibres are arranged in the following three parts:

1. A *vertebral part* from the crura and from the arcuate ligaments. The *right crus* arises from the front of the bodies of the upper three lumbar vertebrae and intervertebral discs; the *left crus* is attached to only the first two vertebrae. The arcuate *ligaments* are a series of fibrous arches, the *medial* being a thickening of the fascia covering psoas major and the *lateral* of the fascia overlying quadratus lumborum. The fibrous medial borders of the two crura form a *median arcuate ligament* over the front of the aorta.
2. A *costal part* is attached to the inner aspect of the lower six ribs and costal cartilages.
3. A *sternal portion* consists of two small slips from the deep surface of the xiphisternum.

The central tendon, into which the muscular fibres are inserted, is trefoil in shape and is partially fused with the undersurface of the pericardium.

The diaphragm receives its entire motor supply from the phrenic nerve (C3, C4, C5), whose long course from the neck follows the embryological migration of the muscle of the diaphragm from the cervical region (*see* the following sections). Injury or operative division of this nerve results in paralysis and elevation of the corresponding half of the diaphragm.

Radiographically, paralysis of the diaphragm is recognized by its elevation and paradoxical movement; instead of descending on inspiration, it is forced upwards by pressure from the abdominal viscera.

The sensory nerve fibres from the central part of the diaphragm also run in the phrenic nerve; hence, irritation of the diaphragmatic pleura (in pleurisy) or of the peritoneum on the undersurface of the diaphragm by subphrenic collections of pus or blood produces referred pain in the corresponding cutaneous area, the shoulder-tip.

The peripheral part of the diaphragm, including the crura, receives sensory fibres from the lower intercostal nerves.

Openings in the diaphragm

The three main openings in the diaphragm (Figs 1.11 and 1.12) are as follows:

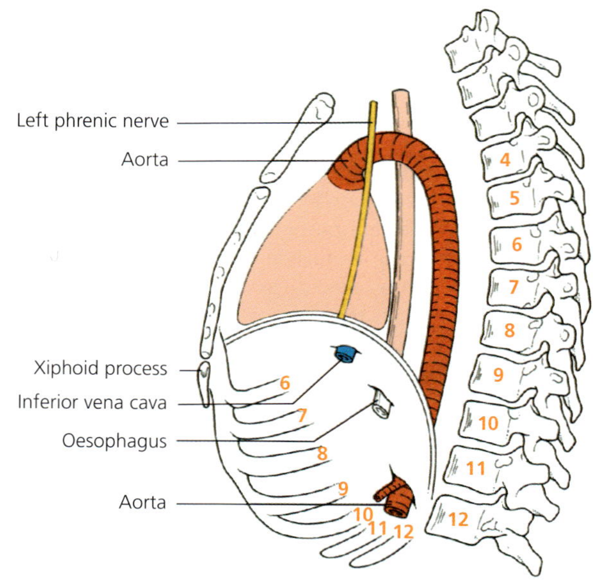

Figure 1.12 Schematic lateral view of the diaphragm to show the levels at which it is pierced by major structures.

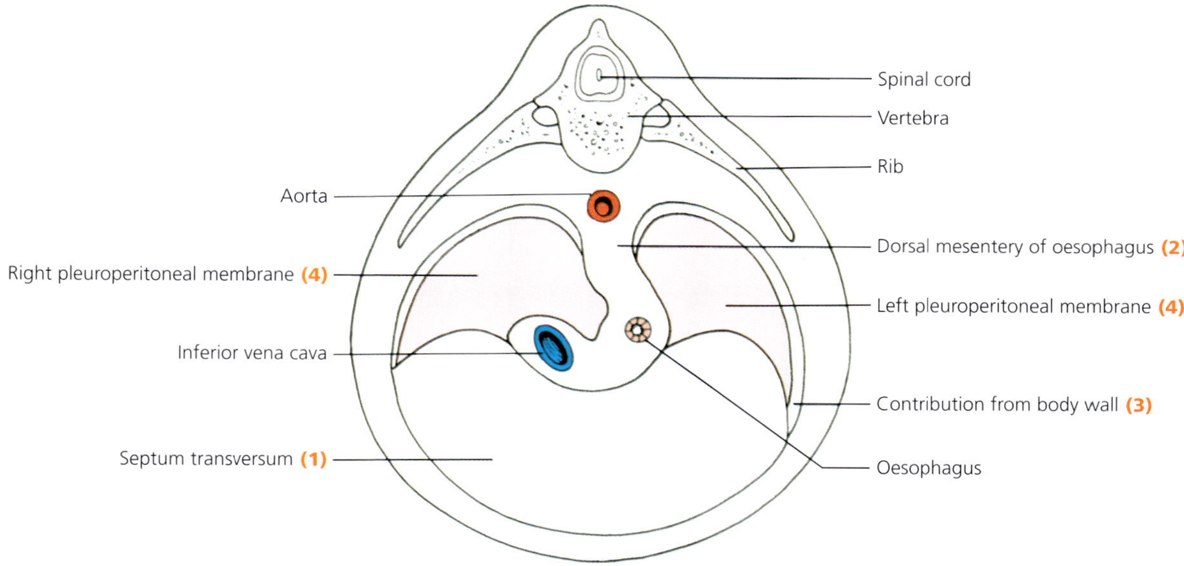

Figure 1.13 The development of the diaphragm, showing the four elements contributing to the diaphragm: (1) septum transversum, (2) dorsal mesentery of the oesophagus, (3) body wall and (4) the pleuroperitoneal membrane.

1. **Aortic opening (at the level of T12):** It is osseoaponeurotic and transmits the abdominal aorta, the thoracic duct and often the azygos vein.
2. **Oesophageal opening (at the level of T10):** It is situated between the muscular fibres of the right crus of the diaphragm and transmits oesophagus, branches of the left gastric artery and vein and the right and left vagus nerves.
3. **Opening for the inferior vena cava (at the level of T8):** It is placed in the central tendon of diaphragm and transmits inferior vena cava and right phrenic nerve.

In addition to these structures, the greater and lesser splanchnic nerves (*see* page 31) pierce the crura and the sympathetic chain passes behind the diaphragm deep to the medial arcuate ligament of the corresponding side.

Development of the diaphragm and the anatomy of diaphragmatic herniae

The diaphragm is formed (Fig. 1.13) in the embryo by fusion of the following:

1. *Septum transversum* (forming the central tendon)
2. *Dorsal oesophageal mesentery*
3. A peripheral rim derived from the *body wall*
4. *Pleuroperitoneal membranes*, which close the foetal communication between the pleural and peritoneal cavities

The septum transversum is the mesoderm which, in early development, lies in front of the head end of the embryo. With the folding off of the head, this mesodermal mass is carried ventrally and caudally to lie in its definitive position at the

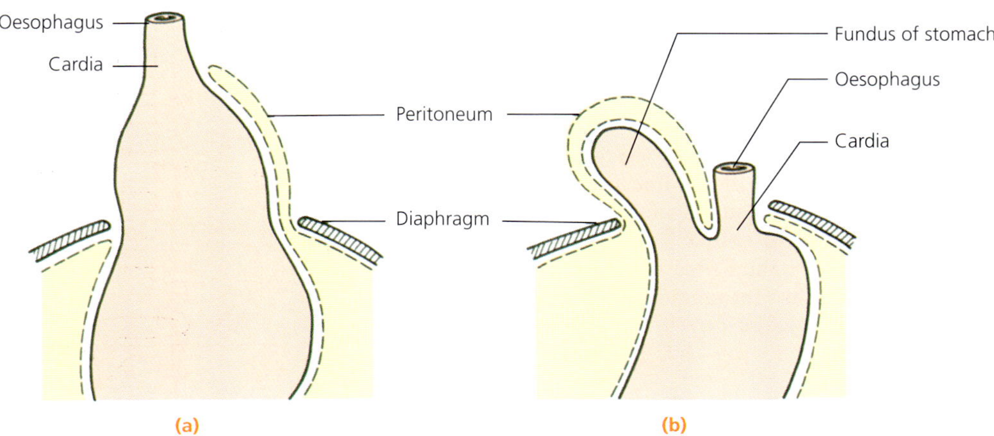

Figure 1.14 (a) A sliding hiatus hernia. (b) A rolling hiatus hernia.

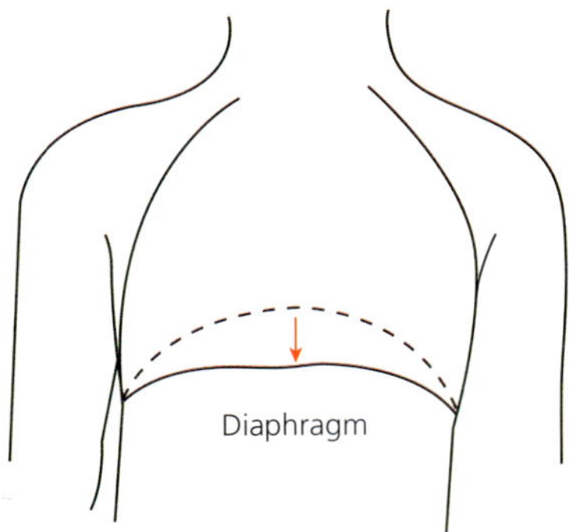

Figure 1.15 Increase in the vertical diameter of the thoracic cavity due to contraction of diaphragm.

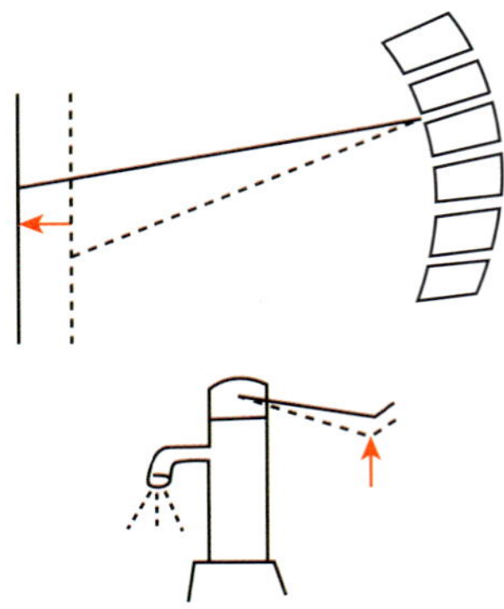

Figure 1.16 Pump handle movement to increase the anteroposterior diameter.

anterior part of the diaphragm. During this migration, the cervical myotomes and nerves contribute muscle and nerve supply, respectively, thus accounting for the long course of the phrenic nerve (C3, C4 and C5) from the neck to the diaphragm.

With such a complex embryological story, one may be surprised to know that congenital abnormalities of the diaphragm are unusual.

However, a number of defects can occur giving rise to a variety of congenital herniae through the diaphragm. These may be the following:

1. Through the foramen of Morgagni – anteriorly between the xiphoid and costal origins
2. Through the foramen of Bochdalek – the unclosed left pleuroperitoneal canal – lying posteriorly (commonest congenital hernia of diaphragm)
3. Through a deficiency of the whole central tendon (occasionally such a hernia may be traumatic in origin)
4. Through a congenitally large oesophageal hiatus

Far more common are the *acquired* hiatus herniae (subdivided into sliding and rolling herniae). These are found in patients usually of middle age in whom weakening and widening of the oesophageal hiatus has occurred (Fig. 1.14).

In the *sliding hernia* the upper stomach and lower oesophagus slide upwards into the chest through the lax hiatus when the patient lies down or bends over; the competence of the cardia is often disturbed and peptic juice can therefore regurgitate into the oesophagus in lying down or bending over. This may be followed by oesophagitis with consequent heartburn, bleeding and, eventually, stricture formation.

In the *rolling hernia* (which is far less common) the cardia remains in its normal position and the cardio-oesophageal junction is intact, but the fundus of the stomach rolls up through the hiatus in front of the oesophagus, hence, the alternative term of para-oesophageal hernia. In such a case there may be epigastric discomfort, flatulence and even dysphagia, but *no* regurgitation because the cardiac mechanism is undisturbed.

Movements of respiration

During inspiration the movements of the chest wall and diaphragm result in an increase in all diameters of the thoracic cavity. This, in turn, brings about an increase in the negative intrapleural pressure and an expansion of the lungs. Conversely, in expiration the relaxation of the respiratory muscles and the elastic recoil of the lungs reduce the thoracic capacity and force air out of the lungs.

The **Quiet inspiration** is brought about almost entirely by active contraction of the diaphragm with very little chest movement. The active contraction of diaphragm leads to increase in the vertical diameter of the thoracic cavity (Fig. 1.15). Confirm this on yourself; your hands on your chest will show minimal movement as you breathe quietly. As respiratory movement grows deeper, the contraction of the intercostal muscles raises the ribs. The 1st rib remains relatively stationary, ribs 2–6 principally increase the anteroposterior diameter of the thorax (the pump handle movement) (Fig. 1.16), while the corresponding action of the lower ribs is to increase the transverse diameter of the thoracic cage (the bucket handle movement) (Fig. 1.17). Again, confirm this on your own chest during deep inspiration. In progressively deeper inspiration, more and more of the diaphragmatic musculature is called into play. On radiographic screening of the chest, the diaphragm will be seen to move approximately 1 in. (2.5 cm) in quiet inspiration and up to 2.5–4 in. (6–10 cm) on deep inspiration.

Normal quiet expiration is brought about by elastic recoil of the elevated ribs and passive relaxation of the contracted

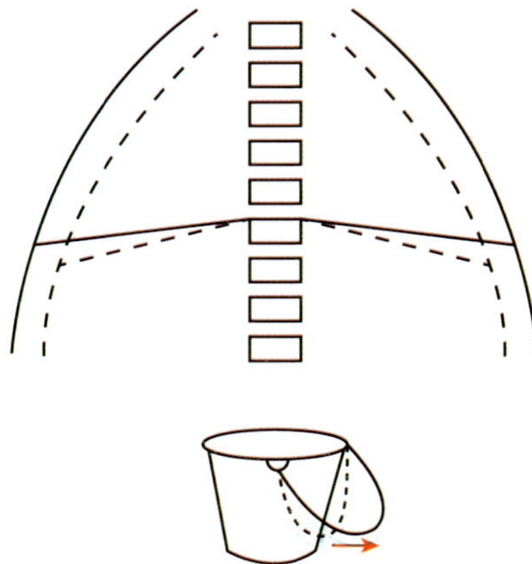

Figure 1.17 Bucket handle movement leading to an increase in transverse diameter of the thoracic cavity.

diaphragm. In deeper expiration, the abdominal muscles have an important part to play – they contract vigorously, compress the abdominal viscera, raise the intra-abdominal pressure and force the relaxed diaphragm upwards. Indeed, diaphragmatic movement accounts for approximately 65% of air exchange, whereas chest movement accounts for the remaining 35%.

In **deep and forced inspiration,** additional '**accessory muscles of respiration**' are called into play. These are the muscles attached to the thorax that are normally used in movements of the arms and the head. Watch an athlete at the end of a run, or observe a severely dyspnoeic patient – he grips his thighs or the table to keep his arms still, holds his head stiffly and uses pectoralis major, serratus anterior, latissimus dorsi and sternocleidomastoid to act 'from insertions to origins' to increase the capacity of the thorax. Observe also that the woman in advanced pregnancy has her diaphragm elevated and splinted by the enlarged foetus – she relies on chest movements in respiration even when she is resting quietly as she sits in the antenatal clinic.

Pleurae

The two pleural cavities are separated from each other by the mediastinum (Fig. 1.2). Each *pleura* consists of two layers: a *visceral layer* intimately related to the surface of the lung, and a *parietal layer* lining the inner aspect of the chest wall, the upper surface of the diaphragm and the sides of the pericardium and mediastinum. The visceral layer is firmly adhered to the underlying lung. In contrast, the parietal pleura is separated from its overlying structures by a loose, thin layer of connective tissue, the extrapleural fascia, which enables the surgeon to strip the parietal pleura easily from the chest wall. The two layers are continuous in front and behind the root of the lung, but below this the pleura hangs down in a loose fold, the *pulmonary ligament*, which forms a 'dead space' for distension of the pulmonary veins. The surface markings of the pleura and lungs have already been described in the section on surface anatomy.

Note that the lungs do not occupy all the available space in the pleural cavity, even in forced inspiration.

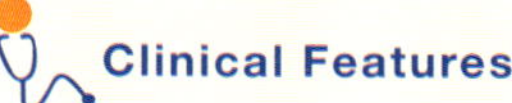

Clinical Features

1 Normally, the two layers of pleura are in close apposition and the space between them is only a potential one. It may, however, fill with air (**pneumothorax**), blood (**haemothorax**) or pus (**empyema**).
2 Since the parietal pleura is segmentally innervated by the somatic intercostal nerves, inflammation of the pleura results in pain referred to the cutaneous distribution of these nerves (i.e. to the thoracic wall or, in the case of the lower nerves, to the anterior abdominal wall, which may mimic an acute abdominal emergency).

Lower respiratory tract

Trachea (Figs 1.18 and 1.19)

The trachea is approximately 4.5 in. (11.5 cm) in length and nearly 1 in. (2.5 cm) in diameter. It commences at the lower border of the cricoid cartilage (C6) and terminates at the level of the sternal angle of Louis (T4/5) by bifurcating into the right and left primary (principal) bronchi. (In the living subject, the level of bifurcation of trachea varies slightly with the phase

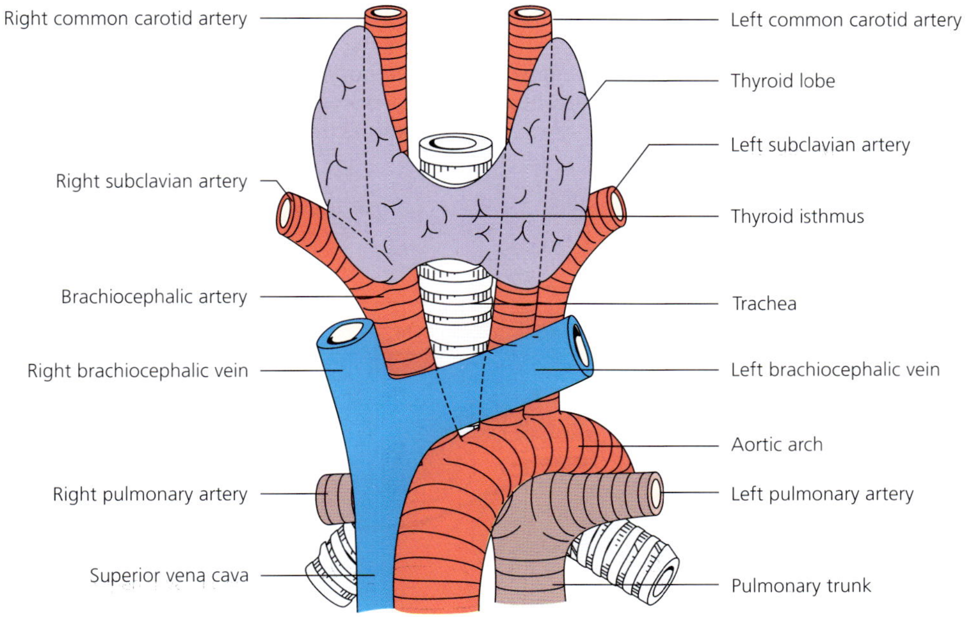

Figure 1.18 Trachea and its anterior relations.

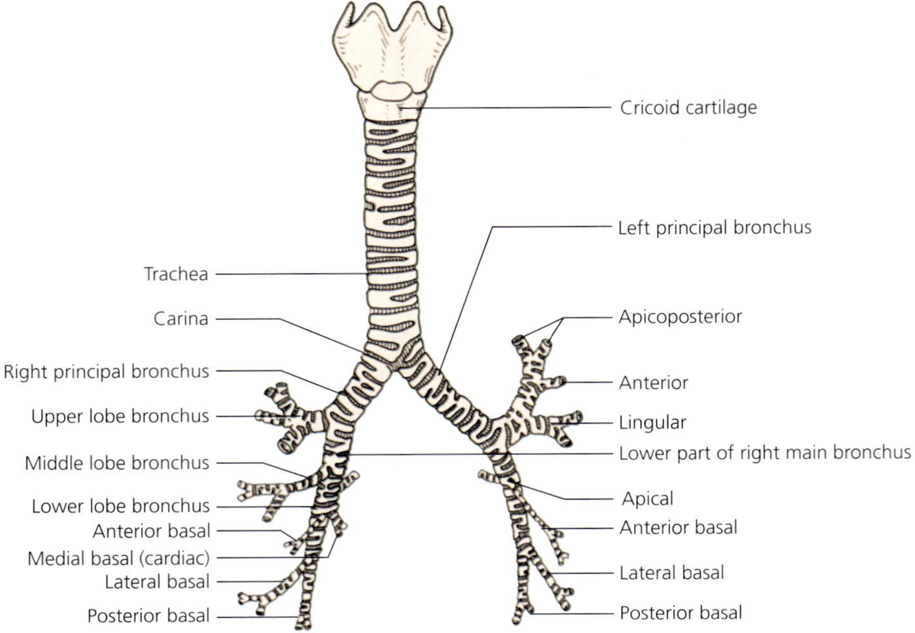

Figure 1.19 The trachea and main bronchi viewed from the front.

of respiration; in deep inspiration it descends to T6 and in expiration it rises to T4.)

Relations

Lying partly in the neck and partly in the thorax (superior mediastinum), its relations are as follows.

In Neck

- **Anteriorly:** Isthmus of the thyroid gland, inferior thyroid veins, sternohyoid and sternothyroid muscles
- **Laterally:** Lobes of the thyroid gland and the common carotid artery
- **Posteriorly:** Oesophagus with the recurrent laryngeal nerve lying in the groove between the oesophagus and trachea (Fig. 1.20)

In thorax

- **Anteriorly:** Commencement of the brachiocephalic artery and left carotid artery, both arising from the arch of the aorta, left brachiocephalic vein and thymus
- **Posteriorly:** Oesophagus and left recurrent laryngeal nerve
- **To the left:** Arch of the aorta, left common carotid and left subclavian arteries, left recurrent laryngeal nerve and pleura
- **To the right:** Vagus, azygos vein and pleura (Fig. 1.21)

Structure

The patency of the trachea is maintained by a series of 15–20 U-shaped hyaline cartilages. Posteriorly, where the cartilage is deficient, the trachea is flattened and its wall completed

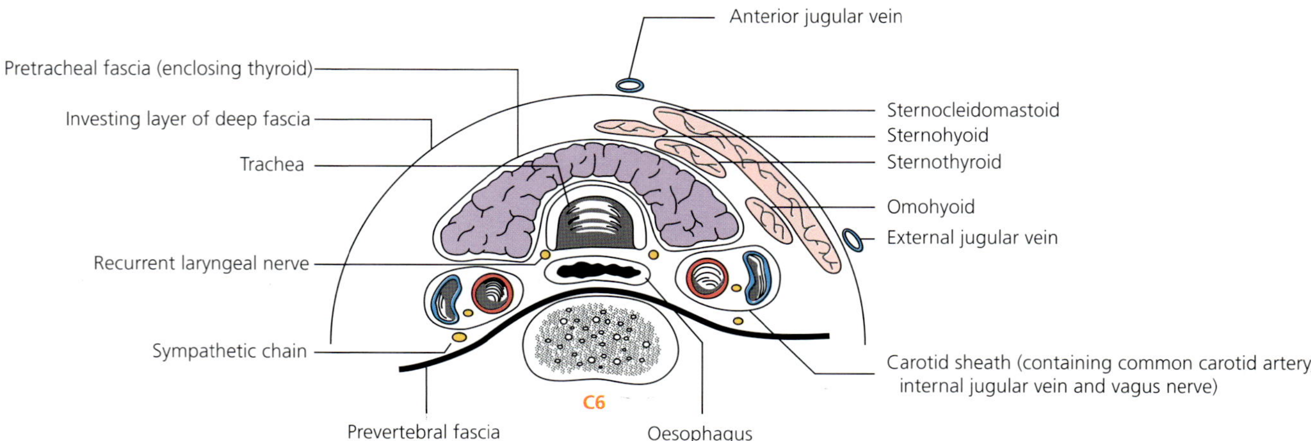

Figure 1.20 Cervical part of the trachea and its relations as seen in transverse section (through the 6th cervical vertebra) (viewed from below).

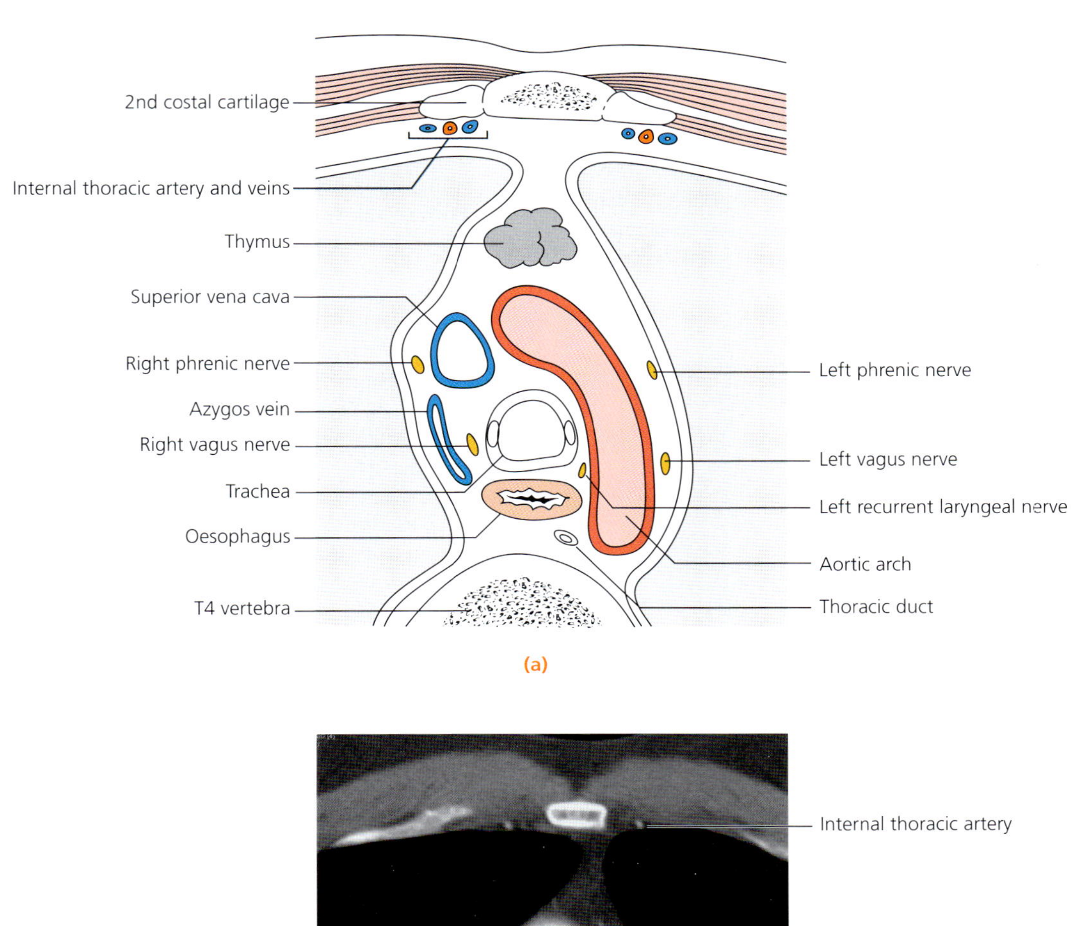

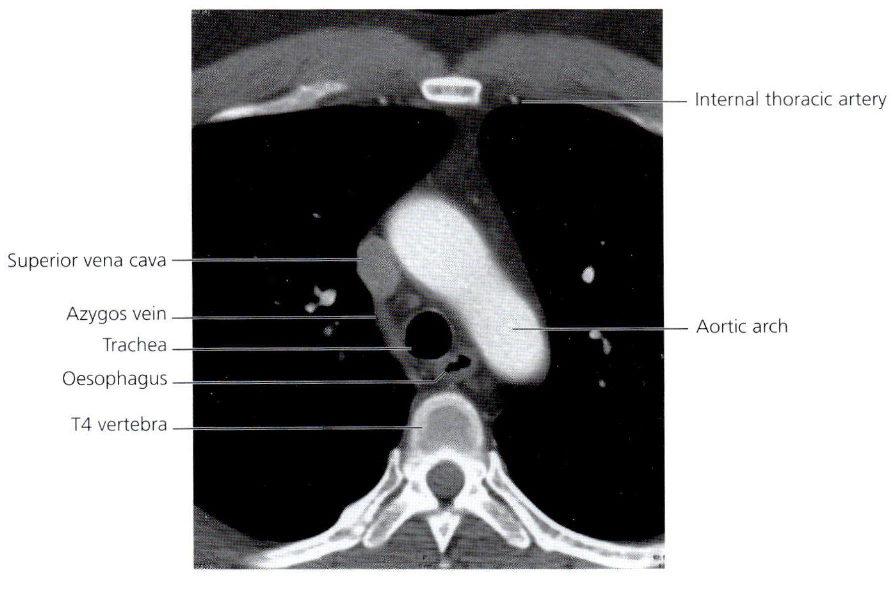

Figure 1.21 **(a)** Thoracic part of the trachea and its relations as seen in transverse section (through the 4th thoracic vertebra) (viewed from below). **(b)** CT scan (axial view) of the superior mediastinum at a level corresponding to that in (a).

by fibrous tissue and a sheet of smooth muscle (trachealis). Within, it is lined by a pseudostratified ciliated columnar epithelium with many goblet cells.

Bronchi (Fig. 1.19)

The *right principal bronchus* is wider, shorter and more vertical than the left. It is approximately 1 in. (2.5 cm) long and passes directly to the root of the lung at T5. Before entering the lung it gives off a branch to the upper lobe of the lung – the *upper lobe bronchus* – and then passes below the pulmonary artery to enter the hilum of the lung. After entering the hilum, it divides into middle and inferior lobar bronchi for the middle and inferior lobes of the lung, respectively. It has two important relations: the azygos vein, which arches over it from behind to reach the superior vena cava, and the pulmonary artery, which lies first below and then anterior to it.

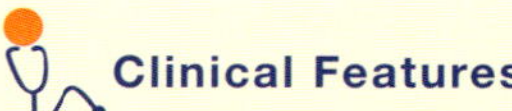

Clinical Features

Radiology

Since trachea contains air, it is more radiotranslucent than the neighbouring structures and is seen in posteroanterior and lateral radiographs as a dark area passing downwards, backwards and slightly to the right. In the elderly, calcification of the tracheal rings may be a source of radiological confusion.

Displacement

The trachea may be compressed or displaced by pathological enlargement of the neighbouring structures, particularly the thyroid gland and the arch of the aorta.

'Tracheal tug'

The intimate relationship between the arch of the aorta and the trachea and left bronchus is responsible for the physical sign known as '**tracheal tug**' characteristic of aneurysms of the aortic arch.

Tracheostomy

Tracheostomy may be required for laryngeal obstruction (diphtheria, tumours, inhaled foreign bodies), for the evacuation of excessive secretions (severe postoperative chest infection in a patient who is too weak to cough adequately) and for long-continued artificial respiration (poliomyelitis, severe chest injuries). It is important to note that respiration is further assisted by considerable reduction of the dead-space air.

The neck is extended and the head held exactly in the midline by an assistant. A vertical incision is made downwards from the cricoid cartilage, passing between the anterior jugular veins. Alternatively, a more cosmetic transverse skin crease incision, placed halfway between the cricoid and suprasternal notch, is employed. A hook is thrust under the lower border of the cricoid to steady the trachea and pull it forwards. The pretracheal fascia is split longitudinally, the isthmus of the thyroid either pushed upwards or divided between clamps and the cartilage of the trachea clearly exposed. A circular opening is then made into the trachea to admit the tracheostomy tube.

In children the neck is relatively short and the left brachiocephalic vein may come up above the suprasternal notch so that dissection is rather more difficult and dangerous. This difficulty is made greater because the child's trachea is softer and more mobile than the adult's and is, therefore, not so readily identified and isolated. Its softness means that care must be taken, in incising the child's trachea, not to let the scalpel plunge through and damage the underlying oesophagus.

In contrast, the trachea may be ossified in the elderly and small bone shears may be required to open into it.

The **golden rule of tracheostomy** – based entirely on anatomical considerations – is *stick exactly to the midline*. If this is not done, major vessels are in jeopardy and it is possible, although the student may not credit it, to miss the trachea entirely.

Cricothyroid puncture is now frequently used in the treatment of emergency upper respiratory obstruction (*see* page 174 and Fig. 5.21.

The *left main bronchus* is nearly 2 in. (5 cm) long and passes downwards and outwards below the arch of the aorta, in front of the oesophagus and descending aorta. Unlike the right, it gives off no branches until it enters the hilum of the lung, which it reaches opposite T6. After entering the hilum, it divides into superior and inferior lobar bronchi for the superior and inferior lobes of the lungs, respectively. The pulmonary artery spirals over the bronchus, lying first anteriorly and then above it.

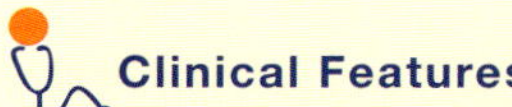

Clinical Features

1. The greater width and more vertical course of the right bronchus accounts for the greater tendency for foreign bodies and aspirated material to pass into the right bronchus (and thence especially into the middle and lower lobes of the right lung) rather than into the left. Note that this also applies to an endotracheal tube which, if too long for the size of the patient, will be pushed down into the right principal bronchus. This must be kept in mind particularly when intubating a baby or child.
2. The inner aspect of the whole of the trachea, the principal and lobar bronchi and the commencement of the first segmental divisions– the territory (segment bronchi) – can be seen at bronchoscopy.
3. Widening and distortion of the angle between the bronchi (the carina) as seen at bronchoscopy is a serious prognostic sign, since it usually indicates carcinomatous involvement of the tracheobronchial lymph nodes around the bifurcation of the trachea.

Lungs (Figs 1.22 and 1.23)

The lungs are organs of respiration. Each lung is conical in shape, having a blunt apex that reaches above the sternal end of the 1st rib, a concave base overlying the diaphragm, an extensive costovertebral surface moulded to the form of the chest wall and a mediastinal surface that is concave to accommodate the pericardium.

Each lung has three borders. The *anterior border* is thin and shorter than the posterior border. In the right lung it is vertical while in the left lung it presents a wide cardiac notch at the level of the 4th costal cartilage. The *posterior border* is thick

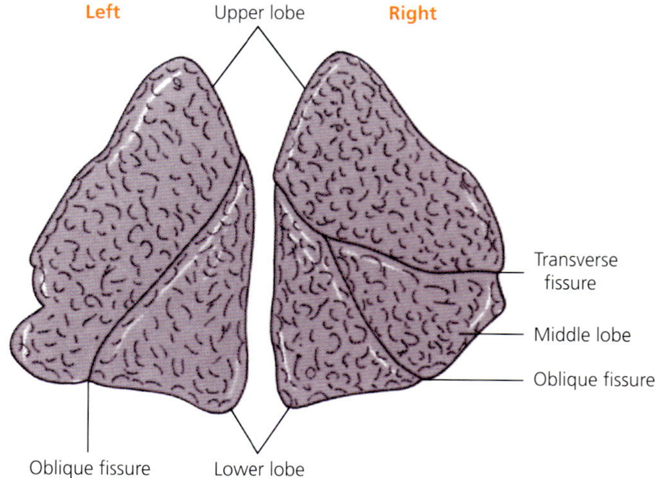

Figure 1.22 The lungs, lateral aspects.

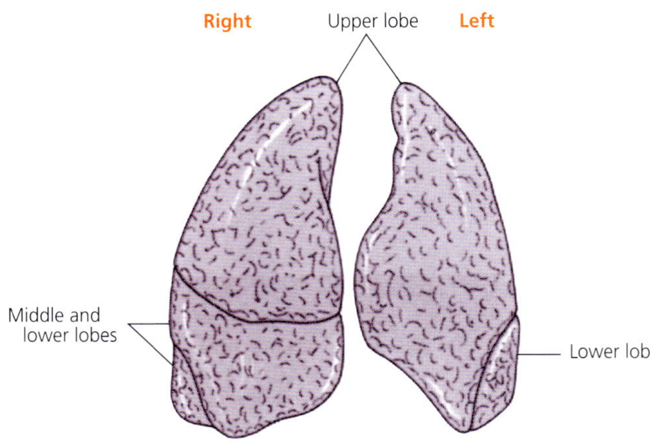

Figure 1.23 The lungs, anterior aspects.

and ill defined. The *inferior border* separates the costovertebral surface from the mediastinal surface.

A tongue-shaped projection of left lung below the cardiac notch is called lingula. It corresponds to the middle lobe of the right lung.

The right lung is somewhat shorter in height than the left; this is because it is pushed upwards by the higher right dome of the diaphragm, that itself is pushed up by the underlying liver. However, although shorter than the left, the right lung is actually the bulkier and heavier of the two because the size of the left lung is reduced by the considerable indentation on its medial aspect produced by the heart.

The right lung is divided into three lobes – the upper, middle and lower – by the oblique and horizontal fissures. The left lung has only an oblique fissure and hence only two lobes – an upper and a lower. There appears to be no physiological advantage in the fact that the lungs are lobed. However, the lobes are of considerable interest:

1. '*Lobar pneumonia*', caused by *Pneumococcus*, affects an individual lobe.
2. A plug of mucus, tumour or an inhaled foreign body may block an individual lobar bronchus and produce a *lobar collapse*, as residual air in the occluded lobe is gradually and progressively absorbed.
3. As each lobe possesses its own bronchus and blood supply, therefore, the surgeon can perform a *lobectomy* in suitable cases.

Blood supply

Mixed venous blood is returned to the lungs by the pulmonary arteries. The nutrition to bronchial tree and lung parenchyma is supplied by the bronchial arteries, which are small arteries. There are three bronchial arteries: one on the right side and two on the left side. The right bronchial artery arises from third right posterior intercostal artery or upper left bronchial artery while the two left bronchial arteries arise from the descending aorta. The *bronchial arteries*, although small, are of great clinical importance. They maintain the blood supply to the lung parenchyma after pulmonary embolism, so that, if the patient recovers, lung function returns to normal.

The *superior* and *inferior pulmonary veins* return oxygenated blood to the left atrium, while the *bronchial veins* drain into the azygos system.

Lymphatic drainage

The lymphatics of the lung drain centripetally from the pleura towards the hilum into the *bronchopulmonary lymph nodes* in the hilum. From these lymph nodes, the efferent lymph channels pass to the *tracheobronchial nodes* at the bifurcation of the trachea, thence to the *paratracheal nodes* and the mediastinal lymph trunks to drain usually directly into the brachiocephalic veins or, rarely, indirectly via the thoracic or right lymphatic duct.

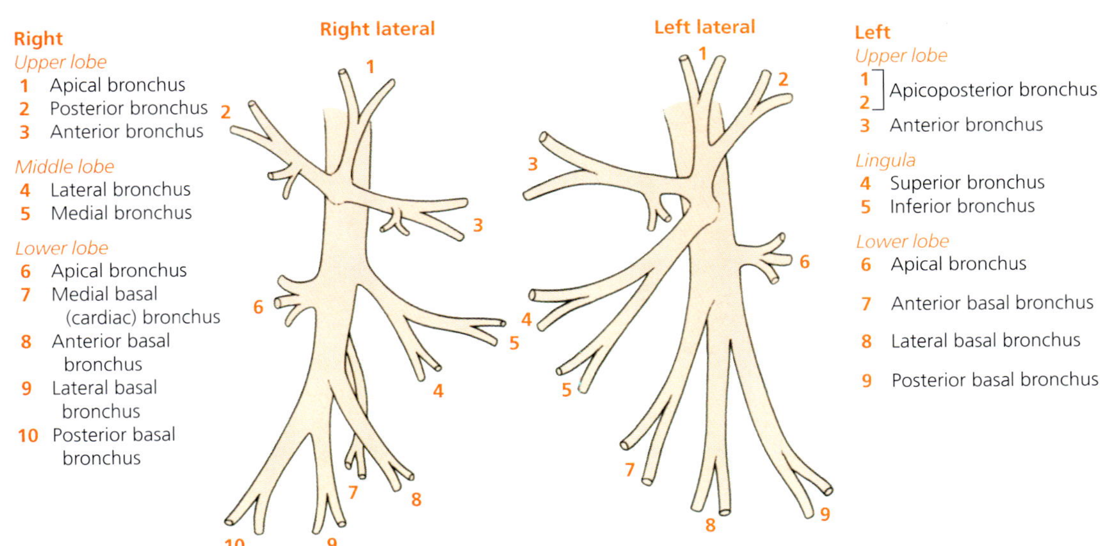

Figure 1.24 The comparison of named divisions of the principal bronchi.

Nerve supply

The innervation of the lung is via the pulmonary plexus at its hilum. This conveys sympathetic (T2–T5 or T6) and parasympathetic (vagus nerve, X) fibres. The sympathetic fibres are bronchodilator to the bronchial muscles, hence the use of sympathomimetic drugs in asthma. The vagal fibres carry signals from stretch receptors in the lungs for cough reflex and provide secretomotor fibres to the mucous glands of the bronchial tree.

Bronchopulmonary segments of the lungs

(Figs 1.24, 1.25 and 1.26)

Knowledge of the finer arrangement of the bronchial tree is an essential prerequisite to intelligent appreciation of lung radiology, to interpretation of bronchoscopy and to the surgical resection of lung segments. Each lobe of the lung is subdivided into a number of bronchopulmonary segments (Figs 1.24 and 1.25). These segments are wedge-shaped with their apices at the hilum and bases at the lung surface; each of these segments is supplied with a segmental bronchus, artery and vein (Fig. 1.26). If excised accurately along their boundaries (which are marked by intersegmental veins), there is little bleeding or alveolar air leakage from the raw lung surface.

The names and arrangements of the bronchi are given in Table 1.1; each bronchopulmonary segment takes its title from that of its supplying segmental bronchus (listed in the right-hand column of the table).

The left upper lobe has a *lingular segment,* supplied by the *lingular bronchus* from the main upper lobe bronchus. This segment is equivalent to the *right middle lobe,* whose bronchus arises as a branch from the main bronchus. Apart from this, differences between the two sides are very slight; on the left, the upper lobe bronchus gives off a combined apicoposterior segmental bronchus and an anterior branch, whereas all three branches are separate on the right side.

On the right also there is a small medial (or cardiac) lower lobe bronchus that is absent on the left, the lower lobes being otherwise mirror images of each other.

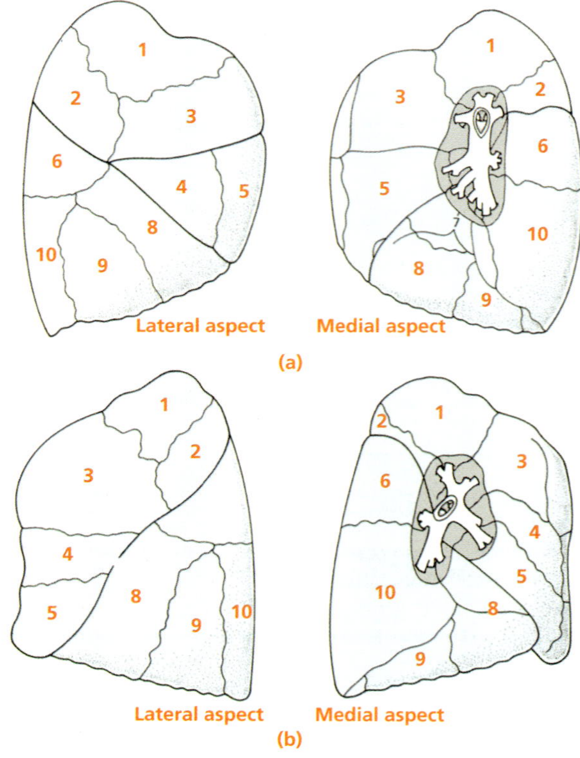

Figure 1.25 **(a)** The segments of the right lung. **(b)** The segments of the left lung.

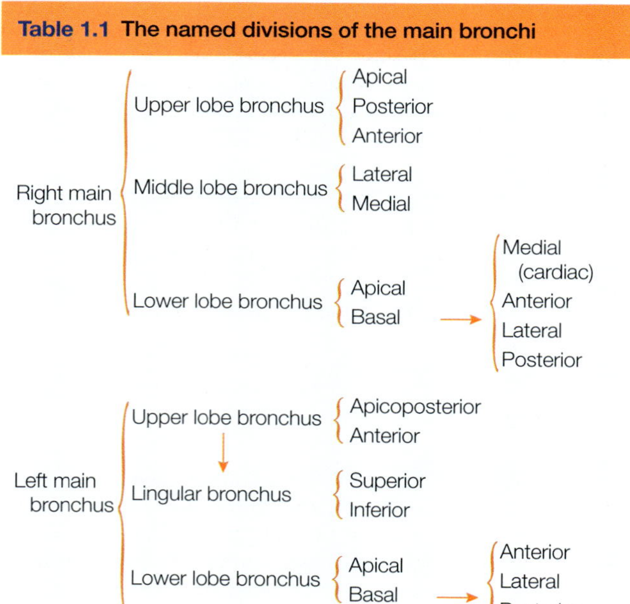

Table 1.1 The named divisions of the main bronchi

Main bronchus	Lobe bronchus	Segmental bronchi	Basal segments
Right main bronchus	Upper lobe bronchus	Apical Posterior Anterior	
	Middle lobe bronchus	Lateral Medial	
	Lower lobe bronchus	Apical Basal →	Medial (cardiac) Anterior Lateral Posterior
Left main bronchus	Upper lobe bronchus ↓	Apicoposterior Anterior	
	Lingular bronchus	Superior Inferior	
	Lower lobe bronchus	Apical Basal →	Anterior Lateral Posterior

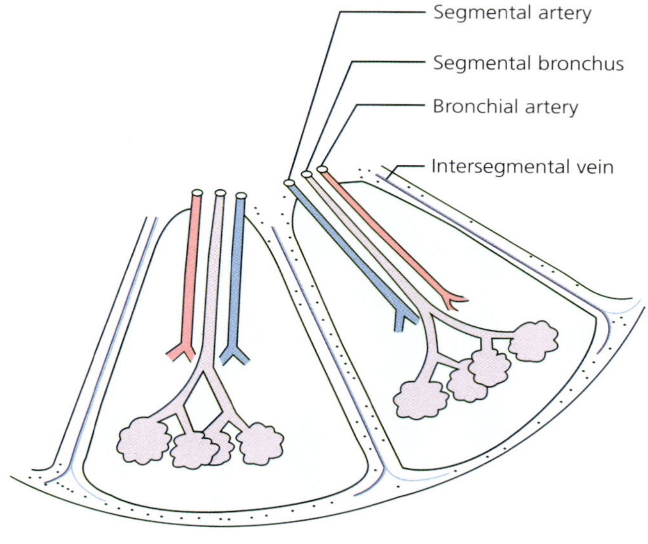

Figure 1.26 The internal structure of bronchopulmonary segment.

Mediastinum

The mediastinum is defined as 'the space within the thoracic cavity which is sandwiched between the two pleural sacs'. For descriptive purposes the mediastinum is divided by a line drawn horizontally from the sternal angle to the lower border of T4 (angle of Louis) into the superior and inferior mediastinum. The inferior mediastinum is further subdivided into the anterior in front of the pericardium, a middle mediastinum containing the pericardium itself with the heart and great vessels and the posterior mediastinum between the pericardium and the lower eight thoracic vertebrae (Fig. 1.27).

Pericardium

The heart and the roots of the great vessels are contained within the conical *fibrous pericardium*, the apex of which is fused with the adventitia of the great vessels and the base with the central tendon of the diaphragm. Anteriorly, it is related to the body of the sternum, to which it is attached by the *sternopericardial ligaments*, the 3rd–6th costal cartilages and the anterior borders of the lungs. Posteriorly, it is related to the oesophagus, descending aorta and vertebra T5–T8, and on either side to the roots of the lungs, the mediastinal pleura and the phrenic nerves.

The *pericardial cavity* is the potential space between the visceral and parietal layers of the pericardium. Just like the pleural and peritoneal cavities, it is lubricated by a film of serous fluid. Following trauma it may fill with blood (haemopericardium).

The inner aspect of the fibrous pericardium is lined by the *parietal layer of serous pericardium*. This, in turn, is reflected around the roots of the great vessels to become continuous with the *visceral layer* or *epicardium*. The lines of pericardial reflexion are marked on the posterior surface of the heart (Fig. 1.28) by the *oblique sinus*, bounded by the inferior vena cava and the four pulmonary veins, which form a recess between the left atrium and the pericardium, and the *transverse sinus* between the superior vena cava and left atrium behind and the pulmonary trunk and aorta in front.

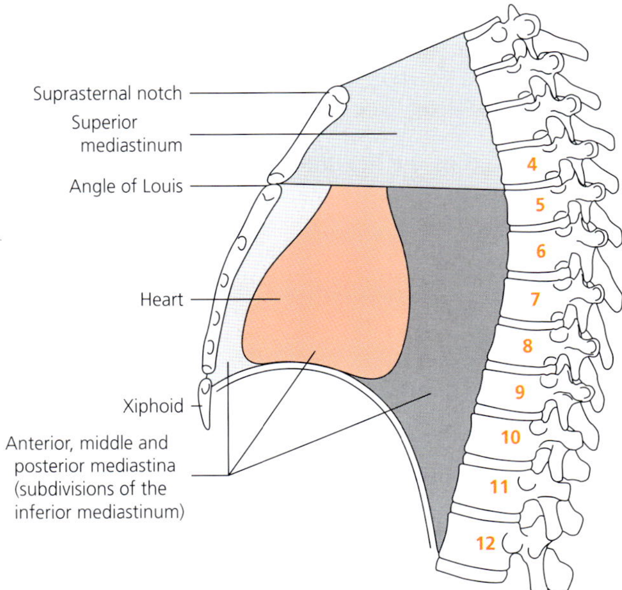

Figure 1.27 The subdivisions of the mediastinum.

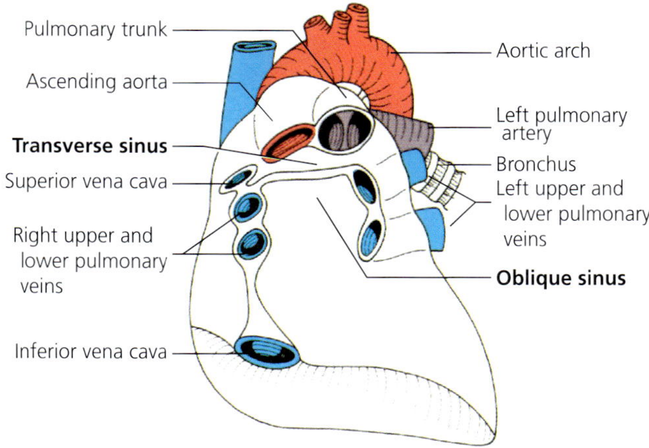

Figure 1.28 The transverse and oblique sinuses of the pericardium. The heart has been removed from the pericardial sac, which is seen in anterior view.

Heart (Fig. 1.29)

The heart is irregularly conical in shape, and it is placed obliquely in the middle mediastinum. Viewed from the front, portions of all the heart chambers can be seen. The right border is formed entirely by the right atrium, the left border partly by the auricular appendage of the left atrium but mainly by the left ventricle and the inferior border chiefly by the right ventricle but also by the lower part of the right atrium and the apex of the left ventricle.

The most of the anterior surface is formed by the right ventricle, which is separated from the right atrium by the *vertical atrioventricular groove* and from the left ventricle by the *anterior interventricular groove*.

The *inferior* or *diaphragmatic surface* consists of the right and left ventricles separated by the posterior interventricular groove and the portion of the right atrium that receives the inferior vena cava.

The *base* or *posterior surface* is quadrilateral in shape and is formed mainly by the left atrium with the openings of the pulmonary veins and, to a lesser extent, by the right atrium.

Chambers of the heart

The human heart possesses four chambers.

Right atrium (Fig. 1.29(a))

The right atrium receives the *superior vena cava* in its upper and posterior part, the *inferior vena cava* and *coronary sinus* in its lower part, and the anterior cardiac vein (draining much of the front of the heart) anteriorly. Running more or less vertically downwards between the venae cavae is a distinct muscular ridge, the *crista terminalis* (indicated on the

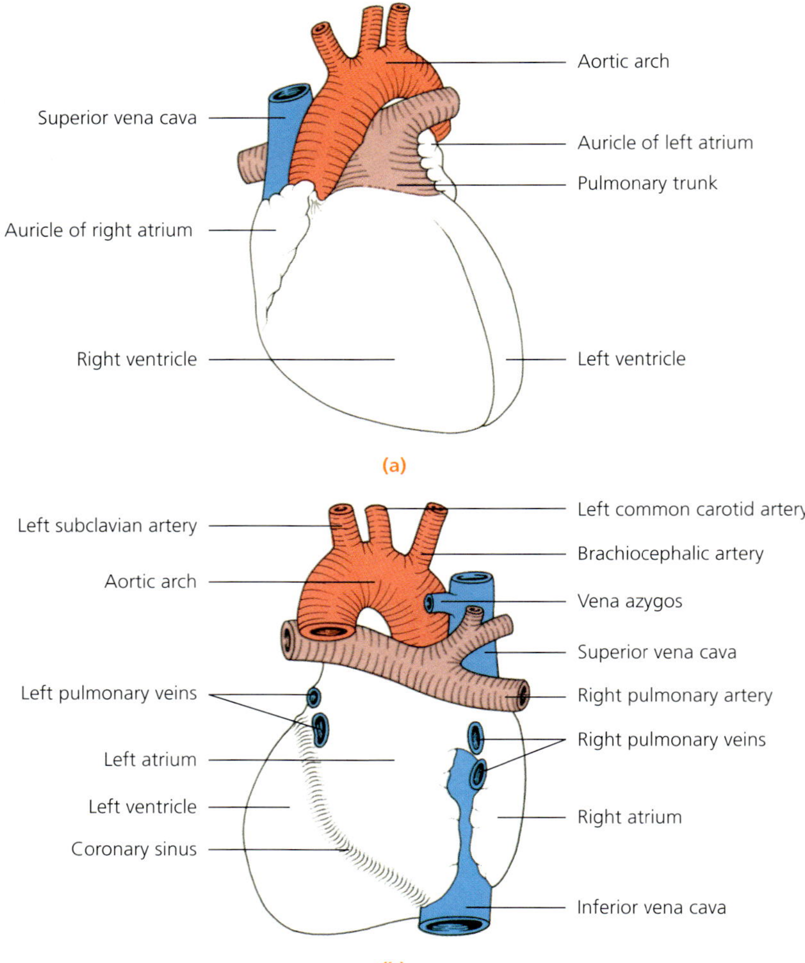

Figure 1.29 The heart: **(a)** anterior and **(b)** posterior aspects.

outer surface of the atrium by a shallow groove – the *sulcus terminalis*). This ridge separates the smooth-walled posterior part of the atrium, derived from the sinus venosus, from the rough-walled anterior portion derived from the true foetal atrium (*see* page 23). The anterior portion is prolonged into the *auricular appendage.*

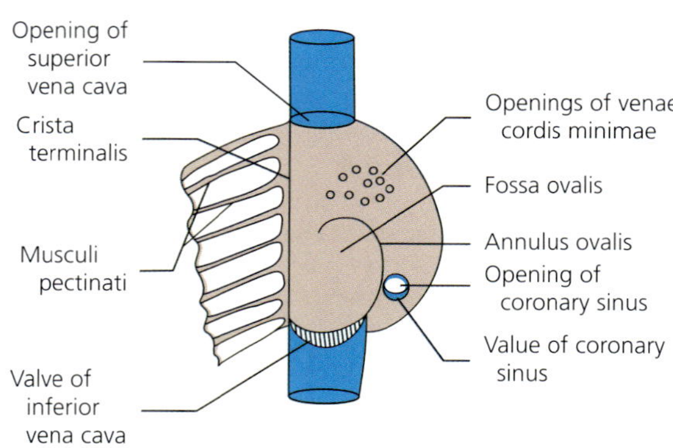

Figure 1.30 The features of the interior of the right atrium.

The trabeculations in the rough-walled part of the atrium are produced by parallel columns of muscle termed *musculi pectinati* (*pectinate muscles*); 'pectinate' comes from the Latin for 'like a comb'. The same term applies to the columns of muscle seen in the auricular appendage of the left atrium.

The openings of the inferior vena cava and the coronary sinus are guarded by rudimentary valves; that of the inferior vena cava being continuous with the *annulus ovalis* around the shallow depression on the atrial septum, the *fossa ovalis,* which marks the site of the foetal *foramen ovale.*

Numerous small veins (venae cordis minimae) open into the smooth part of the right atrium. The features of the interior of the right atrium is shown in Fig. 1.30.

Right ventricle (Fig. 1.31)

The right ventricle is joined to the right atrium by way of the vertically disposed *tricuspid valve,* and with the pulmonary trunk through the pulmonary valve. A muscular ridge, the *infundibuloventricular (supraventricular) crest,* between the atrioventricular and pulmonary orifices, separates the 'inflow' and 'outflow' tracts of the ventricle. The inner aspect of the inflow tract path is marked in the presence of a

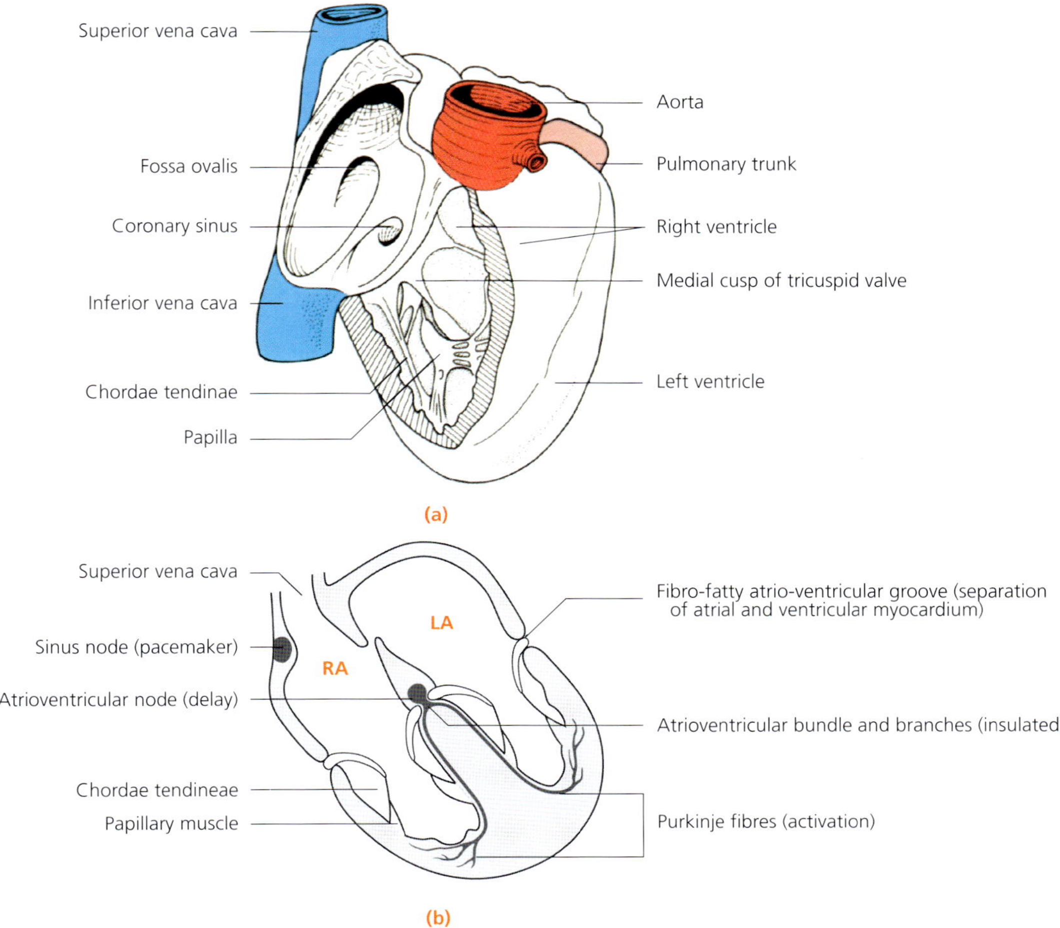

Figure 1.31 (a) The interior of the right atrium and ventricle. **(b)** The conducting system of the heart. LA, left atrium; RA, right atrium.

number of irregular muscular ridges (*trabeculae carneae*), some of them form the *papillary muscles* which project into the lumen of the ventricle and find attachment to the free borders of the cusps of the tricuspid valve by way of the *chordae tendineae*.

When the ventricle contracts in systole, the papillary muscles shorten, the chordae tendineae are pulled upon and the tricuspid valve is prevented from prolapsing into the right atrium. (The same mechanism, of course, takes place with the mitral valve of the left ventricle.) *Rupture of a papillary muscle, following an adjacent myocardial infarction, will allow prolapse of the affected cusp to occur into the atrium at each systole, with consequent acute cardiac failure.*

The *moderator band* is a muscular bundle crossing the ventricular cavity from the interventricular septum to the anterior wall and is of some importance since it conveys the right branch of the atrioventricular bundle to the ventricular muscle.

The outflow tract of the ventricle or *infundibulum* is smooth-walled and is directed upwards and to the right towards the pulmonary trunk. The pulmonary orifice is guarded by the *pulmonary valves*, comprising three semilunar cusps.

The right ventricle receives blood from the right atrium and pumps it into the lungs.

Left atrium

The left atrium is rather smaller than the right but has somewhat thicker walls. On the upper part of its posterior wall it presents the openings of the four pulmonary veins, and on its septal surface there is a shallow depression corresponding to the fossa ovalis of the right atrium. As on the right side, the main part of the cavity is smooth-walled but the surface of the auricle is marked by a number of ridges due to the underlying pectinate muscles. The left atrium receives the oxygenated blood from the lungs and pumps it into the left ventricle.

Left ventricle (Fig. 1.32)

The left ventricle communicates with the left atrium by way of the *mitral valve* (so-called because it vaguely resembles a **bishop's mitre**), which possesses a large anterior and a smaller posterior cusp attached to papillary muscles by chordae tendineae. With the exception of the fibrous *vestibule* immediately below the aortic orifice, the wall of the left ventricle is marked by thick trabeculae carneae.

The term 'cusps' applied to the tricuspid and mitral valves is somewhat misleading. It suggests that, as in the aortic and pulmonary valves, these are individual structures and

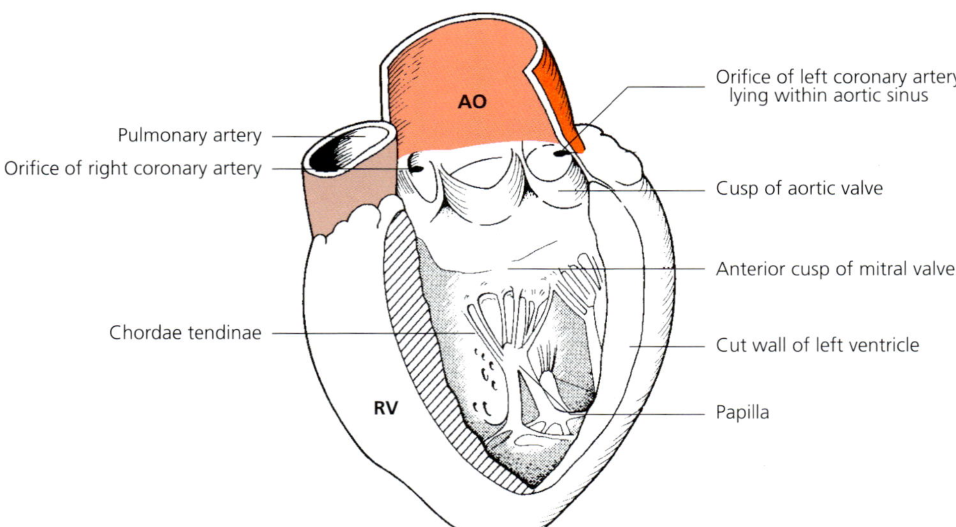

Figure 1.32 The interior of the left ventricle. AO, aorta; RV, right ventricle.

separate from each other (Fig. 1.32). In fact, the tricuspid and mitral valves can be compared to circular curtains that hang down from each atrioventricular orifice, and that descend into the lumen of the ventricle with three drapes on the right side and two drapes on the left, held in place by chordae tendineae.

The aortic orifice is guarded by the three semilunar cusps of the *aortic valve*, immediately above which are the dilated *aortic sinuses*. The mouths of the right and left coronary arteries are seen in the anterior and left posterior sinus, respectively. In diastole, blood refluxing into the aortic sinuses sets up turbulent flow, which helps to close the valve. The same mechanism applies to the pulmonary valve. In addition, on the left, blood refluxes in diastole into the two coronary artery ostia, placed within the sinuses, so that **cardiac perfusion takes place in the ventricular diastolic phase of the cardiac cycle**.

Conducting system of the heart (Fig. 1.31(b))

This consists of specialized cardiac muscle found in the sinuatrial node and in the atrioventricular node and bundle. The heart beat is initiated in the *sinus* (or *sinuatrial*) *node* (the '**pacemaker of the heart**'), situated in the upper part of the crista terminalis just to the right of the opening of the superior vena cava into the right atrium. From there the cardiac impulse spreads throughout the atrial musculature to reach the *atrioventricular node* lying in the atrial septum immediately above the opening of the coronary sinus. The impulse is then conducted to the ventricles by way of the specialized tissue of the *atrioventricular bundle* (*of His*). This bundle divides at the junction of the membranous and muscular parts of the interventricular septum into its right and left branches, which run immediately beneath the endocardium to activate all parts of the ventricular musculature.

Arterial supply to the heart (Fig. 1.33)

The blood supply of the heart is derived from the right and left coronary arteries, whose main branches lie in each of the interventricular and atrioventricular grooves.

The *right coronary artery* arises from the anterior aortic sinus and passes forwards between the pulmonary trunk and the

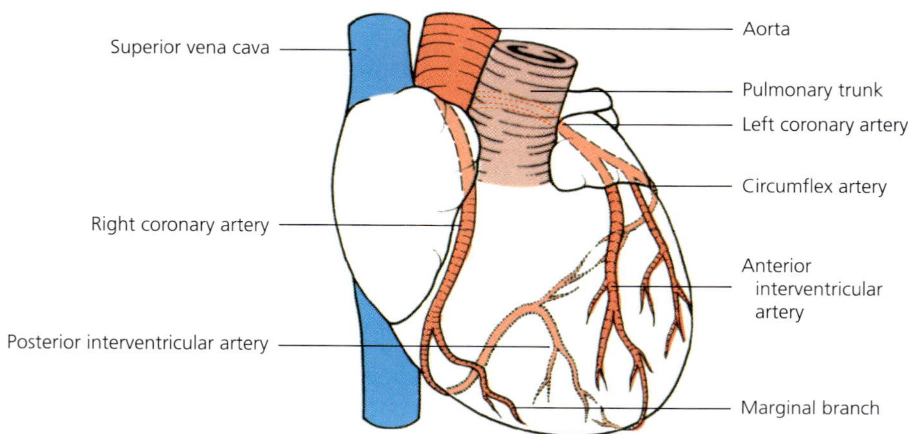

Figure 1.33 The coronary arteries. (Dotted vessels lie posteriorly.)

right atrium to descend in the right part of the atrioventricular groove. At the inferior border of the heart it continues along the atrioventricular groove to anastomose with the left coronary artery at the posterior interventricular groove. It gives off a *marginal branch* along the lower border of the heart and the *posterior interventricular branch* which runs forwards in the interventricular groove on the surface of the heart to anastomose near the apex of the heart with the corresponding branch of the left coronary artery.

The *left coronary artery*, which is larger than the right, arises from the left posterior aortic sinus. Passing first behind and then to the left of the pulmonary trunk, it reaches the left part of the atrioventricular groove, in which it runs laterally round the left border of the heart as the *circumflex artery* to reach the posterior interventricular groove. Its most important branch, given off less than 1 in. (2.5 cm) from its origin, is the *anterior interventricular artery*, which supplies the anterior aspect of both ventricles and passes around the apex of the heart to anastomose with the posterior interventricular branch of the right coronary artery. Note that the sinuatrial node is usually supplied by the right coronary artery, although the left coronary artery takes over this duty in approximately one-third of subjects.

Although anastomoses occur between the terminal branches of the right and left coronary arteries, these are usually inefficient. Thrombosis in one or other of these vessels leads to death of the area of heart muscle supplied (a myocardial infarction).

Venous drainage of the heart (Fig. 1.34)

The bulk of the venous drainage of the heart is achieved by veins that accompany the coronary arteries and open into the right atrium through the coronary sinus (the longest venous channel of the heart). The rest of the venous blood is drained by means of small veins (*venae cordis minimae*) directly into the cardiac cavity.

The *coronary sinus* lies in the posterior atrioventricular groove and opens into the right atrium just to the left of the mouth of the inferior vena cava.

It receives the following:

1. The *great cardiac vein* in the anterior interventricular groove
2. The *middle cardiac vein* in the inferior interventricular groove
3. The *small cardiac vein* accompanying the marginal artery along the lower border of the heart
4. The *oblique vein* descends obliquely on the posterior aspect of the left atrium

The *anterior cardiac veins* (up to three or four in number) cross the anterior atrioventricular groove, drain much of the anterior surface of the heart and open directly into the right atrium.

Nerve supply

The nerve supply of the heart is derived from the vagus (parasympathetic *cardio-inhibitor*) and the cervical and upper three to five thoracic sympathetic ganglia (*cardio-accelerator*) by way of superficial and deep cardiac plexuses.

Development of the heart

The primitive heart is a single tube which soon shows grooves demarcating four swellings, viz *sinus venosus, atrium, ventricle* and *bulbus cordis* from behind forwards. As this tube enlarges it kinks so that its caudal end, receiving venous blood, comes to lie behind its cephalic end with its emerging arteries (Fig. 1.35).

The sinus venosus later absorbs into the atrium and the bulbus becomes incorporated into the ventricle so that, in the fully developed heart, the atria and great veins come to lie posterior to the ventricles and the roots of the great arteries.

The boundary tissue between the primitive single atrial cavity and single ventricle grows out as a *dorsal* and a *ventral endocardial cushion* that meet in the midline, thus dividing the common atrioventricular orifice into a right (tricuspid) and left (mitral) orifice.

The division of the primitive atrium into two is a complicated process but an important one in the understanding of congenital septal defects (Fig. 1.36). A partition, the *septum primum*, grows downwards from the posterior and superior walls of the primitive common atrium to fuse with the endocardial cushions. Before fusion is complete, however, a hole appears in the upper part of this septum which is termed *the foramen secundum in the septum primum.*

A second membrane, the *septum secundum*, then develops to the right of the primum but this is never complete; it has a

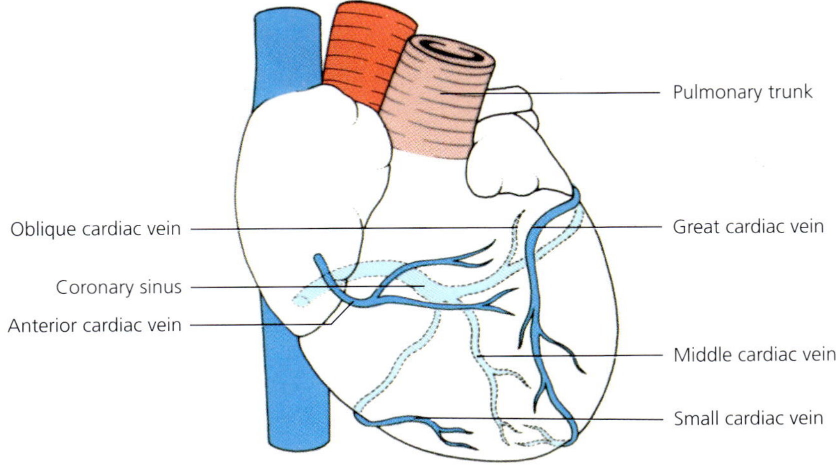

Figure 1.34 The coronary veins. (Dotted vessels lie posteriorly.)

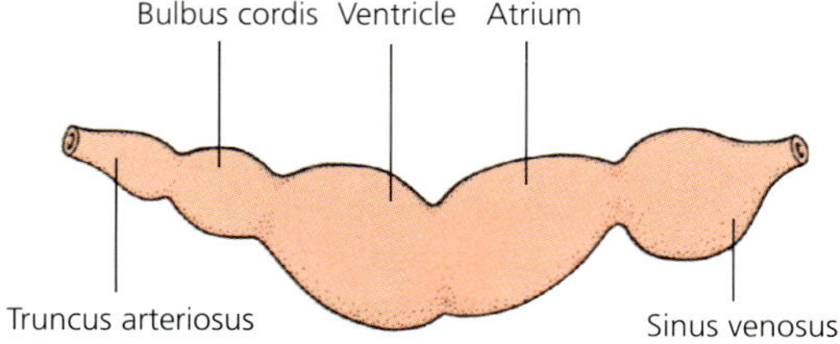

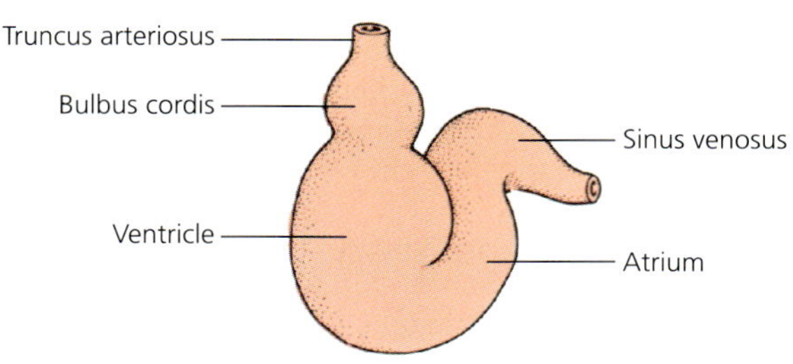

Figure 1.35 The coiling of the primitive heart tube into its definitive form.

free lower edge that does, however, extend low enough for this new septum to overlap the foramen secundum in the septum primum and hence to close it.

The two overlapping defects in the septa form the valve-like *foramen ovale,* which shunts blood from the right to the left heart in the foetus (*see* 'Foetal circulation', page 25). After birth, this foramen usually becomes completely fused, leaving only the fossa ovalis on the septal wall of the right atrium as its memorial. In approximately 10% of adult subjects, however, a probe can still be insinuated through an anatomically patent, although functionally sealed, foramen.

Division of the ventricle is commenced by the upgrowth of a fleshy septum from the apex of the heart towards the endocardial cushions. This stops short of dividing the ventricle completely and thus it has an upper free border, forming a *temporary interventricular foramen.* At the same time, the single truncus arteriosus is divided into the aorta and pulmonary trunk by a spiral septum (hence the spiral relations of these two vessels), which grows downwards to the ventricle and fuses accurately with the upper free border of the ventricular septum. This contributes the small *pars membranacea septi,* which completes the separation of the ventricle in such a way that blood on the left of the septum flows into the aorta and on the right into the pulmonary trunk.

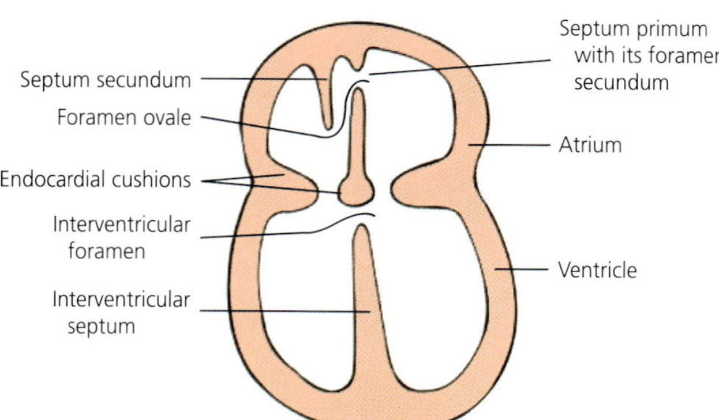

Figure 1.36 The development of the chambers of the heart. (Note: The septum primum and septum secundum that form the interatrial septum, leaving the foramen ovale as a valve-like opening passing between them.)

The primitive *sinus venosus* absorbs into the right atrium so that the venae cavae draining into the sinus come to open separately into this atrium. The smooth-walled part of the adult atrium represents the contribution of the sinus venosus; the pectinate part represents the portion derived from the primitive atrium and is termed the *auricle* or the *auricular appendage* of the right atrium (Fig. 1.29(a)).

Rather similarly, the adult left atrium has a double origin. The original single pulmonary venous trunk entering the left atrium becomes absorbed into it and donates the smooth-walled part of this chamber with the pulmonary veins entering as four separate openings; the trabeculated part of the definitive left atrium is the remains of the original atrial wall. This forms the *auricle* or the *auricular appendage* of the left atrium (Fig. 1.29(a)).

Development of the aortic arches and their derivatives (Fig. 1.37)

Emerging from the bulbus cordis is a common arterial trunk termed the *truncus arteriosus,* from which arise six pairs of aortic arches, equivalent to the arteries supplying the gill clefts of the fish. These arteries curve dorsally around the primitive pharynx on either side and join to form two longitudinally placed dorsal aortae that fuse distally into the descending aorta.

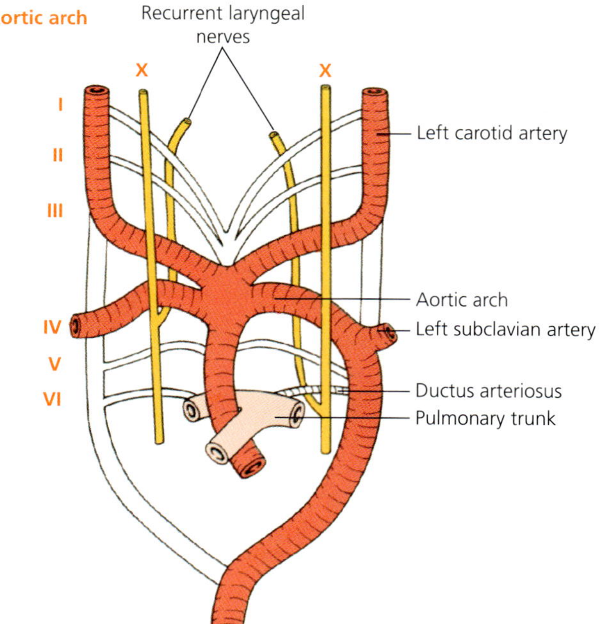

Figure 1.37 The aortic arches and their derivatives. This diagram explains the relationship of the right recurrent laryngeal nerve to the right subclavian artery and the left nerve to the aortic arch and the ligamentum arteriosum (or to a persistent ductus arteriosus).

The 1st and 2nd arches disappear; the 3rd arches become the carotid. The 4th arch on the right becomes the brachiocephalic and right subclavian artery; on the left, it differentiates into the definitive aortic arch, gives off the left subclavian artery and links up distally with the descending aorta.

The 5th arch artery is rudimentary and disappears.

When the truncus arteriosus splits longitudinally to form the ascending aorta and pulmonary trunk, the 6th arch artery, unlike the others, remains linked with the latter and forms the right and left pulmonary arteries. On the left side this arch retains its connection with the dorsal aorta to form the *ductus arteriosus* (the *ligamentum arteriosum* of adult anatomy).

This asymmetrical development of the aortic arches accounts for the different course taken by the recurrent laryngeal nerve on each side. In the early foetus the vagus nerve lies lateral to the primitive pharynx, separated from it by the aortic arches. What are to become the recurrent laryngeal nerves pass medially, caudal to the aortic arches, to supply the developing larynx. With elongation of the neck and caudal migration of the heart, the recurrent nerves are caught up and dragged down by the descending aortic arches. On the right side, the 5th arch and distal part of the 6th arch become absorbed, leaving the nerve to hook round the 4th arch (i.e. the right subclavian artery). On the left side, the nerve remains looped around the persisting distal part of the 6th arch (the ligamentum arteriosum), which is overlapped and dwarfed by the arch of the aorta (Fig. 1.37).

Foetal circulation (Fig. 1.38)

The circulation of the blood in the embryo is a remarkable example of economy in nature and results in the shunting of well-oxygenated blood from the placenta to the brain and the heart, leaving relatively desaturated blood for less essential structures.

The foetal blood is oxygenated in the placenta. The blood is returned from the placenta by the umbilical vein to the inferior vena cava and thence the right atrium, most of it bypassing the liver through the *ductus venosus* (*see* page 56). Relatively, little mixing of oxygenated and deoxygenated blood occurs in the right atrium since the valve overlying the orifice of the inferior vena cava serves to direct the flow of oxygenated blood from that vessel through the *foramen ovale* into the left atrium, while the deoxygenated stream from the superior vena cava is directed through the tricuspid valve into the right ventricle. From the left atrium the oxygenated blood (together with a small amount of deoxygenated blood from the lungs) passes into the left ventricle and hence into the ascending aorta for the supply of the brain and heart via the vertebral, carotid and coronary arteries.

As the lungs of the foetus are inactive, most of the deoxygenated blood from the right ventricle is short-circuited by way of the *ductus arteriosus* from the pulmonary trunk into the descending aorta. This blood supplies the abdominal viscera and the lower limbs and is shunted to the placenta, for oxygenation, along the *umbilical arteries* arising from the internal iliac arteries.

At birth, expansion of the lungs leads to an increased blood flow in the pulmonary arteries; the resulting pressure changes in the two atria bring the overlapping *septum primum* and *septum secundum* into apposition, which effectively closes off the foramen ovale. At the same time active contraction of the muscular wall of the ductus arteriosus results in a functional closure of this arterial shunt and, in the course of the next 2–3 months, its complete obliteration. Similarly, ligature of the

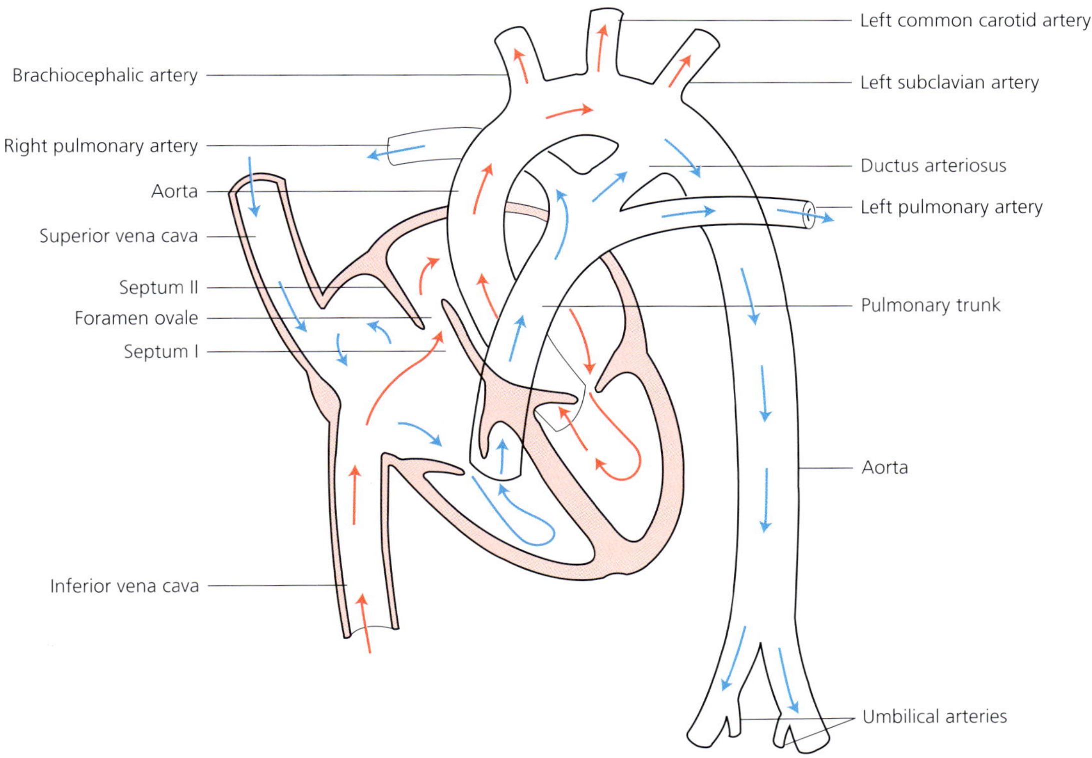

Figure 1.38 The foetal circulation. The red arrows denote oxygenated blood.

umbilical cord is followed by thrombosis and obliteration of the umbilical vessels.

The obliterated umbilical artery is represented by the *medial umbilical ligament*, leading from the superior vesical branch of the internal iliac artery on either side, across the deep aspect of the lower anterior abdominal wall to the umbilicus. The obliterated umbilical vein becomes the *ligamentum teres*, which runs in the free edge of the falciform ligament to the liver (*see* Fig. 2.31).

Congenital abnormalities of the heart and great vessels

The complex development of the heart and major arteries accounts for the multitude of congenital abnormalities that may affect these structures, either alone or in combination.

Dextrocardia

The *dextrorotation of the heart* means that this organ and its emerging vessels lie as a mirror image to the normal anatomy. It may be associated with reversal of all the intra-abdominal organs; one of the authors (H.E.) has seen a student correctly diagnose acute appendicitis as the cause of a patient's severe *left* iliac fossa pain because he found that the apex beat of the heart was on the right side!

Septal defects

At birth, the septum primum and septum secundum are forced together, closing the flap valve of the foramen ovale. Fusion usually takes place approximately 3 months after birth. In approximately 10% of subjects, this fusion may be incomplete. However, the two septa overlap and this patency of the foramen ovale is of no functional significance. If the septum secundum is too short to cover the foramen secundum in the septum primum, an *atrial septal defect* persists after the septum primum and septum secundum are pressed together at birth. This results in an *ostium secundum defect*, which allows shunting of blood from the left to the right atrium. This defect lies high up in the atrial wall and is relatively easy to close surgically. A more serious atrial septal defect results if the septum primum fails to fuse with the endocardial cushions. This *ostium primum defect* lies immediately above the atrioventricular boundary and may be associated with a defect of the pars membranacea septi of the ventricular septum. In such a case, the child is born with both an atrial and ventricular septal defect.

Occasionally, the ventricular septal defect is so huge that the ventricles form a single cavity, giving a *trilocular heart*.

Congenital pulmonary stenosis may affect the trunk of the pulmonary artery, its valve or the infundibulum of the right ventricle. If stenosis occurs in conjunction with a septal defect, the compensatory hypertrophy of the right ventricle (developed to force blood through the pulmonary obstruction) develops a sufficiently high pressure to shunt blood through the defect into the left heart; this mixing of the deoxygenated right heart blood with the oxygenated left-sided blood results in the child being *cyanosed at birth*.

The commonest combination of congenital abnormalities causing cyanosis is *Fallot's tetralogy* (Fig. 1.39). This results from unequal division of the truncus arteriosus by the spiral septum, resulting in a stenosed pulmonary trunk

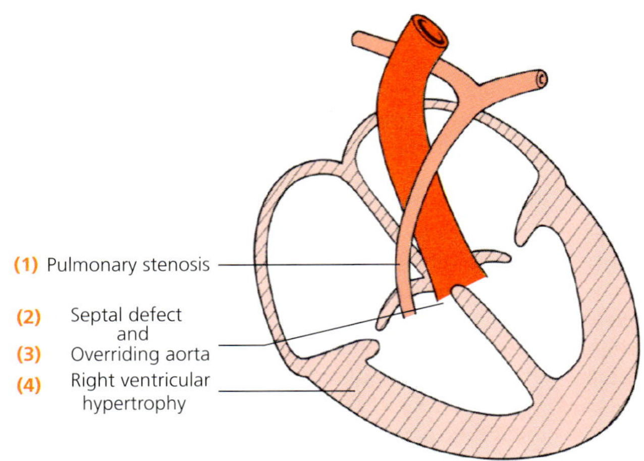

Figure 1.39 The tetralogy of Fallot.

and a wide aorta that overrides the orifices of both the ventricles. The displaced septum is unable to close the interventricular septum, which results in a ventricular septal defect. Right ventricular hypertrophy develops as a consequence of the pulmonary stenosis. Cyanosis results from the shunting of large amounts of unsaturated blood from the right ventricle through the ventricular septal defect into the left ventricle and also directly into the aorta. Thus, the fallot's tetralogy consists of the following four congenital anomalies (Fig. 1.39):

1. Pulmonary stenosis
2. Overriding of aorta
3. Ventricular septal defect
4. Right ventricular hypertrophy

A *persistent ductus arteriosus* (Fig. 1.40(a)) is a relatively common congenital defect of great blood vessels. If left uncorrected, it causes progressive work hypertrophy of the left heart and pulmonary hypertension.

Coarctation of aorta (Fig. 1.40(b)) is thought to be due to an abnormality of the obliterative process that normally occludes the ductus arteriosus. There may be an extensive obstruction of

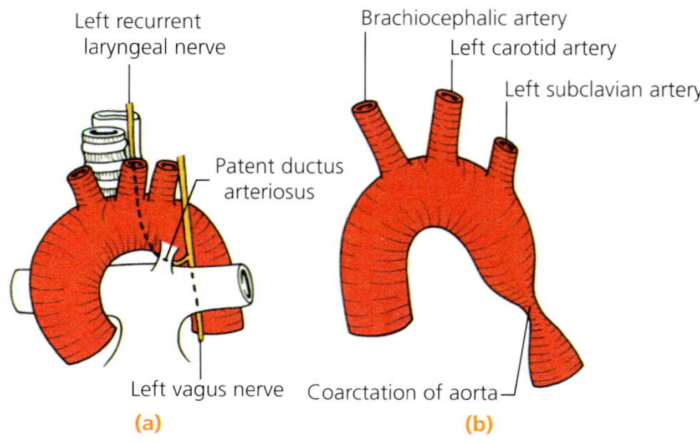

Figure 1.40 **(a)** Persistent ductus arteriosus – showing its close relationship to the left recurrent laryngeal nerve. **(b)** Coarctation of the aorta.

the aorta from the left subclavian artery to the ductus, which is widely patent and maintains the circulation to the lower parts of the body; often, there are multiple other defects and frequently infants so afflicted die at an early age. More commonly, there is a short segment involved in the region of the ligamentum arteriosum or still patent ductus. In these cases, circulation to the lower limbs is maintained via collateral arteries around the scapula anastomosing with the intercostal arteries, and via the link-up between the internal thoracic and inferior epigastric arteries.

Clinically, this circulation may be manifest by *enlarged vessels being palpable around the scapular margins*; radiologically, dilatation of the engorged intercostal arteries results in *notching of the inferior borders of the ribs*.

Abnormal development of the primitive aortic arches may result in the aortic arch being on the right or actually being double. An abnormal right subclavian artery may arise from the dorsal aorta and pass behind the oesophagus – a rare cause of difficulty in swallowing (*dysphagia lusoria*).

Rarely, the division of the truncus into the aorta and pulmonary artery is incomplete, leaving an *aorta–pulmonary window*, the most unusual congenital fistula between the two sides of the heart.

Superior mediastinum

This is bounded in front by the manubrium sterni and behind by the first four thoracic vertebrae (Fig. 1.27). Its *superior limit* is demarcated by a plane of thoracic inlet while its *inferior limit* is demarcated by an imaginary plane passing through the sternal angle in front and the lower border of T4 behind. Above, it is in direct continuity with the root of the neck, and, below, it is continuous with the three subdivisions of the inferior mediastinum. Its principal contents are: the great vessels, trachea, oesophagus, thymus, thoracic duct, vagi, left recurrent laryngeal nerve and the phrenic nerves (Fig. 1.21).

The *arch of the aorta* is directed anteroposteriorly; its three great branches, the *brachiocephalic, left carotid* and *left subclavian arteries*, ascend to the thoracic inlet, the first two forming a 'V' around the trachea. The *brachiocephalic veins* lie in front of the arteries, the left running almost horizontally across the superior mediastinum and the right vertically downwards; the two unite to form the *superior vena cava*. Posteriorly lies the trachea with the oesophagus immediately behind it lying against the vertebral column.

Thymus (Fig. 1.21)

The thymus plays an important role in the immunological defences of the body, by production of thymus-processed lymphocytes (*T-lymphocytes*).

The thymus is a soft, bi-lobed organ that lies in the superior mediastinum, closely related to the left brachiocephalic vein, and extends downwards into the anterior part of the inferior mediastinum.

The gland is large in the foetus and young child, and may extend upwards into the neck even as far as the lower pole of the thyroid gland. It fails to increase much in size after childhood, and thus becomes comparatively smaller in the adult. Moreover, although it is pink and glandular in the foetus and child, it becomes increasingly infiltrated with fat in later years; in adults, it is distinguishable from surrounding fat only by its distinct capsule.

Oesophagus

The oesophagus, which is 10 in. (25 cm) long, extends from the level of the lower border of the cricoid cartilage at the level of the 6th cervical vertebra to the cardiac orifice of the stomach at the level of the 11th thoracic vertebra (Fig. 1.41).

Course and relations

In neck

In the neck it commences in the median plane and deviates slightly to the left as it approaches the thoracic inlet. The trachea and the thyroid gland are its immediate anterior relations, the 6th and 7th cervical vertebrae and the prevertebral muscles covered by prevertebral fascia are behind it and on either side it is related to the common carotid arteries and the recurrent laryngeal nerves. On the left side it is also related to the subclavian artery and the terminal part of the thoracic duct (Fig. 1.20).

In thorax

The thoracic part traverses first the superior and then the posterior mediastinum. From being somewhat over to the left, it returns to the midline at T5 then passes downwards, forwards and to the left to reach the oesophageal opening in the diaphragm at the level of T10 vertebra. For convenience, the relations of this part are given in sequence from above downwards.

Anteriorly, it is crossed by the trachea, the *left bronchus* (which constricts it), the pericardium (separating it from the left atrium) and the diaphragm.

Posteriorly lie the thoracic vertebrae, the thoracic duct, the azygos vein and its tributaries and, near the diaphragm, the descending aorta.

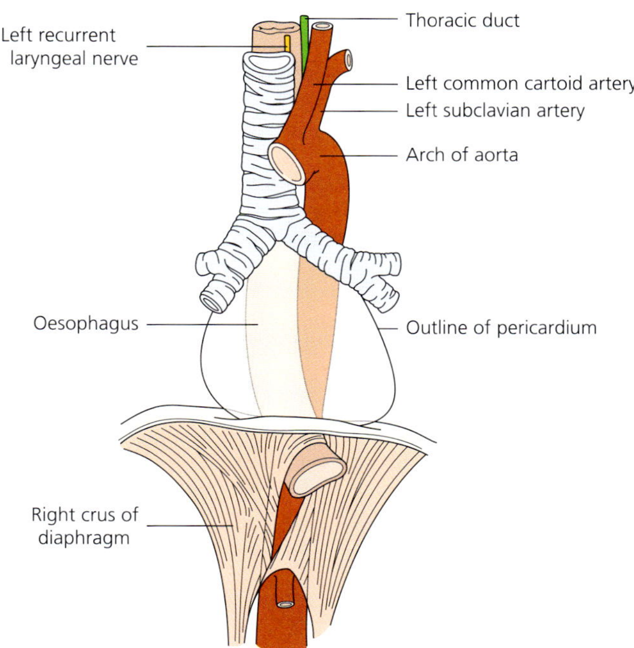

Figure 1.41 The oesophagus and its relations.

On the left side it is related to the left subclavian artery, the terminal part of the aortic arch, the left recurrent laryngeal nerve, the thoracic duct and the left pleura. In the posterior mediastinum it relates to the descending thoracic aorta before this passes posteriorly to the oesophagus above the diaphragm.

On the right side there is the pleura and the azygos vein.

Below the root of the lung the vagi form a plexus on the oesophagus, the left vagus lying anteriorly, the right posteriorly.

In the abdomen, passing forwards through the opening in the right crus of the diaphragm, the oesophagus comes to lie in the oesophageal groove on the posterior surface of the left lobe of the liver, covered by peritoneum on its anterior and left aspects. Behind it is the left crus of the diaphragm. It has a short course of approximately 1.2 in. (3 cm) before it enters the stomach at the cardiac orifice (*see* Fig. 2.13).

Structure

The oesophagus is made of the following:

1. An outer connective tissue sheath of areolar tissue
2. A muscular layer of external longitudinal and internal circular fibres that are striated in the upper two-thirds and smooth in the lower one-third
3. A submucous layer containing mucous glands
4. A stratified squamous epithelium passing abruptly into the columnar epithelium of the stomach

Lower oesophageal sphincter mechanism

There is no anatomical sphincter of thickened circular muscle at the lower end of the human oesophagus, although such a sphincter can be demonstrated in a number of animal species. Nevertheless, a sphincter mechanism clearly exists at the lower end of the oesophagus, as evidenced by the fact that lying down or bending over does not result in gastric contents being refluxed back into the oesophagus. The 'sphincter' can, however, relax to allow vomiting and belching. The lower oesophageal sphincter mechanism is a complex affair, comprising the following:

1. A physiological high-pressure zone at the terminal few centimetres of the oesophagus, which can be demonstrated on oesophageal manometry
2. A pinch-cock effect of the crural sling of the diaphragm (Fig. 1.11)
3. The positive intra-abdominal pressure acting on the short abdominal segment of the oesophagus
4. The valve-like effect of the obliquity of the oesophagogastric angle (*see* Fig. 2.13)
5. The plug-like action of a rosette of mucosal folds (seen on oesophagogastroscopy) at the cardiac orifice

Blood supply, lymphatic drainage and radiology of the oesophagus

Bloody supply

The cervical part is supplied by the inferior thyroid artery, the thoracic part by the branches of the descending thoracic aorta and the abdominal part by the left gastric artery.

Venous drainage

The *veins* from the cervical part drain into the inferior thyroid veins, from the thoracic portion into the azygos vein and from the abdominal portion partly into the azygos and partly into the left gastric veins. The lower end of oesophagus is by far the most important site of the *portocaval anastomoses* (*see* page 53).

Lymphatic drainage

The *lymphatic drainage* is from a peri-oesophageal lymph plexus into the posterior mediastinal nodes, which drain both into the supraclavicular nodes and into nodes around the left gastric vessels. It is not uncommon to be able to palpate hard, fixed supraclavicular nodes in patients with advanced oesophageal cancer.

Radiology of oesophagus

Radiographically, the oesophagus may be studied on films taken after a barium swallow. These show the oesophagus lying in the retrocardiac space just in front of the vertebral column. Anteriorly, the normal oesophagus is indented from above downwards by the three most important structures that cross it – the arch of the aorta, the left bronchus and the left atrium.

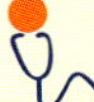

Clinical Features

1 For oesophagoscopy, measurements are made from the upper incisor teeth; the three important levels 7 in. (17 cm), 11 in. (28 cm) and 17 in. (43 cm) corresponding to the commencement of the oesophagus, the point at which it is crossed by the left bronchus and its termination, respectively.

2 These three points also indicate the narrowest parts of the oesophagus: the sites at which, as might be expected, swallowed foreign bodies are most likely to become impacted and strictures are most likely to occur after swallowing corrosive fluids.

3 The anastomosis between the azygos (systemic) and left gastric (portal) venous tributaries in the region of the lower end of the oesophagus is of great importance. In portal hypertension these veins distend into large collateral channels, *oesophageal varices*, which may then rupture with severe haemorrhage (probably as a result of peptic ulceration of the overlying mucosa).

4 Use is made of the close relationship between the oesophagus and the left atrium in determining the degree of left atrial enlargement in mitral stenosis; a barium swallow may show marked backward displacement of the oesophagus caused by the dilated atrium.

5 The oesophagus is crossed solely by the vena azygos on the right side. This is, therefore, the side of election to approach the oesophagus surgically.

Development of the oesophagus

The oesophagus develops from the distal part of the primitive foregut. From the floor of the foregut also differentiate the larynx and trachea, first as a groove (the *laryngotracheal groove*) which then converts into a tube, a bud on each side of which develops and ramifies into the lung.

This close relationship between the origins of the oesophagus and trachea accounts for the relatively common malformation in which the upper part of the oesophagus ends blindly while the lower part opens into the lower trachea at the level of T4 (*oesophageal atresia with tracheo-oesophageal fistula*). Less commonly, the upper part of the oesophagus opens into the trachea, or oesophageal atresia occurs without concomitant fistula into the trachea. Rarely, there is a tracheo-oesophageal fistula without atresia (Fig. 1.42).

Thoracic duct (Fig. 1.43 and *see* Fig. 5.30)

The *cisterna chyli* lies between the abdominal aorta and right crus of the diaphragm. It drains lymphatics from the abdomen and the lower limbs, then passes upwards through the aortic opening to become the *thoracic duct*. This ascends behind the oesophagus, inclines to the left of the oesophagus at the level of T5, then runs upwards behind the carotid sheath, arches laterally at the level of the transverse process of C7. Finally, it descends over the subclavian artery and drains into the commencement of the left brachiocephalic vein at the junction between left subclavian and left internal jugular veins (*see* Fig. 5.30).

The left *jugular, subclavian* and *mediastinal lymph trunks*, draining the left side of the head and neck, upper limb and thorax, respectively, usually join the thoracic duct, although they may open directly into the adjacent large veins at the root of the neck.

The thoracic duct thus usually drains the whole lymphatic field below the diaphragm and the left half of the lymphatics field above it.

On the right side, the *right subclavian, jugular* and *mediastinal trunks* may open independently into the great veins. Usually, the subclavian and jugular trunks first join into a *right lymphatic duct*; this may be joined by the mediastinal trunk so that all three then have a common opening into the origin of the right brachiocephalic vein.

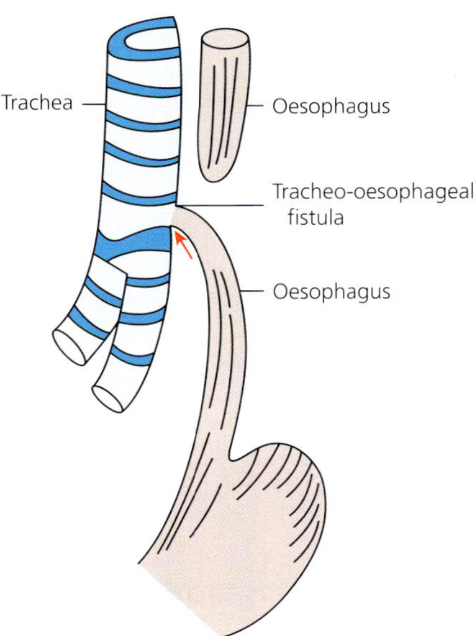

Figure 1.42 The usual form of tracheo-oesophageal fistula. The upper oesophagus ends blindly; the lower oesophagus communicates with the trachea at the level of the 4th thoracic vertebra.

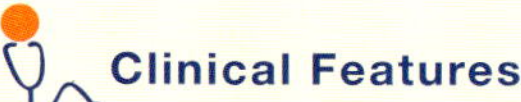

Clinical Features

1 The lymphatics may become blocked by infection and fibrosis due to *Microfilaria bancrofti*. This usually results in lymphoedema of the legs and scrotum, but occasional involvement of the main channels of the trunk and thorax is followed by chylous ascites, chyluria and chylous pleural effusion.
2 The thoracic duct may be damaged during block dissection of the neck. If noticed at operation, the injured duct should be ligated; lymph then finds its way into the venous system by anastomosing channels. If the accident is missed, there follows an unpleasant chylous fistula in the neck.
3 Tears of the thoracic duct have also been reported as a complication of fractures of the thoracic vertebrae to which, in its lower part, the duct is closely related. It may also be damaged in mobilizing the oesophagus at oesophagectomy. Such injuries are followed by a chylothorax.

Thoracic sympathetic trunk (Fig. 1.44(a) and (b))

The sympathetic chain lies immediately lateral to the mediastinum behind the parietal pleura.

Descending from the cervical chain, it crosses the following:

- The neck of the 1st rib
- The heads of the 2nd–10th ribs
- The bodies of the 11th and 12th thoracic vertebrae

It then passes behind the medial arcuate ligament of the diaphragm to continue as the lumbar sympathetic trunk.

The thoracic chain bears a ganglion for each spinal nerve; the first frequently joins the inferior cervical ganglion to form the *stellate ganglion*. Each ganglion receives a white

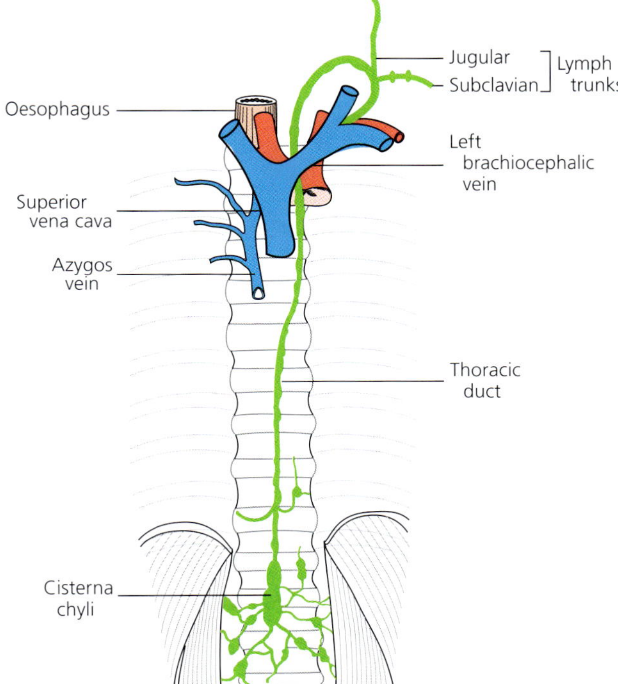

Figure 1.43 The course of the thoracic duct.

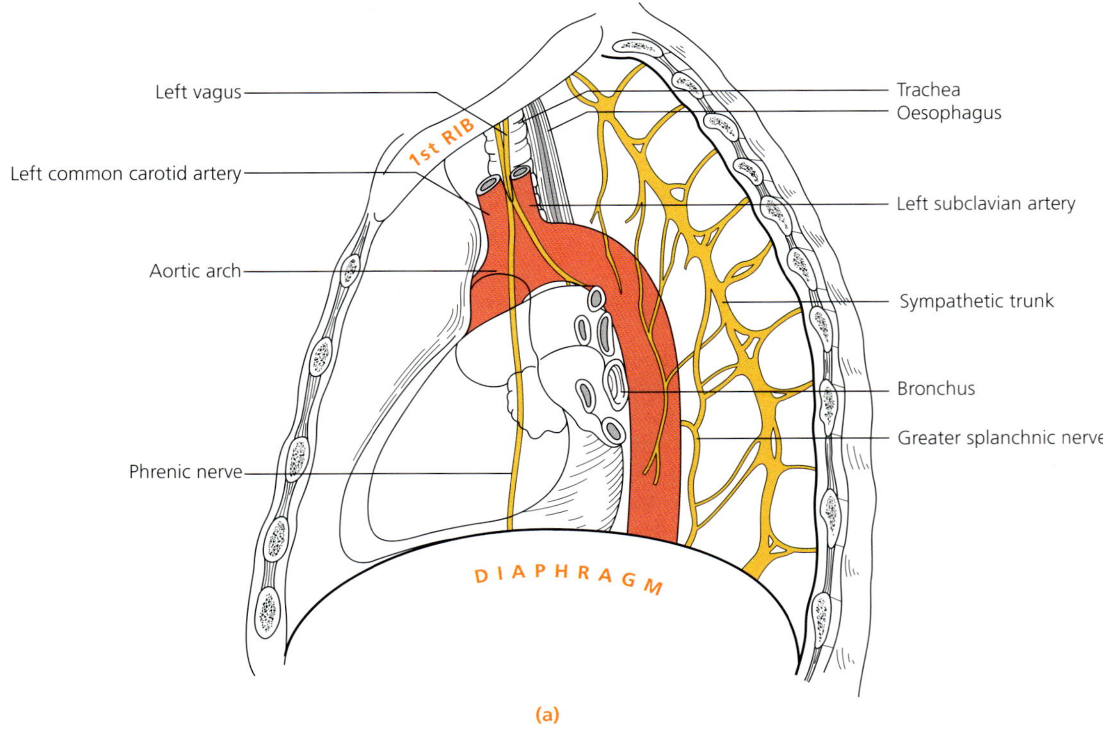

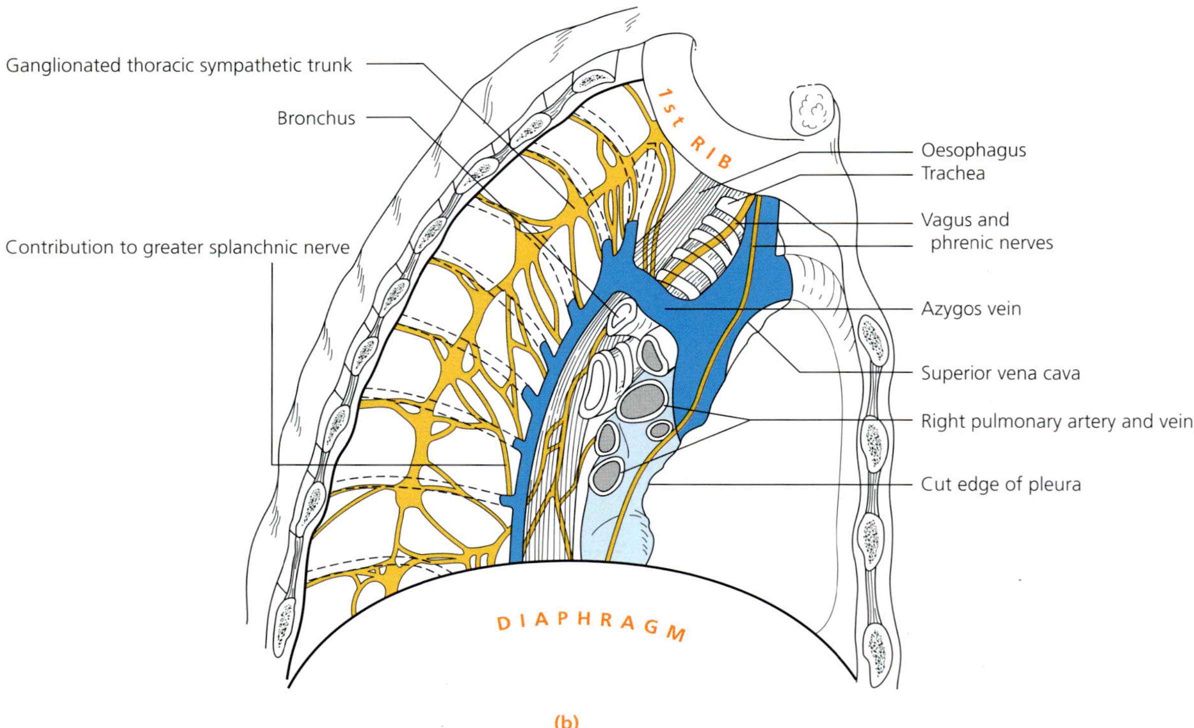

Figure 1.44 **(a)** The left thoracic sympathetic trunk with a display of the left mediastinum. **(b)** The right thoracic sympathetic trunk with a display of the right mediastinum.

ramus communicans containing preganglionic fibres from its corresponding spinal nerve and donates back a grey ramus, bearing postganglionic fibres.

Branches

1. Sympathetic fibres are distributed to the skin with each of the thoracic spinal nerves.
2. Postganglionic fibres from T1–T5 are distributed to the thoracic viscera – the heart and great vessels, the lungs and the oesophagus.
3. Mainly preganglionic fibres from T5–T12 form the *splanchnic nerves*, which pierce the crura of the diaphragm and pass to the coeliac, superior mesenteric, inferior mesenteric and renal ganglia, from which they are relayed as postganglionic fibres to the abdominal viscera. These splanchnic nerves are classically divided into the following three:
   - *Greater splanchnic (T5–T10)*
   - *Lesser splanchnic (T10–T11)*
   - *Least splanchnic (T12)*

However, although these fibres do indeed arise from the T5–T12 ganglia, their exact arrangement is very variable.

The splanchnic nerves lie medial to the sympathetic trunk on the bodies of the thoracic vertebrae and are quite easily visible through the parietal pleura. (For their distribution, *see* page 240.)

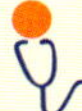

Clinical Features

A high spinal anaesthetic will produce temporary hypotension by paralysing the sympathetic (vasoconstrictor) preganglionic outflow from spinal segment T5 downwards, passing to the abdominal viscera.

On the examination of a chest radiograph

The following features should be examined in every radiograph of the chest.

'Centering' and density of film

The sternal ends of the two clavicles should be equidistant from the shadow of the vertebral spines. The assessment of the density of the film can be learned only by experience, but in a 'normal' film the bony cage should be clearly outlined and the larger vessels in the lung fields clearly visible.

General shape

Any abnormalities in the general form of the thorax (scoliosis, kyphosis and the barrel chest of emphysema, for example) should always be noted before other abnormalities are described.

Bony cage

The thoracic vertebrae should be examined first, then each of the ribs in turn (counting conveniently from their posterior ends and comparing each one with its fellow of the opposite side), and finally clavicles and scapulae. Unless this procedure is carried out systematically, important diagnostic clues (e.g. the presence of a cervical rib or notching of the ribs by enlarged anastomotic vessels) are liable to be missed.

The domes of the diaphragm

These should be examined for height and symmetry and the nature of the cardiophrenic and costophrenic angles observed.

The mediastinum

The outline of the mediastinum should be traced systematically. Special note should be made of the size of the heart, of mediastinal shift and of the vessels and nodes at the hilum of the lung.

Lung fields

Again, systematic examination of the lung fields visible in each intercostal space is necessary if slight differences between the two sides are not to be overlooked.

Abnormalities

When this scheme has been carefully followed, any abnormalities in the bony cage, the mediastinum or lung fields should now be apparent. They should then be defined anatomically as accurately as possible and checked, where necessary, by reference to a film taken from a different angle.

Radiographic appearance of the heart

For the appearance of the heart as seen at fluoroscopy, reference should be made to a standard work in radiology or cardiology. In the present account, only the more important features of the heart and great vessels that can be seen in standard posteroanterior and oblique lateral radiographs of the chest will be described.

The heart and great vessels in anteroposterior radiographs (Fig. 1.45)

The greater part of the 'mediastinal shadow' in an anteroposterior film of the chest is formed by the heart and great vessels. These should be examined as follows.

Size and shape of the heart

Normally, the transverse diameter should not exceed half the total width of the chest, but since it varies widely with bodily build and the position of the heart, these factors must also be assessed. The *shape* of the cardiac shadow also varies a good deal with the position of the heart, being long and narrow in a vertically disposed heart and broad and rounded in the so-called horizontal heart.

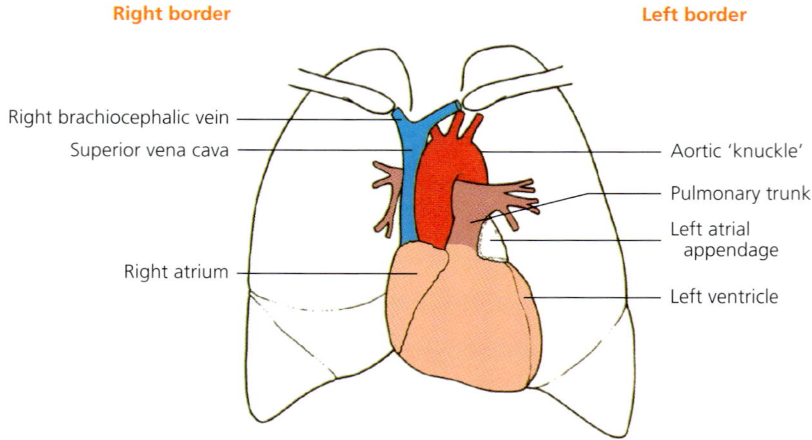

Figure 1.45 The tracing of a chest radiograph to show the composition of the right and left borders of the mediastinal shadow.

The cardiac outline

Each 'border' of the cardiac shadow should be examined in turn. The *right border* of the mediastinal shadow is formed from above downwards by the right brachiocephalic vein, the superior vena cava and the right atrium. Immediately above the heart, the *left border* of the mediastinal shadow presents a well-marked projection, the *aortic knuckle*, which represents the arch of the aorta seen 'end-on'. Beneath this there are, successively, the shadows due to the pulmonary trunk (or the infundibulum of the right ventricle), the auricle of the left atrium and the left ventricle. The shadow of the inferior border of the heart blends centrally with that of the diaphragm, but on either side the two shadows are separated by the well-defined cardiophrenic angles.

Part II

The abdomen and pelvis

Surface anatomy and surface markings

Examination of the patient's abdomen requires not only skill and gentleness but also detailed knowledge of its anatomy.

Look at your own abdomen in the mirror with your muscles tensed, or examine a muscular patient. The midline *linea alba* is evident, and, even more obvious, the linea semilunaris on either side (*see* Fig. 2.1). The tendinous intersections of the rectus at the level of the umbilicus and halfway between the umbilicus and xiphoid are responsible for the six-pack appearance of the tensed rectus muscles in a well-developed subject.

You should be able to identify the following landmarks on yourself or the patient (Fig. 2.2).

The *xiphoid* can be felt in the floor of epigastric fossa. The *costal margin* extends from the 7th costal cartilage at the xiphoid to the tip of the 12th rib (although the latter is often difficult to feel); this margin bears a distinct step, which is the tip of the 9th costal cartilage. The infrasternal/subcostal angle is formed between the right and left costal margins.

The *iliac crest* ends in front at the *anterior superior iliac spine* from which the *inguinal ligament* (*Poupart's ligament*) passes downwards and medially to the *pubic tubercle*. Identify this tubercle by direct palpation and also by running the fingers along the adductor longus tendon (tensed by flexing, abducting and externally rotating the thigh) to its origin just inferior to the tubercle.

In the male feel the firm *vas deferens* between the finger and thumb as it lies within the spermatic cord in the scrotal neck. Trace the vas upwards and note that it passes medial to the pubic tubercle and thence through the *external inguinal ring*, which can be felt by invaginating the scrotal skin with the fingertip.

Vertebral levels (Fig. 2.2(a))

The important vertebral levels are as mentioned below:

- **T9:** *The xiphoid* process is felt in the subcostal/infrasternal angle.
- **L1:** *The transpyloric plane of Addison*, as originally described, lies halfway between the suprasternal notch of the sternum and the top of the pubic symphysis. No clinician uses this, and a useful approximation is that the line lies a hand's breadth below the xiphoid. This plane passes through the tips of 9th costal cartilages, pylorus, the neck of pancreas, the duodenojejunal flexure, the fundus of the gall bladder, and the hila of the kidneys. It also corresponds to the level of termination of the spinal cord.
- **L3:** The *subcostal plane* is a horizontal plane at the level of the lowest part of the costal margin, which is the inferior margin of the 10th rib. It passes through the origin of the inferior mesenteric artery.
- **L4:** The *supracristal plane (supracristal line) at the level of the summits of the iliac crests.* This corresponds to the level of the bifurcation of the aorta. It is also a useful landmark in performing a lumbar puncture, since it is well below the level of the termination of the spinal cord, which is approximately at L1 (*see* page 217 and Fig. 6.13).
- The *umbilicus* is an inconstant landmark. In the healthy adult it lies at the junction of the L3 and L4 vertebrae. It is lower in the infant and, naturally, when the abdomen is pendulous. It is higher in late pregnancy.

Surface markings of individual viscera (Fig. 2.2(b))

The abdominal viscera are inconstant in their position but the surface markings of the following structures are of clinical value.

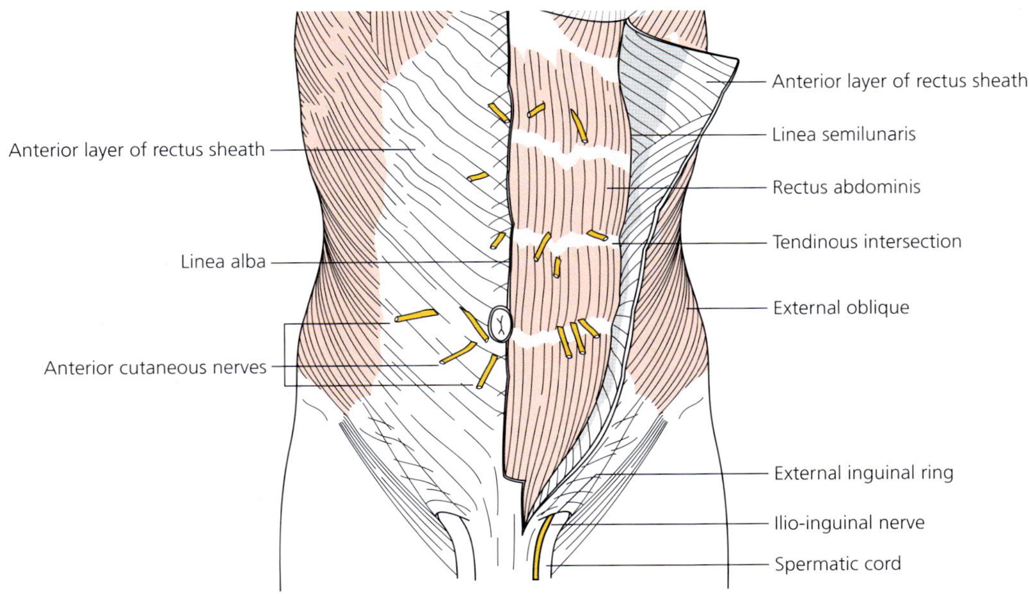

Figure 2.1 Anterior abdominal wall. The anterior rectus sheath on the left side has been reflected laterally.

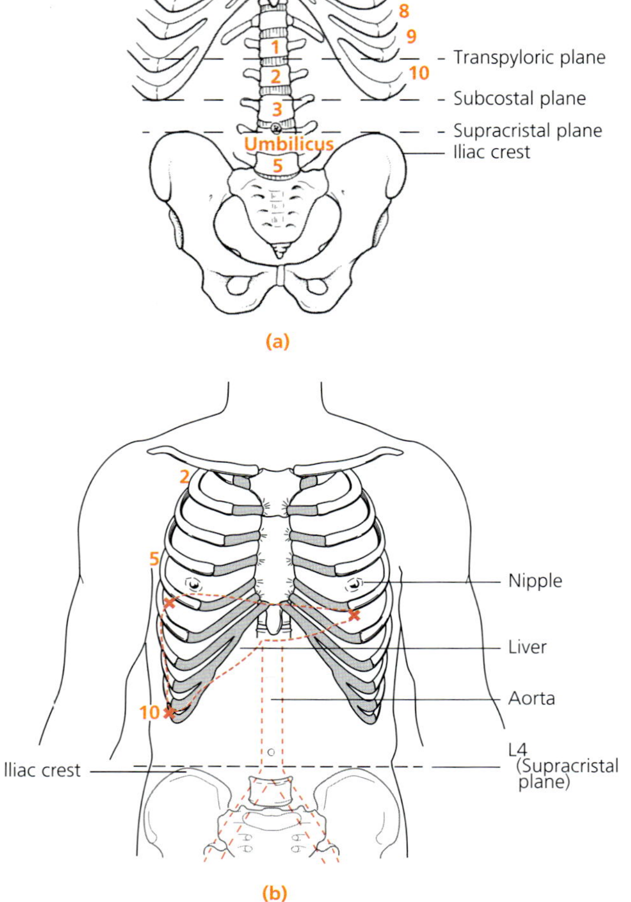

Figure 2.2 **(a)** Boundaries, bony landmarks and vertebral levels of the abdomen. **(b)** The surface markings of the liver and aorta. X's mark the outline of the liver which reaches from the right 5th intercostal space in the midaxillary line to the left 5th intercostal space in mid clavicular line, and lower margin right 10th rib in the midaxillary line. The aorta bifurcates at L4 which is in line with the iliac crests.

Liver

Mark the position of the right 10th rib in the midaxillary line (the costal border); mark the 5th right intercostal space in the midaxillary line; mark the left 5th intercostal space in the midclavicular line. Join these three points to outline the position of the normal liver. The liver is not palpable in a normal subject.

Spleen

This underlies the 9th, 10th and 11th ribs posteriorly on the left side commencing 2 in. (5 cm) from the midline. It is approximately the size of the subject's cupped hand. The spleen must be enlarged to at least two times its normal size to be clinically palpable – so an easily felt spleen is enormously enlarged.

Gall bladder

The fundus of the gall bladder corresponds to the point where the lateral border of the right rectus abdominis cuts the costal margin; this is at the tip of the 9th right costal cartilage, easily detected as a distinct 'step' when the fingers are run along the costal margin.

Pancreas

The transpyloric plane defines the level of the neck of the pancreas, which overlies the vertebral column. From this landmark, the head can be imagined passing downwards and to the right, the body and tail passing upwards and to the left.

Aorta

The pulsations of the aorta can be felt in thin-built subjects by firm downward palpation of the abdomen in the midline. Because of the lumbar lordosis, the lower part of the aorta is pushed forwards and is therefore more readily felt than its upper part. These pulsations terminate at the level of the aortic bifurcation at L4 (Fig. 2.2).

Kidneys

The lower pole of the normal right kidney may sometimes be felt in the thin subject on deep inspiration. Anteriorly, the hilum of the kidney lies in the transpyloric plane four fingerbreadths from the midline. Posteriorly, the upper pole of the kidney lies deep to the 12th rib. The right kidney normally extends approximately 1 in. (2.5 cm) lower than the left. Using these landmarks, the kidney outlines can be projected onto either the anterior or posterior aspects of the abdomen.

Fasciae and muscles of the abdominal wall

Fasciae of the abdominal wall

There is no deep fascia over the anterior abdominal wall, only the superficial fascia. (If there were, we would presumably be unable to take a deep breath or enjoy a large meal!) This, in the lower abdomen, forms a *superficial fatty layer* (*of Camper*) and a deeper *fibrous layer* (*of Scarpa*). The fatty layer is continuous with the superficial fascia of the rest of the body, but the fibrous layer blends with the deep fascia of the upper thigh along the

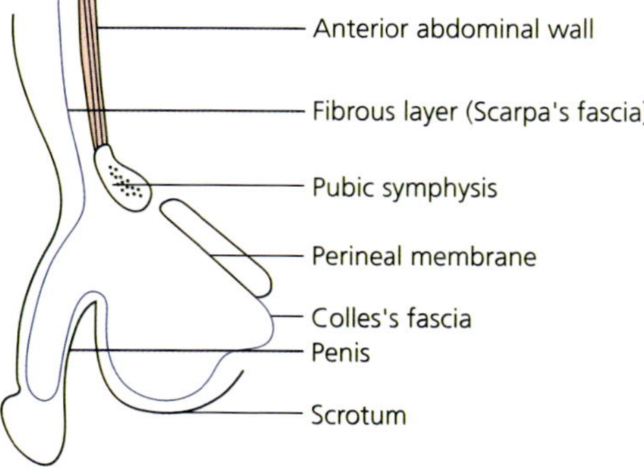

Figure 2.3 Disposition of superficial fascia of anterior abdominal wall in sagittal section.

Holden's line and extends into the penis and scrotum (or labia majora) and into the perineum as *Colles' fascia* (Fig. 2.3). In the perineum it is attached, behind, to the perineal body and posterior margin of the perineal membrane and, laterally, to the ischiopubic rami. It is because of these attachments that a rupture of the urethral bulb in perineum may lead to extravasation of urine into the perineum, scrotum and penis and then into the lower abdomen deep to the fibrous layer of superficial fascia (Scarpa's fascia) but there would be no extravasation of urine downwards into the thighs due to the attachment of the Scarpa's fascia to the deep fascia of the upper thigh.

Nerve supply

The segmental nerve supply of the abdominal muscles and the overlying skin is derived from T7–L1. This distribution can be mapped out approximately if it is remembered that the umbilicus is supplied by T10 and the groin and scrotum by L1 (via the ilio-inguinal and iliohypogastric nerves – *see* Fig. 3.26).

Muscles of the anterior abdominal wall

On either side of the midline, there are four large muscles in the anterior abdominal wall, viz. rectus abdominis, external oblique, internal oblique and transverse abdominis.

The *anterior muscles* of the abdominal wall comprise two strap muscles called rectus abdominis. These are of considerable surgical importance because their anatomy forms the basis of abdominal incisions.

The *rectus abdominis muscle* (Fig. 2.1) arises by two tendinous heads: (a) lateral head from lateral 1 in. (2.5 cm) of pubic crest and (b) medial head from the anterior pubic ligament. It is inserted on the front of the thoracic wall on a 3 in. (7.5 cm) horizontal line from the 5th, 6th and 7th costal cartilages. At the tip of the xiphoid, at the umbilicus and halfway between, are three constant *transverse tendinous intersections*; below the umbilicus there is sometimes a fourth. These intersections are seen only on the anterior aspect of the muscle and here they adhere to the anterior rectus sheath. Posteriorly they are not in evidence and, in consequence, the rectus muscle is completely free behind. At each intersection, vessels from the superior epigastric artery and vein pierce the rectus.

The sheath in which the rectus lies is called the rectus sheath. It is formed, to a large extent, by the aponeurotic expansions of the lateral abdominal muscles (Fig. 2.4) as follows:

a. Above the costal margin, the anterior sheath comprises the external oblique aponeurosis only; posteriorly lie the costal cartilages.
b. From the costal margin to a point halfway between the umbilicus and pubis, the external oblique and the anterior lamina of the internal oblique aponeurosis form the anterior sheath. Posteriorly lie the posterior lamina of this split internal oblique aponeurosis and the aponeurosis of transversus abdominis.
c. Below a point halfway between the umbilicus and pubis, all the aponeuroses pass in front of the rectus so that the anterior sheath here comprises the tendinous expansions of all three oblique muscles blended together. The posterior wall at this level is made up of the only other structures available – the transversalis fascia (the thickened extraperitoneal fascia of the lower abdominal wall) and the peritoneum.

The posterior junction between (b) and (c) is marked by the *arcuate line of Douglas*, which is the lower border of the posterior aponeurotic part of the rectus sheath. At this point the inferior epigastric artery and vein (from the external iliac vessels) enter the sheath, pass upwards and anastomose with the superior epigastric vessels, which are terminal branches of the internal thoracic artery and vein. The rectus sheaths fuse in the midline to form the *linea alba* stretching from the xiphoid to the pubic symphysis.

The *lateral muscles of the abdominal wall comprise* three flat muscles (the external and internal oblique and the transversus abdominis). These correspond to the three layers of muscle of the chest wall – external, internal and innermost intercostals – and, like them, have their neurovascular bundles running between the second and third layer. They are clinically important in making up the rectus sheath and the inguinal canal, and also because they must be divided in making lateral abdominal incisions.

Their attachments can be remembered when one bears in mind that they fill the space between the costal margin above, the iliac crest below, and the lumbar muscles covered

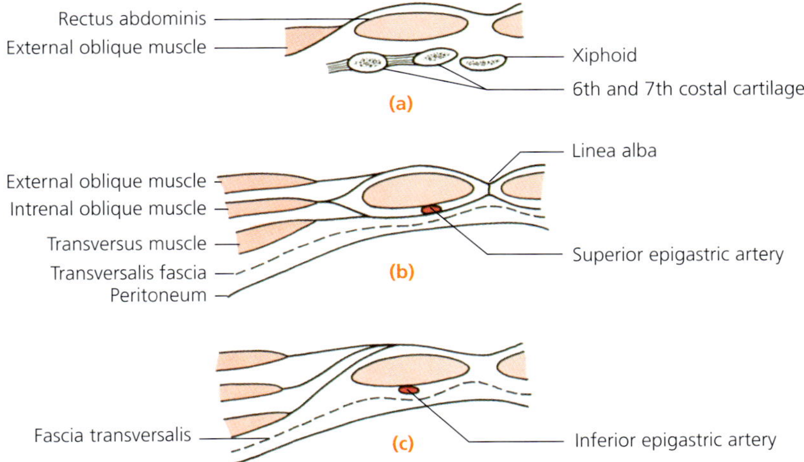

Figure 2.4 The composition of the rectus sheath shown in transverse section **(a)** above the costal margin, **(b)** above the arcuate line and **(c)** below the arcuate line.

by lumbar fascia behind. Medially, as already noted, they constitute the rectus sheath and thence blend into the linea alba from xiphoid to pubic crest.

The *obliquus externus abdominis* (external oblique) arises from the outer surfaces of the lower eight ribs and fans out into the xiphoid, linea alba, the pubic crest, pubic tubercle and the anterior half of the iliac crest.

From the pubic tubercle to the anterior superior iliac spine its lower border forms the aponeurotic *inguinal ligament of Poupart*.

The *obliquus internus abdominis* (internal oblique) arises from the lumbar fascia, the anterior two-thirds of the iliac crest and the lateral two-thirds of the inguinal ligament. It is inserted into the lowest six costal cartilages, linea alba and the pubic crest.

The *transversus abdominis* arises from the lowest six costal cartilages (interdigitating with the diaphragm), the lumbar fascia, the anterior two-thirds of the iliac crest and the lateral one-third of the inguinal ligament; it is inserted into the linea alba and the pubic crest.

The fibres of external oblique pass downwards and forwards, the internal oblique upwards and forwards and the transversus transversely. Note also that the external oblique has its posterior border free but the deeper two muscles both arise posteriorly from the lumbar fascia.

Anatomy of abdominal incisions

Incisions to expose the intraperitoneal structures represent a compromise on the part of the surgeon. On the one hand, he requires maximum access; on the other hand, he wishes to leave a scar which lies, if possible, in a skin crease, and which will have done minimal damage to the muscles of the abdominal wall and to their nerve supply.

The nerve supply to the lateral abdominal muscles forms a richly communicating network so that cuts across the lines of fibres of these muscles, with division of one or two nerves, produce no clinical ill effects. The segmental nerve supply to the rectus, however, has little cross-communication and damage to these nerves must, if possible, be avoided.

The copious anastomoses between the blood vessels supplying the abdominal muscles make damage to these by operative incisions of no practical importance.

Midline incision

The midline incision is made through the linea alba. Superiorly, this is a relatively wide fibrous structure, but below the umbilicus it becomes almost hairline and the surgeon may experience difficulty in finding the exact point of cleavage between the recti at this level. Being made of fibrous tissue only, it provides an almost bloodless line along which the abdomen can be opened rapidly and, if necessary, from one end to the other.

Paramedian incision

The paramedian incision is a vertical incision placed 1 in. (2.5 cm) to 1.5 in. (4 cm) lateral, and parallel, to the midline; the anterior rectus sheath is opened, the rectus displaced laterally and the posterior sheath, together with peritoneum, then incised. This incision has the advantage that, on suturing the peritoneum, the rectus slips back into place to cover and protect the peritoneal scar.

The adherence of the anterior sheath to the rectus muscle at its tendinous intersections means that the sheath must be dissected off the muscle at each of these sites, and at each of these a segmental vessel requires division. Having done this, the rectus is easily slid laterally from the posterior sheath from which it is quite free. The posterior sheath and the peritoneum form a tough membrane down to halfway between the pubis and umbilicus, but it is much thinner and more fatty below this where, as we have seen, it loses its aponeurotic component and is made up of only transversalis fascia and peritoneum. The inferior epigastric vessels are seen passing under the arcuate line of Douglas in the posterior sheath and usually require division in a low paramedian incision.

Transrectus incision

Occasionally, the rectus abdominis muscle is split in the line of the paramedian incision. The rectus receives its nerve supply laterally and the muscle medial to the incision must, in consequence, be deprived of its innervation and undergo atrophy; it is an incision therefore best avoided.

Subcostal incision

The subcostal (Kocher) incision is used on the right side in biliary surgery, and on the left in exposure of the spleen. The skin incision commences at the midline and extends parallel to, and 1 in. (2.5 cm) below, the costal margin.

The anterior rectus sheath is opened, the rectus cut and the posterior sheath with underlying adherent peritoneum incised. The small 8th intercostal nerve branch to the rectus is sacrificed but the larger and more important 9th nerve, in the lateral part of the wound, is preserved. The divided rectus muscle is held by the intersections above and below and retracts very little. It subsequently heals by fibrous tissue. This incision is valuable in the patient with the wide subcostal angle. Where this angle is narrow, the paramedian incision is usually preferred.

Muscle split or gridiron incision to the appendix

The gridiron incision is used in appendicectomy. The oblique skin incision centred at *McBurney's point* (two-thirds of the way laterally along the line from the umbilicus to the anterior superior iliac spine) is now less popular than an almost transverse incision in the line of the skin crease forwards from, and 1 in. (2.5 cm) above, the anterior spine.

The aponeurosis of the external oblique is incised in the line of its fibres (obliquely downwards and medially); the internal oblique and transversus muscles are then split in the line of their fibres, and retracted without their having to be divided. On closing the incision, these muscles snap together again, leaving a virtually undamaged abdominal wall.

Transverse and oblique incisions

Incisions cutting through the lateral abdominal muscles do not damage their richly anastomosing nerve supply and heal without weakness. They are useful, for example, in exposing the sigmoid colon or the caecum or, by displacing the peritoneum medially, extraperitoneal structures such as the ureter, sympathetic chain and the external iliac vessels.

Pfannenstiel incision

This is a useful incision in gynaecological surgery, Caesarian section and open extraperitoneal exposure of the prostate and urinary bladder in the retropubic space. A curving transverse incision is made approximately 2 in. (5 cm) above the pubic symphysis. The anterior rectus sheath is incised on either side in the line of the skin incision and the underlying rectus abdominis muscle, with the small triangular pyramidalis muscle, is dissected off the sheath on either side, retracted laterally and the peritoneum opened in the midline. Care is taken not to damage the bladder; first, by emptying it by catheterization before surgery and, second, by commencing the incision of the peritoneum at the upper end of the exposed peritoneum. The healed incision, lying in a skin crease and just within the line of the pubic hair, is invisible.

Thoraco-abdominal incisions

An upper paramedian or upper oblique abdominal incision can be extended through the 8th or 9th intercostal space, the diaphragm incised and an extensive exposure achieved of both the upper abdomen and thorax. This is used, for example, on the left in removing growths of the upper stomach or lower oesophagus and on the right in resection of the right lobe of the liver.

Paracentesis abdominis

Intraperitoneal fluid collections can be evacuated via a cannula inserted through the abdominal wall. The bladder having been first emptied with a catheter, the cannula is introduced on a trocar either through the midline (where the linea alba is relatively bloodless) or lateral to McBurney's point (where there is no danger of wounding the inferior epigastric vessels). The coils of gut are not in danger in this procedure because they are mobile and are pushed away by the tip of the trocar. These two landmarks are also used for insertion of cannulae for laparoscopic surgery.

Inguinal canal (Fig. 2.5)

The inguinal canal is an oblique passage in the lower part of the anterior abdominal wall. This canal represents the oblique passage taken through the lower abdominal wall by the testis and cord (the round ligament in the female).

The canal is 1.5 in. (4 cm) long. It passes downwards and medially from the internal to the external inguinal rings and lies parallel to, and immediately above, the inguinal ligament.

Questions on the anatomy of this region are probably asked more often than any other in examinations because of its importance in the diagnosis and treatment of hernias.

Boundaries (Relations)

The boundaries of inguinal canal are as mentioned below:

- **Anteriorly:** The skin, superficial fascia and the external oblique aponeurosis cover the full length of the canal; the internal oblique covers its lateral one-third
- **Posteriorly:** The *conjoint tendon* forms the posterior wall of the canal medially, the transversalis fascia laterally. (The conjoint tendon represents the fused common insertion of the internal oblique and transversus into the pubic crest and pectineal line. The transversalis fascia is the name given to the extraperitoneal fascia which, in the lower abdomen, is much thickened.)
- **Above:** Arched lowest fibres of the internal oblique and transversus abdominis
- **Below:** Lies the inguinal ligament

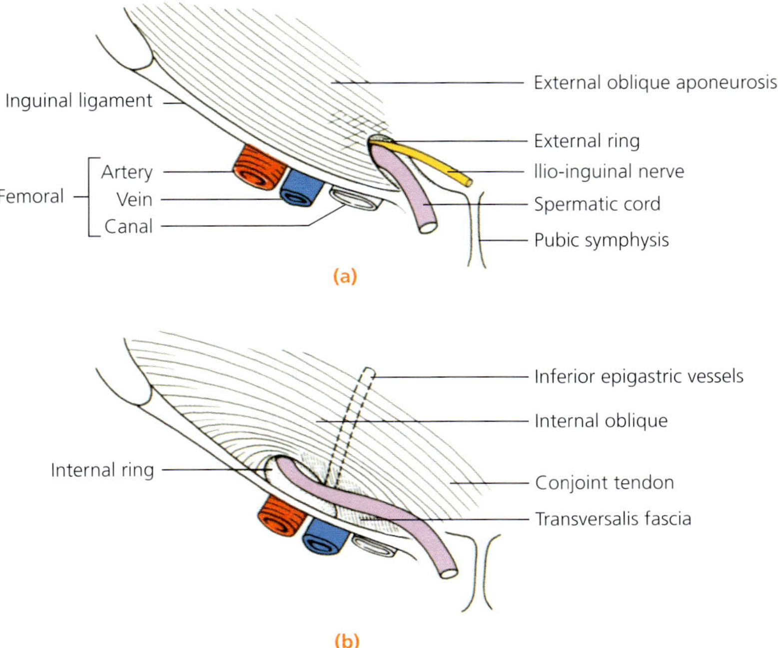

Figure 2.5 The right inguinal canal **(a)** with the external oblique aponeurosis intact and **(b)** with the aponeurosis laid open.

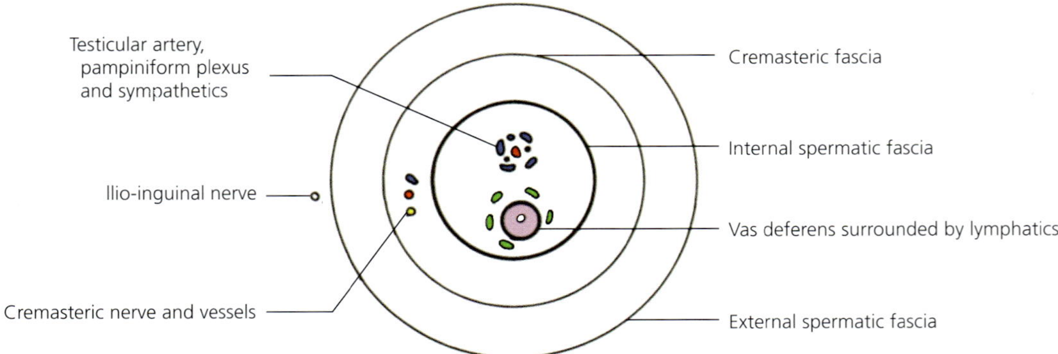

Figure 2.6 Scheme of the spermatic cord and its contents, in transverse section.

Inguinal rings

The *internal (or deep) ring* represents the point at which the spermatic cord pushes through the transversalis fascia, dragging from it a covering which forms the *internal spermatic fascia*. This ring is oval in shape and is situated 1/2 in. (1.25 cm) above the mid-inguinal points. It is demarcated medially by the inferior epigastric vessels passing upwards from the external iliac artery and vein.

The *external (or superficial) ring* is a V-shaped defect in the external oblique aponeurosis and lies immediately above and medial to the pubic tubercle. As the cord traverses this opening, it carries the *external spermatic fascia* from the ring's margins.

In the male, the inguinal canal transmits the spermatic cord and the ilio-inguinal nerve. In the female, the canal is a much smaller affair – it is still made up of the three layers of fascia described below, but transmits only the round ligament of the uterus (which represents the gubernaculum testis of the male embryo, *see* page 72) together with the ilio-inguinal nerve.

Spermatic cord

The *spermatic cord* comprises the following (Fig. 2.6):

- **Three layers of fascia:** The *external spermatic*, from the external oblique aponeurosis; the *cremasteric*, from the internal oblique aponeurosis (containing muscle fibres termed the *cremaster muscle*); the *internal spermatic*, from the transversalis fascia
- **Three arteries:** The testicular (from the aorta); the cremasteric (from the inferior epigastric artery); the artery of the vas (from the inferior vesical artery)
- **Three veins:** The pampiniform plexus of veins (draining the right testis into the inferior vena cava and the left into the left renal vein), and the cremasteric vein and vein of the vas, which accompany their corresponding arteries
- **Three nerves:** The nerve to the cremaster (from the genitofemoral nerve); sympathetic fibres from the T10 and T11 spinal segments; the ilio-inguinal nerve (strictly, *on* and not *in* the cord)
- **Three other structures:** The vas deferens; lymphatics of the testis, which pass to the para-aortic lymph nodes; and, pathologically present as the third structure, a patent processus vaginalis in patients with an indirect inguinal hernia

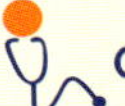

Clinical Features

An *indirect inguinal hernia* passes through the internal ring, along the canal and then, if large enough, emerges through the external ring and descends into the scrotum. If reducible, such a hernia can be completely controlled by pressure with the fingertip over the internal ring, which lies 0.5 in. (1.25 cm) above the point where the femoral artery passes under the inguinal ligament, i.e. 0.5 in. (1.25 cm) above the femoral pulse. This pulse can be felt at the mid-inguinal point, halfway between the anterior superior iliac spine and the symphysis pubis (*see* Fig. 4.6).

If the hernia protrudes through the external ring, it can be felt to lie above and medial to the pubic tubercle, and is thus differentiated from a femoral hernia emerging from the femoral canal, which lies below and lateral to this landmark (*see* Fig. 4.32).

A *direct inguinal hernia* pushes its way directly forwards through the posterior wall of the inguinal canal in the region of inguinal triangle (Hesselbach's triangle) bounded medially by the lateral border of rectus abdominis and laterally by inferior epigastric artery. Since it lies medial to the internal ring, it is not controlled by digital pressure applied immediately above the femoral pulse. Occasionally, a direct hernia becomes large enough to push its way through the external ring and then into the neck of the scrotum. This is so unusual that one can usually assume that a scrotal hernia is an indirect hernia.

The only certain way of determining the issue is at operation; the inferior epigastric vessels demarcate the medial edge of the internal ring, therefore an indirect hernia sac will pass lateral and a direct hernia medial to these vessels. Quite often both a direct and an indirect hernia coexist; they bulge through on each side of the inferior epigastric vessels like the legs of a pair of pantaloons.

Peritoneal cavity

The endothelial lining of the primitive coelomic cavity of the embryo becomes the thoracic pleura and the abdominal peritoneum. Each is invaginated by ingrowing viscera that thus come to be covered by a serous membrane and to be packed snugly into a serous-lined cavity, the visceral and parietal layer, respectively.

In the male, the peritoneal cavity is completely closed, but in the female it is perforated by the openings of the uterine

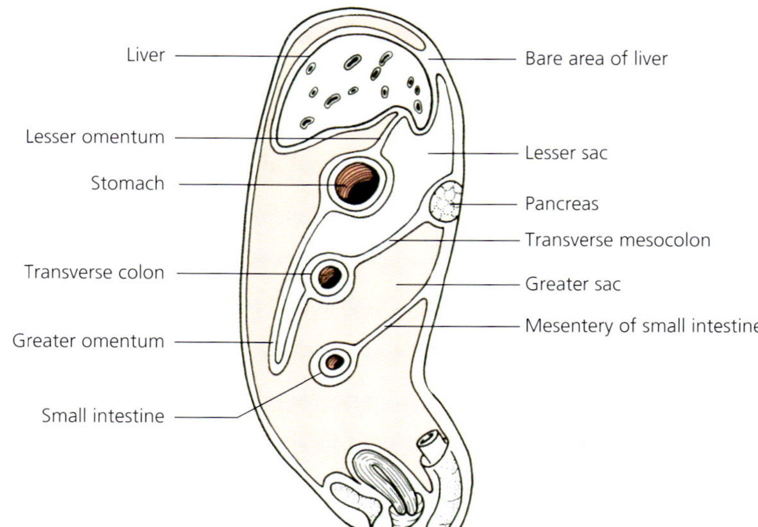

Figure 2.7 The peritoneal cavity in longitudinal (sagittal) section (female).

tubes, which constitute a possible pathway of infection from the exterior.

To revise the complicated attachments of the peritoneum, it is best to start at one point and trace this membrane in an imaginary round-trip of the abdominal cavity, aided by Figs 2.7 and 2.8. A convenient point of departure is the parietal peritoneum of the anterior abdominal wall below the umbilicus. At this level the membrane is smooth apart from the shallow ridges formed by the median umbilical fold (the obliterated foetal urachus passing from the bladder to the umbilicus), the medial umbilical folds (the obliterated umbilical arteries passing to the umbilicus from the internal iliac arteries) and the lateral umbilical folds (the peritoneum covering the inferior epigastric vessels).

A cicatrix can usually be felt and seen at the posterior aspect of the umbilicus, and from this the *falciform ligament* sweeps upwards and slightly to the right of the midline to the liver. In the free border of this ligament lies the *ligamentum teres* (the obliterated foetal left umbilical vein), which passes into the groove between the quadrate lobe and left lobe of the liver (*see* Fig. 2.31).

Elsewhere, the peritoneum sweeps over the inferior aspect of the diaphragm, to be reflected onto the liver (leaving a bare

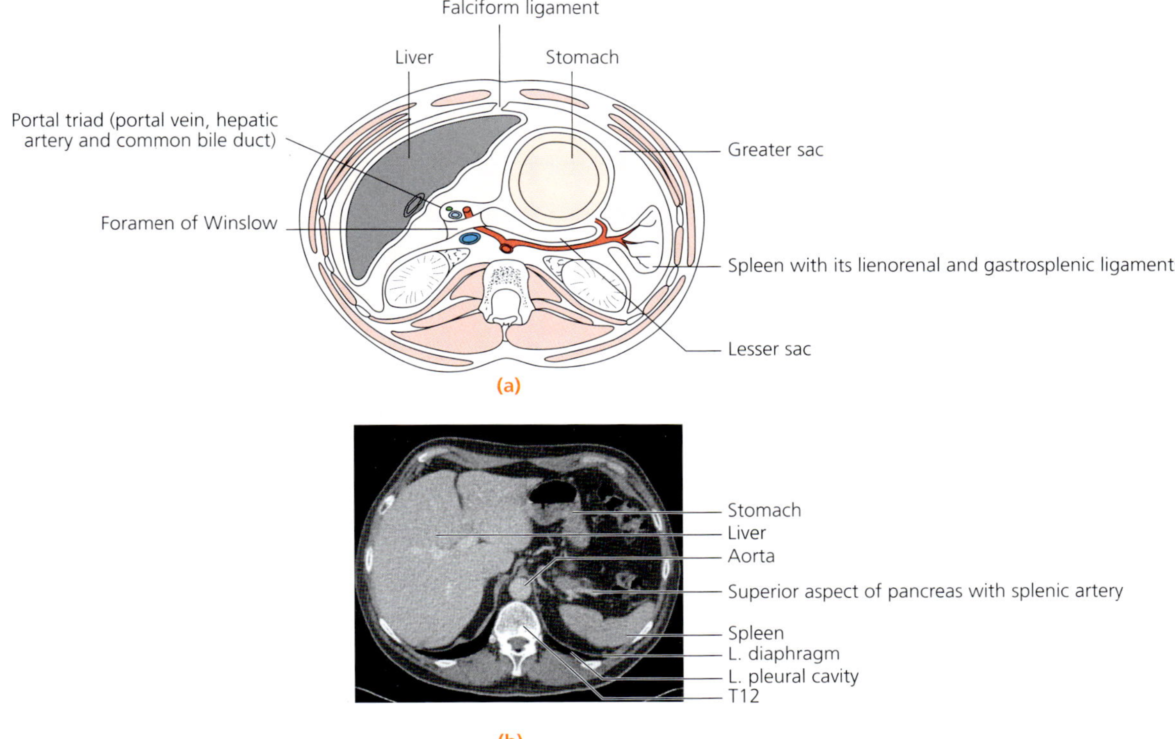

Figure 2.8 **(a)** The peritoneal cavity in transverse section (through the foramen of Winslow), seen from below. **(b)** The corresponding CT scan through T12.

area demarcated by the *upper* and *lower coronary ligaments* of the liver) and onto the right margin of the abdominal oesophagus. After enclosing the liver (for further details, *see* page 56), the peritoneum descends from the porta hepatis as a double sheet, the *lesser omentum*, to the lesser curve of the stomach. Here, it again splits to enclose this organ, reforms at its greater curve, then loops much downwards and then up again to attach to the length of the transverse colon, forming the apron-like *greater omentum*.

The transverse colon, in turn, is enclosed within this peritoneum, which then passes upwards and backwards as the transverse mesocolon to the posterior abdominal wall, where it is attached along the anterior aspect of the pancreas.

At the base of the transverse mesocolon, this double peritoneal sheet divides once again; the upper leaf passes upwards over the posterior abdominal wall to reflect onto the liver (at the bare area), the lower leaf passes over the lower part of the posterior abdominal wall to cover the pelvic viscera and to link up once again with the peritoneum of the anterior wall. This posterior layer is, however, interrupted by its being reflected along an oblique line running from the duodenojejunal flexure, above and to the left, to the ileocaecal junction, below and to the right, to form the *mesentery of the small intestine*.

The mesentery of the small intestine, the lesser and greater omenta and mesocolon all carry the vascular supply and lymph drainage of their contained viscera.

The *lesser sac* (Fig. 2.8) is the extensive pouch lying behind the lesser omentum and the stomach and projecting downwards (although usually this space is obliterated) between the layers of the greater omentum. Its left wall is formed by the spleen attached by the *gastrosplenic* and splenorenal (*lienorenal*) *ligaments*. The right extremity of the sac opens into the main peritoneal cavity via the *epiploic foramen* or *foramen of Winslow* (Fig. 2.9), whose boundaries are as follows:

- **Anteriorly:** The free edge of the lesser omentum, containing the common bile duct to the right, the hepatic artery to the left and the portal vein posteriorly
- **Posteriorly:** The inferior vena cava
- **Inferiorly:** The first part of the duodenum, over which runs the hepatic artery before this ascends into the anterior wall of the foramen
- **Superiorly**: The caudate process of the caudate lobe of the liver

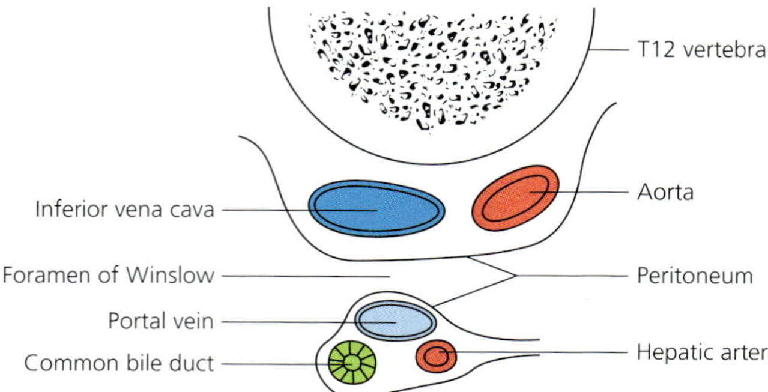

Figure 2.9 The foramen of Winslow in transverse section (viewed from above).

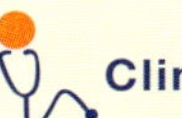

Clinical Features

1 Occasionally a loop of intestine passes through the foramen of Winslow into the lesser sac and becomes strangulated by the edges of the foramen. Notice that none of these important boundaries can be incised to release the strangulation; the bowel must be decompressed by a needle to allow its reduction.

2 It is important to the surgeon that the hepatic artery can be compressed between his index finger within the foramen of Winslow and his thumb on its anterior wall. If the cystic artery is torn during cholecystectomy, haemorrhage can be controlled by this manoeuvre (named after James Pringle), which then enables the damaged vessel to be identified and secured.

Intraperitoneal fossae

A number of fossae occur within the peritoneal cavity in which loops of bowel may become caught and strangulated. Those of importance are as follows:

1. **Lesser sac:** Which communicates with greater sac via the foramen of Winslow
2. **Paraduodenal fossa:** Between the duodenojejunal flexure and the inferior mesenteric vessels
3. **Retrocaecal fossa:** In which the appendix frequently lies
4. **Intersigmoid fossa:** Formed by the inverted 'V' attachment of the mesosigmoid

Subphrenic spaces (Fig. 2.10)

Below the diaphragm are a number of potential spaces formed in relation to the attachments of the liver. One or more of these spaces may become filled with pus (a subphrenic abscess) walled off inferiorly by adhesions. There are five subdivisions of clinical importance.

The *right* and *left subphrenic spaces* lie between the diaphragm and the liver, separated from each other by the falciform ligament.

The *right* and *left subhepatic spaces* lie below the liver. The right is the *pouch of Morison* and is bounded by the posterior abdominal wall behind and by the liver above. It communicates anteriorly with the right subphrenic space around the anterior margin of the right lobe of the liver and below both open into the general peritoneal cavity from which infection may track, for example, from a perforated appendix or a perforated peptic ulcer. The left subhepatic space is the lesser sac, which communicates with the right through the foramen of Winslow. It may fill with fluid as a result of a perforation in the posterior wall of the stomach or from an inflamed or injured pancreas to form a *pseudocyst of the pancreas*.

The *right extraperitoneal space* lies between the bare area of the liver and the diaphragm. It may become involved in retroperitoneal infections or directly from a liver abscess.

Posterior subphrenic abscesses are drained by an incision below, or through the bed of, the 12th rib. A finger is then passed upwards and forwards between the liver and diaphragm to open into the abscess cavity. An anteriorly placed collection of pus below the diaphragm can alternatively be drained via an incision placed below and parallel to the costal

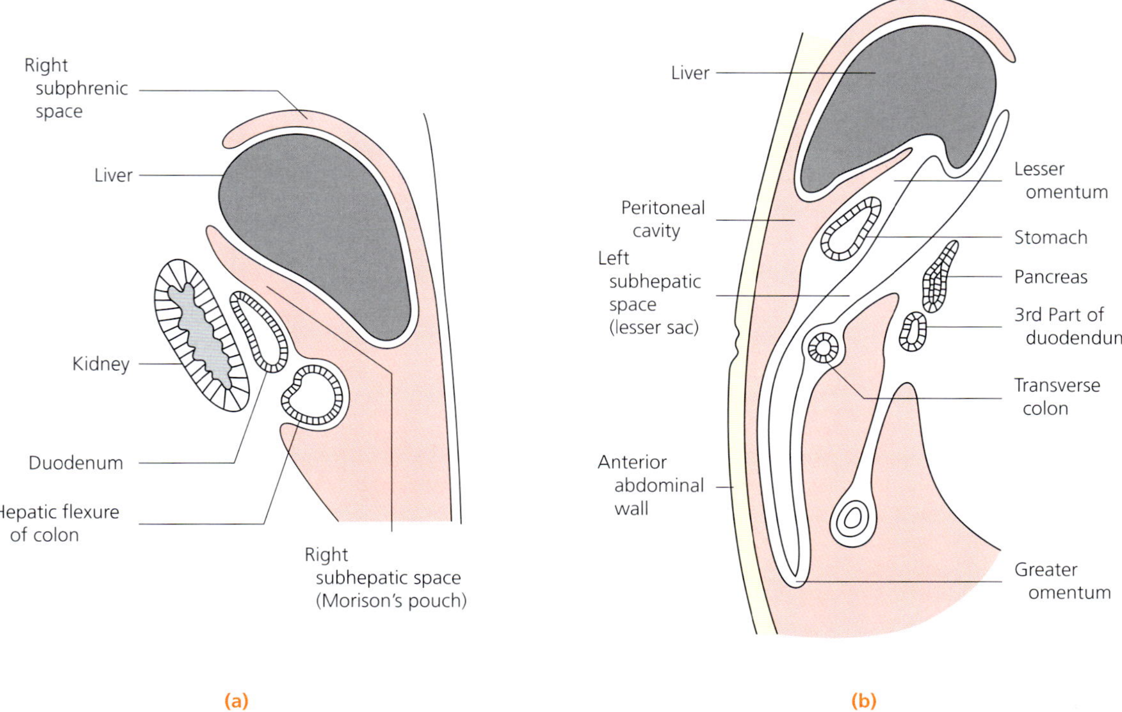

Figure 2.10 The anatomy of **(a)** the right and **(b)** the left subphrenic spaces in sagittal section.

margin. Nowadays, intra-abdominal fluid collections can often be drained percutaneously under ultrasound or CT control.

Gastrointestinal tract

Stomach

The stomach is a muscular bag and forms the widest and most distensible part of the digestive tube. It is roughly J-shaped, although its size and shape vary considerably. It tends to be high and transverse in the obese short subject and to be elongated in the asthenic individual; even in the same person, its shape depends on whether it is full or empty, on the position of the body and on the phase of respiration. The stomach has *two surfaces* – the anterior and posterior; *two curvatures* – the greater and lesser; and *two orifices* – the cardia and pylorus (Fig. 2.11).

The stomach projects to the left, above the level of the cardiac orifice (or *cardia*), to form the dome-like gastric *fundus*, demarcates from the oesophagus by a *cardiac notch*. Along the lesser curve is a distinct notch, the *incisura angularis*. Between the cardiac orifice and the incisura is the body of the stomach, while the area between the incisura and the pylorus is the pyloric antrum. The junction of the pylorus with the duodenum is marked by a constriction externally and also by a constant vein that crosses it on the front, the prepyloric *vein of Mayo*.

It is the body of the stomach that bears the HCl-secreting parietal cells. The antrum secretes the enzyme gastrin and its secretion is alkaline.

The thickened *pyloric sphincter* is easily felt and surrounds the lumen of the *pyloric canal*. The pyloric sphincter is an anatomical structure as well as a physiological mechanism. The cardia, on the other hand, although competent (gastric contents do not flow out of your mouth if you stand on your head), is not demarcated by a distinct anatomical sphincter. The exact nature of the cardiac sphincter action is still not fully understood, but the following mechanisms have been suggested, each supported by some experimental and clinical evidence.

1. The mucosal folds at the oesophagogastric junction act as a valve.
2. The acute angle of entry of the oesophagus into the stomach produces a valve-like effect.

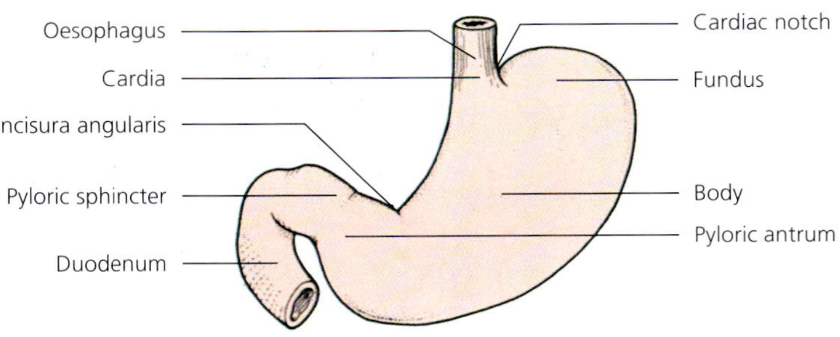

Figure 2.11 The stomach and its subdivisions.

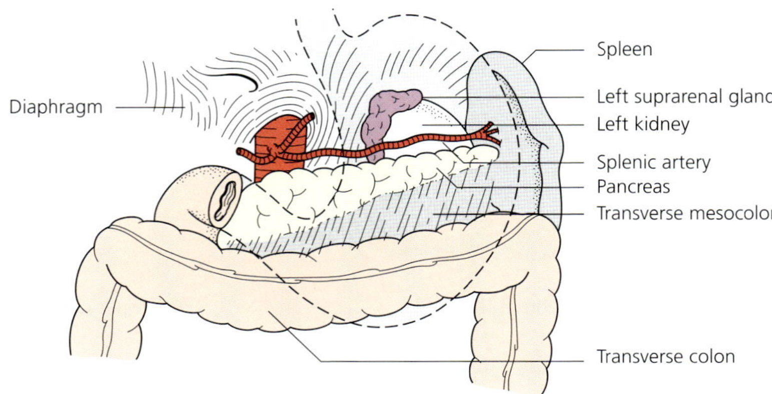

Figure 2.12 The posterior relations of the stomach; the stomach (indicated by the broken line) is superimposed upon its bed.

3. The circular muscle of the lower oesophagus is a physiological, as distinct from an anatomical, sphincter.
4. The arrangement of the muscle fibres of the stomach around the cardia either acts as a sphincter or else maintains the acute angle of entry of the oesophagus into the stomach.
5. The right crus of the diaphragm acts as a 'pinch-cock' to the lower oesophagus as it pierces this muscle.
6. The positive intra-abdominal pressure compresses the walls of the short segment of the intra-abdominal oesophagus.

Relations (Fig. 2.12)

These are as follows:

- **Anteriorly:** The abdominal wall, the left costal margin, the diaphragm and the left lobe of the liver
- **Posteriorly:** The lesser sac, which separates the stomach from the pancreas, transverse mesocolon, left kidney, left suprarenal, the spleen and the splenic artery
- **Superiorly:** The left dome of the diaphragm

The lesser omentum is attached along the lesser curvature of the stomach; the greater omentum along the greater curvature. These omenta contain the vascular and lymphatic supply of the stomach.

Arterial supply

The *arterial supply* (Fig. 2.13) to the stomach is extremely rich and comprises the following:

- **The left gastric artery:** From the coeliac axis
- **The right gastric artery:** From the hepatic artery
- **The right gastro-epiploic artery:** From the gastroduodenal branch of the hepatic artery
- **The left gastro-epiploic artery:** From the splenic artery
- **The short gastric arteries:** From the splenic artery

The corresponding veins drain into the portal system.

Lymphatic drainage

The *lymphatic drainage* of the stomach accompanies its blood vessels. The stomach can be divided into the following three drainage zones (Fig. 2.14).

- **Area I:** The superior two-thirds of the stomach drain along the left and right gastric vessels to the aortic nodes.
- **Area II:** The right two-thirds of the inferior one-third of the stomach drain along the right gastro-epiploic vessels to the subpyloric nodes and thence to the aortic nodes.
- **Area III:** The left one-third of the greater curvature of the stomach drains along the short gastric and splenic vessels lying in the gastrosplenic and splenorenal ligaments, then, via the *suprapancreatic nodes*, to the aortic group.

This extensive lymphatic drainage and the technical impossibility of its complete removal is one of the serious problems in dealing with stomach cancer. Involvement of the nodes along the splenic vessels can be dealt with by removing the spleen, the gastrosplenic and splenorenal ligaments and the body and tail of the pancreas. Lymph nodes among the gastro-epiploic

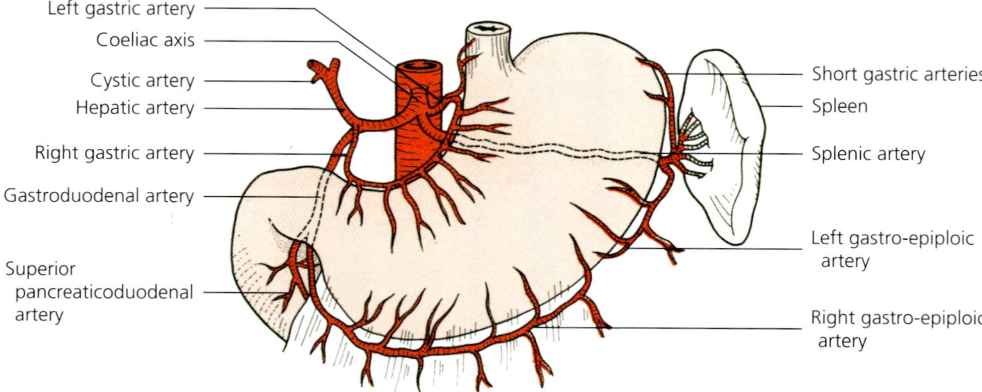

Figure 2.13 The arterial supply of the stomach.

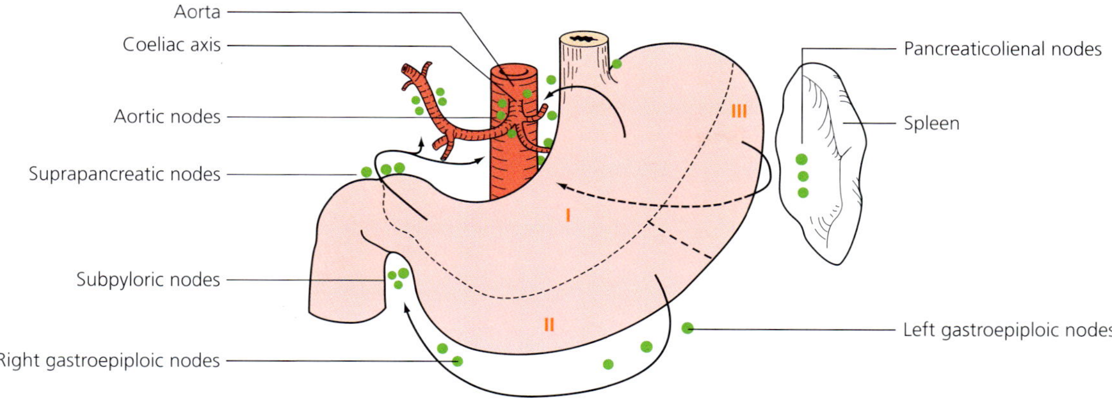

Figure 2.14 The lymph drainage of the stomach.

- Area I drains along the right and left gastric vessels to the aortic nodes.
- Area II drains to the subpyloric and thence aortic nodes via lymphatics along the right gastro-epiploic vessels.
- Area III drains via lymphatics along the splenic vessels to the suprapancreatic nodes and thence to the aortic nodes.

vessels are removed by excising the greater omentum. However, involvement of the nodes around the aorta and the head of the pancreas may render the growth incurable.

Nerve Supply

The stomach is supplied by both parasympathetic and sympathetic fibres.

Parasympathetic/Vagal supply to the stomach (Fig. 2.15)

It is derived from vagi. The anterior and posterior vagi enter the abdomen through the oesophageal hiatus. The anterior nerve lies close to the stomach wall but the posterior, and larger, nerve is at a little distance from it. The anterior vagus supplies branches to the cardia and lesser curve of the stomach and also a large hepatic branch. The posterior vagus gives branches to both the anterior and posterior aspects of the body of the stomach but the bulk of the nerve forms the coeliac branch. This runs along the left gastric artery to the coeliac ganglion for distribution to the intestine, as far as the mid-transverse colon, and the pancreas.

The exact means by which the vagal fibres reach the stomach is of considerable practical importance to the surgeon. The gastric divisions of both the anterior and posterior vagi reach the stomach at the cardia and descend along the lesser curvature between the anterior and posterior layers of peritoneal attachments of the lesser omentum (the **anterior and posterior nerves of Latarjet**). The stomach is innervated by terminal branches from the anterior and posterior gastric nerves and it is, therefore, possible to divide those branches that supply the acid-secreting body of the stomach and yet preserve the pyloric innervation (**highly selective vagotomy**, *see* below).

The vagus constitutes the motor and secretory nerve supply for the stomach. When divided, in the operation of *vagotomy*, the neurogenic (reflex) gastric acid secretion is abolished but the stomach is, at the same time, rendered atonic so that it empties only with difficulty; because of this, total vagotomy must always be accompanied by some sort of drainage procedure, either a pyloroplasty (to enlarge the pyloric exit and render the pyloric sphincter incompetent) or a gastrojejunostomy (to drain the stomach into the proximal small intestine). Drainage can be avoided if the nerve of Latarjet is preserved, thus maintaining the innervation and function of the pyloric antrum (highly selective vagotomy).

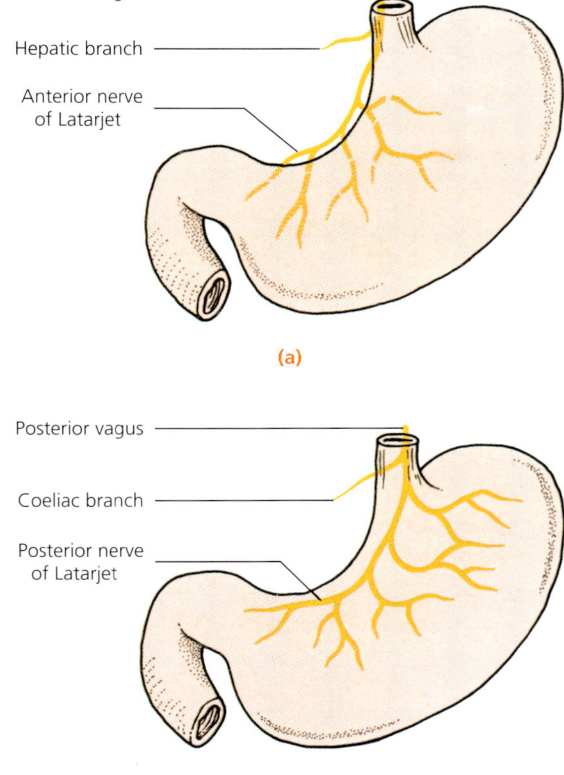

Figure 2.15 The vagal supply to the stomach: **(a)** anterior vagus and **(b)** posterior vagus.

Sympathetic supply

It is by sympathetic fibres derived from T6 to T10 spinal segments. These fibres are motor to pyloric sphincter but inhibitory to the rest of the stomach. They also provide pathways for pain sensations from the stomach.

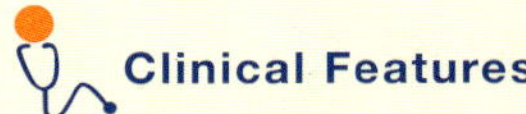

Clinical Features

1 A posterior gastric ulcer or cancer may erode the pancreas, giving pain referred to the back. Ulceration into the splenic artery – a direct posterior relation – may cause torrential haemorrhage.

2 There may be adhesions across the lesser sac that bring the transverse mesocolon into intimate relationship with the stomach or greater omentum. In these circumstances, the middle colic vessels are in danger of damage during mobilization of the stomach for gastrectomy.

3 *Radiology of the stomach* (Fig. 2.16). A plain erect X-ray film of the abdomen reveals a bubble of air below the left diaphragm; this is gas in the stomach fundus. After the subject has swallowed radio-opaque contrast fluid, for example barium sulphate (called barium meal), the stomach can be seen and its position, movements and outline studied. The wide variations in the position and shape of the stomach that we have already mentioned have come to light principally as a result of such investigations.

By tipping the subject head-down, the opaque meal can be made to impinge against the cardia; incompetence of this sphincter mechanism will be demonstrated by seeing barium regurgitate into the oesophagus.

In X-ray film taken after the barium meal, the first part of the duodenum is seen as a triangular shadow – **the duodenal cap.**

4 *Gastroscopy.* The mucosa of the air-inflated stomach can be inspected in the living subject through the gastroscope. With the modern fibre-optic instrument the whole of the gastric mucosa can be viewed, the duodenum examined, and the common bile duct and the pancreatic duct cannulated for retrograde contrast-enhanced radiological study.

Duodenum

The duodenum is the shortest, widest and most fixed part of the small intestine. It curves in a C around the head of the pancreas and is 10 in. (25 cm) long (roughly equal to the width of 12 fingers). The term duodenum is derived from the Greek word 'dodeca dactylous', meaning 12 fingers. At its origin from the pylorus it is completely covered with peritoneum for approximately 1 in. (2.5 cm), but then becomes a retroperitoneal organ, only partially covered by serous membrane.

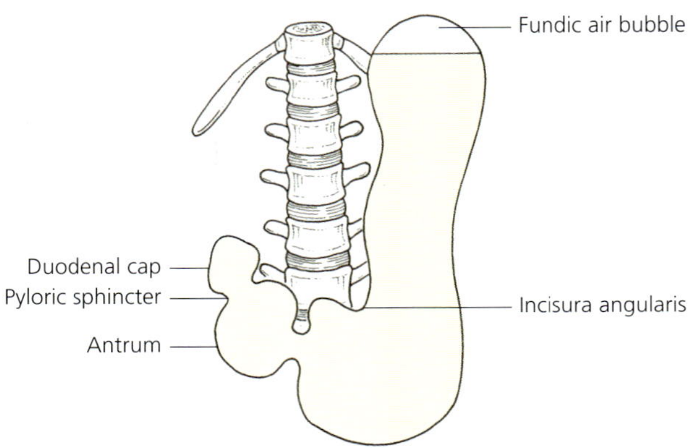

Figure 2.16 Tracing of a barium meal radiograph of the stomach.

Relations (Figs 2.17 and 2.18)

For descriptive purposes, the duodenum is divided into four parts.

The **first part** (2 in. (5 cm)) ascends from the gastroduodenal junction, overlapped by the liver and gall bladder. Immediately posterior to it lie the portal vein, common bile duct and gastroduodenal artery, which separate it from the inferior vena cava.

The **second part** (3 in. (7.5 cm)) descends in a curve around the head of the pancreas. It is crossed by the transverse colon and lies on the right kidney and ureter. Halfway along, its posteromedial aspect enters the common opening of the bile duct and the *main pancreatic duct (of Wirsung)* onto an eminence called the *duodenal papilla.* This common opening is guarded by the *sphincter of Oddi.* The *accessory pancreatic duct (of Santorini)* opens into the duodenum a little above the papilla.

The **third part** (4 in. (10 cm)) runs transversely to the left, crossing the inferior vena cava, the aorta and the 3rd lumbar vertebra. It is itself crossed anteriorly by the root of the mesentery and the superior mesenteric vessels. Its upper border hugs the pancreatic head.

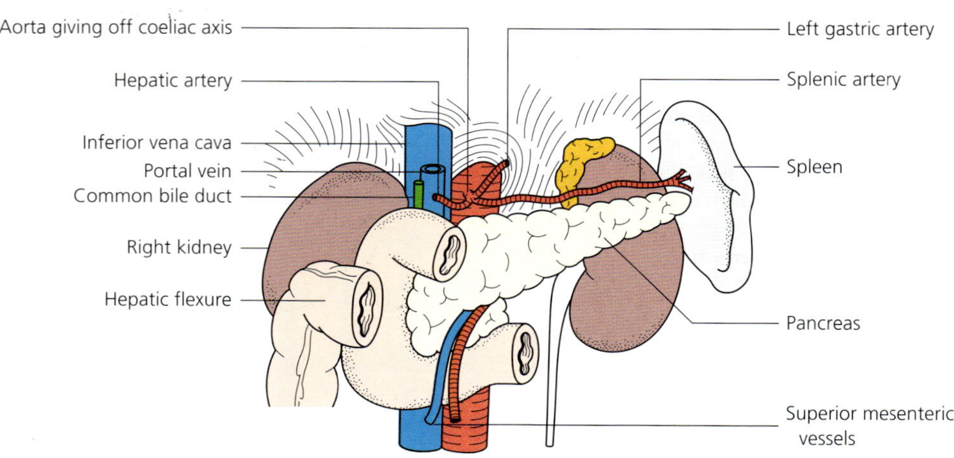

Figure 2.17 The relations of the duodenum.

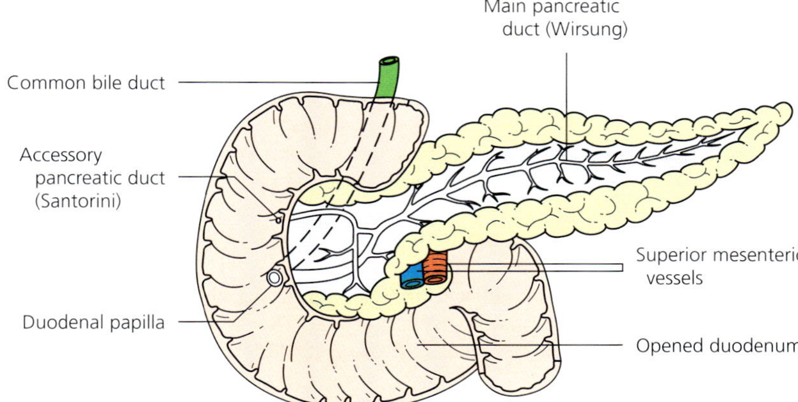

Figure 2.18 The duodenum and pancreas dissected to show the pancreatic ducts and their orifices.

The **fourth part** (1 in. (2.5 cm)) ascends upwards and to the left to end at the duodenojejunal junction. It is surprisingly easy for the surgeon to confuse this with the ileocaecal junction, a mistake which may be disastrous. He confirms the identity of the duodenojejunal junction (the duodenal termination) by the presence of the *suspensory ligament of Treitz*, which is a well-marked peritoneal fold descending from the right crus of the diaphragm to the duodenal termination, and by visualizing the inferior mesenteric vein, which descends from behind the pancreas immediately to the left of the duodenojejunal junction.

Blood supply

The duodenum is supplied by superior and inferior pancreaticoduodenal arteries. The superior pancreaticoduodenal artery arises from the gastroduodenal artery; the inferior pancreaticoduodenal artery originates as the first branch of the superior mesenteric artery. These vessels both lie in the curve between the duodenum and the head of the pancreas, supplying both structures. Interestingly, their anastomosis represents the site of the junction of the foregut (supplied by the coeliac artery) and the midgut (supplied by the superior mesenteric artery), at the level of the duodenal papilla (*see* page 46 and Fig. 2.18).

Clinical Features

1 The first part of the duodenum is overlapped by the liver and gall bladder, either of which may adhere to, or even be eroded by, a duodenal ulcer. Moreover, a gallstone may be extruded from the fundus of a chronically inflamed gall bladder into the duodenum. The gallstone may then impact in the lower ileum as it traverses the gut to produce intestinal obstruction (*gallstone ileus*).

2 The pancreas, as the duodenum's most intimate relation, is readily invaded by a posterior duodenal ulcer. This should be suspected if the patient's pain radiates into the dorsolumbar region. Erosion of the gastroduodenal artery by such an ulcer results in severe haemorrhage.

3 Extensive dissection of a duodenum, scarred by severe ulceration, may damage the common bile duct, which passes behind the first part of the duodenum approximately 1 in. (2.5 cm) from the pylorus.

(*Continued ...*)

(*... continued*)

4 The hepatic flexure of the colon crosses the second part of the duodenum and the latter may be damaged during a right hemicolectomy. Similarly, the right kidney lies directly behind this part of the duodenum, which may be injured in performing a right nephrectomy.

5 *Radiology of the duodenum.* Within a few minutes of swallowing a barium meal, the first part of the duodenum becomes visible as a triangular shadow termed the *duodenal cap* (Fig. 2.16). Every few seconds the duodenum contracts, emptying this cap, which promptly proceeds to fill again. It is in this region that the great majority of duodenal ulcers occur; an actual ulcer crater may be visualized, filled with barium, or deformity of the cap, produced by scar tissue, may be evident. The rest of the duodenum can also be seen, the shadow being floccular owing to the rugose arrangement of the mucosa.

6 *Mobilization of the duodenum,* together with the head of the pancreas and termination of the common bile duct, is performed by incising the peritoneum lateral to the second part of the duodenum and developing the avascular plane between these structures and the posterior abdominal wall – Kocher's manoeuvre (*see also* page 54).

Small intestine (jejunum and ileum)

The *length* of the small intestine varies from 10 to 33 ft. (3–10 m) in different subjects; the average is some 24 ft. (6.5 m). Resection of up to one-third or even half of the small intestine is compatible with a perfectly normal life, and survival has been reported with only 18 in. (45 cm) of small intestine preserved.

The small intestine is suspended from the posterior abdominal wall by a broad fan-shaped fold of peritoneum called mesentery.

The *mesentery* of the small intestine has a 6 in. (15 cm) origin from the posterior abdominal wall, which commences at the duodenojejunal junction to the left of the 2nd lumbar vertebra, and passes obliquely downwards to the right sacro-iliac joint; it contains the superior mesenteric vessels, the lymph nodes draining the small gut and autonomic nerve fibres.

The upper two-fifth of the small intestine is termed the *jejunum*; the remainder three-fifth is the *ileum*. There is no sharp distinction between the two and this division is a conventional one only. The bowel does, however, change its character from above downwards, the following points enabling the surgeon to determine the level of a loop of small intestine at operation.

1. The jejunum has a thicker wall as the circular folds of mucosa (*valvulae conniventes*) are larger and thicker more proximally.
2. The proximal small intestine is of greater diameter than the distal.
3. The jejunum tends to lie at the umbilical region; the ileum in the suprapubic region and pelvis.
4. The mesentery becomes thicker and more fat-laden from above downwards.
5. The mesenteric vessels form only one or two arcades to the jejunum, with long and relatively infrequent terminal branches passing to the gut wall. The ileum is supplied by shorter and more numerous terminal vessels arising from complete series of three, four or even five arcades (Fig. 2.19).

Large intestine

The large intestine extends from the ileocaecal junction to the anal orifice. It is subdivided, for descriptive purposes, into the following:

- Caecum with the appendix vermiformis
- Ascending colon (5–8 in. (12–20 cm))
- Hepatic flexure
- Transverse colon (18 in. (45 cm))
- Splenic flexure
- Descending colon (9–12 in. (22–30 cm))
- Sigmoid colon (5–30 in. (12–76 cm), average 15 in. (38 cm))
- Rectum (5 in. (12 cm))
- Anal canal (1.5 in. (4 cm))

The large bowel may vary considerably in length in different subjects; the average is approximately 5 ft. (1.5 m). The three cardinal features of the colon are: (a) appendices epiploicae, (b) taenia coli and (c) sacculations.

The colon (but not the appendix, caecum, rectum or anal canal) bears characteristic fat-filled peritoneal tags called *appendices epiploicae* scattered over its surface. These are especially numerous in the sigmoid colon. Their function, if any, is obscure but they may undergo torsion, which is an unusual cause of *acute abdominal pain*.

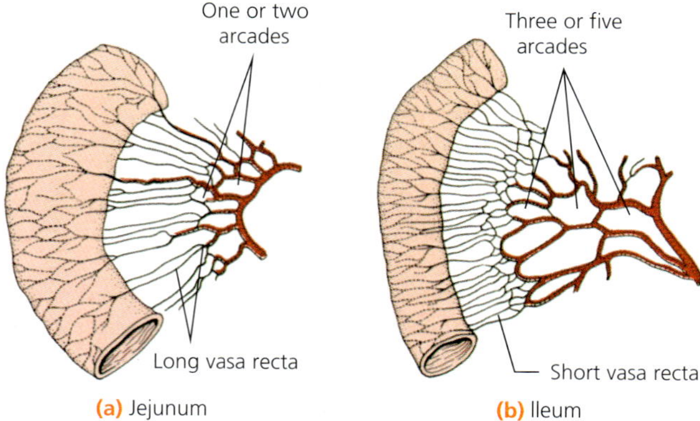

Figure 2.19 The simple arterial arcades of the jejunum **(a)** compared with the complex arcades of the ileum **(b)**.

The colon and caecum (but not the appendix, rectum or anal canal) are marked by the *taeniae coli*. These are three flattened bands commencing at the base of the appendix and running the length of the large intestine to end at the rectosigmoid junction. They represent the great bulk of the longitudinal muscle of the large bowel; because the taeniae are approximately 12 in. (30 cm) shorter than the gut to which they are attached, the colon becomes condensed into its typical sacculated shape. These sacculations may be seen in a plain radiograph of the abdomen when the large bowel is distended and appear as incomplete septa projecting into the gas shadow. The radiograph of distended small intestine, in contrast, characteristically has complete transverse lines across the bowel shadow owing to the transverse mucosal folds of the valvulae conniventes.

Peritoneal attachments

The transverse colon and sigmoid colon are completely peritonealized (the former being readily identified by its attachment to the greater omentum). The ascending and descending colon have no mesocolon but adhere directly to the posterior abdominal wall (although exceptionally the ascending colon may have a mesocolon). The caecum may or may not be completely peritonealized, and the appendix, although usually free within its own mesentery, occasionally lies extraperitoneally behind the caecum and ascending colon or adheres to the posterior wall of these structures.

The rectum is extraperitoneal on its posterior aspect in its upper third, posteriorly and laterally in its middle third and completely extraperitoneal in its lower third as it sinks below the pelvic peritoneum.

Appendix

The appendix arises from the posteromedial aspect of the caecum approximately 1 in. (2.5 cm) below the ileocaecal valve; its length ranges from 0.5 in. (1.25 cm) to 9 in. (22 cm). In the foetus it is a direct outpouching of the caecum, but differential overgrowth of the lateral caecal wall results in its medial displacement.

Positions

The position of the appendix is extremely variable – more so than that of any other organ (Fig. 2.20(a) and (b)). The positions are often compared to that of the hour hand of a clock. Most frequently (75% of cases) the appendix lies behind the caecum (retrocaecal/12 o'clock position). The appendix is usually quite free in this position, although occasionally it lies beneath the peritoneal covering of the caecum. If the appendix is very long, it may actually extend behind the ascending colon and abut against the right kidney or the duodenum; in these cases, its distal portion lies extraperitoneally.

In approximately 20% of cases, the appendix lies just below the caecum (subcecal/6 o'clock position) or else hangs down into the pelvis (pelvic/4 o'clock position). Less commonly, it passes in front of or behind the terminal ileum (splenic/2 o'clock position), or lies in front of the caecum or in the right paracolic gutter (paracolic/11 o'clock position). Sometimes it may pass horizontally towards sacral promontory (promontoric/3 o'clock position).

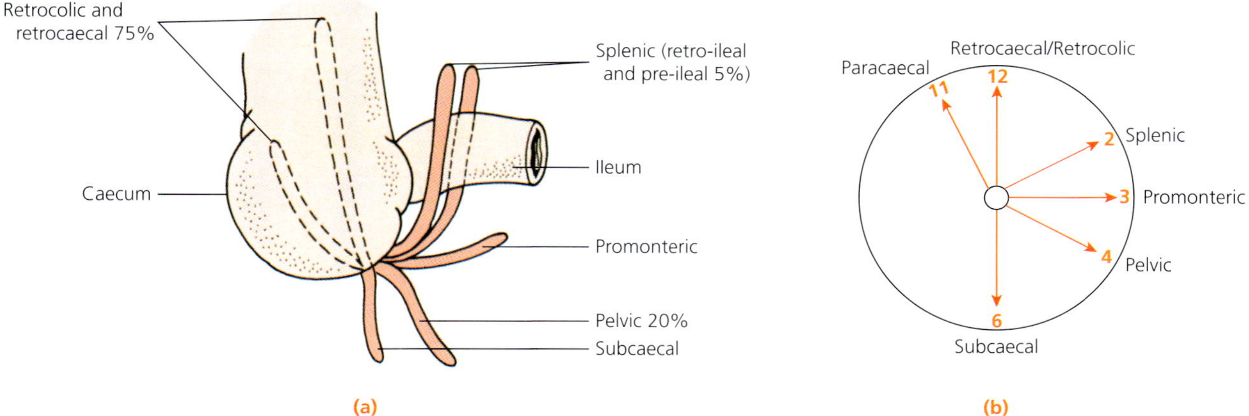

Figure 2.20 **(a)** The positions in which the appendix may lie together with their approximate incidence. **(b)** Positions of appendix according to a clock.

A long appendix has been known to ulcerate into the duodenum or perforate into the *left* paracolic gutter. It may well be said that 'the appendix is the only organ in the body that has no anatomy'.

The mesentery of the appendix, containing the *appendicular artery,* a branch of the ileocolic artery, descends behind the ileum as a triangular fold (Fig. 2.21). Another peritoneal sheet, the *ileocaecal fold,* passes to the appendix or to the base of the caecum from the front of the ileum. The ileocaecal fold is termed the *bloodless fold of Treves* although, in fact, it often contains a vessel and, if cut, proves far from bloodless.

The appendix mesentery, containing the appendicular vessels, is firmly tied and divided, the appendix base tied, the appendix removed and its stump invaginated into the caecum.

Clinical Features

1 The inflammation of appendix is called appendicitis. The pain is first felt in the umbilical region (referred pain) because both appendix and umbilicus are supplied by the T10 spinal segment. The McBurney's point is the site of maximum tenderness as it corresponds to the base of the appendix.

2 The lumen of the appendix is relatively wide in the infant and is frequently completely obliterated in the elderly. Since obstruction of the lumen is the usual precipitating cause of acute appendicitis it is not unnatural, therefore, that appendicitis should be uncommon at the two extremes of life.

3 The appendicular artery represents the entire vascular supply of the appendix. It runs first in the edge of the appendicular mesentery and then, distally, along the wall of the appendix. Acute infection of the appendix may result in thrombosis of this artery with rapid development of gangrene and subsequent perforation. This is in contrast to acute cholecystitis, where the rich collateral vascular supply from the liver bed ensures the rarity of gangrene of the gall bladder even if the cystic artery becomes thrombosed.

4 *Appendicectomy* is usually performed through a muscle-splitting grid-iron incision in the right iliac fossa (*see* 'Anatomy of abdominal incisions', page 38). The caecum is delivered into the wound and, if the appendix is not immediately visible, it is located by tracing the taeniae coli along the caecum – they fuse

(*Continued ...*)

(*... continued*)

at the base of the appendix. When the caecum is extraperitoneal it may be difficult to bring the appendix up into the incision; this is facilitated by first mobilizing the caecum by incising the almost avascular peritoneum along its lateral and inferior borders.

Rectum

The rectum is the distal part of the large intestine. It is 5 in. (12 cm) in length. It commences anterior to the third segment of the sacrum and ends at the level of the apex of the prostate or, in the female, at the level of the lower end of the intrapelvic vagina, where it pierces levator ani and leads into the anal canal.

The rectum is straight in lower mammals (hence its name) but is curved in man to fit into the sacral hollow. Moreover, it presents, externally, a series of three lateral inflexions, marked on the inside by the *valves of Houston,* projecting left, right and left from above downwards.

Relations (Figs 2.22 and 2.23)

The main relations of the rectum are important. They must be visualized in carrying out a rectal examination, they provide the key to the local spread of rectal growths and they are important in operative removal of the rectum.

Posteriorly lie the sacrum and coccyx and the middle sacral artery, which are separated from it by extraperitoneal connective tissue containing the rectal vessels and lymphatics. The lower sacral nerves, emerging from the anterior sacral

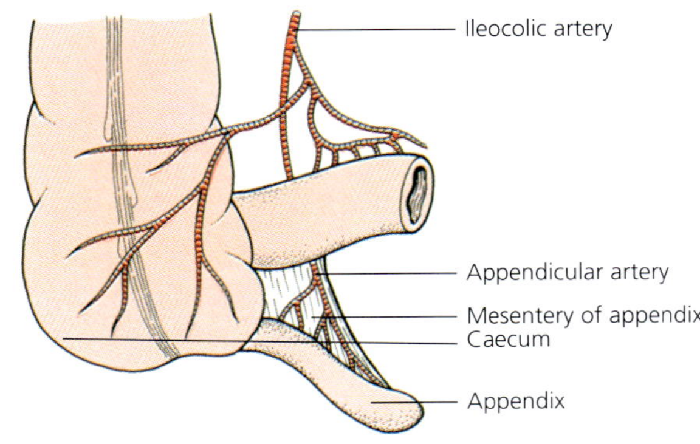

Figure 2.21 The blood supply of the appendix.

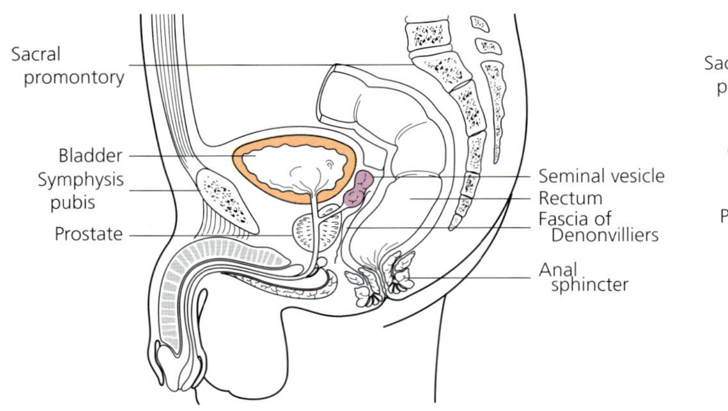

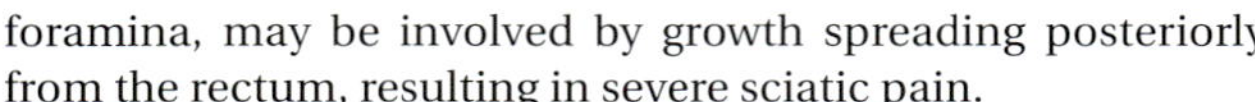
Figure 2.22 Sagittal section of the rectum and its related viscera in the male.

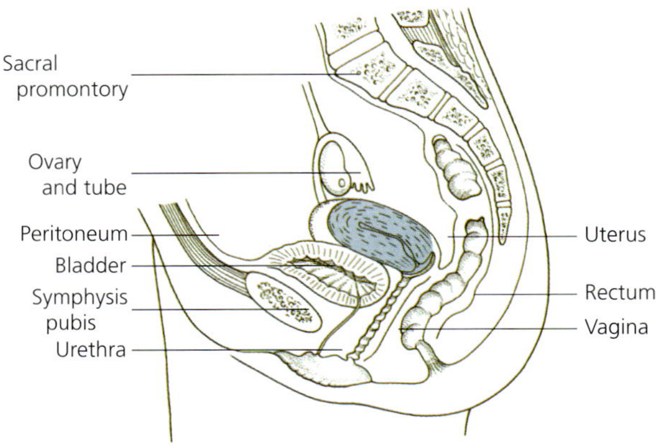

Figure 2.23 Sagittal section of the rectum and its related viscera in the female.

foramina, may be involved by growth spreading posteriorly from the rectum, resulting in severe sciatic pain.

Anteriorly, the upper two-thirds of the rectum are covered by peritoneum and relate to coils of small intestine which lie in the cul-de-sac of the pouch of Douglas between the rectum and the bladder or the uterus. In front of the lower one-third lie the prostate, bladder base and seminal vesicles in the male, or the vagina in the female. A layer of fascia (*Denonvilliers*) separates the rectum from the anterior structures and forms the plane of dissection which must be sought when performing excision of the rectum. Laterally, the rectum is supported by the levator ani.

Arterial supply

The rectum is supplied by *superior rectal artery* (a continuation of inferior mesenteric artery), *middle rectal artery* (a branch of anterior division of internal iliac artery) and *median sacral artery* (a branch from aorta near its lower end).

Venous drainage

It is done by the *superior rectal vein* which continues upwards as the inferior mesenteric vein to drain into the portal system, and *middle rectal vein* which drains into the internal iliac vein (caval system).

Lymphatic drainage

The lymph vessels from the upper half of the rectum drains into *pararectal, sigmoid* and *inferior mesenteric nodes,* while those from the lower half drain into *internal iliac nodes.*

Anal canal (Fig. 2.24)

The anal canal is the terminal part of the large intestine. It is 1.5 in. (4 cm) long and is directed downwards and backwards from the rectum to end at the anal orifice. The mid-anal canal

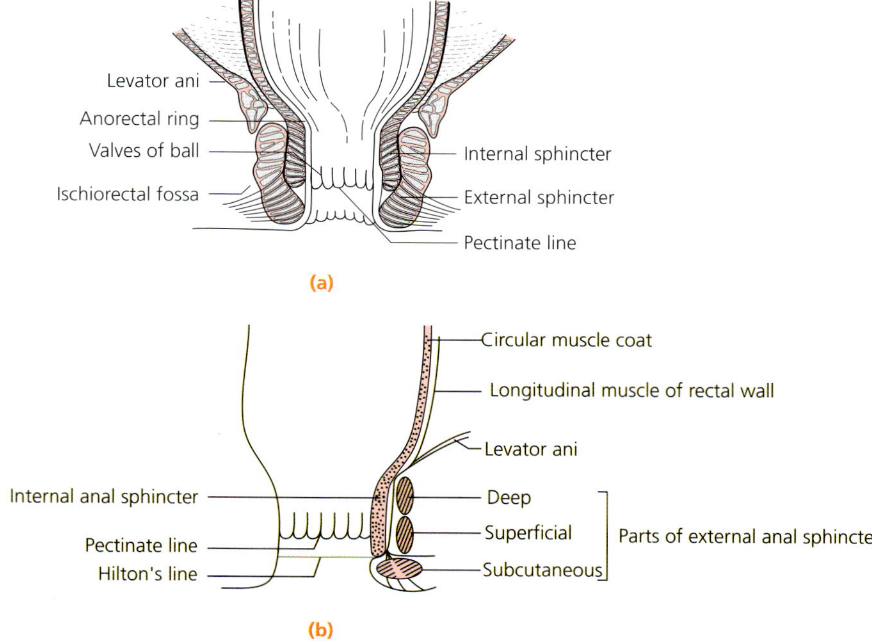

Figure 2.24 **(a)** The sphincters of the anus. **(b)** Subdivisions of external anal sphincter.

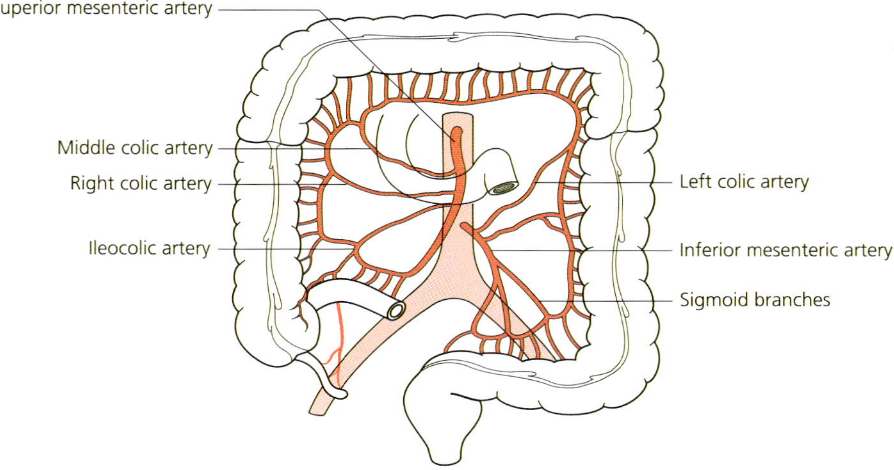

Figure 2.25 The superior and inferior mesenteric arteries and their branches.

represents the junction between the endoderm of the hindgut and the ectoderm of the cutaneous invagination termed the *proctodaeum*. Failure of breakdown of the separating membrane results in *imperforate anus*.

1. The lower half is lined by squamous epithelium and the upper half by columnar epithelium; the latter presents vertical columns of mucosa (*the columns of Morgagni*) connected at their distal extremities by valve-like folds (*the valves of Ball*). A carcinoma of the upper anal canal is thus an adenocarcinoma, whereas that arising from the lower part is a squamous cell carcinoma.
2. The blood supply of the upper half of the anal canal is from the superior rectal artery, derived from the inferior mesenteric artery (*see* Fig. 2.25), and its corresponding superior rectal vein, which drains into the inferior mesenteric vein, which, in turn, enters the splenic vein and thus drains into the portal vein (*see* Fig. 2.26). In contrast, the blood supply of the lower anal canal and the surrounding perianal skin is from the inferior rectal vessels, derived from the internal pudendal and, ultimately, the internal iliac artery and vein. The two venous systems communicate and therefore form one of the important sites of anastomoses between the portal and systemic venous systems (i.e. portocaval anastomosis).
3. The lymphatics above this mucocutaneous junction drain along the superior rectal vessels to the lumbar nodes, whereas, below this line, drainage is to the inguinal nodes. A carcinoma of the rectum that invades the lower anal canal may thus metastasize to the groin nodes.
4. The nerve supply to the upper anal canal is by autonomic fibres (both sympathetic and parasympathetic) via the autonomic plexuses; the lower part is supplied by the somatic inferior rectal nerve, a terminal branch of the pudendal nerve (*see* Fig. 2.59(b)). (The lower canal is, therefore, sensitive to the prick of a hypodermic needle, whereas injection of an internal haemorrhoid with sclerosant fluid, by passing a needle through the mucosa of the upper part of the canal, is painless.)

Anal sphincter

Forming the walls of the anal canal is a rather complicated muscle arrangement which constitutes a powerful sphincter mechanism (Fig. 2.24(a)). This comprises the following:

- *The internal anal sphincter*, of involuntary muscle, which continues above with the circular muscle coat of the rectum
- *The external anal sphincter*, of voluntary muscle, which surrounds the internal sphincter and which extends further downwards and curves medially to occupy a position below and slightly lateral to the lower rounded edge of the internal sphincter, close to the skin of the anal orifice. It consists of the following three parts: subcutaneous, superficial and deep (Fig. 2.24(b)). The lowermost, or subcutaneous, portion of the external sphincter is traversed by a fan-shaped expansion of the longitudinal muscle fibres of the anal canal that continue above with the longitudinal muscle of the rectal wall. The superficial part surrounds the lower part of the internal sphincter. The deep part surrounds the upper part of the internal sphincter. At its upper end the external sphincter fuses with the fibres of levator ani

In carrying out a digital rectal examination, the ring of muscle on which the flexed finger rests just over 1 in. (2.5 cm) from the anal margin is the *anorectal ring*. This represents the deep part of the external sphincter where this blends with the internal sphincter and levator ani, and demarcates the junction between the anal canal and the rectum.

The anal canal is related posteriorly to the fibrous tissue between it and the coccyx (the anococcygeal body), laterally to the *ischioanal fossa* on either side, containing fat, and anteriorly to the perineal body, which separates it from the bulb of the urethra in the male and the lower vagina in the female. Note that the *ischiorectal fossa* is now often referred to, more accurately, as the *ischioanal fossa* – it relates to the anal canal rather than the rectum.

Rectal examination

The following structures can be palpated by the finger passed *per rectum* in the normal patient:

1. **Both sexes:** The anorectal ring (*see* above), coccyx and sacrum, ischioanal fossae, ischial spines
2. **Male:** Prostate, rarely the healthy seminal vesicles
3. **Female:** Perineal body, cervix, occasionally the ovaries

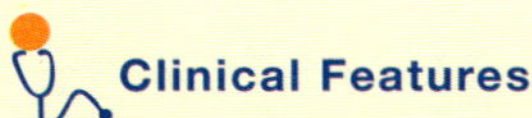

Clinical Features

Haemorrhoids

The internal *haemorrhoids (piles)* are sustained, pathological engorgements of the submucosal arteriovenous cushions (anastomoses) that are normally present in the upper half of the anal canal. Initially contained within the anal canal (**1st degree**), they gradually enlarge until they prolapse on defecation (**2nd degree**) and finally remain prolapsed through the anal orifice (**3rd degree**). Anatomically, each pile comprises: a venous plexus draining into one of the superior rectal veins; terminal branches of the corresponding superior rectal artery; and a covering of anal canal mucosa and submucosa. There are arteriovenous anastomoses between the vessels; hence, bleeding from piles is characteristically bright red. The external piles occur below the pectinate line and are, therefore, painful. The so-called 'thrombosed external pile' is a small tense haematoma at the anal margin caused by rupture of a subcutaneous vein and is much better termed a *perianal haematoma*.

Perianal abscesses (Fig. 2.26)

These may be localized beneath the anal mucosa (*submucous*), beneath perianal skin (*subcutaneous*) or occupy the ischioanal fossa (ischioanal abcess). Occasionally, abscesses lie in the pelvirectal space above levator ani, alongside the rectum, in an extraperitoneal location.

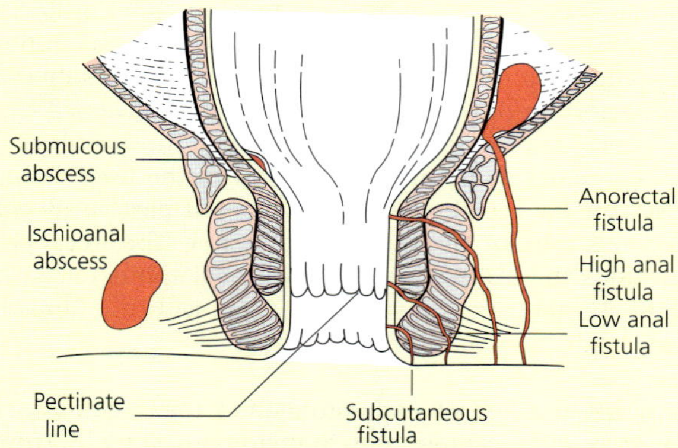

Figure 2.26 The anatomy of perianal fistulae and abscesses.

Fistulae (Fig. 2.26)

Anal fistulae usually result from rupture of perianal abscesses. They are classified anatomically as mentioned below:

- *Submucous* – confined to the tissues immediately below the anal mucosa
- *Subcutaneous* – confined to the perianal skin
- *Low level* – passing through the lower part of the superficial sphincter (most common)
- *High level* – passing through the deeper part of the superficial sphincter
- *Anorectal* – which has its track passing above the anorectal ring and which may or may not open into the rectum

In laying open *fistulae in ano*, it is essential to preserve the *anorectal ring* if faecal incontinence is to be avoided. The lower part of the sphincter, on the other hand, can be divided quite safely without this risk.

(Continued ...)

(... continued)

Fissure *in ano*

This is a tear in the anal mucosa; over 90% occur posteriorly in the midline. The anatomical basis for this probably lies in the insertion of the superficial component of the external anal sphincter posteriorly into the coccyx; between the two limbs of the 'V' thus formed, the mucosa is relatively unsupported and may therefore be torn by a hard faecal mass at this site.

Abnormalities which can be detected include the following:

1. **Within the lumen:** Faecal impaction, foreign bodies
2. **In the wall**: Rectal growths, strictures, granulomata, etc., but *not* haemorrhoids unless these are thrombosed
3. **Outside the rectal wall:** Pelvic bony tumours, abnormalities of the prostate or seminal vesicle, distended bladder, uterine or ovarian enlargement, collections of fluid or neoplastic masses in the pouch of Douglas

Do not be deceived by foreign objects placed in the vagina. The commonest are a tampon or a pessary. During parturition, dilatation of the cervical os can be assessed by rectal examination since it can be felt quite easily through the rectal wall.

Arterial supply of the intestine

The alimentary tract develops from the fore-, mid- and hindgut; the arterial supply to each is discrete, although anastomosing with its neighbour. The foregut comprises the stomach and duodenum as far as the entry of the bile duct and is supplied by branches of the *coeliac axis*, which arises from the aorta at the T12 vertebral level (Fig. 2.13).

The midgut extends from mid-duodenum to the proximal two-third of the transverse colon and is supplied by the *superior mesenteric artery* (Fig. 2.25) arising from the aorta at the level of L1. Its branches are as follows:

1. **Inferior pancreaticoduodenal artery**
2. **Jejunal and ileal branches:** Supplying the bulk of the small intestine
3. **Ileocolic artery:** Supplying the terminal ileum, caecum and the commencement of the ascending colon and giving off an *appendicular branch* to the appendix; the latter branch is the most commonly ligated intra-abdominal artery
4. **Right colic artery:** Supplying the ascending colon
5. **Middle colic artery:** Supplying the transverse colon

The hindgut receives its supply from the *inferior mesenteric artery* (Fig. 2.25), arising from the aorta at L3 and giving the following branches:

1. **Left colic artery:** Supplying the descending colon
2. **Sigmoid branches:** Supplying the sigmoid
3. **Superior rectal artery:** Supplying the rectum

Each branch of the superior and inferior mesenteric artery anastomoses with its neighbour above and below so that there is, in fact, a continuous vascular arcade situated along the concavity of the whole length of the colon. It is also termed as the *marginal artery of Drummond*.

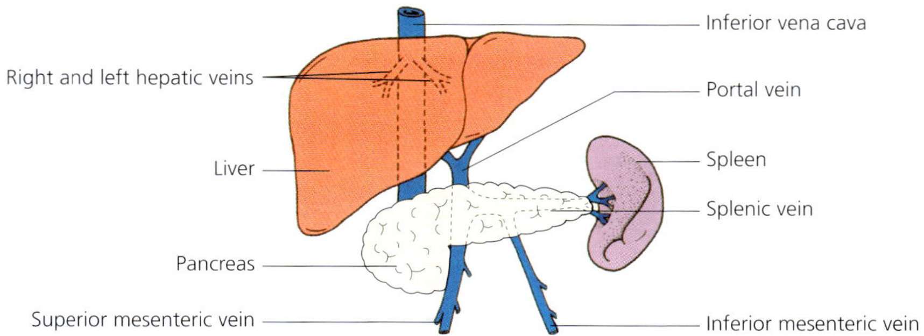

Figure 2.27 The composition of the portal system.

Portal system of veins

The portal venous system drains blood to the liver from the abdominal part of the alimentary canal (excluding the anal canal), the spleen, the pancreas and the gall bladder and its ducts.

The distal tributaries of this system correspond to, and accompany, the branches of the coeliac and the superior and inferior mesenteric arteries enumerated above; only proximally (Fig. 2.27) does the arrangement differ.

The *inferior mesenteric vein* ascends above the point of origin of its artery to enter the splenic vein behind the pancreas.

The *superior mesenteric vein* joins the splenic vein behind the neck of the pancreas in the transpyloric plane to form the *portal vein*, which ascends behind the first part of the duodenum into the anterior wall of the foramen of Winslow and thence to the porta hepatis. Here the portal vein divides into right and left branches and breaks up into capillaries running between the lobules of the liver. These capillaries drain into the radicles of the hepatic vein through which they empty into the inferior vena cava.

Portacaval anastomosis (connections between the portal and systemic) venous systems

Normally, portal venous blood traverses the liver as described above and empties into the systemic venous circulation via the hepatic vein and inferior vena cava. This pathway may be blocked by a variety of causes, which are classified into the following:

- Prehepatic, e.g. thrombosis or congenital obliteration of the portal vein
- Hepatic, e.g. cirrhosis of the liver
- Posthepatic, e.g. congenital stenosis of the hepatic veins

If obstruction from any of these causes occurs, the portal venous pressure rises (*portal hypertension*) and collateral pathways open up between the portal and systemic venous systems.

These sites of portacaval anastomosis/communications are as follows:

1. **Lower end of oesophagus:** Between the oesophageal branch of the left gastric vein and the oesophageal veins of the azygos system. In portal hypertension, the collateral pathways open up and may form oesophageal varices. These *oesophageal varices* are the cause of the severe haematemeses that maybe fatal.
2. **Anal canal:** Between the superior rectal branch of the inferior mesenteric vein and the inferior rectal veins draining into the internal iliac vein via its internal pudendal tributary. In portal hypertension, the opening of collateral pathway may form haemorrhoids.
3. **Posterior abdominal wall:** Between the portal tributaries in the mesentery and mesocolon and the retroperitoneal veins communicating with the renal, lumbar and phrenic veins.
4. **Umbilicus:** Between the portal branches in the liver and the veins of the abdominal wall via veins passing along the falciform ligament from the umbilicus (which may result in the formation of a cluster of dilated veins which radiate from the navel and which are called the *caput medusae*).
5. **Bare area of the liver:** Between the portal branches in the liver and the veins of the diaphragm across the bare area of the liver.

A striking feature of operations upon patients with portal hypertension is the extraordinary dilatation of every available channel between the two systems that renders such procedures tedious and bloody.

Lymph drainage of the intestine (Fig. 2.28)

The arrangement of lymph nodes is relatively uniform throughout the small and large intestine. Numerous small nodes lying near, or even on, the bowel wall (epiploic/paracolic nodes) drain to intermediately placed and rather larger nodes along the vessels in the mesentery or mesocolon (intermediate nodes) and thence to clumps of nodes situated near the origins of the superior and inferior mesenteric arteries (proximal nodes). From these, efferent vessels link up to drain into the *cisterna chyli*.

The lymphatic drainage field of each segment of bowel corresponds fairly accurately to its blood supply. High ligation of the vessels to the involved segment of bowel with removal of a wide surrounding segment of mesocolon will, therefore, remove the lymph nodes draining the area. Division of the middle colic vessels and a resection of a generous wedge of transverse mesocolon, for example, would be performed for a growth of transverse colon.

Structure of the alimentary canal

The alimentary canal is made up of mucosa demarcated by the *muscularis mucosae* from the *submucosa*, the *muscle coat* and the *serosa* – the last being absent where the gut is extraperitoneal.

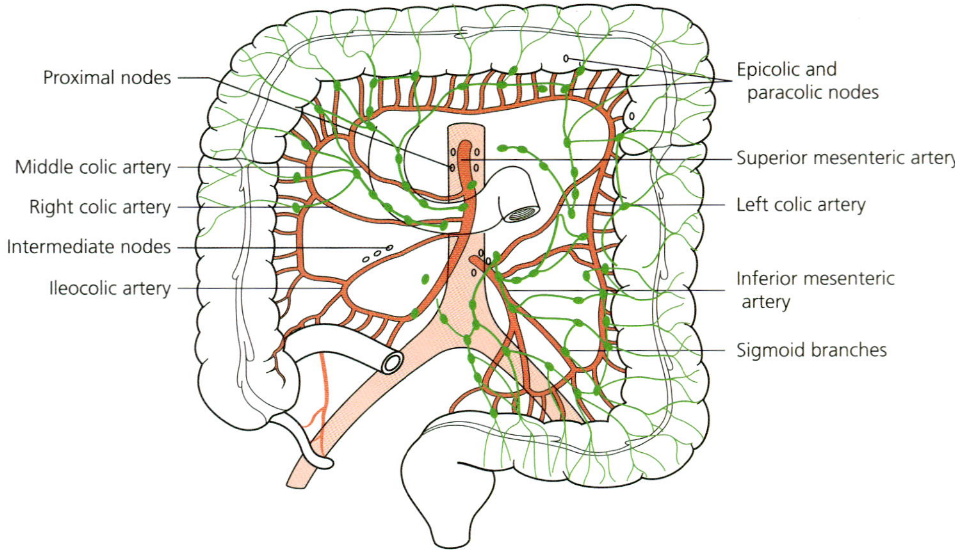

Figure 2.28 Lymph nodes of the large intestine.

The oesophageal mucosa and that of the lower anal canal is stratified squamous epithelium; elsewhere, it is columnar. At the cardio-oesophageal junction this transition is quite sharp, although occasionally columnar epithelium may line the lower oesophagus.

The gastric mucosa bears simple crypt-like glands projecting down to the muscularis mucosae. The pyloric antrum secretes an alkaline juice containing mucus and the hormone gastrin. The body of the stomach secretes pepsin and also HCl, the latter from the *oxyntic cells* lying sandwiched deeply between the surface cells. The stomach mucosa also produces intrinsic factor.

The mucosa of the duodenum and small intestine, as well as bearing crypt-like glands, projects into the bowel lumen in villous processes which greatly increase its surface area. The duodenum is distinguished by its crypts extending deep through the muscularis mucosae and opening into an extensive system of mucous acini in the submucosa termed *Brunner's glands.*

The mucosa of the large intestine is lined almost entirely by mucus-secreting goblet cells; there are no villi. The muscle coat of the alimentary tract is made up of an inner circular layer and an outer longitudinal layer. In the upper two-thirds of the oesophagus and at the anal margin this muscle is voluntary; elsewhere it is involuntary. The stomach wall is reinforced by an innermost oblique coat of muscle and the colon is characterized by the condensation of its longitudinal layer into three *taeniae coli.*

The autonomic nerve plexuses of Meissner and Auerbach lie, respectively, in the submucosal layer and between the circular and longitudinal muscle coats.

Development of the intestine and its congenital abnormalities (Fig. 2.29)

The primitive endodermal tube of the gut is divided into foregut, midgut and hindgut.

1. The *foregut* (supplied by the coeliac axis) extending as far as the entry of the bile duct into the duodenum
2. The *midgut* (supplied by the superior mesenteric artery) continuing as far as the junction of medial proximal two-third and the distal one-third of the transverse colon
3. The *hindgut* (supplied by the inferior mesenteric artery) extending thence to the ectodermal part of the anal canal

At an early stage rapid proliferation of the gut wall obliterates its lumen and this is followed by subsequent recanalization.

The foregut becomes rotated with the development of the lesser sac so that the original right wall of the stomach comes to form its posterior surface and the left wall its anterior surface. The vagi rotate with the stomach and therefore lie anteriorly and posteriorly to it at the oesophageal hiatus.

This rotation swings the duodenum to the right and the mesentery of this organ then blends with the peritoneum of the posterior abdominal wall – this blending process is termed *zygosis.*

The midgut enlarges rapidly in the 5 week foetus, becomes too large to be contained within the abdomen and herniates into the umbilical cord. The apex of this herniated bowel is continuous with the vitello-intestinal duct and the yolk sac, but this connection, even at this early stage of foetal life, is already reduced to a fibrous strand.

The axis of this herniated loop of gut is formed by the superior mesenteric artery, which demarcates a cephalic and a caudal limb. The cephalic element develops into the proximal small intestine; the caudal segment differentiates into the terminal 2 ft. (62 cm) of ileum, the caecum and the colon as far as the junction of the middle and left thirds of the transverse colon.

A bud that develops on the caudal segment indicates the site of subsequent formation of the caecum; it may well be that this bud delays the return of the caudal limb in favour of the cephalic gut during the subsequent reduction of the herniated bowel.

At 10 weeks this return of the bowel into the abdominal cavity commences. The midgut loop first rotates anticlockwise through 90°.

The cephalic limb returns first, passing upwards and to the left into the space left available by the bulky liver. In doing so,

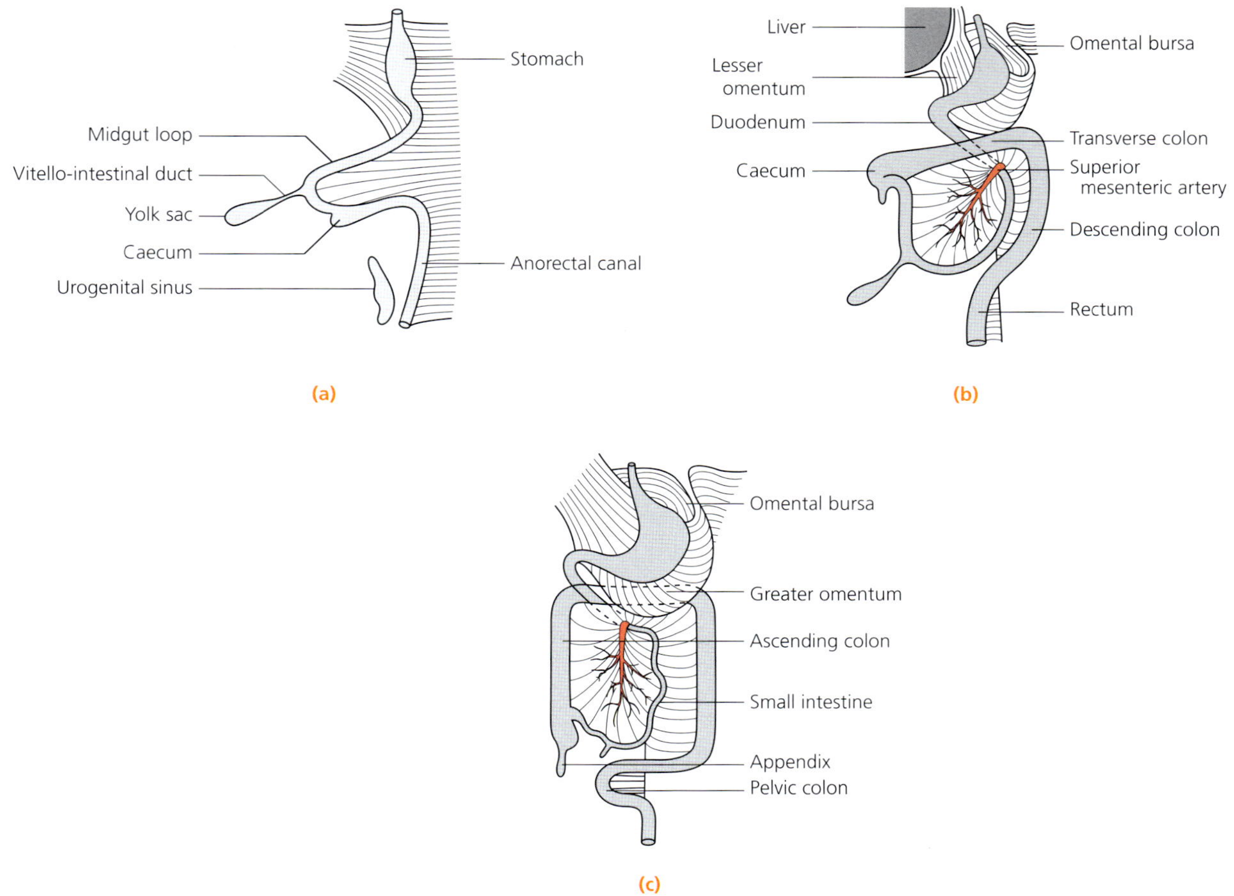

Figure 2.29 Stages in rotation of the bowel. **(a)** The prolapsed midgut loop, seen in lateral view. **(b)** The midgut returns to the abdomen. **(c)** The caecum descends to its definitive position. Note the completion of stomach rotation with the formation of the lesser sac (omental bursa).

this midgut passes *behind* the superior mesenteric artery (which thus comes to cross the third part of the duodenum) and also pushes the hindgut – the definitive distal colon – over to the left.

When the caudal limb returns, it lies in the only space remaining to it, superficial to, and above, the small intestine with the caecum lying immediately below the liver.

The caecum then descends into its definitive position in the right iliac fossa, dragging the colon with it. The transverse colon thus comes to lie in front of the superior mesenteric vessels and the small intestine.

Finally, the mesenteries of the ascending and descending parts of the colon blend with the posterior abdominal wall peritoneum by *zygosis*. This embryological fusion of peritoneal surfaces is of major surgical importance. Thus, in mobilizing the right or left colon, an incision is made along this avascular line of zygosis lateral to the bowel, allowing it to be mobilized with its mesocolon and blood supply. In a similar fashion, the duodenum, head of pancreas and termination of the common bile duct can be mobilized bloodlessly by incising the peritoneum along the right border of the duodenum – Kocher's manoeuvre (*see* page 47). Further mobilization of the third part of the duodenum, together with its second part and the pancreas, allows exposure of the abdominal aorta as far proximally as the level of its crossing by the left renal vein (*see* Fig. 2.71).

Numerous anomalies may occur in the highly complex developmental process as follows:

1. *Atresia* or *stenosis of the bowel* may result from failure of recanalization of the lumen. Another cause of this may be damage to the blood supply to the bowel within the foetal umbilical hernia with consequent ischaemic changes. *Imperforate anus – see* page 50.
2. *Meckel's diverticulum* represents the remains of the embryonic vitello-intestinal duct (communication between the primitive midgut and yolk sac) and is, therefore, always on the anti-mesenteric border of the bowel. As an approximation to the truth it can be said to occur in 2% of subjects, twice as often in males as in females, to be situated at 2 ft. (62 cm) from the ileocaecal junction and to be 2 in. (5 cm) long. In fact, it may occur anywhere from 6 in. (15 cm) to 12 ft. (3.5 m) from the terminal ileum and may vary from a tiny stump to a 6 in. (15 cm) long sac. Occasionally, the diverticulum ends in a whip-like solid strand.

As well as a diverticulum – the commonest form – this duct may persist as a fistula or band connecting the intestine to the umbilicus, as a cyst hanging from the anti-mesenteric border of the ileum or as a 'raspberry tumour' at the umbilicus, formed by the red mucosa of a persistent umbilical extremity of the diverticulum pouting at the navel (Fig. 2.30).

The mucosa lining the diverticulum may contain islands of peptic epithelium with oxyntic (acid secreting) cells. Peptic ulceration of adjacent intestinal epithelium may then occur with haemorrhage or perforation.

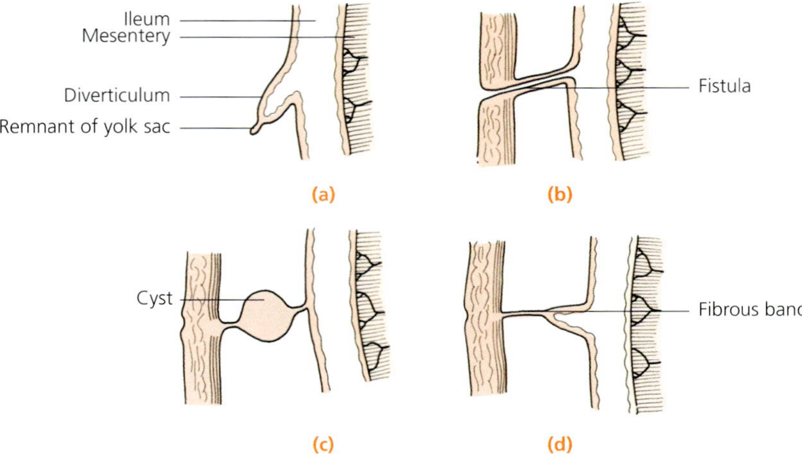

Figure 2.30 Abnormalities associated with persistence of the vitello-intestinal tract. **(a)** Meckel's diverticulum. **(b)** Patent vitello-intestinal duct. **(c)** Cyst within a fibrous cord passing from the anti-mesenteric border of the intestine to the umbilicus. **(d)** Meckel's diverticulum with a terminal filament passing to the umbilicus.

3. The caecum may fail to descend; the peritoneal fold which normally seals it in the right iliac fossa passes, instead, across the duodenum and causes a neonatal intestinal obstruction. The mesentery of the small intestine in such a case is left as a narrow pedicle, which allows volvulus of the whole small intestine to occur (*volvulus neonatorum*).
4. Occasionally, reversed rotation occurs, in which the transverse colon comes to lie *behind* the superior mesenteric vessels with the duodenum in front of them; this may again be accompanied by extrinsic duodenal obstruction due to a peritoneal fold.
5. *Exomphalos* is persistence of the midgut herniation at the umbilicus after birth.

Gastrointestinal adnexae: liver, gall bladder and its ducts, pancreas and spleen

Liver (Fig. 2.31)

This is the largest organ in the body mainly situated in the right upper quadrant of the abdomen. It weighs about 1500 g. It is related by its domed *upper surface* to the diaphragm, which separates it from the pleura, lungs, pericardium and heart. Its *postero-inferior (or visceral) surface* overlaps the abdominal oesophagus, the stomach and the duodenum, the hepatic flexure of the colon and the right kidney and suprarenal, besides carrying the gall bladder.

The liver is divided into a larger right and small left lobe, separated superiorly by the falciform ligament and postero-inferiorly by an 'H'-shaped arrangement of fossae and grooves (Fig. 2.31(b) and (c)) as mentioned below:

- **Anteriorly and to the right:** The fossa for the gall bladder
- **Posteriorly and to the right:** The groove in which the inferior vena cava lies embedded
- **Anteriorly and to the left:** The fissure containing the ligamentum teres
- **Posteriorly and to the left:** The fissure for the ligamentum venosum

The cross-bar of the 'H' is formed by the *porta hepatis*. Two subsidiary lobes are marked out on the visceral aspect of the liver between the limbs of this 'H' – the *quadrate lobe* in front and the *caudate lobe* behind.

The *ligamentum teres* is the obliterated remains of the left umbilical vein which, *in utero*, brings blood from the placenta back into the foetus. The *ligamentum venosum* is the fibrous remnant of the foetal *ductus venosus* which shunts oxygenated blood from this left umbilical vein to the inferior vena cava, short-circuiting the liver. It is easy enough to realize, then, that the grooves for the ligamentum teres, ligamentum venosum and inferior vena cava, representing as they do the pathway of a foetal venous trunk, are continuous in the adult. *See also* 'The foetal circulation', page 25.

Lying in the **porta hepatis** (which is 2 in. (5 cm) long) are:

1. **Common hepatic duct:** Anteriorly
2. **Hepatic artery:** In the middle
3. **Portal vein:** Posteriorly

As well as these, autonomic nerve fibres (sympathetic from the coeliac axis and parasympathetic from the vagus), lymphatic vessels and lymph nodes are found there.

Peritoneal attachments

The liver is enclosed in peritoneum except for a small posterior bare area, demarcated by the peritoneum from the diaphragm reflected onto it as the upper and lower layers of the *coronary ligament*. To the right, these fuse to form the *right triangular ligament*.

The *falciform ligament* ascends to the liver from the umbilicus, somewhat to the right of the midline, and bears the ligamentum teres in its free border. The ligamentum teres passes into its fissure in the inferior surface of the liver while the falciform ligament passes over the dome of the liver and then divaricates. Its right limb joins the upper layer of the coronary ligament and its left limb stretches out as the long narrow *left triangular ligament* which, when traced posteriorly and to the right, joins the lesser omentum in the upper end of the fissure for the ligamentum venosum.

The *lesser omentum* arises from the fissures of the porta hepatis and the ligamentum venosum and passes as a sheet to be attached along the lesser curvature of the stomach and first inch of the first part of the duodenum.

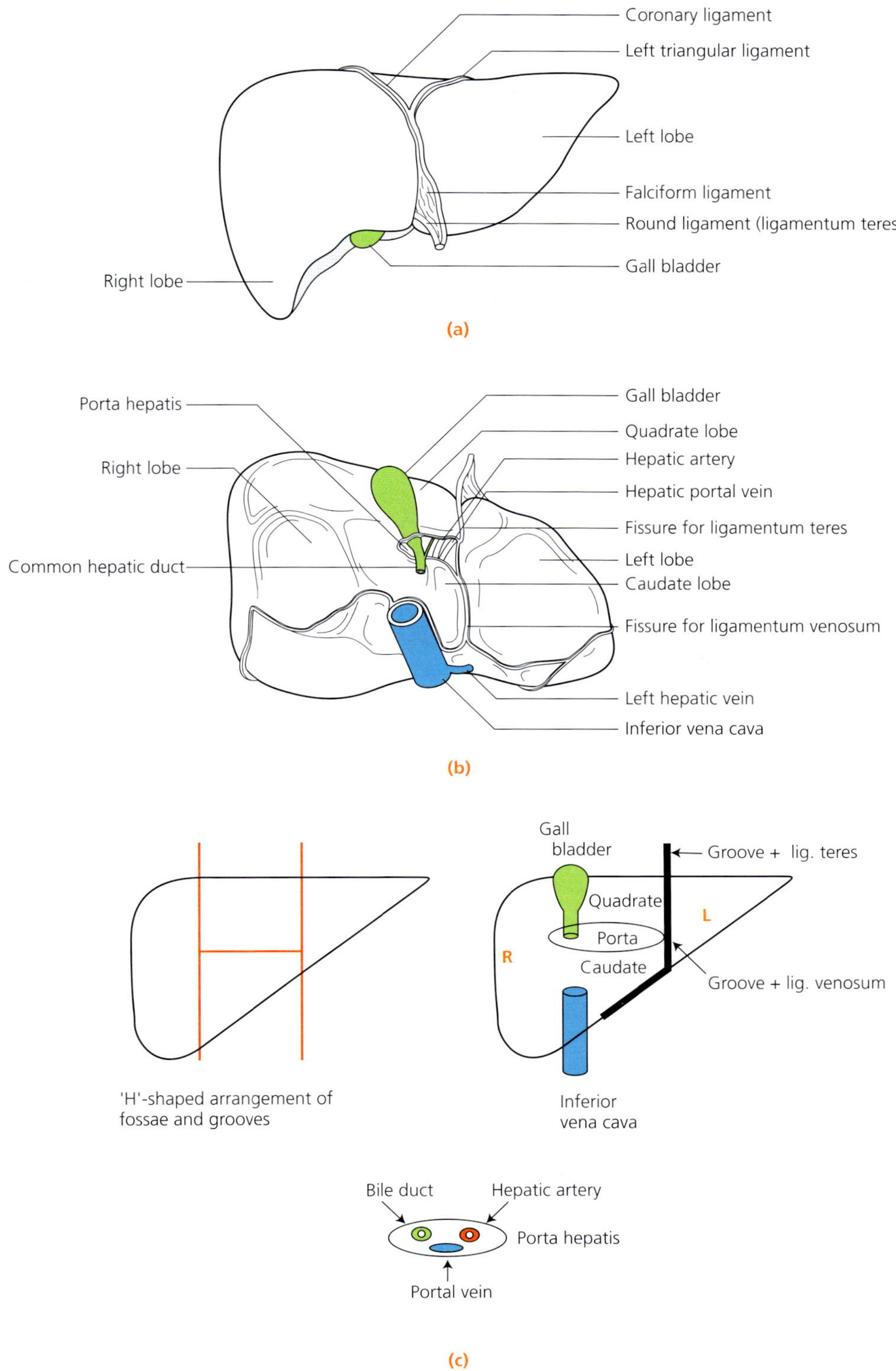

Figure 2.31 The liver and its subdivisions: **(a)** Anterior aspect. **(b)** Inferior aspect. **(c)** 'H'-shaped arrangement of fossae and grooves on the posteroinferior surface.

Structure

The liver is made up of lobules, each with a solitary central vein that is a tributary of the hepatic vein, which, in turn, drains into the inferior vena cava. In the spaces between the lobules, termed *portal canals*, lie branches of the hepatic artery (bringing systemic blood) and the portal vein, both of which drain into the central vein by means of sinusoids traversing the lobule.

Branches of the *hepatic duct* also lie in the portal canals and receive fine bile capillaries from the liver lobules.

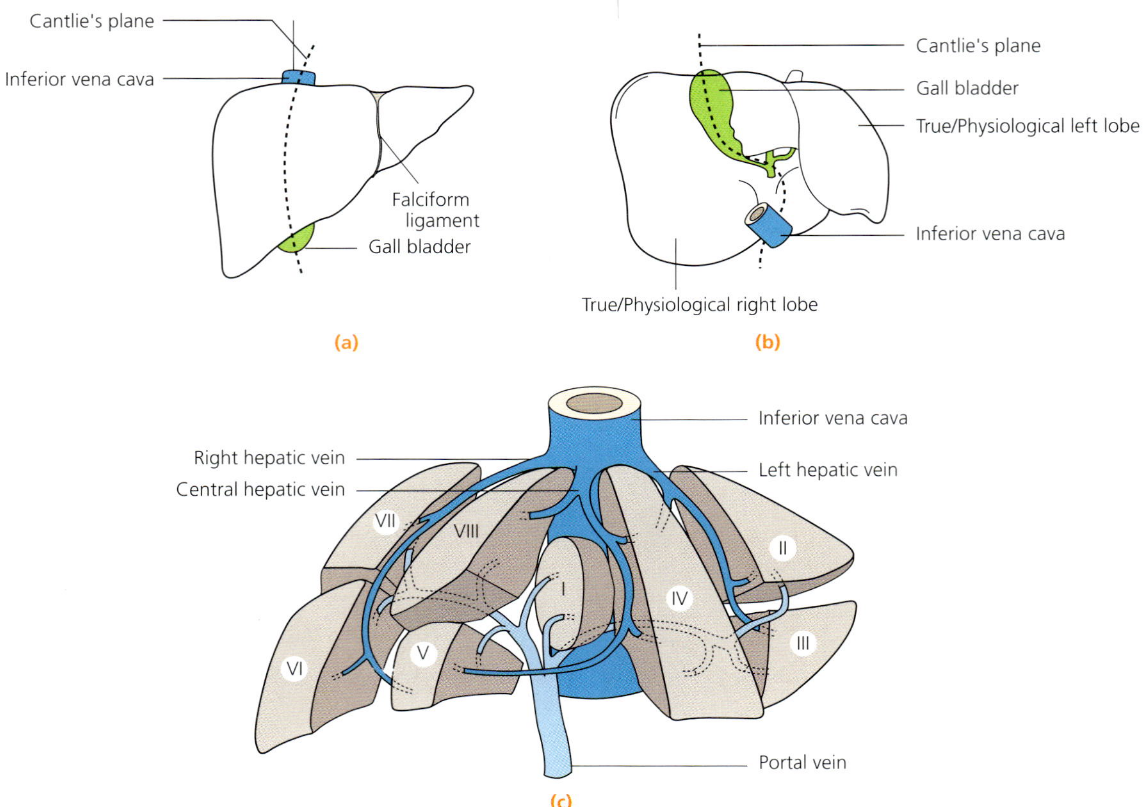

Figure 2.32 The morphological/physiological right and left lobes of the liver shown separated by the dotted line: **(a)** anterior and **(b)** inferior aspect. Note that the quadrate lobe is morphologically a part of the left lobe while the caudate lobe belongs to both the right and left lobes. **(c)** Further segmental divisions of the liver.

Segmental anatomy

The gross anatomical division of the liver into a right and left lobe, demarcated by a line passing from the attachment of the falciform ligament on its anterior surface to the fissures for the ligamentum teres and ligamentum venosum on its posteroinferior surface, is simply a gross anatomical descriptive term with no morphological significance. Studies of the distribution of the hepatic blood vessels and ducts have indicated that the true morphological and physiological division of the liver is into right and left lobes (also called true lobes of the liver) demarcated by a plane (Cantlie's plane) that passes through the fossa of the gall bladder and the fossa of the inferior vena cava. Although these two lobes are not differentiated by any visible line on the dome of the liver, each has its own arterial and portal venous blood supply and separate biliary drainage. This morphological division lies to the right of the gross anatomical plane and in this the quadrate lobe comes to be part of the left morphological lobe of the liver while the caudate lobe divides partly to the left and partly to the right lobe (Fig. 2.32).

The true right and left lobes of the liver can be further subdivided into a number of segments, four for each lobe (Fig. 2.32(c)). The student need not learn the details of these, but of course to the hepatic surgeon, carrying out a partial resection of the liver, knowledge of these segments, with their individual blood supply and biliary drainage, is of great importance.

At the hilum of the liver, the hepatic artery, portal vein and bile duct each divide into right and left branches and there is little or no anastomosis between the divisions on the two sides

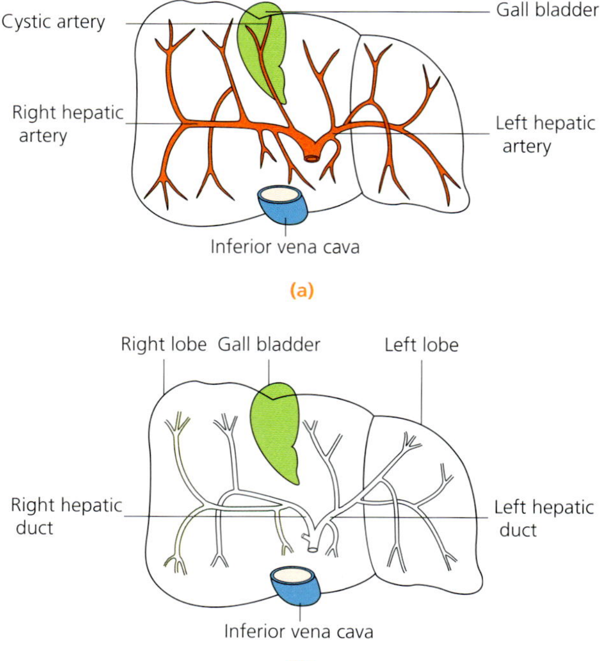

Figure 2.33 **(a)** Distribution of hepatic arteries. **(b)** Distribution of hepatic biliary ducts. Note that the quadrate lobe is supplied exclusively by the left hepatic artery and drained by the left hepatic duct. The caudate lobe is supplied by each.

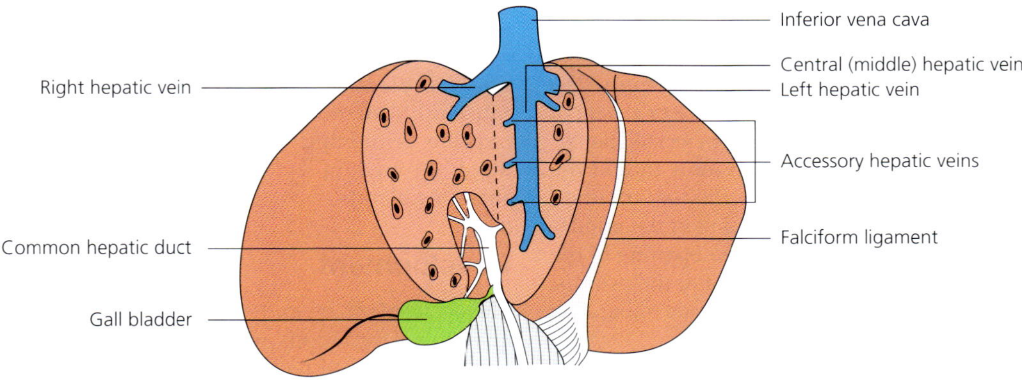

Figure 2.34 Liver split open to demonstrate the hepatic veins and their tributaries.

(Fig. 2.33). From the region of the porta hepatis, the branches pass laterally and spread upwards and downwards throughout the liver substance, defining the morphological left and right lobes.

Hepatic veins (Fig. 2.32(c) and 2.34)

These veins are massive and their distribution is somewhat different from that of the portal, hepatic arterial and bile duct systems already described. There are three major hepatic veins, comprising a right, a central and a left. These pass upwards and backwards to drain into the inferior vena cava at the superior margin of the liver. Their terminations are somewhat variable but usually the central hepatic vein enters the left hepatic vein near its termination. In other specimens it may drain directly into the cava. In addition, small hepatic venous tributaries run directly backwards from the substance of the liver to enter the vena cava more distally to the main hepatic veins. Although these are not of great functional importance they obtrude upon the surgeon during the course of a right hepatic lobectomy.

The three principal hepatic veins have three zones of drainage corresponding roughly to the right, the middle and the left thirds of the liver. The plane defined by the falciform ligament corresponds to the boundary of the zones drained by the left and middle hepatic veins. Unfortunately for the surgeon, the middle hepatic vein lies just at the line of the principal plane of the liver between its right and left morphological lobes and it is this fact which complicates the operation of right or left hepatic resection (Fig. 2.34).

Extrahepatic biliary apparatus

(Fig. 2.35)

The extrahepatic biliary apparatus consists of gallbladder and biliary duct system outside the liver. It is responsible for the collection of bile from the liver, its storage and concentration in the gallbladder and its transmission from the gallbladder to the second part of the duodenum.

The *right* and *left hepatic ducts* fuse in the porta hepatis to form the *common hepatic duct* (1.5 in. (4 cm)). This joins with the *cystic duct* (1.5 in. (4 cm)), draining the gall bladder, to form the *common bile duct* (4 in. (10 cm)). The common bile duct

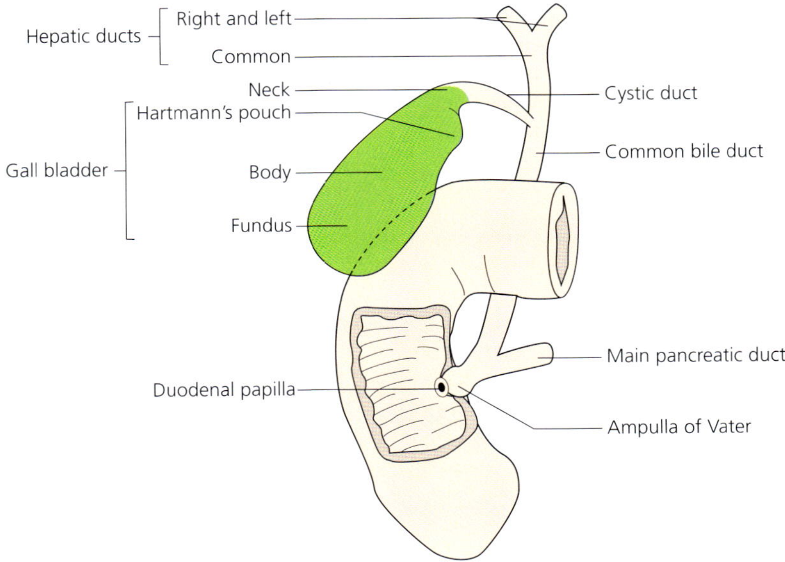

Figure 2.35 Extrahepatic biliary apparatus. (The anterior wall of the second part of the duodenum has been removed.)

commences approximately 1 in. (2.5 cm) above the duodenum, then passes behind it to open at a papilla on the medial aspect of the second part of the duodenum. In this course the common duct either lies in a groove in the posterior aspect of the head of the pancreas or is actually buried in its substance.

As a rule, the common duct termination joins that of the main pancreatic duct (of Wirsung) in a dilated common vestibule, the *ampulla of Vater*, whose opening in the duodenum is guarded by the *sphincter of Oddi*. The opening of the main pancreatic duct is located 8–10 cm distal to the pylorus. Occasionally, the bile and pancreatic ducts open separately into the duodenum.

The common hepatic duct and the supraduodenal part of the common bile duct lie in the free edge of the lesser omentum, where they are related as follows (Fig. 2.9):

- **Bile duct:** Anterior to the right
- **Hepatic artery:** Anterior to the left
- **Portal vein:** Posterior
- **Inferior vena cava:** Still more posterior, separated from the portal vein by the foramen of Winslow

Gall bladder (Fig. 2.35)

The gall bladder normally holds approximately 50 mL of bile and acts as a bile concentrator and reservoir. It lies in a fossa separating the right and quadrate lobes of the liver and is related inferiorly to the duodenum and transverse colon. (An inflamed gall bladder may occasionally ulcerate into either of these structures.)

For descriptive purposes, the organ is divided into the fundus, body and neck, the last opening into the cystic duct. In dilated and pathological gall bladders there is frequently a pouch present on the ventral aspect just proximal to the neck termed *Hartmann's pouch* in which gallstones may become lodged.

Blood supply (Fig. 2.36)

The gall bladder is supplied by the cystic artery (a branch usually of the right hepatic artery), which lies in the triangle made by the liver, the cystic duct and the common hepatic duct (Calot's triangle). Other vessels derived from the hepatic artery pass to the gall bladder from its bed in the liver. Interestingly, there is no accompanying vein to the cystic artery. Small veins pass from the gall bladder through its bed directly into tributaries of the right portal vein within the liver.

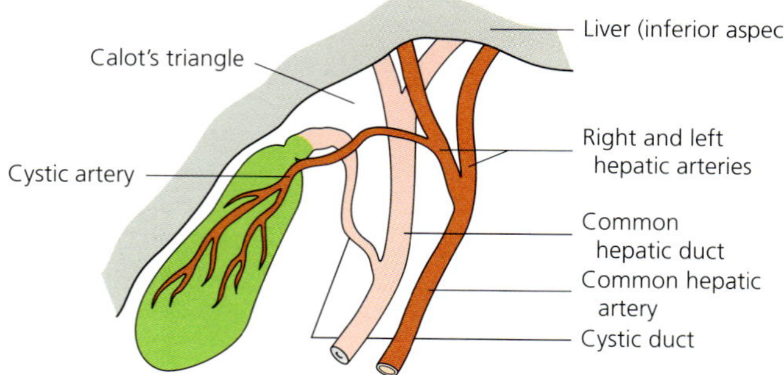

Figure 2.36 The arterial supply of the gall bladder and Calot's triangle.

Structure

The gall bladder wall and the sphincter of Oddi contain muscle, but there are only scattered muscle fibres throughout the remaining biliary duct system. The mucosa is lined throughout by columnar cells and bears mucus-secreting glands.

Development

The gall bladder and ducts are subject to numerous anatomical variations which are best understood by considering their embryological development. An endodermal diverticulum (hepatic bud) grows out from the caudal part of the foregut (ventral wall of the future duodenum) which differentiates into the hepatic ducts and the liver (*see* Fig. 2.38). Another diverticulum from the side of the hepatic duct bud forms the gall bladder and cystic duct. Some variations are shown in Fig. 2.37.

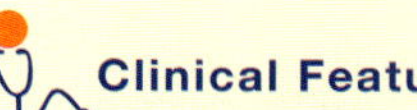

Clinical Features

1 Errors in gall bladder surgery are frequently the result of failure to appreciate the variations in the anatomy of the biliary system; it is important, therefore, before dividing any structures and removing the gall bladder, to have all three biliary ducts clearly identified, together with the cystic and hepatic arteries. The cystic artery is constantly found in Calot's triangle (Fig. 2.36), formed by the cystic duct, the common hepatic duct and the inferior aspect of the liver.

2 Haemorrhage during cholecystectomy may be controlled by compressing the hepatic artery (which gives off the cystic branch) between the finger and thumb where it lies in the anterior wall of the foramen of Winslow (Pringle's manoeuvre) (Fig. 2.9).

3 Gangrene of the gall bladder is rare because even if the cystic artery becomes thrombosed in acute cholecystitis there is a rich secondary blood supply coming in from the liver bed. Gangrene may occur in the unusual event of a gall bladder on an abnormally long mesentery undergoing torsion, which will destroy both its sources of blood supply.

4 Stones in the common duct can usually be removed endoscopically using a Dormia basket introduced after dividing the sphincter of Oddi. At other times, the common bile duct is explored via an incision in its supraduodenal portion. Sometimes a stone impacted at the ampulla of Vater must be approached via an incision in the second part of the duodenum. This last approach is also used when it is necessary to divide the sphincter of Oddi or to remove a tumour arising at the termination of the common bile duct.

Pancreas (Figs 2.17 and 2.18)

The pancreas is a soft, lobulated and elongated gland which lies retroperitoneally in roughly the transpyloric plane. It is an exoendocrine gland. Its exocrine part secretes pancreatic juice, while its endocrine part secretes hormones, viz. insulin, etc. For descriptive purposes it is divided into the head, neck, body and tail.

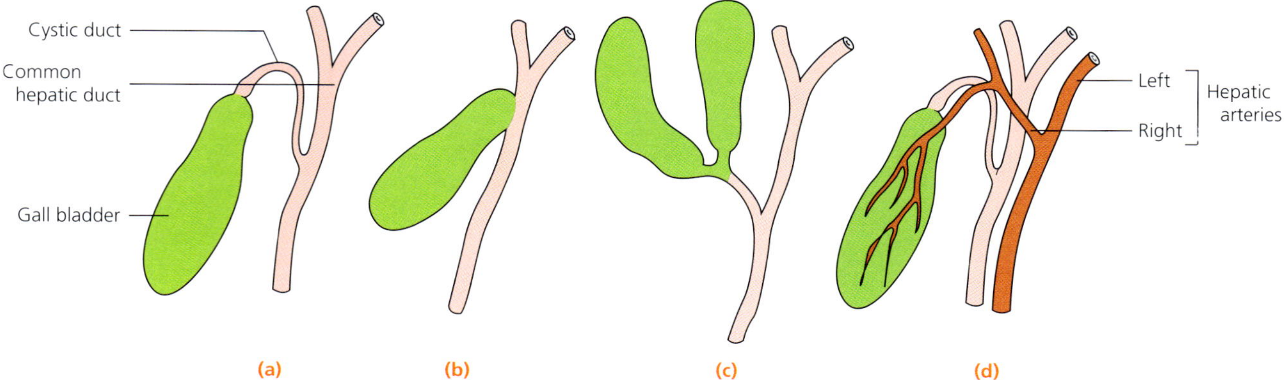

Figure 2.37 Some variations in biliary anatomy. **(a)** A long cystic duct joining the hepatic duct low down behind the duodenum. **(b)** Absence of the cystic duct – the gall bladder opens directly into the common hepatic duct. **(c)** A double gall bladder, the result of a rare bifid embryonic diverticulum from the hepatic duct. **(d)** The right hepatic artery crosses *in front* of the common hepatic duct; this occurs in 25% of cases.

Relations

The head lies in the C-curve of the duodenum and sends out the *uncinate process*, inferiorly and to the left, which hooks posteriorly to the superior mesenteric vessels as these travel from behind the pancreas into the root of the mesentery.

Posteriorly lie the inferior vena cava, the commencement of the portal vein, the aorta, the superior mesenteric vessels, the crura of the diaphragm, the coeliac plexus, the left kidney and the suprarenal gland. The tortuous splenic artery runs along the upper border of the pancreas. The splenic vein runs behind the gland, receives the inferior mesenteric vein and joins the superior mesenteric to form the portal vein behind the pancreatic neck (Fig. 2.26).

To complete this list of important posterior relationships, the common bile duct either lies in a groove in the right extremity of the gland or is embedded in its substance, as it passes to open into the second part of the duodenum.

Anteriorly lies the stomach separated by the lesser sac. To the left, the pancreatic tail lies against the hilum of the spleen.

Blood supply

Blood is supplied from the splenic and the pancreaticoduodenal arteries derived from coeliac and superior mesenteric arteries; the corresponding veins drain into the portal system.

Lymphatic drainage

The lymphatics drain into nodes which lie along its upper border, in the groove between its head and the duodenum, and along the root of the superior mesenteric vessels.

Structure

The pancreas macroscopically is lobulated and is contained within a fine capsule; these lobules are made up of alveoli of serous secretory cells draining via their ductules into the principal ducts. Between these alveoli lie the insulin-secreting *islets of Langerhans*.

The *main duct of the pancreas (Wirsung)* (Fig. 2.18) runs the length of the gland and usually opens at the summit of the ampulla of Vater along with the common bile duct; very occasionally, it drains separately into the duodenum.

The *accessory duct* (*of Santorini*) passes from the lower part of the head, in front of the main duct, communicates with it, and then opens into the duodenum above it. Occasionally it is absent.

Development (Fig. 2.38)

The pancreas develops from two buds: a larger *dorsal bud* (diverticulum) from the endodermal lining of the duodenum and a smaller *ventral bud* (outpouching) from the side of the common bile duct adjacent to the duodenal wall. The ventral bud swings round posteriorly to fuse with the lower aspect of the dorsal bud, trapping the superior mesenteric vessels between the two parts.

The ducts of the two formative segments of the pancreas then communicate; that of the smaller takes over the main pancreatic flow to form the main duct, leaving the original duct of the larger portion of the gland distal to communication as the accessory duct.

Clinical Features

1 Rarely, the two developing segments of the pancreas completely surround the second part of the duodenum (**'annular pancreas'**) and may produce duodenal obstruction.
2 Note from the posterior relations of the pancreas that a neoplasm of the head of the pancreas will produce obstructive jaundice by compressing the common bile duct. An extensive growth in the body of the gland may cause portal or inferior vena caval obstruction.
3 Anterior to the pancreas lies the stomach, separated from it by the lesser sac. This sac may become closed off and distended with fluid either from perforation of a posterior gastric ulcer or from the outpouring of fluid in acute pancreatitis, forming a ***pseudocyst of the pancreas***. Such a collection may almost fill the abdominal cavity.

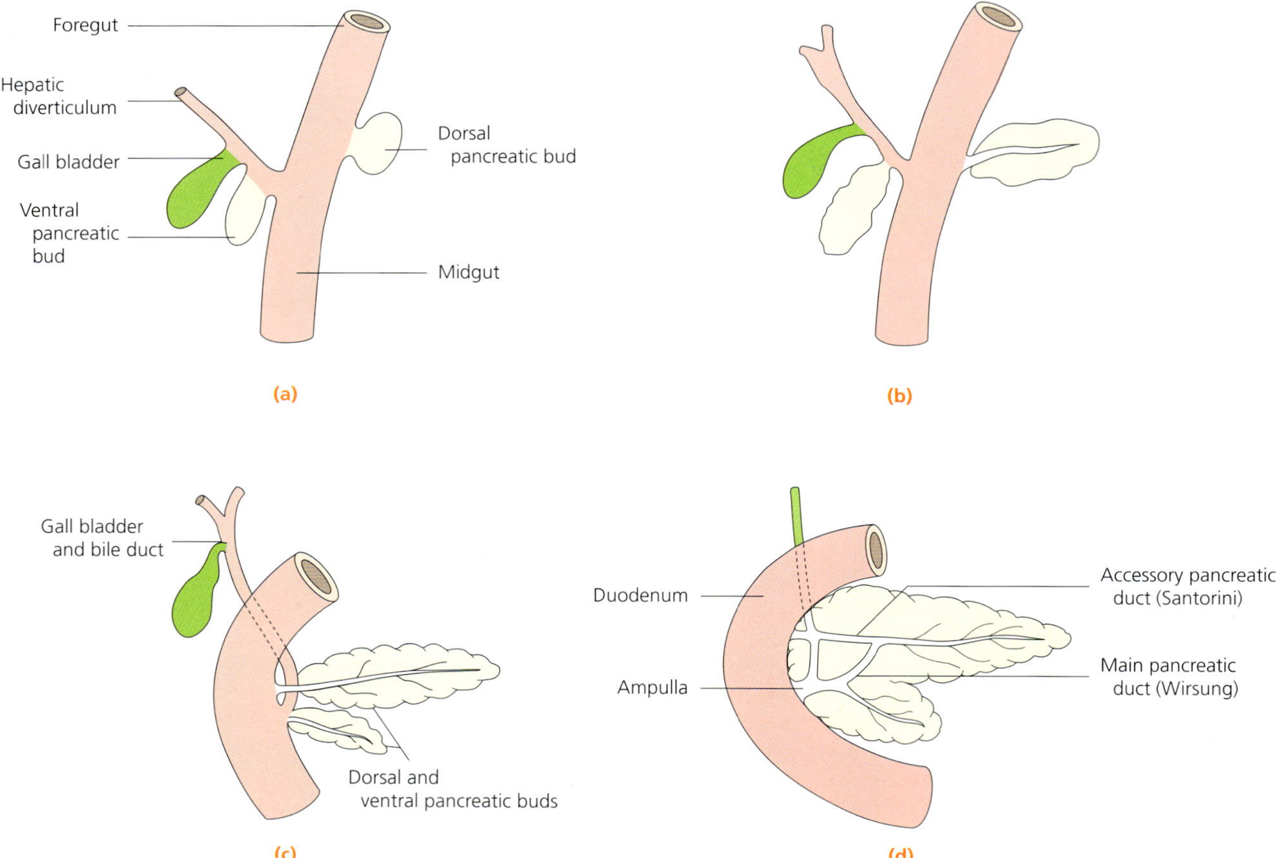

Figure 2.38 (a–d) Development of the intestinal adnexae.

Spleen

The spleen is a wedge-shaped lymphoid organ situated mainly in the left hypochondrium. It is approximately equal to the size of the cupped hand. It forms the left lateral extremity of the lesser sac. Passing from it are the *gastrosplenic ligament* to the greater curvature of stomach (carrying the short gastric and left gastro-epiploic vessels) and the *splenorenal ligament* to the posterior abdominal wall (carrying the splenic vessels and the tail of the pancreas).

The spleen has an expanded anterior end and a round posterior end. It has superior, inferior and intermedial borders. The superior border is characteristically notched. It also presents two surfaces: a smooth convex diaphragmatic surface and a concave irregular visceral surface.

Relations (Fig. 2.39)

These are as follows:

a. **Diaphragmatic surface**
   - The left diaphragm, separating it from the pleura, left lung and the 9th, 10th and 11th ribs

b. **Visceral surface**
   - **Anteriorly:** The stomach
   - **Inferiorly:** The splenic flexure of the colon
   - **Medially:** The left kidney

The tail of the pancreas abuts against the hilum of the spleen through which vessels and nerves enter and leave this organ.

Blood supply

The splenic artery is one of the three main branches of the coeliac axis. While the splenic artery appears perfectly straight in lower animals and even the human infant, in human adults it is tortuous: the only artery to display this feature within the body cavities. The splenic artery is thus easily identified on an aortogram or enhanced CT, as it is the only tortuous artery to be seen in the abdomen. The cause or significance of this is unknown. The splenic vein is joined by the superior mesenteric to form the portal vein. (Note that the splenic vessels are also the principal source of blood supply to the pancreas. This important fact is often forgotten in the heat of an oral examination. It would be easier for candidates if these vessels were more accurately named the 'pancreatico-splenic artery and vein').

Structure

The spleen represents the largest accumulation of reticulo-endothelial tissue in the body. It has a thin fibrous capsule, to which the peritoneum adheres intimately. The fibrous tissue of the capsule extends into the spleen to form a series of trabeculae between which lies the splenic pulp.

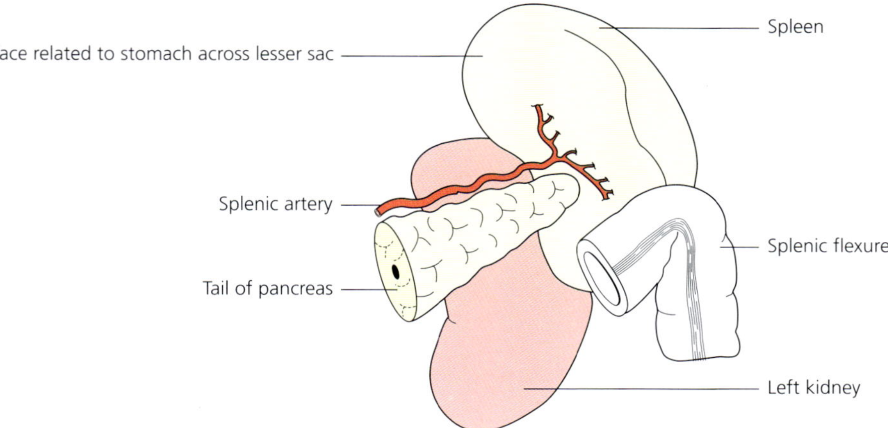

Figure 2.39 The spleen and its immediate relations.

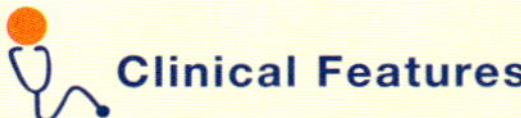

Clinical Features

1 In performing a splenectomy the close relationship of the pancreatic tail to the hilum and splenic pedicle must be remembered; it is easily wounded.
2 Note the close proximity of the lower ribs, the lowest part of the left lung and pleural cavity, the left diaphragm, the left kidney and the spleen; injuries to the left upper abdomen may damage any combination of these structures. Similarly, a stab wound of the posterior left chest may penetrate the diaphragm and tear the spleen. The spleen, with its thin tense capsule, is the commonest in-tra-abdominal viscus to be ruptured by blunt trauma.
3 Accessory spleens (one or more) may occur most commonly near the hilum, but also in the tail of the pancreas, the mesentery of the spleen, the omentum, the small bowel mesentery, the ovary and even the testis. They occur in approximately one in 10 subjects and, if left behind, may result in persistence of symptoms following splenectomy for congenital acholuric jaundice or thrombocytopenic purpura.
4 Splenomegaly (enlargement of spleen) may occur in a number of diseases, viz. malaria, chronic myeloid leukaemia, etc. In this condition, splenic notches are palpable just below the left costal margin. In cases of massive splenomegaly, it projects towards the right iliac fossa in the direction of the axis of the 10th rib.

Urinary tract

Kidneys

The kidneys are a pair of excretory organs. They lie retroperitoneally on the posterior abdominal wall; the right kidney is 0.5 in. (1.2 cm) lower than the left, presumably because of its downward displacement by the bulk of the liver. Each measures approximately 4.5 in. (11 cm) long, 2.5 in. (6 cm) wide and 1.5 in. (4 cm) thick.

Relations (Figs 2.40 and 2.41)

These are as follows:

- **Posteriorly:** The diaphragm (separating pleura), quadratus lumborum, psoas, transversus abdominis, the 12th rib and three nerves – the subcostal (T12), iliohypogastric and ilio-inguinal (L1). In addition to this, the left kidney being higher is also related to the 11th rib.
- **Anteriorly:** The right kidney is related to the liver, the second part of the duodenum (which may be opened accidentally in performing a right nephrectomy) and the ascending colon. In front of the left kidney lie the stomach, the pancreas and its vessels, the spleen and the descending colon. The suprarenals sit on each side as a cap on the kidney's upper pole.

The medial aspect of the kidney presents a deep vertical slit, the *hilum*, which transmits, from before backwards, the renal vein, the renal artery, the renal pelvis and, usually, a subsidiary branch of the renal artery. Lymphatics and nerves

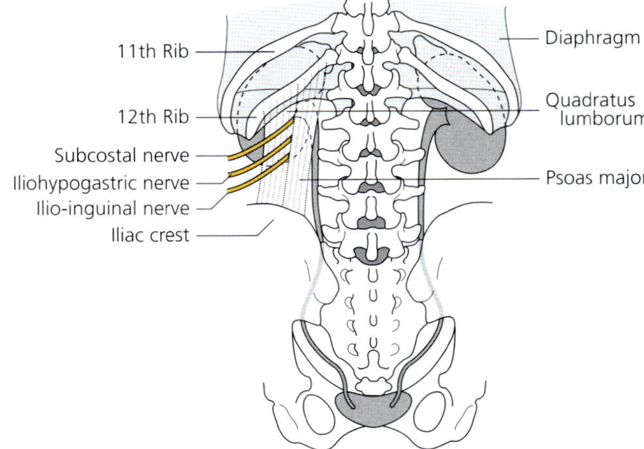

Figure 2.40 The posterior relations of the kidney (viewed from behind).

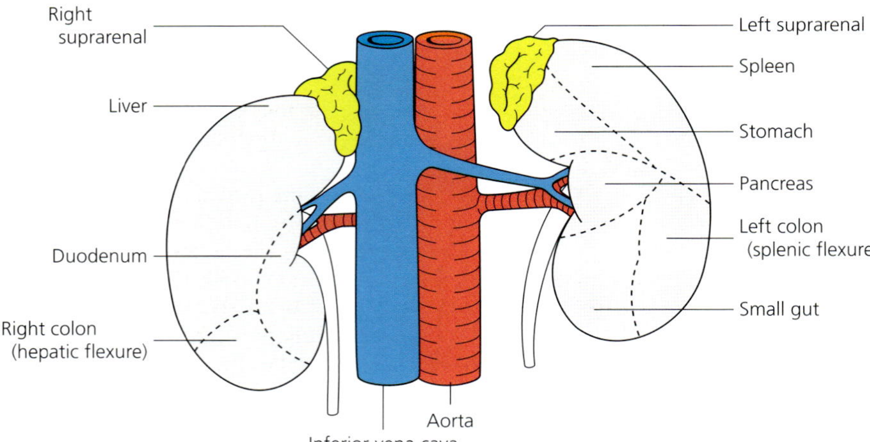

Figure 2.41 The anterior relations of the kidneys.

also enter the hilum, the latter being sympathetic, mainly vasomotor, fibres.

The *renal pelvis* is subject to considerable anatomical variations (Fig. 2.42); it may lie completely outside the substance of the kidney (even to the extent of having part of the major calyces extrarenal) or may be almost buried in the renal hilum. All gradations exist between these extremes. If a calculus is lodged in the renal pelvis, its removal is comparatively simple when this is extrarenal, and it is correspondingly difficult when the pelvis is hidden within the substance of the kidney.

Within the kidney, the renal pelvis receives two or three *major calyces*, each of which receives a number of *minor calyces*. Each of these, in turn, is indented by a papilla of renal tissue and it is here that the collecting tubules of the kidney discharge urine into the conducting part of the urinary tract.

The kidneys lie in an abundant fatty cushion (*perinephric fat*) contained in the *renal fascia* (Fig. 2.43). Above, the renal fascia blends with the fascia on the undersurface of the diaphragm, leaving a separate compartment for the suprarenal (which is thus easily separated and left behind in performing a nephrectomy). Medially, the fascia blends with the sheaths of the aorta and inferior vena cava. Laterally, it is continuous with the transversalis fascia. Only inferiorly does it remain relatively open – tracking around the ureter into the pelvis.

The kidney has, in fact, three capsules from outside to inside. These are as follows:

1. Fascial capsule (renal fascia)
2. Fatty capsule (perinephric fat)
3. True capsule: The fibrous capsule is a thin membrane which strips readily from the normal kidney surface but adheres firmly to an organ that has been inflamed

Blood supply

The *renal artery* derives directly from the aorta. The *renal vein* drains directly into the inferior vena cava. The *left renal vein* passes in front of the aorta immediately below the origin of the superior mesenteric artery. The *right renal artery* passes behind the inferior vena cava.

Lymph drainage

Lymphatics drain directly to the para-aortic lymph nodes.

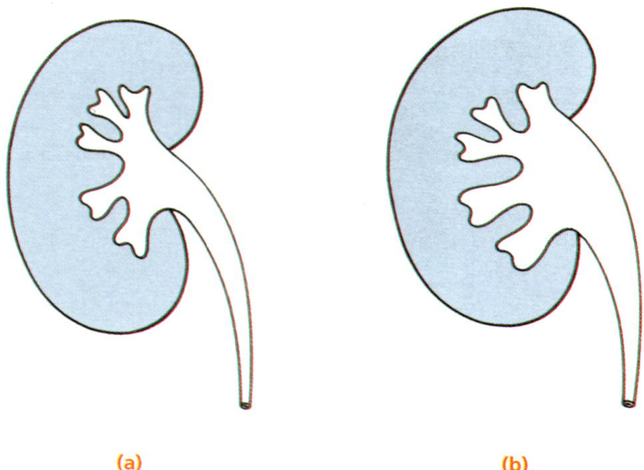

Figure 2.42 Variations in the renal pelvis. **(a)** The pelvis is buried within the renal parenchyma – pyelolithotomy difficult. **(b)** The pelvis protrudes generously – pyelolithotomy easy.

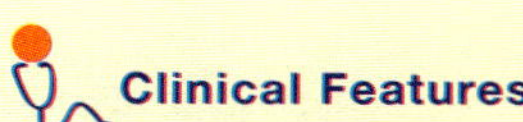

Clinical Features

1 The highly vascular kidney is not infrequently ruptured by closed trauma, e.g. a kick in the loin. The capsule is torn and blood extravasates into the perinephric fat space. This is usually tamponaded by the renal fascia, and the bleeding controlled. Only if this fascial layer tears does haemorrhage continue and surgery – often nephrectomy – become mandatory. The midline attachment of the renal fascia prevents extravasation to the opposite side.

2 In hypermobility of the kidney ('floating kidney'), this organ can be moved up and down in its fascial compartment but not from side to side. To a lesser degree, it is in this plane that the normal kidney moves during respiration.

3 *Renal angle:* It is an angle between the lower border of the 12th rib and the outer border of an erector spinae. It overlies on the kidney; hence, the tenderness in kidney is elicited by pressing the angle with the thumb.

(Continued ...)

(... *continued*)

4 *Exposure of the kidney via the loin:* An oblique incision is usually favoured midway between the 12th rib and the iliac crest, extending laterally from the lateral border of erector spinae. Latissimus dorsi and serratus posterior inferior are divided and the free posterior border of external oblique is identified, enabling this muscle to be split along its fibres. Internal oblique and transversus abdominis are then divided, revealing peritoneum anteriorly, which is pushed forwards. The renal fascial capsule is then brought clearly into view and is opened. The subcostal nerve and vessels are usually encountered in the upper part of the incision and are preserved. If more room is required, the lateral edge of quadratus lumborum may be divided and also the 12th rib excised, care being taken to push up, but not to open, the pleura, which crosses the medial half of the rib.

Ureter

The ureter is a narrow thick–walled muscular tube which transports urine from kidney to the urinary bladder. It is 10 in. (25 cm) long and comprises its abdominal, pelvic and intravesical portions.

The *abdominal ureter* lies on the medial edge of psoas major (which separates it from the tips of the transverse processes of L2–L5) and then crosses into the pelvis at the bifurcation of the common iliac artery in front of the sacro-iliac joint. Anteriorly, the right ureter is covered at its origin by the second part of the duodenum and then lies lateral to the inferior vena cava and behind the posterior peritoneum. It is crossed by the testicular (or ovarian), right colic and ileocolic vessels. The left ureter is crossed by the testicular (or ovarian) and left colic vessels and then passes above the pelvic brim, behind the mesosigmoid and sigmoid colon to cross the common iliac artery immediately above its bifurcation.

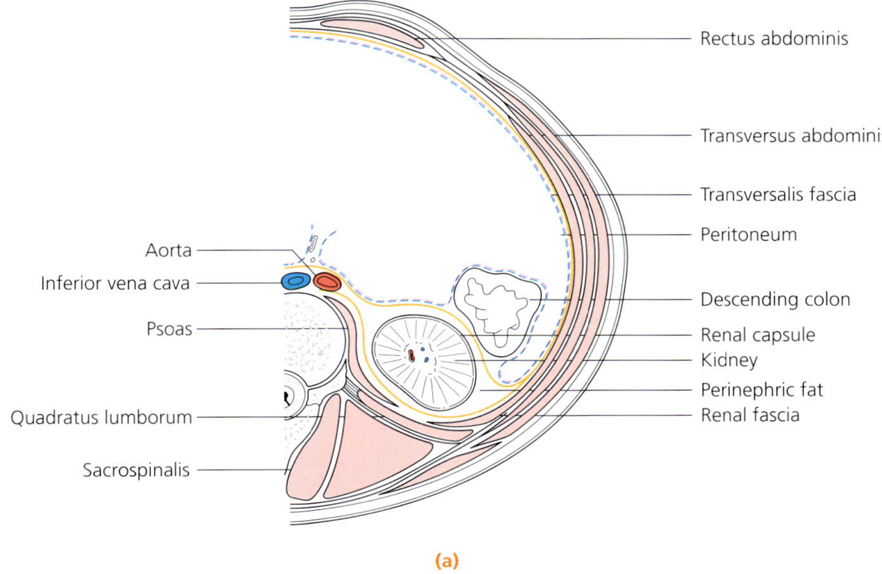

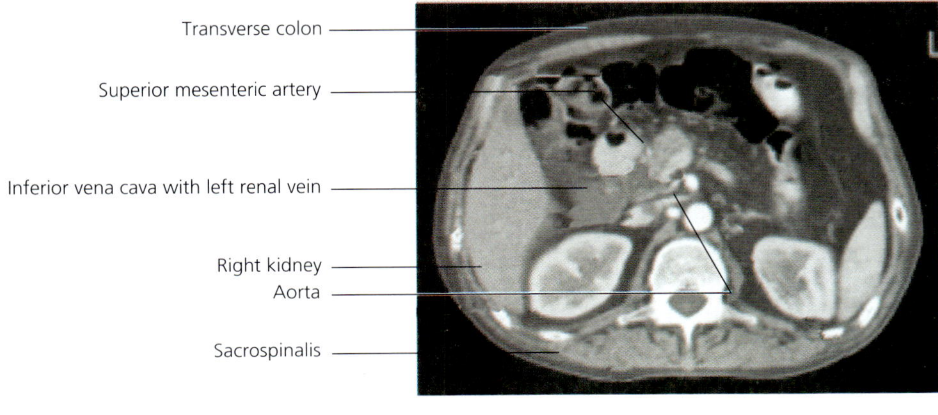

Figure 2.43 **(a)** Transverse section (seen from below) demonstrating the fascial compartments of the kidney. **(b)** CT scan of the same region. Note that CT scans, by convention, are viewed from below, so that the aorta, for example, is seen on the right side. The blood vessels have been enhanced by an intravenous injection of contrast; CT: Computed tomography.

The *pelvic ureter* runs on the lateral wall of the pelvis in front of the internal iliac artery to just in front of the ischial spine; it then turns forwards and medially to enter the bladder. In the male, it lies above the seminal vesicle near its termination and is crossed superficially by the vas deferens (*see* Fig. 2.47). In the female, the ureter passes above the lateral fornix of the vagina 0.5 in. (1.25 cm) lateral to the supravaginal portion of the cervix and lies below the broad ligament and uterine vessels (*see* Fig. 2.65).

The *intravesical ureter* passes obliquely through the wall of the bladder for 0.75 in. (2 cm); the vesical muscle and obliquity of this course produce, respectively, a sphincteric and valve-like arrangement at the termination of this duct.

Blood supply

The ureter receives a rich segmental blood supply from all available arteries along its course: the aorta, and the renal, testicular (or ovarian), internal iliac and inferior vesical arteries.

Clinical Features

1 The ureter is readily identified in life by its thick muscular wall which is seen to undergo worm-like (vermicular) writhing movements, particularly if gently stroked or squeezed.
2 Throughout its abdominal and the upper part of its pelvic course, it adheres to the overlying peritoneum (through which it can be seen in the thin subject), and this fact is used in exposing the ureter – as the parietal peritoneum is dissected upwards, the ureter comes into view sticking to its posterior aspect.
3 The ureter is relatively narrowed at three sites as mentioned below:
   - At the junction of the renal pelvis and ureter (pelvi-ureteric junction)
   - At the pelvic brim and
   - At the ureteric orifice (narrowest of all)

   A ureteric calculus is likely to lodge at one of these three levels.
4 Renal colic: It is a severe spasmodic pain due to ureteric stone. It starts in the loin and radiates to the groin and inner aspect of the thigh. Note, the pain is referred to T11 to L2 segments which also supply the ureter.

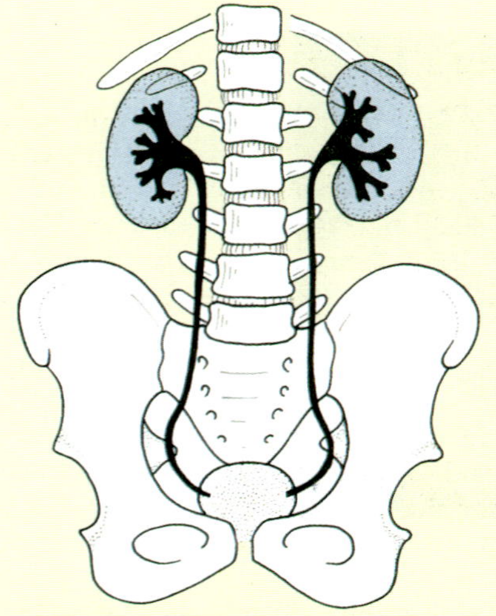

Figure 2.44 Drawing from an intravenous pyelogram to show the relationship of the ureters to the bony landmarks.

(Continued ...)

(... continued)

5 In searching for a ureteric stone on a plain radiograph of the abdomen, one must imagine the course of the ureter in relation to the bony skeleton (Fig. 2.44). It lies along the tips of the transverse processes, crosses in front of the sacro-iliac joint, swings out to the ischial spine and then passes medially to the bladder. An opaque shadow along this line is suspicious of calculus. This course of the ureter is readily studied by examining a radiograph showing a radio-opaque ureteric catheter *in situ*. A ureter is likely to be ligated inadvertently with uterine artery during hysterectomy, as it lies 2 cm lateral to the cervix and is crossed by the uterine artery from the lateral to the medial side.

Embryology and congenital abnormalities of the kidney and ureter (Fig. 2.45)

The kidney and ureter are mesodermal in origin and develop in an unusual manner of considerable interest to the comparative anatomist.

The *pronephros*, of importance in the lower vertebrates, is transient in humans, but the distal part of its duct receives the tubules of the next renal organ to develop, the *mesonephros*, and now becomes the *mesonephric* or *Wolffian duct*. The mesonephros itself then disappears except for some of its ducts, which form the efferent tubules of the testis. For further details of the fates of the mesonephros and mesonephric duct, *see* page 87.

A diverticulum then appears at the lower end of the mesonephric duct which develops into the *metanephric duct*; on top of the latter a cap of tissue differentiates to form the definitive kidney or *metanephros*. The metanephric duct develops into the ureter, pelvis, calyces and collecting tubules; the metanephros into the glomeruli and the proximal part of the renal duct system.

The mesonephric duct now loses its renal connection, atrophies in the female (remaining only as the epoöphoron) but persists in the male, to become the epididymis and vas deferens.

The kidney first develops in the pelvis and then migrates upwards. Its blood supply is first obtained from the common

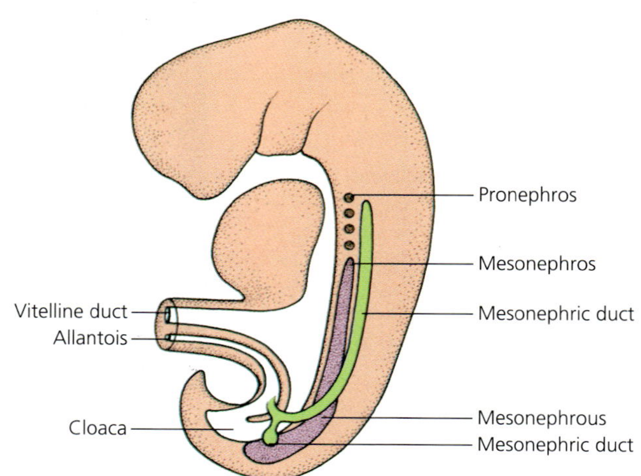

Figure 2.45 Development of the pro-, meso- and metanephric systems (after Langman).

iliac artery but, during migration, a series of vessels form to supply it, only to involute again when the renal artery takes over this duty.

Developmental abnormalities (Fig. 2.46)

These are as follows:

1. It is common for one or more distally placed arteries to persist (*aberrant renal arteries*) and one may even run to the kidney from the common iliac artery.
2. Occasionally the kidney will fail to migrate cranially, resulting in a persistent *pelvic kidney*.
3. The two metanephric masses may fuse in development, forming a *horseshoe kidney* linked across the midline.
4. In one in 2400 births there is complete failure of development of one kidney (*congenital absence of the kidney*).
5. *Congenital polycystic kidneys* (which are nearly always bilateral) are believed to result from failure of metanephric tissue to link up with some of the metanephric duct collecting tubules; blind ducts therefore form which subsequently become distended with fluid. This theory of origin does not explain their occasional association with multiple cysts of the liver, pancreas, lung and ovary.
6. The mesonephric duct may give off a double metanephric bud so that two ureters may develop on one or both sides. These ureters may fuse into a single duct anywhere along their course or open separately into the bladder (where the *upper* ureter enters *below* the *lower* ureter).

Rarely, the extra ureter may open ectopically into the vagina or urethra resulting in urinary incontinence.

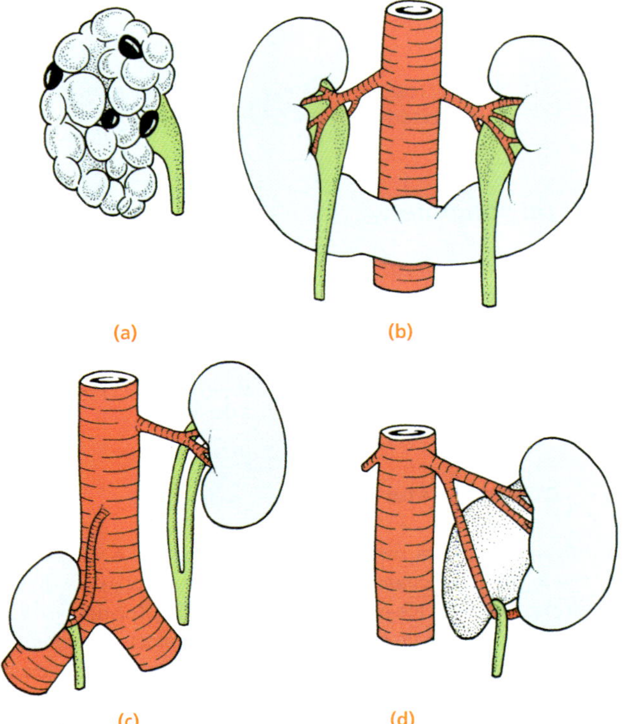

Figure 2.46 Renal abnormalities. (a) Polycystic kidney. (b) Horseshoe kidney. (c) Pelvic kidney (right) and double ureter (left). (d) Aberrant renal artery and associated hydronephrosis.

Urinary bladder (Figs 2.22, 2.23 and 2.47)

The urinary bladder is a muscular reservoir of urine, situated immediately behind the pubic bones. The bladder capacity in the normal adult is variable, the average being approximately 300 mL. In cases of retention of urine, the adult bladder distends from the pelvic cavity into the abdomen, stripping the peritoneum upwards from the anterior abdominal wall. The surgeon utilizes this fact in carrying out an extraperitoneal incision or suprapubic puncture into the bladder. In children up to the age of approximately 3 years, the pelvis is relatively small and the bladder is, in fact, intra-abdominal although still extraperitoneal.

Relations

These are as follows:

- **Anteriorly:** The pubic symphysis
- **Superiorly:** The bladder is covered by peritoneum with coils of small intestine and sigmoid colon lying against it. In the female, the body of the uterus flops against its posterosuperior aspect
- **Posteriorly:** In the male the rectum, the termination of the vasa deferentia and the seminal vesicles; in the female, the vagina and the supravaginal part of the cervix
- **Laterally:** The levator ani and obturator internus

The **neck of the bladder** fuses with the prostate in the male; in the female it lies directly on the pelvic fascia surrounding the short urethra.

The muscle coat of the bladder is formed by a criss-cross arrangement of bundles; when these undergo hypertrophy in chronic obstruction (due to an enlarged prostate, for example) they account for the typical trabeculated 'open weave' appearance of the bladder wall, readily seen through a cystoscope.

The circular component of the muscle coat condenses as an (involuntary) *internal urethral sphincter* around the internal orifice. This can be destroyed without incontinence providing the external sphincter remains intact (as occurs in prostatectomy).

Cystoscopy

The interior of the bladder and its three orifices (the internal meatus and the two ureters) are easily inspected by means of a cystoscope. The ureteric orifices lie 1 in. (2.5 cm) apart in the empty bladder, but, when this is distended for cystoscopic examination, the distance increases to 2 in. (5 cm). The submucosa and mucosa of most of the bladder are only loosely adherent to the underlying muscle and are thrown into folds when the bladder is empty, smoothing out during distension of the organ. Over the *trigone*, the triangular area bounded by the ureteric orifices and the internal meatus, the mucosa is adherent and remains smooth even in the empty bladder.

Between the ureters, a raised fold of mucosa can be seen that is called the *interureteric ridge*, which is produced by an underlying bar of muscle.

A slight elevation immediately above the urethral orifice, produced by the median lobe of prostate, is called *uvula vesicae*.

Blood supply

Blood is supplied from the superior and inferior vesical branches of the internal iliac artery. The vesical veins form a plexus which drains into the internal iliac vein.

Lymph drainage

Lymphatics drain alongside the vesical blood vessels to the iliac and then para-aortic nodes.

Nerve supply

Efferent parasympathetic fibres from S2 to S4 accompany the vesical arteries to the bladder. They convey motor fibres to the muscles of the bladder wall and inhibitory fibres to its internal sphincter. Sympathetic efferent fibres are said to be inhibitory to the bladder muscles and motor to its sphincter, although they may be mainly vasomotor in function, so that normal filling and emptying of the bladder are probably controlled exclusively by its parasympathetic innervation. The external sphincter is made up of striated muscle. It is also concerned in the control of micturition and is supplied by the pudendal nerve (S2, S3, S4). Sensory fibres from the bladder, which are stimulated by distension, are conveyed in both the sympathetic and parasympathetic nerves, the latter pathway being the more important.

Urethra

Male urethra (Fig. 2.47(b))

The male urethra is a common passage for urine and semen. It is 8 in. (20 cm) long and extends from the neck of the bladder to the external meatus on the tip of glans penis. It is divided into three parts: prostatic, membranous and spongy.

The *prostatic urethra* (1.25 in. (3 cm)), as its name implies, traverses the prostate. Its posterior wall bears a longitudinal elevation termed the *urethral crest*, on each side of which is a shallow depression, the *prostatic sinus*, into which the 15–20 prostatic ducts empty. At approximately the middle of the crest is a prominence termed the *colliculus seminalis* (*verumontanum*) into which opens the *prostatic utricle*. This is a blind tract, approximately 0.25 in. (0.5 cm) long, running downwards from the substance of the median lobe of the prostate. It is believed to represent the male equivalent of the vagina, a remnant of the paramesonephric duct (*see* page 87). On either side of the orifice of the prostatic utricle open the *ejaculatory ducts*, formed by the union of the duct of the seminal vesicle and the terminal part of the vas deferens. It is the widest and the most dilatable part.

The *membranous urethra* (0.75 in. (2 cm)) pierces the external sphincter urethrae (the voluntary sphincter of the bladder) and the fascial perineal membrane which covers the superficial aspect of the sphincter. It is the least dilatable part.

The *spongy urethra* (6 in. (15 cm)) traverses the corpus spongiosum of the penis. It first passes upwards and forwards to lie below the pubic symphysis and then in its flaccid state bends downwards and forwards. It presents two dilatations as mentioned below:

a. Intrabulbar fossa in the bulb of the penis
b. Navicular fossa in the glans penis

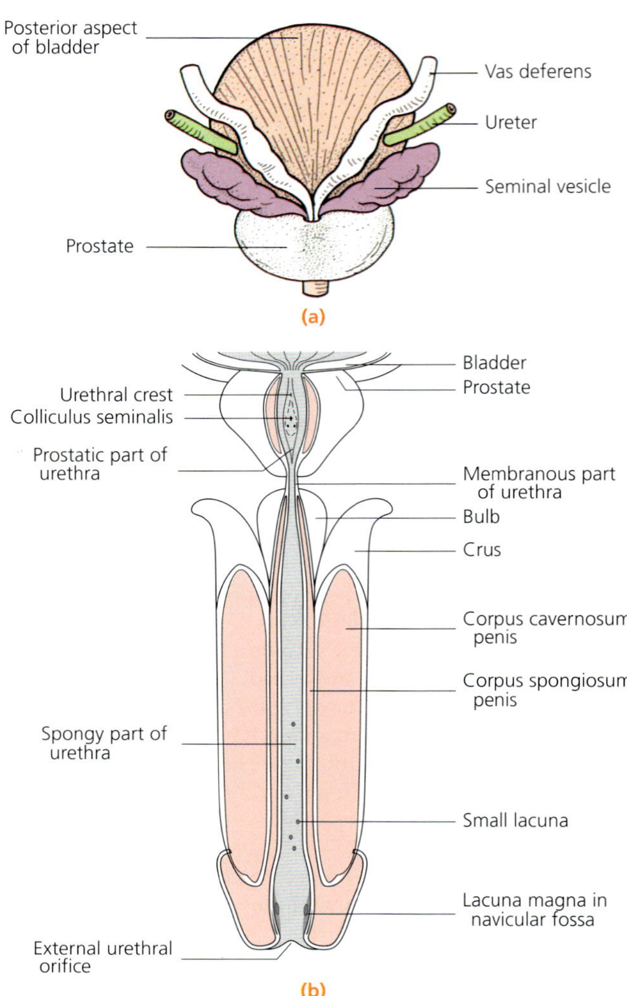

Figure 2.47 **(a)** The prostate, seminal vesicles and vasa shown in a posterior view of the bladder. **(b)** The prostate and urethra in vertical section.

Urethral sphincters

The *internal urethral sphincter* (sphincter vesicae) is involuntary in nature and controls the neck of the bladder and prostatic urethra above the openings of the ejaculatory ducts. The *external urethral sphincter* (sphincter urethrae) is voluntary in nature and controls the membranous part of the urethra. It is responsible for voiding of the urine.

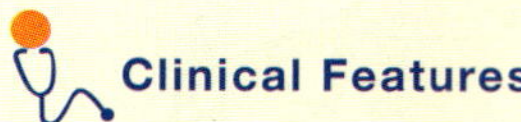

Clinical Features

1 Where the urethra passes beneath the pubis is a common site for it to be ruptured by a fall astride a sharp object, which crushes it against the edge of the symphysis. (a) The rupture of urethra above the urogenital diaphragm (i.e. prostatic urethra) leads to the extravasation of urine in retropubic periprostatic and perirectal spaces. (b) The rupture of urethra below the urogenital diaphragm (i.e. bulbous part of spongy urethra) leads to the extravasation of urine in superficial perineal pouch.

(Continued ...)

(... *continued*)

2 The external orifice is the narrowest part of the urethra and a calculus may lodge there. Immediately within the meatus, the urethra dilates into a terminal fossa whose roof bears a mucosal fold (the *lacuna magna*), which may catch the tip of a catheter. Instruments should always be introduced into the urethra beak downwards for this reason.

Female urethra

The female urethra is 1.5 in. (4 cm) long; it traverses the sphincter urethrae and lies immediately in front of, indeed embedded in the wall of, the vagina. Its external meatus opens 1 in. (2.5 cm) behind the clitoris. The sphincter urethrae in the female is a tenuous structure and vesical control appears to depend mainly on the intrinsic sphincter of condensed circular muscle fibres of the bladder.

Mucosa of the urinary tract

The renal pelvis and calyceal system, ureter, bladder and urethra are lined by a transitional epithelium as far as the entry of the ejaculatory ducts in the prostatic urethra. This is conveniently termed the *uroepithelium* or urothelium since it has a uniform appearance and is subject to the same pathological processes, e.g. the development of papillomata. The remainder of the urethra has a columnar lining except at its termination, where the epithelium becomes squamous.

Radiology of the urinary tract

The renal contours can often be identified on a soft-tissue radiograph of the abdomen. Intravenous injection of iodine-containing compounds excreted by the kidney will produce an outline of the calyces and the ureter (intravenous urogram). When the injection medium enters the bladder, a cystogram is obtained (Fig. 2.44).

Further information can be obtained by passing a catheter up the ureter through a cystoscope and injecting radio-opaque fluid to fill the pelvis and calyx system (retrograde pyelogram). Similarly, injection of such fluid into the urethra or bladder may be used for the radiographic study of these viscera.

The kidneys are beautifully delineated in transverse section on CT scans (Fig. 2.43(b), and *see* Figs 2.73 and 2.74).

Male genital organs

Prostate (Fig. 2.47)

The prostate is a pyramidal-shaped, fibromuscular and glandular organ, 1.25 in. (3 cm) long, which surrounds the prostatic urethra. It resembles the size and shape of a chestnut. The secretions of this gland along with those of seminal vesicles form the bulk of the seminal fluid.

Relations (Fig. 2.22)

- **Superiorly:** The prostate is continuous with the neck of the bladder. The urethra enters the upper aspect of the prostate near its anterior border
- **Inferiorly:** The apex of the prostate rests on the external sphincter of the bladder, which lies within the deep perineal pouch
- **Anteriorly:** Lies the pubic symphysis separated by the extraperitoneal fat of the *cave of Retzius* or *retropubic space*. Close against the prostate in this space lies the prostatic plexus of veins. Near the apex of the prostate, the *puboprostatic ligament* (a condensation of fibrous tissue) passes forwards to the pubis
- **Posteriorly:** Lies the rectum separated by *the fascia of Denonvilliers*
- **Laterally:** Lies levator ani

The ejaculatory ducts enter the upper posterior part of the gland to open into the urethra at the *colliculus seminalis* or verumontanum, one on either side of the prostatic utricle, dividing off a *median prostatic lobe* lying between these three ducts. In benign prostatic hypertrophy (but not in the normal prostate), a shallow posterior *median groove* (which can be felt on rectal examination) further divides the prostate into left and right *lobes*. Anterior to the urethra, the prostate consists of a narrow isthmus only.

Prostatic capsules (Fig. 2.48)

Anatomically, these are two in number, but pathologically, these are three in number, as mentioned below:

1. **True capsule:** It is a thin fibrous sheath which surrounds the gland.
2. **False capsule:** It is a condensed extraperitoneal fascia which continues into the fascia surrounding the bladder and with the fascia of Denonvilliers posteriorly. Between layers 1 and 2 lies the prostatic venous plexus.
3. **Pathological capsule:** When benign 'adenomatous' hypertrophy of the prostate takes place, the normal peripheral part of the gland becomes compressed into a capsule around this enlarging mass (Fig. 2.48). In performing an enucleation of the prostate, the plane between the adenomatous mass and this compressed peripheral tissue is entered, the 'tumour' enucleated and a condensed rim of prostate tissue, lying deep to the true capsule, left behind. The prostatic venous plexus, lying external to this, is thus undisturbed.

Lobes

Anatomically, these are five in number as mentioned below:

- **Median/Middle lobe:** It is a wedge-shaped part behind the urethra and above the ejaculatory ducts.
- **Posterior lobe:** It lies behind the lower part of the urethra and below the ejaculatory duct.
- **Right and left lateral lobes:** These are one on either side of the urethra.
- **Anterior lobe:** It lies in front of the urethra.

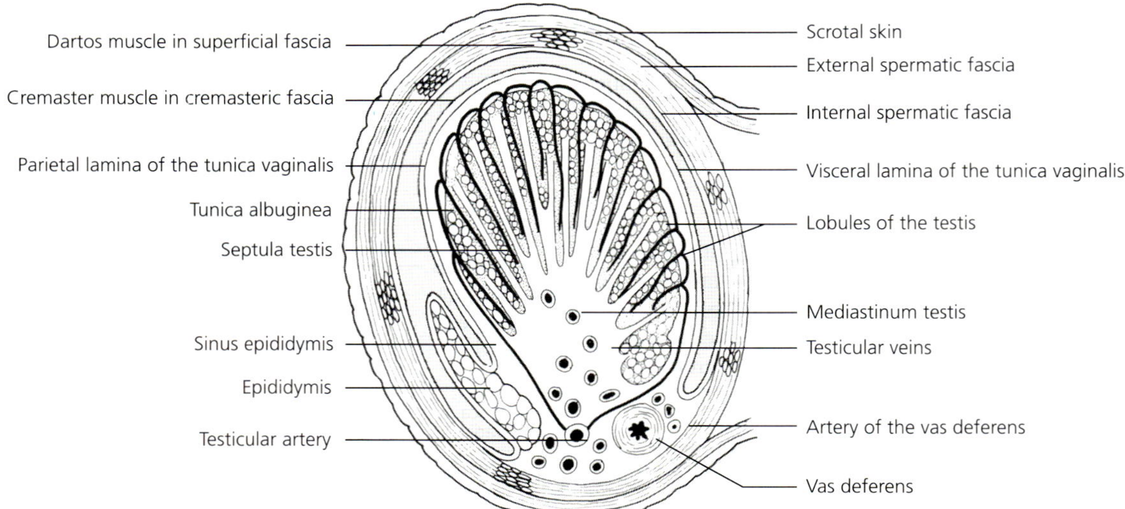

Figure 2.50 Transverse section of the testis.

Development of the testis

This is important and is the key to several features which are of clinical interest.

The testis arises from a germinal ridge of mesoderm in the posterior wall of the abdomen just medial to the mesonephros (Fig. 2.45), and links up with the epididymis and vas, which differentiate from the mesonephric duct. As the testis enlarges, it also undergoes a caudal migration according to Table 2.1.

A mesenchymal strand, the *gubernaculum testis*, extends from the caudal end of the developing testis along the course of its descent to blend into the scrotal fascia. The exact role of this structure in the descent of the testis is not known; theories are that it acts as a guide (*gubernaculum* = rudder) or that its swelling dilates the inguinal canal and scrotum.

In the third foetal month, a prolongation of the peritoneal cavity invades the gubernacular mesenchyme and projects into the scrotum as the *processus vaginalis*. The testis slides into the scrotum posterior to this, projects into it and is therefore clothed front and sides with peritoneum. About the time of birth this processus obliterates, leaving the testis covered by the tunica vaginalis. Very rarely, fragments of adjacent developing organs – spleen or suprarenal – are caught up and carried into the scrotum along with the testis.

Notice that, from the anatomical point of view, a hydrocele (apart from one of the cord) must surround the front and sides of the testis since the tunica vaginalis bears this relationship to it. A *cyst of the epididymis*, in contrast, arises from the efferent ducts of the epididymis and must therefore lie above and behind the testis. This point enables the differential diagnosis between these two common scrotal cysts to be made confidently.

Table 2.1 Descent of the testis

3rd Month (of foetal life)	Reaches the iliac fossa
7th Month	Traverses the inguinal canal
8th Month	Reaches the external ring
9th Month	Rescends into the scrotum

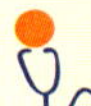

Clinical Features

1 The testis arises at the level of the mesonephros at the level of the L2/3 vertebrae and drags its vascular, lymphatic and nerve supply from this region. Pain from the kidney is often referred to the scrotum and, conversely, testicular pain may radiate to the loin.

2 When searching for secondary lymphatic spread from a neoplasm of the testis, the upper abdomen must be palpated carefully for enlarged para-aortic nodes; because of cross-communications, these may be present on either side. Mediastinal and cervical nodes may also become involved. It is the beginner's mistake to feel for nodes in the groin; these are only involved if the tumour has ulcerated the scrotal skin and hence invaded scrotal lymphatics which drain to the inguinal nodes.

3 Varicocele is a condition in which there is dilatation and elongation of the pampiniform plexus of veins. Rarely, a rapidly developing *varicocele* (dilatation of the pampiniform plexus of veins) is said to be a presenting sign of a tumour of the left kidney which, by invading the renal vein, blocks the drainage of the left testicular vein. Most examples of varicocele are idiopathic; why the vast majority are on the left side is unknown, but theories are that the left testicular vein is compressed by a loaded sigmoid colon, obstructed by angulation at its entry into the renal vein or even that it is put into spasm by adrenaline (epinephrine)-rich blood entering the renal vein from the suprarenal vein!

4 The testis may fail to descend and may rest anywhere along its course (imperfect descent/cryptorchidism) – intra-abdominally, within the inguinal canal, at the external ring or high in the scrotum. Failure to descend must be carefully distinguished from retraction of the testis; it is common in children for contraction of the cremaster muscle to draw the testis up into the superficial inguinal pouch – a potential space deep to the superficial fascia over the external ring. Gentle pressure from above, or the relaxing effect of a hot bath, coaxes the testis back into the scrotum in such cases.

Occasionally the testis descends, but into an unusual (*ectopic*) position; most commonly, the testis passes laterally

(*Continued ...*)

(... *continued*)

2 The external orifice is the narrowest part of the urethra and a calculus may lodge there. Immediately within the meatus, the urethra dilates into a terminal fossa whose roof bears a mucosal fold (the *lacuna magna*), which may catch the tip of a catheter. Instruments should always be introduced into the urethra beak downwards for this reason.

Female urethra

The female urethra is 1.5 in. (4 cm) long; it traverses the sphincter urethrae and lies immediately in front of, indeed embedded in the wall of, the vagina. Its external meatus opens 1 in. (2.5 cm) behind the clitoris. The sphincter urethrae in the female is a tenuous structure and vesical control appears to depend mainly on the intrinsic sphincter of condensed circular muscle fibres of the bladder.

Mucosa of the urinary tract

The renal pelvis and calyceal system, ureter, bladder and urethra are lined by a transitional epithelium as far as the entry of the ejaculatory ducts in the prostatic urethra. This is conveniently termed the *uroepithelium* or urothelium since it has a uniform appearance and is subject to the same pathological processes, e.g. the development of papillomata. The remainder of the urethra has a columnar lining except at its termination, where the epithelium becomes squamous.

Radiology of the urinary tract

The renal contours can often be identified on a soft-tissue radiograph of the abdomen. Intravenous injection of iodine-containing compounds excreted by the kidney will produce an outline of the calyces and the ureter (intravenous urogram). When the injection medium enters the bladder, a cystogram is obtained (Fig. 2.44).

Further information can be obtained by passing a catheter up the ureter through a cystoscope and injecting radio-opaque fluid to fill the pelvis and calyx system (retrograde pyelogram). Similarly, injection of such fluid into the urethra or bladder may be used for the radiographic study of these viscera.

The kidneys are beautifully delineated in transverse section on CT scans (Fig. 2.43(b), and *see* Figs 2.73 and 2.74).

Male genital organs

Prostate (Fig. 2.47)

The prostate is a pyramidal-shaped, fibromuscular and glandular organ, 1.25 in. (3 cm) long, which surrounds the prostatic urethra. It resembles the size and shape of a chestnut. The secretions of this gland along with those of seminal vesicles form the bulk of the seminal fluid.

Relations (Fig. 2.22)

- **Superiorly:** The prostate is continuous with the neck of the bladder. The urethra enters the upper aspect of the prostate near its anterior border
- **Inferiorly:** The apex of the prostate rests on the external sphincter of the bladder, which lies within the deep perineal pouch
- **Anteriorly:** Lies the pubic symphysis separated by the extraperitoneal fat of the *cave of Retzius* or *retropubic space*. Close against the prostate in this space lies the prostatic plexus of veins. Near the apex of the prostate, the *puboprostatic ligament* (a condensation of fibrous tissue) passes forwards to the pubis
- **Posteriorly:** Lies the rectum separated by *the fascia of Denonvilliers*
- **Laterally:** Lies levator ani

The ejaculatory ducts enter the upper posterior part of the gland to open into the urethra at the *colliculus seminalis* or verumontanum, one on either side of the prostatic utricle, dividing off a *median prostatic lobe* lying between these three ducts. In benign prostatic hypertrophy (but not in the normal prostate), a shallow posterior *median groove* (which can be felt on rectal examination) further divides the prostate into left and right *lobes*. Anterior to the urethra, the prostate consists of a narrow isthmus only.

Prostatic capsules (Fig. 2.48)

Anatomically, these are two in number, but pathologically, these are three in number, as mentioned below:

1. **True capsule:** It is a thin fibrous sheath which surrounds the gland.
2. **False capsule:** It is a condensed extraperitoneal fascia which continues into the fascia surrounding the bladder and with the fascia of Denonvilliers posteriorly. Between layers 1 and 2 lies the prostatic venous plexus.
3. **Pathological capsule:** When benign 'adenomatous' hypertrophy of the prostate takes place, the normal peripheral part of the gland becomes compressed into a capsule around this enlarging mass (Fig. 2.48). In performing an enucleation of the prostate, the plane between the adenomatous mass and this compressed peripheral tissue is entered, the 'tumour' enucleated and a condensed rim of prostate tissue, lying deep to the true capsule, left behind. The prostatic venous plexus, lying external to this, is thus undisturbed.

Lobes

Anatomically, these are five in number as mentioned below:

- **Median/Middle lobe:** It is a wedge-shaped part behind the urethra and above the ejaculatory ducts.
- **Posterior lobe:** It lies behind the lower part of the urethra and below the ejaculatory duct.
- **Right and left lateral lobes:** These are one on either side of the urethra.
- **Anterior lobe:** It lies in front of the urethra.

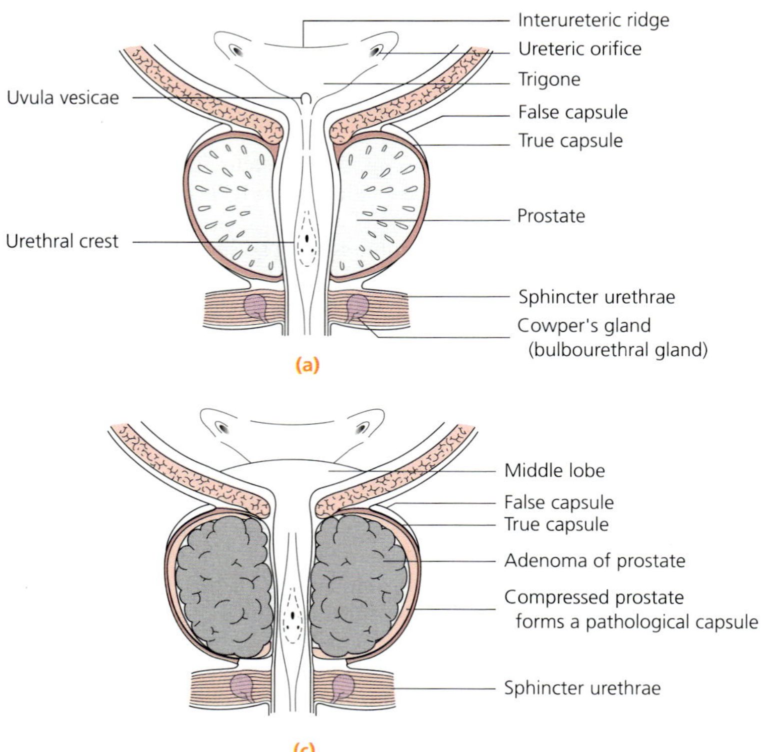

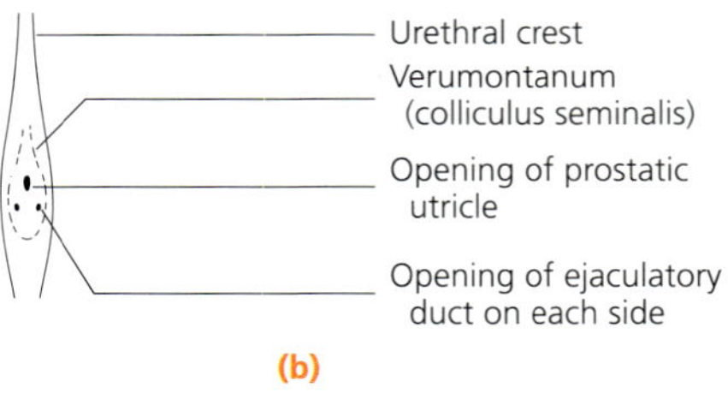

Figure 2.48 The surgical anatomy of prostatectomy. **(a)** The normal prostate in vertical section. **(b)** Detail of the prostatic urethra. **(c)** A prostatic adenoma (benign hypertrophy) compresses the normal prostatic tissue into a false capsule.

Blood supply

The arterial supply is derived from the inferior vesical artery (a branch of the internal iliac artery), a branch entering the prostate on each side at its lateral extremity.

The veins form a prostatic plexus, which receives the dorsal vein of the penis and drains into the internal iliac vein on each side. Some of the venous drainage passes to the plexus of veins lying in front of the vertebral bodies and within the neural canal. These veins are valveless and constitute the *valveless vertebral veins of Batson*. This communication may explain the readiness with which carcinoma of the prostate spreads to the pelvic bones and vertebrae.

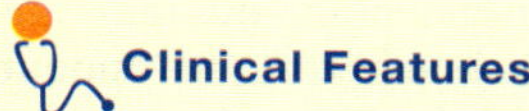

Clinical Features

1 Prostatectomy for benign prostatic hyperplasia (BPH) involves removal of the hyperplastic mass of glandular tissue from the surrounding normal prostate, which is compressed as a thin rim around it – a false pathological capsule (Fig. 2.48). This is usually performed transurethrally by means of an operating cystoscope armed with a cutting diathermy loop. During this procedure, the verumontanum (colliculus seminalis) is an important landmark. The surgeon keeps the resection above this structure in order not to damage the urethral sphincter. If the prostate is very enlarged, open prostatectomy is indicated. The gland is approached retropubically, the capsule incised transversely and the hyperplastic mass of gland enucleated. The median lobe of prostate is commonly involved in benign

(Continued ...)

(... continued)

hypertrophy of prostate, while primary carcinoma of prostate commonly begins in the posterior lobe.

2 After the age of 45 years some degree of prostatic hyperplasia is all but invariable; it is as much a sign of ageing as greying of the hair. Usually the lateral lobes are affected, and such enlargement is readily detected on rectal examination. The median lobe may also be involved in this process or may be enlarged without the lateral lobes being affected. In such an instance, symptoms of prostatic obstruction may occur (because of the valve-like effect of this hypertrophied lobe lying over the internal urethral orifice) without prostatic enlargement being detectable on rectal examination.

   Anterior to the urethra the prostate consists of a narrow fibromuscular isthmus containing little, if any, glandular tissue. Benign glandular hypertrophy of the prostate, therefore, never affects this part of the organ.

3 The *metastasis of carcinoma prostate* occurs in the vertebral column and skull through vertebral venous plexus.

4 The fascia of Denonvilliers is important surgically; in excising the rectum, it is the plane to be sought after in order to separate off the prostate and urethra without damaging these structures. A carcinoma of the prostate only rarely penetrates this fascial barrier so that ulceration into the rectum is very unusual.

Scrotum

The scrotum is the musculocutaneous bag/pouch which contains the testes epididymes and their coverings, and the lower ends of spermatic cords. In cryptorchidism, not unnaturally, this pouch is not well developed.

The skin of the scrotum is thin, pigmented, rugose and marked by a longitudinal median raphe. It is richly endowed with sebaceous glands, and consequently a common site for sebaceous cysts, which are often multiple. The subcutaneous tissue contains no fat but does contain the involuntary *dartos muscle*.

Layers of scrotum

The scrotum is considered as the outpouching of the lower part of the anterior abdominal wall; hence, all the layers of the anterior abdominal wall continue in it except the transverse abdominis. The layers of the scrotum from superficial to deep are skin, dartos muscle, external spermatic fascia, cremasteric fascia and internal spermatic fascia.

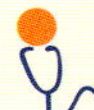

Clinical Features

The scrotal subcutaneous tissue is continuous with the fasciae of the abdominal wall and perineum and therefore extravasations of urine or blood deep to this plane will gravitate into the scrotum. The scrotum is divided by a septum into right and left compartments but this septum is incomplete superiorly so extravasations of fluid into this sac are always bilateral.

The lax tissues of the scrotum and its dependent position cause it to fill readily with oedema fluid in cardiac or renal failure. Such a condition must be carefully differentiated from extravasation or from a scrotal swelling due to a hernia or hydrocele.

Testis and epididymis (Figs 2.49 and 2.50)

The testis is the male gonad. It is a firm, mobile, oval organ and lies in the scrotum. The left testis lies at a lower level than the right within the scrotum; rarely, this arrangement is reversed. Each testis is contained by a white fibrous capsule, the *tunica albuginea*, and each is invaginated anteriorly into a double serous covering, the *tunica vaginalis*, just as the intestine is invaginated anteriorly into the peritoneum.

Along the posterior border of the testis, rather to its lateral side, lies the *epididymis*, which is divided into an expanded head, a body and a pointed tail inferiorly. Medially, there is a distinct groove, the *sinus epididymis*, between it and the testis. The epididymis is covered by the tunica vaginalis except at its posterior margin, which is free or, so to say, 'extraperitoneal'.

The testis and epididymis each bear at their upper extremities a small stalked body, termed, respectively, the *appendix testis* and *appendix epididymis* (*hydatid of Morgagni*). The appendix testis is a remnant of the upper end of the paramesonephric (Müllerian) duct; the appendix epididymis is a remnant of the mesonephros. These structures, being stalked, are liable to undergo torsion.

Blood supply

The testicular artery arises from the aorta at the level of the renal vessels. It anastomoses with the artery to the vas, supplying the vas deferens and epididymis, which arises from the inferior vesical branch of the internal iliac artery. This cross-connection means that ligation of the testicular artery is not necessarily followed by testicular atrophy.

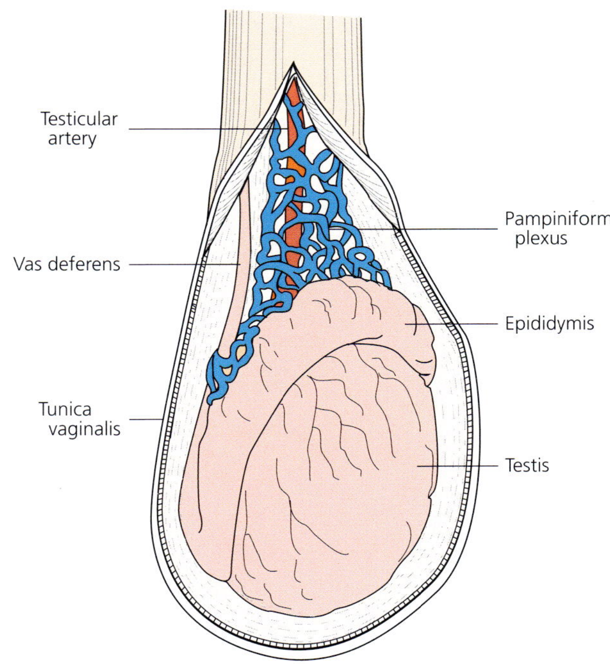

Figure 2.49 Testis and epididymis.

The pampiniform plexus of veins becomes a single vessel, the testicular vein, in the region of the internal ring. On the right, this drains into the inferior vena cava; on the left, into the renal vein.

Lymph drainage

The lymphatic drainage of the testis obeys the usual rule: it accompanies the venous drainage and thus passes to the para-aortic lymph nodes at the level of the renal vessels. Free communication occurs between the lymphatics on either side; there is also a plentiful anastomosis with the para-aortic intrathoracic nodes and, in turn, with the cervical nodes, so that spread of malignant disease from the testis to the nodes at the root of the neck is not rare.

Nerve supply

T10 and T11 sympathetic fibres via the renal and aortic plexus. These convey afferent (pain) fibres – hence referred pain from the testis to the umbilicus, loin and groin.

Structure

The testis is divided into 200–300 lobules, each containing one to three *seminiferous tubules*. Each tubule is some 2 ft. (62 cm) in length when teased out, and is thus obviously coiled and convoluted to pack away within the testis. The tubules anastomose posteriorly into a plexus termed the *rete testis* from which approximately a dozen fine *efferent ducts* arise, pierce the tunica albuginea at the upper part of the testis and pass into the head of the epididymis, which is actually formed by these efferent ducts coiled within it. The efferent ducts fuse to form a considerably convoluted single tube that constitutes the body and tail of the epididymis; unravelled, it is the length of a cricket pitch.

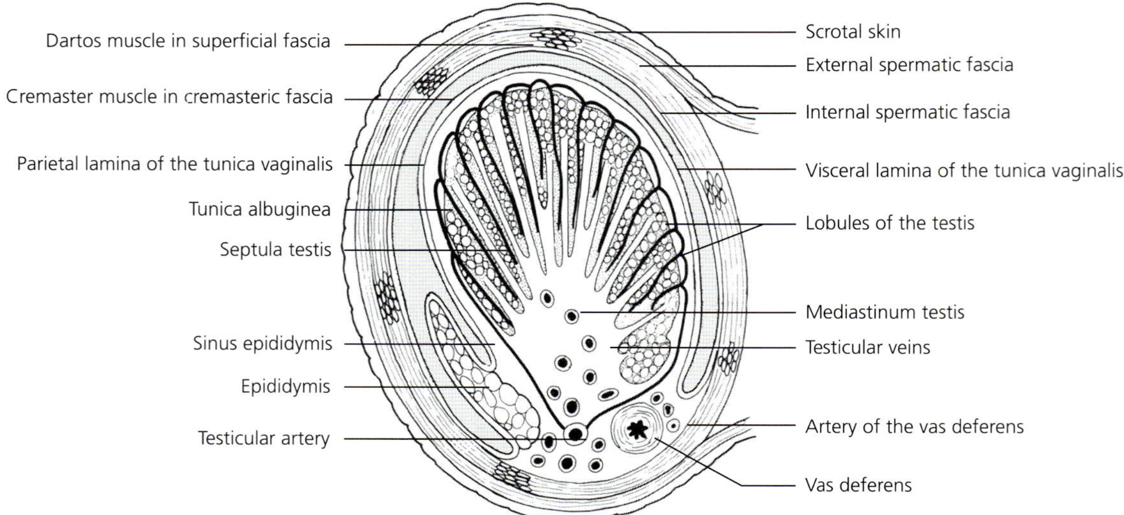

Figure 2.50 Transverse section of the testis.

Development of the testis

This is important and is the key to several features which are of clinical interest.

The testis arises from a germinal ridge of mesoderm in the posterior wall of the abdomen just medial to the mesonephros (Fig. 2.45), and links up with the epididymis and vas, which differentiate from the mesonephric duct. As the testis enlarges, it also undergoes a caudal migration according to Table 2.1.

A mesenchymal strand, the *gubernaculum testis*, extends from the caudal end of the developing testis along the course of its descent to blend into the scrotal fascia. The exact role of this structure in the descent of the testis is not known; theories are that it acts as a guide (*gubernaculum* = rudder) or that its swelling dilates the inguinal canal and scrotum.

In the third foetal month, a prolongation of the peritoneal cavity invades the gubernacular mesenchyme and projects into the scrotum as the *processus vaginalis*. The testis slides into the scrotum posterior to this, projects into it and is therefore clothed front and sides with peritoneum. About the time of birth this processus obliterates, leaving the testis covered by the tunica vaginalis. Very rarely, fragments of adjacent developing organs – spleen or suprarenal – are caught up and carried into the scrotum along with the testis.

Notice that, from the anatomical point of view, a hydrocele (apart from one of the cord) must surround the front and sides of the testis since the tunica vaginalis bears this relationship to it. A *cyst of the epididymis*, in contrast, arises from the efferent ducts of the epididymis and must therefore lie above and behind the testis. This point enables the differential diagnosis between these two common scrotal cysts to be made confidently.

Table 2.1 Descent of the testis

3rd Month (of foetal life)	Reaches the iliac fossa
7th Month	Traverses the inguinal canal
8th Month	Reaches the external ring
9th Month	Rescends into the scrotum

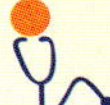

Clinical Features

1 The testis arises at the level of the mesonephros at the level of the L2/3 vertebrae and drags its vascular, lymphatic and nerve supply from this region. Pain from the kidney is often referred to the scrotum and, conversely, testicular pain may radiate to the loin.

2 When searching for secondary lymphatic spread from a neoplasm of the testis, the upper abdomen must be palpated carefully for enlarged para-aortic nodes; because of cross-communications, these may be present on either side. Mediastinal and cervical nodes may also become involved. It is the beginner's mistake to feel for nodes in the groin; these are only involved if the tumour has ulcerated the scrotal skin and hence invaded scrotal lymphatics which drain to the inguinal nodes.

3 Varicocele is a condition in which there is dilatation and elongation of the pampiniform plexus of veins. Rarely, a rapidly developing *varicocele* (dilatation of the pampiniform plexus of veins) is said to be a presenting sign of a tumour of the left kidney which, by invading the renal vein, blocks the drainage of the left testicular vein. Most examples of varicocele are idiopathic; why the vast majority are on the left side is unknown, but theories are that the left testicular vein is compressed by a loaded sigmoid colon, obstructed by angulation at its entry into the renal vein or even that it is put into spasm by adrenaline (epinephrine)-rich blood entering the renal vein from the suprarenal vein!

4 The testis may fail to descend and may rest anywhere along its course (imperfect descent/cryptorchidism) – intra-abdominally, within the inguinal canal, at the external ring or high in the scrotum. Failure to descend must be carefully distinguished from retraction of the testis; it is common in children for contraction of the cremaster muscle to draw the testis up into the superficial inguinal pouch – a potential space deep to the superficial fascia over the external ring. Gentle pressure from above, or the relaxing effect of a hot bath, coaxes the testis back into the scrotum in such cases.

Occasionally the testis descends, but into an unusual (*ectopic*) position; most commonly, the testis passes laterally

(Continued ...)

(... continued)

after leaving the external ring to lie superficial to the inguinal ligament, but it may be found in front of the pubis, in the perineum or in the upper thigh. In these cases (unlike the undescended testis), the cord is long and replacement into the scrotum without tension presents no surgical difficulty.

5 Abnormalities of the obliteration of the processus vaginalis lead to a number of extremely common surgical conditions, of which the *indirect inguinal hernia* is the most important.

This variety of hernia may be present at birth or develop in later life; in the latter circumstance, it is probable that the processus vaginalis has persisted as a narrow empty sac and that development of the hernia results from some sudden strain due to a cough, straining at micturition or at stool, which forces abdominal contents into this peritoneal recess.

In infants, the sac frequently has the testis lying in its wall (congenital inguinal hernia), but this is unusual in older patients.

6 Hydrocele is a condition in which closed-off tunica vaginalis become distended with fluid. It may be idiopathic (primary) or secondary to disease in the underlying testis. The anatomical classification of hydroceles is into the following groups (Fig. 2.51):

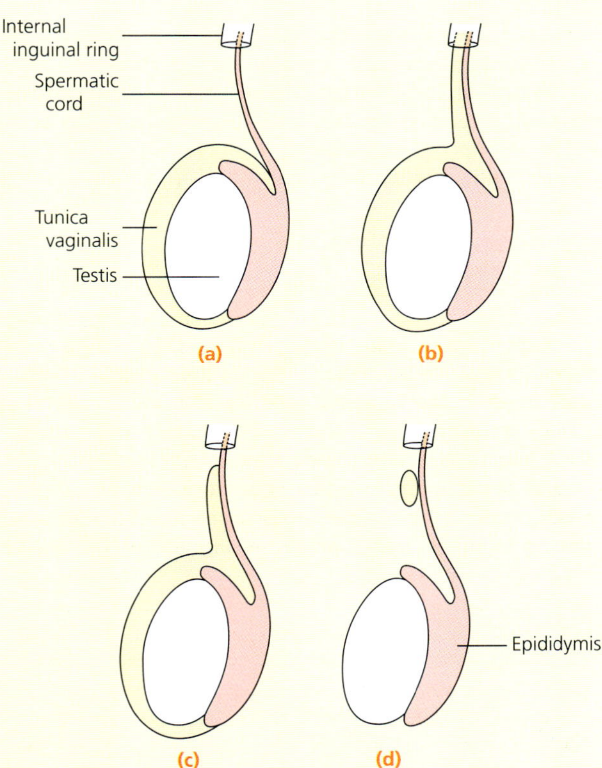

Figure 2.51 Types of hydrocele. (a) Vaginal hydrocele, (b) congenital hydrocele, (c) infantile hydrocele, (d) hydrocele of the cord. (The tube at the upper end of each diagram represents the internal inguinal ring. Yellow, hydrocele; brown, vas and epididymis.)

- **Vaginal:** Confined to the scrotum and so called because it distends the tunica vaginalis
- **Congenital:** Communicating with the peritoneal cavity
- **Infantile:** Extending upwards to the internal ring
- **Hydrocele of the cord:** Confined to the cord

Vas deferens (ductus deferens) (Fig. 2.47)

The vas deferens is a thick-walled muscular tube which transports spermatozoa from epididymis to the ejaculatory duct.

This tube is 18 in. (45 cm) long (a distance which one may remember is also the length of the thoracic duct, the spinal cord and the femur, and the distance from the incisor teeth to the cardiac end of the stomach).

The vas passes from the tail of the epididymis to traverse the scrotum and inguinal canal and so comes to lie upon the side wall of the pelvis. Here, it lies immediately below the peritoneum of the lateral wall, extends almost to the ischial tuberosity then turns medially to the base of the bladder. Here, it joins the more laterally placed seminal vesicle to form the *ejaculatory duct*, which traverses the prostate to open into the prostatic urethra at the verumontanum on either side of the utricle.

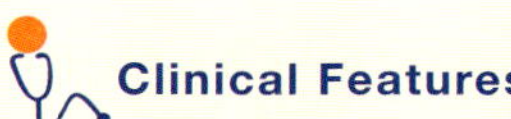

1 Infection may track from the bladder and urethra along the vas to the epididymis (*acute epididymitis*).
2 The operation of bilateral *vasectomy* is a common procedure for male sterilization. The vas is identified by its very firm consistency, which, in coaching days, was likened to whipcord but which today might, more aptly, be compared to fine plastic tubing.

Seminal vesicles

These are coiled sacculated tubes 2 in. (5 cm) long which can be unravelled to three times that length. They lie, one on each side, extraperitoneally at the bladder base, lateral to the termination of the vasa. Each has common drainage with its neighbouring vas via the ejaculatory duct (Fig. 2.47). In spite of their name, they do not act as receptacles for semen, although their secretion does contribute considerably to the seminal fluid.

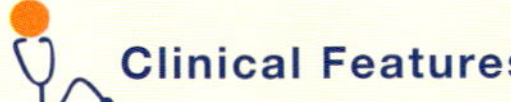

The vesicles can be felt on rectal examination if enlarged; this occurs typically in tuberculous infection.

Bony and ligamentous pelvis

The pelvis is made up of the innominate bones, the sacrum and the coccyx, bound to each other by dense ligaments.

Os innominatum (Fig. 2.52)

Examine the bone and revise the following structures.

The *ilium* with its *iliac crest* running between the *anterior* and *posterior superior iliac spines*; below each of these are the corresponding *inferior spines*. Well-defined ridges on its lateral surface are the strong muscle markings of the glutei. Its inner aspect bears the large *auricular surface*, which articulates with the sacrum. The *iliopectineal line* runs forwards from the apex of the auricular surface and demarcates the *true* from the *false pelvis*.

The pubis comprises the body and the superior and inferior pubic rami.

The *ischium* has a vertically disposed *body*, bearing the *ischial spine* on its posterior border that demarcates an upper (greater) and lower (lesser) sciatic notch. The inferior pole of the body bears the *ischial tuberosity*, then projects forwards almost at right angles into the *ischial ramus* to meet the inferior pubic ramus.

The *obturator foramen* lies bounded by the body and rami of the pubis and the body and ramus of the ischium.

All three bones fuse at the *acetabulum*, which forms the socket for the femoral head, for which it bears a wide crescentic articular surface.

The pelvis is tilted in the erect position so that the plane of its inlet is at an angle 60° to the horizontal. (To place a pelvis into this position, hold it against a wall so that the anterior superior spine and the top of the pubic symphysis both touch it.)

Sacrum (Fig. 2.53)

The sacrum is made up of five fused vertebrae and is roughly triangular. The anterior border of its upper part is termed the *sacral promontory* and is readily felt at laparotomy.

Its anterior aspect presents a *central mass*, a row of four *anterior sacral foramina* on each side (transmitting the upper four sacral anterior primary rami), and, lateral to these, the *lateral masses* of the sacrum. The superior aspect of the lateral mass on each side forms a fan-shaped surface termed the *ala*.

Note that the central mass is roughly rectangular – the triangular shape of the sacrum is due to the rapid shrinkage in size of the lateral masses of the sacrum from above down.

Posteriorly lies the *sacral canal*, continuing the vertebral canal, bounded by short pedicles, strong laminae and diminutive spinous processes. Perforating through from the sacral canal is a row of four *posterior sacral foramina* on each side. Inferiorly, the canal terminates in the *sacral hiatus*, which transmits the 5th sacral nerve. On either side of the lower extremity of the hiatus lie the *sacral cornua*. These can easily be palpated by the finger immediately above the natal cleft.

On its lateral aspect, the sacrum presents an *auricular facet* for articulation with the corresponding surface of the ilium.

The 5th lumbar vertebra may occasionally fuse with the sacrum in whole or in part (sacralization of L5); alternatively, the 1st sacral segment may be partially or completely separated from the rest of the sacrum (lumbarization of S1). The posterior arch of the sacrum is occasionally bifid.

Note that the dural sheath terminates distally at the second piece of the sacrum. Beyond this the sacral canal is filled with the fatty tissue of the extradural space, the cauda equina and the filum terminale. (For sacral block, *see* page 78.)

Coccyx

The coccyx is made up of three to five fused vertebrae articulating with the sacrum; occasionally, the first segment remains separate. It represents, of course, the tail of more primitive animals.

Inlet and outlet of pelvis

The *pelvic inlet* is bounded posteriorly by the sacral promontory, anteriorly by the pubic symphysis (upper margin) and on each side by the linea terminalis. The *pelvic outlet* is bounded anteriorly by the inferior margin of pubic symphysis, posteriorly by the coccyx and on each side by pubic arch, ischial tuberosity and sacrotuberous ligament.

Functions of the pelvis

1. It protects the pelvic viscera.
2. It supports the weight of the body, which is transmitted through the vertebrae, thence through the sacrum, across the sacro-iliac joints to the innominate bones and then to the femora in the standing position or to the ischial tuberosities when sitting. (The sacro-iliac joint is reinforced for this task as will be described below.)
3. During walking the pelvis swings from side to side by a rotatory movement at the lumbosacral articulation, which occurs together with similar movements of the lumbar

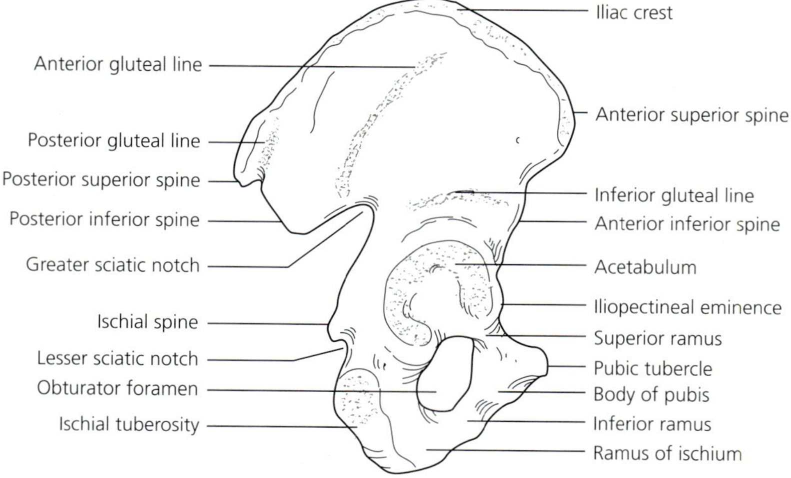

Figure 2.52 Lateral view of the os innominatum.

intervertebral joints. Even if the hip joints are fixed, this swing of the pelvis enables the patient to walk reasonably well.

4. As with all but a few small bones in the hand and foot, the pelvis provides attachments for muscles.
5. In the female it provides bony support for the birth canal.

Joints and ligamentous connections of the pelvis

The *symphysis pubis* is the name given to the secondary cartilaginous joint between the pubic bones. Each pubic bone is covered by a layer of hyaline cartilage and is connected across the midline by a dense layer of fibrocartilage. The centre of the latter may break down to form a cleft-like joint space which, however, is not seen before the first decade and which is not lined by a synovial membrane.

The joint is surrounded and strengthened by fibrous ligaments, especially above and below.

The *sacro-iliac joints* are the articulations between the auricular surfaces of the sacrum and ilium on each side and are true synovium-lined and cartilage-covered joints.

The sacrum 'hangs' from these joints supported by the extremely dense *posterior sacro-iliac ligaments* lying posteriorly to the auricular joint surfaces. These support the whole weight of the body, tending to drag the sacrum forwards into the pelvis and, not surprisingly, are the strongest ligaments in the body.

Their action is assisted by an interlocking of the grooves between the auricular surfaces of the sacrum and ilium.

The *sacrotuberous ligament* passes from the ischial tuberosity to the side of the sacrum and coccyx.

The *sacrospinous ligament* passes from the ischial spine to the side of the sacrum and coccyx.

The following two ligaments help to define two important exits from the pelvis:

1. **The greater sciatic foramen:** Formed by the sacrospinous ligament and the greater sciatic notch
2. **the lesser sciatic foramen:** Formed by the sacrotuberous ligament and the lesser sciatic notch

Note: There is a useful surface landmark in this region – the dimple constantly seen on each side immediately above the buttock – which defines the following:

1. The posterior superior iliac spine
2. The centre of the sacro-iliac joint
3. The level of the second sacral segment
4. The level at which the dural sheath of the spinal meninges terminates

Differences between the male and female pelvis (Fig. 2.54)

The pelvis demonstrates a large number of sex differences associated principally with two features: first, the heavier build and stronger muscles in the male, accounting for the stronger bone structure and better defined muscle markings in this sex;

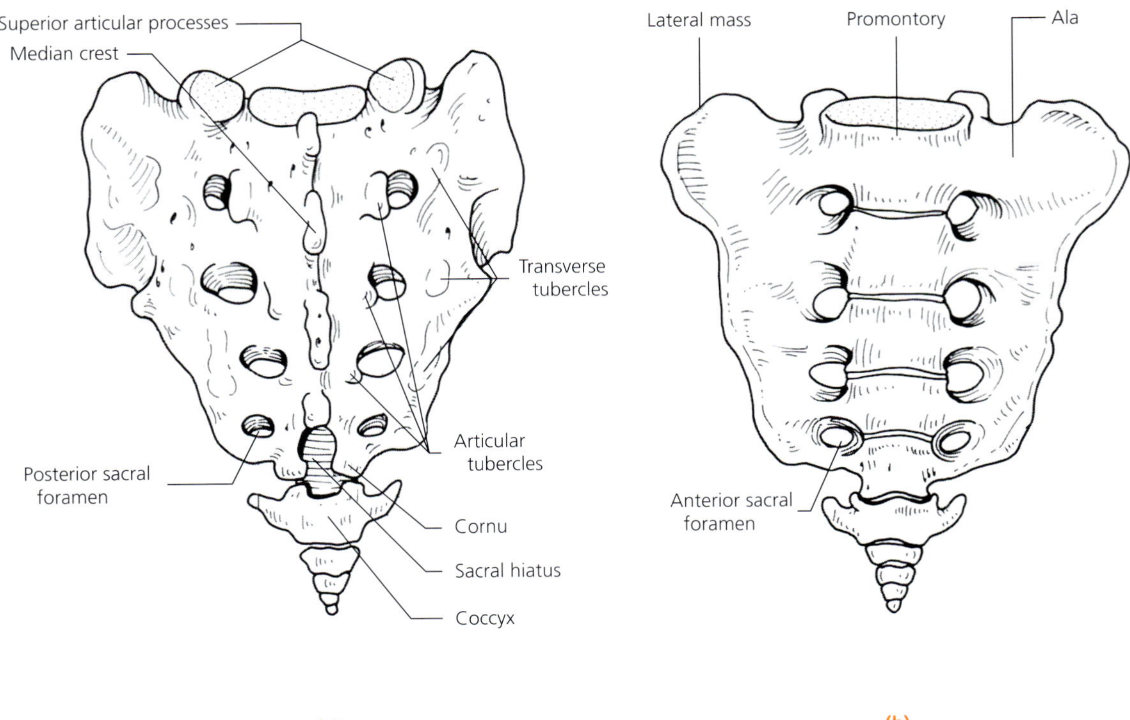

Figure 2.53 The sacrum in: **(a)** posterior and **(b)** anterior views.

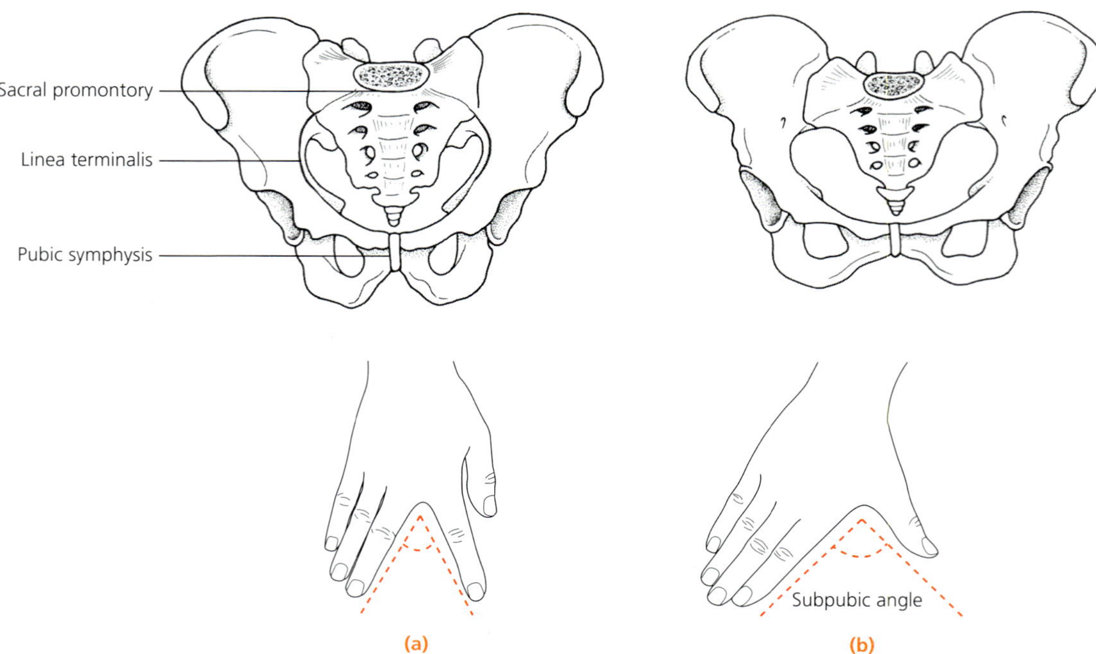

Figure 2.54 (a) Male and (b) female pelvis compared.

second, the comparatively wider and shallower pelvic cavity in the female, correlated with its role as the bony part of the birth canal.

The sex differences are summarized in Table 2.2.

When looking at a radiograph of the pelvis, the sex is best determined by the following three features:

1. The pelvic inlet, which is heart-shaped in the male, oval in the female
2. The angle between the inferior pubic rami, which is narrow in the male, wide in the female. In the former, it corresponds almost exactly to the angle between the index and middle fingers when these are held apart; in the latter, the

Table 2.2 Comparison of male and female pelvis

	Male	Female
General structure	Heavy and thick	Light and thin
Joint surfaces	Large	Small
Muscle attachments	Well marked	Rather indistinct
False pelvis	Deep	Shallow
Pelvic inlet	Heart shaped	Oval
Pelvic canal	'Long segment of a short cone', i.e. long and tapered	'Short segment of a long cone', i.e. short with almost parallel sides
Pelvic outlet	Comparatively small	Comparatively large
1st Piece of sacrum	The superior surface of the body occupies nearly half the width of the sacrum	Oval superior surface of the body occupies approximately one-third of the width of the sacrum
Sacrum	Long, narrow, with smooth concavity	Short, wide, flat, curving forwards in the lower part
Sacro-iliac articular facet (auricular surface)	Extends well down the 3rd piece of the sacrum	Extends down only to the upper border of the 3rd piece
Subpubic angle (between inferior pubic rami)	'The angle between the middle and index fingers'	'The angle between the thumb and the index finger'
Inferior pubic ramus	Presents a strong everted surface for attachment of the crus of the penis	This marking is not present
Acetabulum	Large	Small
Ischial tuberosities	Inturned	Everted
Obturator foramen	Round	Oval

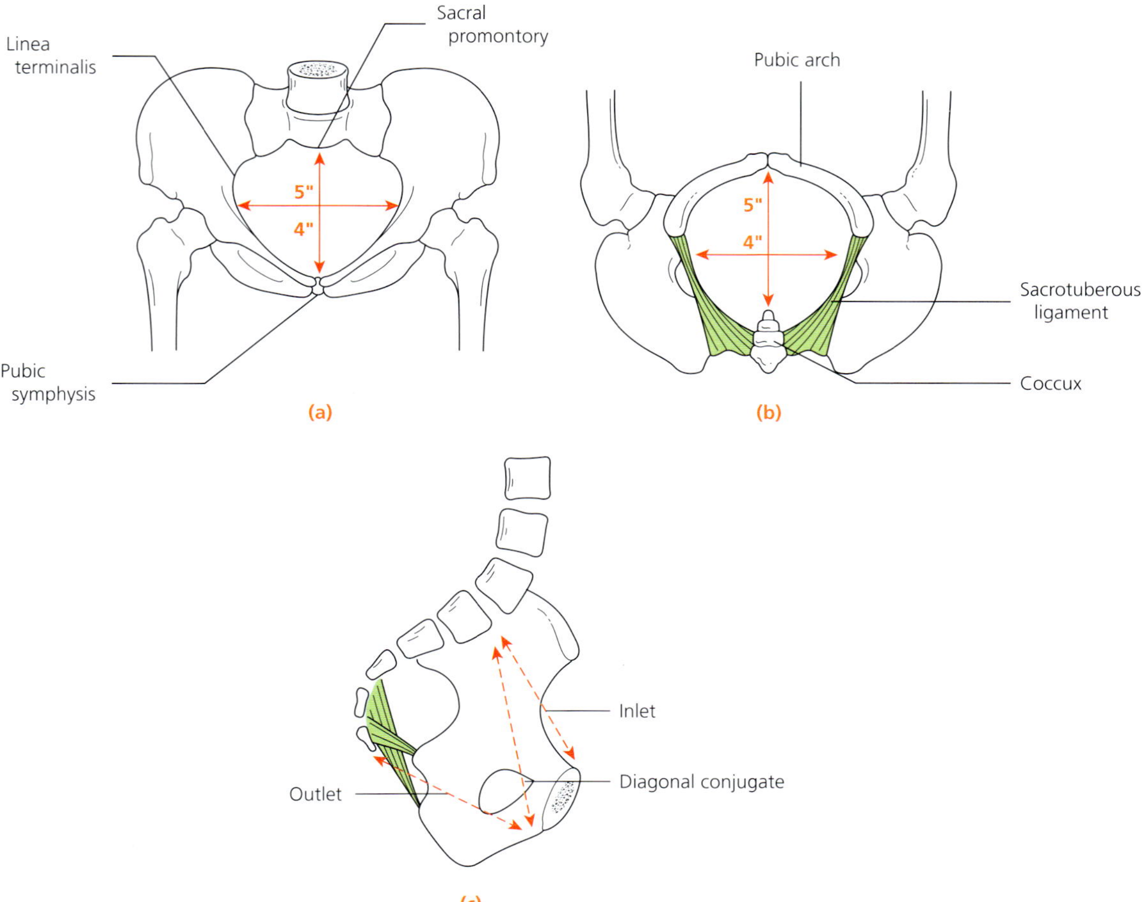

Figure 2.55 The measurements of the female pelvis. **(a)** The inlet and **(b)** the outlet. **(c)** Lateral view to show the diagonal conjugate.

angle equals that between the fully extended thumb and the index finger. This is a particularly reliable feature

3. The soft-tissue shadow of the penis and scrotum can usually be seen or, if not, the dense shadow of the lead screen used to shield the testes from harmful radiation

Obstetrical pelvic measurements (Fig. 2.55)

The figures for the measurements of the inlet, mid-cavity and outlet of the true pelvis are readily committed to memory in the form shown in Table 2.3.

The *transverse diameter of the outlet* is assessed clinically by measuring the distance between the ischial tuberosities along a plane passing across the anus; the *anteroposterior outlet diameter* is measured from the pubis to the sacrococcygeal joint. The most useful measurement clinically is, however, the *diagonal conjugate* – from the lower border of the pubic symphysis to the promontory of the sacrum. This normally measures 5 in. (12.5 cm); from the practical point of view, it is not possible in the normal pelvis to reach the sacral promontory on vaginal examination either readily or without discomfort to the patient.

Another useful clinical guide is the *subpubic arch*: the examiner's four knuckles (i.e. his clenched fist) should rest comfortably between the ischial tuberosities below the pubic symphysis.

Note that these measurements are all of the bony pelvis; the 'dynamic pelvis' of the birth canal, in fact, is narrowed by the pelvic musculature, the rectum and the thickness of the uterine wall. Today accurate imaging techniques enable exact measurements to be made of the bony pelvis.

Table 2.3 Obstetrical pelvic measurements

	Transverse	Oblique	Anteroposterior
Inlet	5 in. (12.5 cm)	4.5 in. (11.5 cm)	4 in. (10 cm)
Mid-pelvis	4.5 in. (11.5 cm)	4.5 in. (11.5 cm)	4.5 in. (11.5 cm)
Outlet	4 in. (10 cm)	4.5 in. (11.5 cm)	5 in. (12.5 cm)

Variations of the pelvic shape (Fig. 2.56)

The shapes of the female pelvis may be subdivided (after Caldwell and Moloy) as follows.

1. Normal and its variants
   - **Gynaecoid:** Normal (most common variety in Caucasian women)
   - **Android:** The masculine type of pelvis
   - **Platypelloid:** Shortened in the anteroposterior diameter, increased in the transverse diameter (the 'non-rachitic flat pelvis')

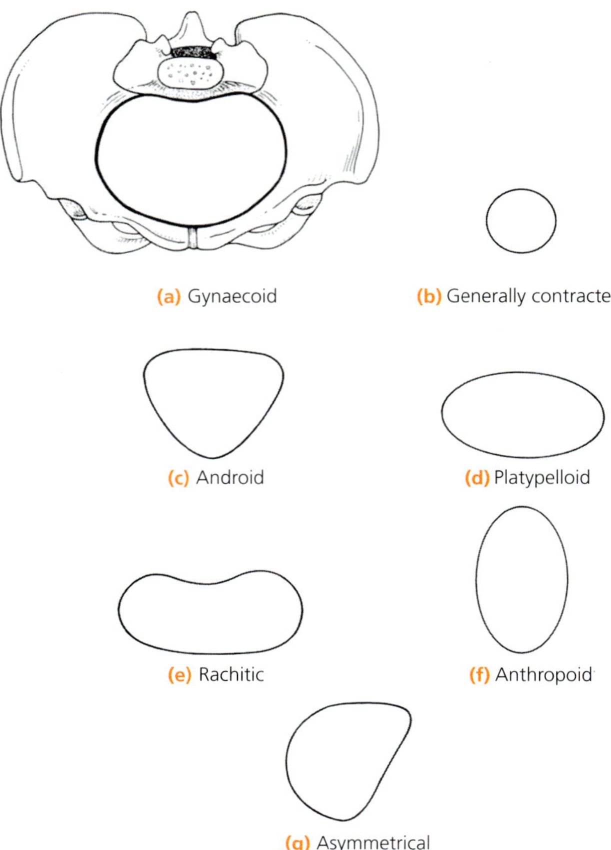

Figure 2.56 Pelvic variations and abnormalities – shown as diagrammatic outlines of the pelvic inlet.

- **Anthropoid:** Resembling that of an anthropoid ape with a much lengthened anteroposterior diameter and a shortened transverse diameter

2. Symmetrically contracted pelvis
   - That of a small woman but with a symmetrical shape
3. Rachitic flat pelvis
   - The sacrum is rotated so that the sacral promontory projects forwards and the coccyx tips backwards. The anteroposterior diameter of the inlet is therefore narrowed, but that of the outlet is increased. This deformity is typical of rickets, the result of vitamin D deficiency
4. Asymmetrical pelvis
   - Asymmetry can be due to a variety of causes such as scoliosis, longstanding hip disease (e.g. congenital dislocation), poliomyelitis, pelvic fracture, congenital abnormality due to thalidomide and the *Naegele pelvis*, which is due to the congenital absence of one wing of the sacrum or its destruction by disease

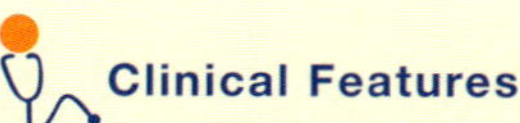

Clinical Features

Fractures of the pelvis

These may be isolated lesions due to a localized blow or may be displacements of part of the pelvic ring due to compression injuries. Lateral compression usually results in fractures through both

(Continued ...)

(... continued)

pubic rami on each side, or both rami on one side with dislocation at the symphysis; anteroposterior compression may be followed by dislocation at the symphysis or fractures through the pubic rami accompanied by dislocation at the sacro-iliac joint.

Displacement of part of the pelvic ring must, of course, mean that the ring has been broken in two places.

Falls upon the leg may force the head of the femur through the acetabulum, the so-called central dislocation of the hip. Isolated fractures may be produced by local trauma, especially to the iliac wing, sacrum and pubis.

Associated with pelvic fractures one must always consider soft-tissue injuries to the bladder, urethra and rectum, which may be penetrated by spicules of bone or torn by wide displacements of the pelvic fragments.

Occasionally in these pelvic displacements the iliolumbar branch of the internal iliac artery is ruptured as it crosses above the sacro-iliac joint; this may be followed by a severe or even fatal extraperitoneal haemorrhage.

Sacral (caudal) anaesthesia

The sacral hiatus, between the last piece of sacrum and coccyx, can be entered by a needle which pierces the skin, fascia and the tough posterior sacrococcygeal ligament to enter the sacral canal. The hiatus can be defined by palpating the sacral cornua on either side (Fig. 2.53) immediately above the natal cleft.

Anaesthetic solutions injected here will spread readily in the semi-liquid extradural fat to bathe the spinal roots emerging from the dural sheath, which terminates at the level of the 2nd sacral segment. The perineal anaesthesia can be used for low forceps delivery, episiotomy and repair of a perineal tear.

Muscles of the pelvic floor and perineum

The canal of the bony and ligamentous pelvis is closed by a diaphragm of muscles and fasciae, which the rectum, urethra in male and, rectum urethra and vagina in the female must pierce to reach the exterior. The muscles are divided into (1) the *pelvic diaphragm*, formed by the levator ani and the coccygeus; and (2) the *muscles* of (a) the anterior (urogenital) perineum and (b) the posterior (anal) perineum.

Levator ani (Fig. 2.57) is the largest and most important muscle of the pelvic floor. It arises from the posterior aspect of the body of the pubic bone, the fascia of the side wall of the pelvis (covering obturator internus) and the spine of the ischium. From this wide origin it sweeps down in a series of loops as mentioned below:

1. To form a sling around the prostate (*levator prostatae*) or vagina (*sphincter vaginae*), inserting into the perineal body
2. To form a sling around the rectum and also insert into, and reinforce the deep part of, the anal sphincter at the anorectal ring (*puborectalis*)
3. The posterior fibres are attached to the sides of the coccyx and to a median fibrous raphe, which stretches between the apex of the coccyx and the anorectal junction

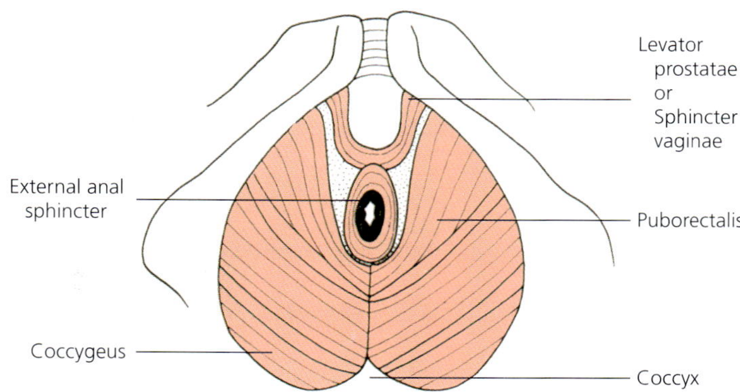

Figure 2.57 Levator ani – inferior aspect. It forms the 'diaphragm of the pelvis'.

(Note that the *coccygeus* is in the same tissue plane as levator ani. It corresponds almost exactly with the sacrospinous ligament, which it overlies, and the latter is commonly regarded as a degenerate part of the muscle. The muscle is well developed and the ligament is often missing in those mammals with a mobile tail.)

The muscle acts as the principal support of the pelvic floor, has a sphincter action on the rectum and vagina and assists in increasing intra-abdominal pressure during defecation, micturition and parturition.

Its deep aspect is related to the pelvic viscera and its perineal aspect forms the inner wall of the ischioanal fossa (*see* below).

Anterior (urogenital) perineum (Figs 2.58 and 2.59)

A line joining the ischial tuberosities passes just in front of the anus. Between this line and the ischiopubic inferior rami lies the urogenital part of the perineum or the ***urogenital triangle***.

Attached to the sides of this triangle is a tough fascial sheet termed the *perineal membrane*, which is pierced by the urethra in the male and by the urethra and the vagina in the female. Deep to this membrane is the external *sphincter* of the urethra consisting of voluntary muscle fibres surrounding the membranous urethra; these are competent even when the internal sphincter has been completely destroyed. In the female, the superficial sphincter is also pierced by the vagina.

Enclosing the deep aspect of the external sphincter is a second fascial sheath (comprising areolar tissue on the deep aspect of levator ani), so that this muscle is, in fact, contained within a fascial capsule that is termed the *deep perineal pouch*. This pouch contains, in addition, the deep transverse perineal muscles and, in the male, the two *bulbo-urethral glands of Cowper*, whose ducts pass forwards to open into the bulbous urethra. Superficial to the perineal membrane is the *superficial perineal pouch*, which contains the following in the male:

1. The *bulbospongiosus muscle* covering the corpus spongiosum, which, in turn, surrounds the urethra (the distal corpus spongiosum expands into the glans penis)
2. The *ischiocavernosus muscle* on each side, arising from the ischial ramus and covering the corpus cavernosum. The urethra is thus enclosed in a spongy sheath supported by a cavernous tube on each side containing thin-walled venous sinuses which become engorged with blood when erection occurs
3. The superficial transverse perineal muscle, running transversely from the perineal body to the ischial ramus. It is of no functional importance but is seen during perineal excision of the rectum

In the female the same muscles are present, although much less well developed, and the bulbospongiosus is pierced by the vagina.

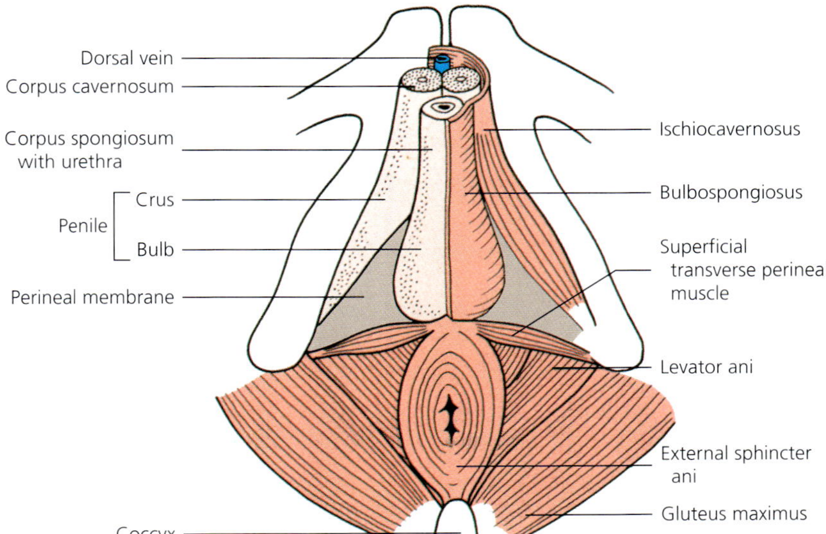

Figure 2.58 The male perineum – on the right side the muscles of the anterior perineum have been dissected away.

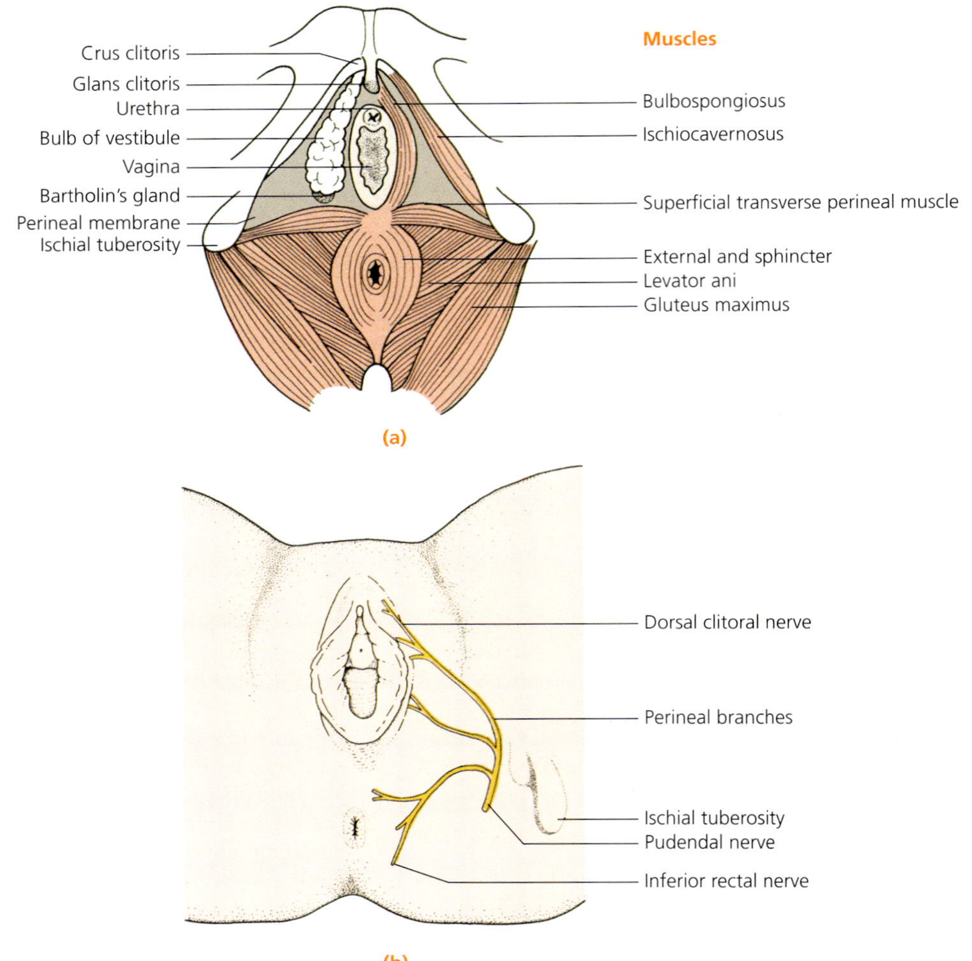

Figure 2.59 **(a)** The female perineum – on the right side the muscles of the anterior perineum have been dissected away. **(b)** Distribution of the pudendal nerve to the female perineum.

Perineal body (central perineal tendon)

This fibromuscular node lies in the midline at the junction of the anterior and posterior perineum. It is the point of attachment for the anal sphincters, the bulbospongiosus, the transverse perineal muscles and fibres of levator ani.

Posterior (anal) perineum (Figs 2.59 and 2.60)

This is the triangle lying between the ischial tuberosities on each side and the coccyx. It comprises the anal canal with its external sphincter, levator ani and, at each side, the ischioanal fossa.

Ischioanal fossa (Fig. 2.60)

It is of considerable surgical importance because of its great tendency to become infected. Its boundaries are as follows:

- **Laterally**: The fascia over obturator internus (i.e. the side wall of the pelvis); contained in this wall within a fascial tunnel termed the *pudendal* or *Alcock's canal* are the pudendal

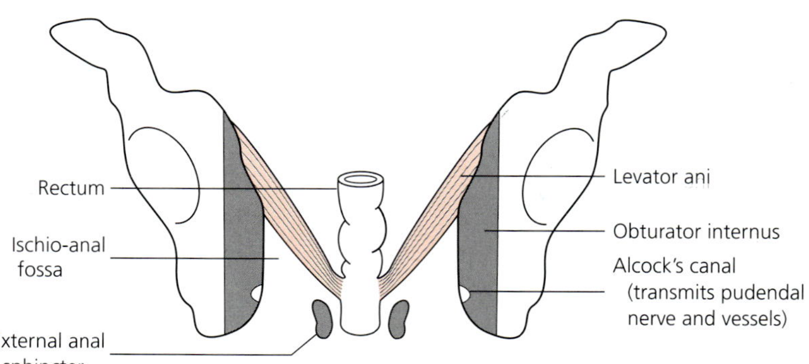

Figure 2.60 The ischiorectal fossa (more accurately called the ischio-anal fossa).

vessels and nerve which give off, respectively, the inferior rectal vessels and nerve, which supply the external sphincter and perianal skin, then pass forwards to supply the perineal tissues

- **Medially**: The fascia over levator ani and the external anal sphincter
- **Posteriorly**: The sacrotuberous ligament covered posteriorly by gluteus maximus
- **Anteriorly**: The urogenital perineum
- **Floor**: Skin and subcutaneous fat

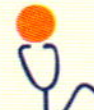

Clinical Features

1 The content of the ischioanal fossa is coarsely lobulated fat. It is important to note that the ischioanal fossae communicate with each other behind the anal canal – infection in one may therefore pass to the other.

Infection of this space may occur from boils or abrasions of the perianal skin, or from lesions within the rectum and anal canal, especially infection of the branched anal glands, approximately six in number, which lie immediately above the valves of Ball (*see* page 50 and Fig. 2.24). Occasionally, it may follow from pelvic infection bursting through levator ani or, rarely, via the bloodstream. The fossa contains no important structures and can, therefore, be incised without fear when infected.

2 The pudendal nerves can be blocked in Alcock's canal on either side to give useful regional anaesthesia in obstetrical forceps delivery (Fig. 2.59 and *see* page 150).

3 *Injury to the perineal body* weakens the pelvic floor and may lead to the prolapse of the uterus. *Episiotomy*, a relaxing incision given frequently in the posterior vaginal wall to ease the delivery of the baby and prevent tearing of the perineal body.

Female genital organs

Vulva

The *vulva* (or *pudendum*) is the term applied to the female external genitalia.

The *labia majora* are the prominent hair-bearing folds extending back from the *mons pubis* to meet posteriorly in the midline of the perineum. They are the equivalent of the male scrotum.

The *labia minora* lie between the labia majora as lips of soft skin which meet posteriorly in a sharp fold, the *fourchette*. Anteriorly, they split to enclose the *clitoris*, forming an anterior *prepuce* and posterior *frenulum*.

The *vestibule* is the area enclosed by the labia minora and contains the *urethral orifice* (which lies immediately behind the clitoris) and the *vaginal orifice*.

The vaginal orifice is guarded in the virgin by a thin mucosal fold, the *hymen*, which is perforated to allow the egress of the menses, and may have an annular, semilunar, septate or cribriform appearance. Rarely, it is imperforate and menstrual blood distends the vagina (haematocolpos). At first coitus the hymen tears, usually posteriorly or posterolaterally, and after childbirth nothing is left of it but a few tags termed *carunculae myrtiformes*.

Bartholin's glands (the greater vestibular glands) are a pair of lobulated, pea-sized, mucus-secreting glands lying deep to the posterior parts of the labia majora. They are impalpable when healthy but become obvious when inflamed or distended. Each drains by a duct 1 in. (2.5 cm) long which opens into the groove between the hymen and the posterior part of the labium minus.

Anteriorly, each gland is overlapped by the *bulb of the vestibule* – a mass of cavernous erectile tissue equivalent to the bulbus spongiosum of the male. This tissue passes forwards, under cover of bulbospongiosus, around the sides of the vagina to the roots of the clitoris.

Vagina (Fig. 2.61)

The vagina is a fibromuscular tube which surrounds the cervix of the uterus, then passes downwards and forwards through the pelvic floor to open into the vestibule. It forms the female organ of copulation.

The cervix projects into the anterior part of the vault of the vagina so that the continuous gutter surrounding the cervix is shallow anteriorly (where the vaginal wall is 3 in. (7.5 cm) in length) and is deep posteriorly (where the wall is 4 in. (10 cm) long). This continuous gutter is, for convenience of description, divided into the anterior, posterior and lateral *fornices*.

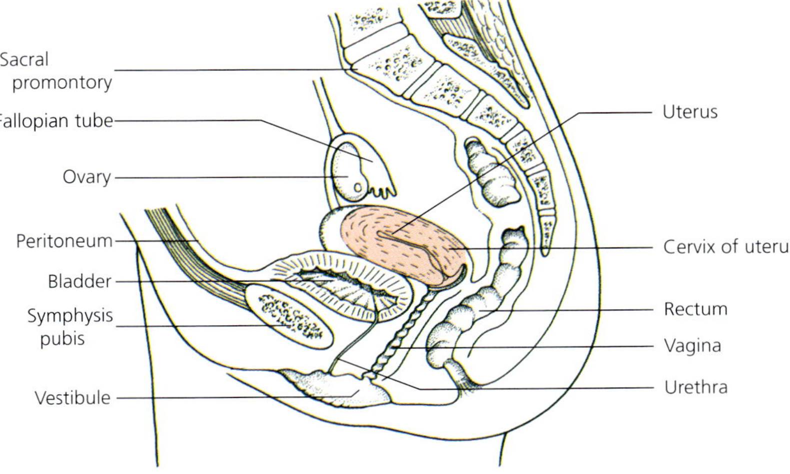

Figure 2.61 Sagittal section of the uterus and its relations.

Clinical Features

At childbirth the introitus may be enlarged by making an incision in the perineum (*episiotomy*). This starts at the fourchette and extends posterolaterally on the right side for 1.5 in. (3 cm). The skin, vaginal epithelium, subcutaneous fat, perineal body and superficial transverse perineal muscle are incised. After delivery the episiotomy is carefully sutured in layers.

Relations

- **Anteriorly:** The base of the bladder and the urethra (which is embedded in the anterior vaginal wall).
- **Posteriorly:** From below upwards, the anal canal (separated by the perineal body), the rectum and then the peritoneum of the pouch of Douglas, which covers the *upper quarter of the posterior vaginal wall.*
- **Laterally:** Levator ani, pelvic fascia and the *ureters*, which lie *immediately above the lateral fornices.*

The amateur abortionist (or inexperienced gynaecologist) without a knowledge of anatomy fails to realize that the uterus passes upwards and forwards from the vagina; he pushes the instrument or IUCD (intra-uterine contraceptive device), with the intention of inserting the device in the cervix, directly backwards through the posterior fornix. To make matters worse, this is the only part of the vagina which is covered by peritoneum; the peritoneal cavity is thus entered and peritonitis follows.

Blood supply

Arterial supply is from the internal iliac artery via its vaginal, uterine, internal pudendal and middle rectal branches.

A venous plexus drains via the vaginal vein into the internal iliac vein.

Lymphatic drainage (*see* Fig. 2.66)

- *Upper third* to the external and internal iliac nodes
- *Middle third* to the internal iliac nodes
- *Lower third* to the superficial inguinal nodes

Structure

A stratified squamous epithelium lines the vagina and the vaginal cervix; it contains no glands and is lubricated partly by cervical mucus and partly by desquamated vaginal epithelial cells. In nulliparous women the vaginal wall is rugose, but it becomes smoother after childbirth. The rugae of the anterior wall are situated transversely; this allows for filling of the bladder and for intercourse. In contrast, the rugae on the posterior wall run longitudinally. This allows for sideways stretching to accommodate a rectum distended with stool and for the passage of the foetal head.

Beneath the epithelial coat is a thin connective tissue layer separating it from the muscular wall, which is made up of a criss-cross arrangement of involuntary muscle fibres. This muscle layer is ensheathed in a fascial capsule that blends with adjacent pelvic connective tissues, so that the vagina is firmly supported in place.

In old age the vagina shrinks in length and diameter. The cervix projects far less into it so that the fornices all but disappear.

Uterus (Figs 2.61 and 2.62)

The uterus is a pear-shaped organ, 3 in. (7.5 cm) in length, made up of the *fundus, body* and *cervix*. The *Fallopian (uterine) tubes* enter into each superolateral angle (the *cornu*), above which lies the fundus.

The body of the uterus narrows to a waist termed the *isthmus*, continuing into the *cervix* which is embraced about its middle by the vagina; this attachment delimits a supravaginal and vaginal part of the cervix.

The isthmus is 1.5 mm wide. The anatomical *internal os* marks its junction with the uterine body but its mucosa is histologically similar to the endometrium. The isthmus is that part of the uterus which becomes the lower segment in pregnancy.

The cavity of the uterine body is triangular in coronal section, but in the sagittal plane it is no more than a slit. This cavity communicates via the internal os with the *cervical canal*, which, in turn, opens into the vagina by the *external os*.

The nulliparous external os is circular, but after childbirth it becomes a transverse slit with an anterior and a posterior lip.

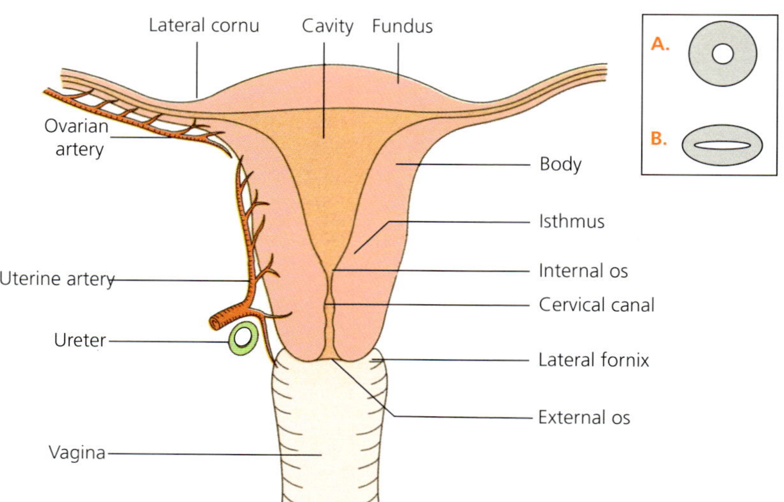

Figure 2.62 Coronal section of the uterus and vagina. Note the important relationships of the ureter and uterine artery. The inset on the right side shows the shape of external os **(A)** in nulliparous and **(B)** after birth.

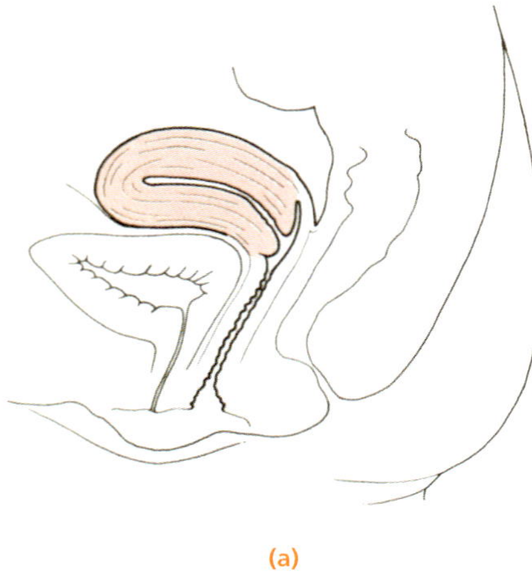

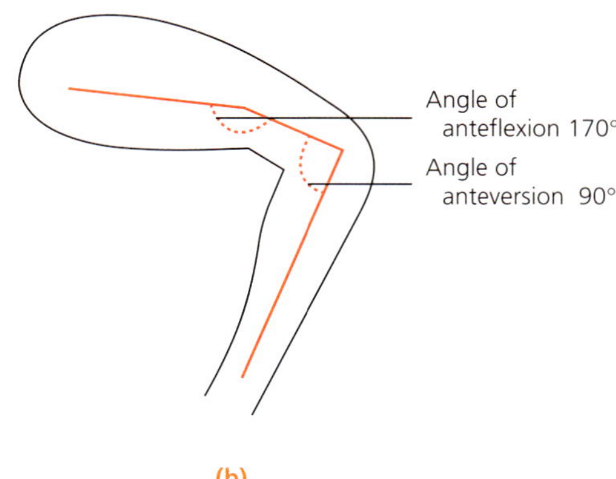

(a) (b)

Figure 2.63 Position of uterus. **(a)** Normal anteflexed and anteverted position of uterus. **(b)** Angles of anteflexion and anteversion.

The non-pregnant cervix has the firm consistency of the nose; the pregnant cervix has the soft consistency of the lips.

In foetal life the cervix is considerably larger than the body; in childhood (the *infantile uterus*) the cervix is still twice the size of the body but, during puberty, the uterus enlarges to its adult size and proportions by relative overgrowth of the body. The adult uterus is bent forwards on itself at about the level of the internal os to form an angle of 170°; this is termed *anteflexion of the uterus*. Moreover, the axis of the cervix forms an angle of 90° with the axis of the vagina – *anteversion of the uterus*. The uterus thus lies in an almost horizontal plane (Fig. 2.63).

In *retroversion of the uterus*, the axis of the cervix is directed upwards and backwards. Normally, on vaginal examination the lowermost part of the cervix to be felt is its anterior lip; in retroversion, either the os or the posterior lip becomes the presenting part.

In *retroflexion* the axis of the body of the uterus passes upwards and backwards in relation to the axis of the cervix.

Frequently these two conditions co-exist. They may be mobile and symptomless – as a result of distension of the bladder or purely as a development anomaly. Indeed, mobile retroversion is found in a quarter of the female population and may be regarded as a normal variant. Less commonly, they are fixed, the result of adhesions, previous pelvic infection, endometriosis or the pressure of a tumour in front of the uterus (Fig. 2.64).

Relations

- **Anteriorly:** The body is related to the uterovesical pouch of peritoneum and lies either on the superior surface of the bladder or on coils of intestine. The supravaginal cervix is related directly to the bladder, separated only by connective tissue. The infravaginal cervix has the anterior fornix immediately in front of it
- **Posteriorly:** Lies the pouch of Douglas, with coils of intestine within it
- **Laterally:** The broad ligament and its contents (*see* below); *the ureter lies approximately 0.5 in. (1.2 cm) lateral to the supravaginal cervix*

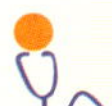

Clinical Features

The most important single practical relationship in this region is that of the ureter to the supravaginal cervix. At this point, the ureter lies just above the level of the lateral fornix, below the uterine vessels as these pass across within the broad ligament (Fig. 2.65). In performing a hysterectomy, the ureter may be accidentally divided in clamping the uterine vessels, especially when the pelvic anatomy has been distorted by a previous operation, a mass of fibroids, infection or malignant infiltration.

(Continued ...)

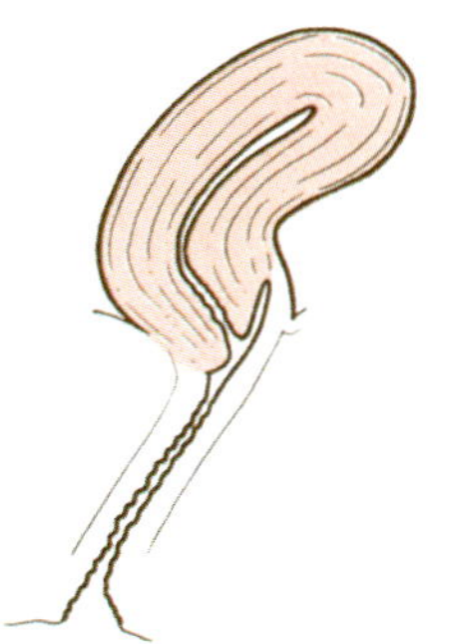

(a) Retroflexion (uterus still anteverted)

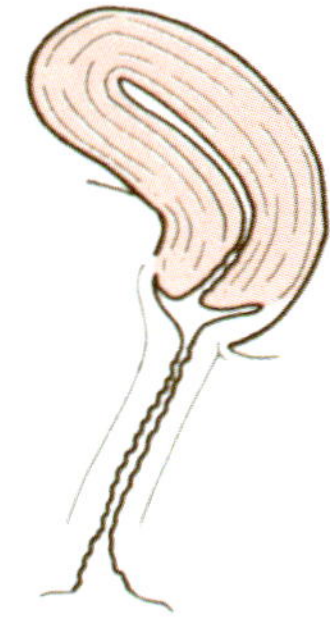

(b) Retroversion (uterus still anteflexed)

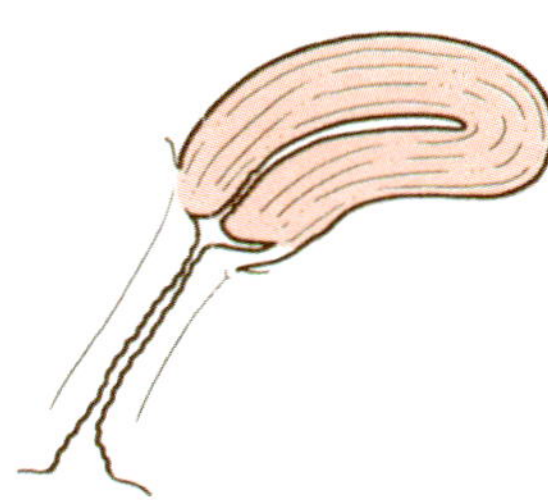

(c) Retroversion and retroflexion

Figure 2.64 Variations in uterine position and their terminology.

(... continued)

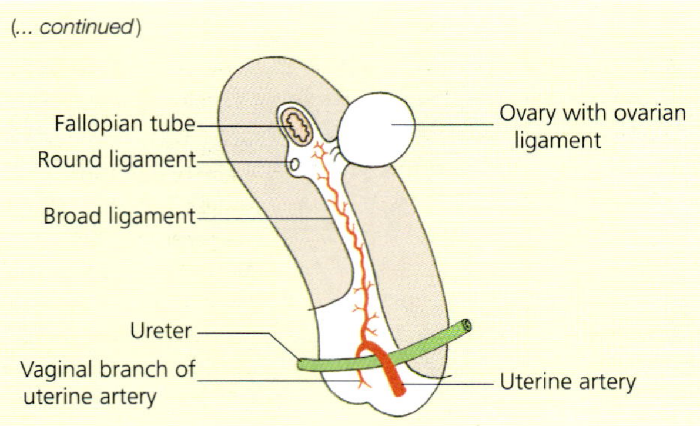

Figure 2.65 Lateral view of the uterus (schematic) to show the composition of the broad ligament, the relations of the ureter and uterine artery, and the peritoneal covering of the uterus (pink).

The ureter is readily infiltrated by lateral extension of a carcinoma of the uterus; bilateral hydronephrosis with uraemia is a frequent mode of termination of this disease.

The close relationship of the ureter to the lateral fornix is best appreciated by realizing that a ureteric stone at this site can be palpated on vaginal examination. (This is the answer to the examination question: 'When can a stone in the ureter be felt?')

Blood supply

The *uterine artery* (from the internal iliac) runs in the base of the broad ligament and crosses above and at right angles to the ureter to reach the uterus at the level of the internal os (Fig. 2.65). The artery then ascends in a tortuous manner alongside the uterus, supplying the corpus, and then anastomoses with the *ovarian artery*. The uterine artery also gives off a descending branch to the cervix and branches to the upper vagina. The veins accompany the arteries and drain into the internal iliac veins, but they also communicate via the pelvic plexus with the veins of the vagina and bladder.

Lymph drainage (Fig. 2.66)

1. The fundus (together with the ovary and Fallopian tube) drains along the ovarian vessels to the aortic nodes – apart from some lymphatics, which pass along the round ligament to the inguinal nodes.
2. The body drains via the broad ligament to nodes lying alongside the external iliac vessels.
3. The cervix drains in three directions – laterally, in the broad ligament, to the external iliac nodes; posterolaterally along the uterine vessels to the internal iliac nodes; and posteriorly along the recto-uterine folds to the sacral nodes.

Always examine the inguinal nodes in a suspected carcinoma of the corpus uteri – they may be involved by lymphatic spread along the round ligament.

Structure

The body of the uterus is covered with peritoneum except where this is reflected off at two sites, anteriorly onto the bladder at the uterine isthmus and laterally at the broad ligaments. Anteriorly, the peritoneum is only loosely adherent to the supravaginal cervix; this allows for bladder distension. The muscle wall is thick and made up of a criss-cross of involuntary fibres mixed with fibro-elastic connective tissue.

The *mucosa* is applied directly to muscle with no submucosa intervening. The mucosa of the body of the uterus is the *endometrium*, made up of a single layer of cuboidal ciliated cells forming simple tubular glands which dip down to the underlying muscular wall. Below this epithelium is a stroma of connective tissue containing blood vessels and round cells.

The cervical canal epithelium is made up of tall columnar cells which form a series of complicated branching glands; these secrete an alkaline mucus that forms a protective '*cervical plug*' filling the canal.

The vaginal aspect of the cervix is covered with a stratified squamous epithelium continuous with that of the vagina.

The mucosa of the corpus undergoes extensive changes during the menstrual cycle, which may be briefly summarized thus as the following:

1. First 4 days: Desquamation of its superficial two-thirds with bleeding
2. Subsequent 2–3 days: Rapid reconstitution of the raw mucosal surface by growth from the remaining epithelial cells in the depths of the glands
3. By the 14th day the endometrium has reformed; this is the end of the *proliferative phase*
4. From the 14th day until the menstrual flow commences is the *secretory phase*; the endometrium thickens, the glands lengthen and distend with fluid and the stroma becomes oedematous and stuffed with white cells.

At the end of this phase, three layers can be defined as follows:

1. A compact superficial zone
2. A spongy middle zone – with dilated glands and oedematous stroma
3. A basal zone of inactive non-secreting tubules

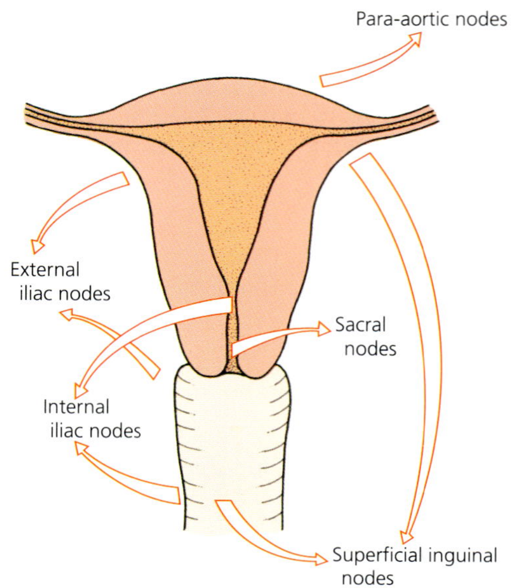

Figure 2.66 Lymph drainage of the uterus and vagina.

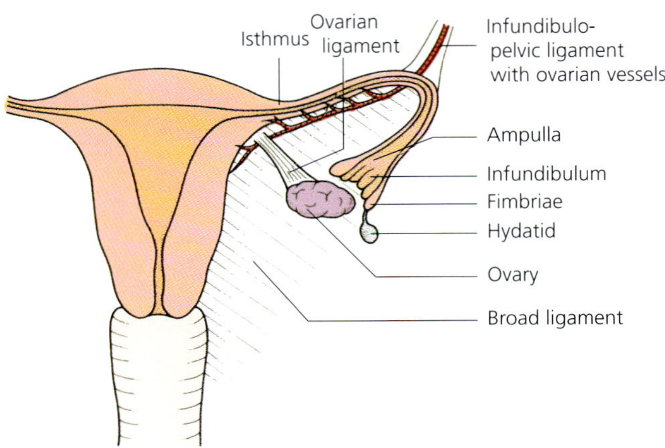

Figure 2.67 The Fallopian tube, ovary and broad ligament (viewed from behind).

With degeneration of the corpus luteum there is shrinkage of the endometrium, the arteries retract and coil, producing ischaemia of the middle and superficial zones, which then desquamate. It is probable that spasm of the vessels in the basal layer (which remains non-desquamated) prevents the woman bleeding to death.

Only very slight desquamation and bleeding takes place in the mucosa of the cervical canal.

Fallopian tubes (Fig. 2.67)

The Fallopian, or uterine, tubes are approximately 4 in. (10 cm) long; they lie in the free edge of the broad ligaments and open into the cornu of the uterus. Each comprises the following four parts:

1. **The infundibulum:** The bugle-shaped extremity extending beyond the broad ligament and opening into the peritoneal cavity by the *ostium*. Its mouth is fimbriated and overlies the ovary, to which one long fimbria actually adheres (*fimbria ovarica*)
2. **The ampulla:** Wide, thin-walled and tortuous
3. **The isthmus:** Narrow, straight and thick-walled
4. **The interstitial part:** Which pierces the uterine wall

Structure

Apart from the interstitial part, the tube is clothed in peritoneum. Beneath this is a muscle of outer longitudinal and inner circular fibres.

The mucosa is formed of columnar, mainly ciliated cells and lies in longitudinal ridges, each of which is thrown into numerous folds.

The ova are propelled to the uterus along this tube, partly by peristalsis and partly by cilial action.

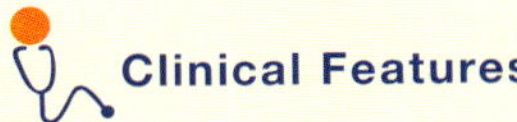

Clinical Features

1 Note that the genital canal in the female is the only direct communication into the peritoneum from the exterior and is a potential pathway for infection (e.g. in gonorrhoea).

(Continued ...)

(... continued)

2 The fertilized ovum may implant ectopically, i.e. in a site other than the endometrium of the corpus uteri called ectopic pregnancy. When this occurs in the Fallopian tube it is called, according to the exact site, fimbrial, ampullary, isthmic or interstitial, of which the ampullary is the commonest and interstitial the rarest.

As the ectopic embryo enlarges, it may abort into the peritoneal cavity (where rarely it continues to grow as a *secondary abdominal pregnancy*), or else ruptures the tube. This second fate is particularly likely to occur in the narrow and relatively non-distensible isthmus; rupture is usually into the peritoneal cavity but may rarely occur into the broad ligament.

Ovary (Fig. 2.67)

The ovary is a female gonad. It is an almond-shaped organ, 1.5 in. (4 cm) long, attached to the back of the broad ligament by the *mesovarium*. The ovary has two other attachments: the *infundibulopelvic ligament* (sometimes called the *suspensory ligament of the ovary*), along which pass the ovarian vessels, sympathetic nerves and lymphatics from the side wall of the pelvis, and the *ovarian ligament*, which passes to the cornu of the uterus.

Relations

The ovary is usually described as lying on the side wall of the pelvis opposite the *ovarian fossa*, which is a depression bounded by the external iliac vessels in front and the ureter and internal iliac vessels behind and which contains the obturator nerve. However, the ovary is extremely variable in its position and is frequently found prolapsed into the pouch of Douglas in perfectly normal women.

The ovary, like the testis, develops from the genital ridge and then descends into the pelvis. In the same way as the testis, it therefore drags its blood supply and lymphatic drainage downwards with it from the posterior abdominal wall.

Blood supply, lymph drainage and nerve supply

Blood supply is from the ovarian artery, which arises from the aorta just below the level of the renal arteries. The ovarian vein drains, on the right side, to the inferior vena cava and, on the left, to the left renal vein, exactly comparable to the venous drainage of the testis.

Lymphatics pass to the aortic nodes at the level of the renal vessels, following the general rule that lymphatic drainage accompanies the venous drainage of an organ.

Nerve supply is from the aortic plexus (T10 and T11); hence, referral of ovarian pain to the umbilicus, loin and groin. These are sympathetic (pain-conducting) afferent fibres.

All these structures pass to the ovary in the infundibulopelvic ligament.

Structure

The ovary has no peritoneal covering; the serosa ends at the mesovarian attachment. It consists of a connective tissue stroma containing *Graafian follicles* at various stages of development, *corpora lutea* and *corpora albicantia* (hyalinized, regressing corpora lutea, which take several months to absorb completely).

The surface of the ovary in young children is covered with a so-called 'germinal epithelium' of cuboidal cells. It is now known, however, that the primordial follicles develop in the ovary in early foetal life and do not differentiate from these cells. In adult life, in fact, the epithelial covering of the ovary disappears, leaving only a fibrous capsule termed the *tunica albuginea*.

After the menopause the ovary becomes small and shrivelled; in old age, the follicles disappear completely.

Endopelvic fascia and the pelvic ligaments (Fig. 2.68)

Pelvic fascia is the term applied to the connective tissue floor of the pelvis covering levator ani and obturator internus. The *endopelvic fascia* is the extraperitoneal cellular tissue of the uterus (the *parametrium*), vagina, bladder and rectum. Within this endopelvic fascia are the following three important condensations of connective tissue called ligaments, which sling the pelvic viscera from the pelvic walls.

1. The ***cardinal ligaments*** (transverse cervical, or Mackenrodt's ligaments), which pass laterally from the cervix and upper vagina to the side walls of the pelvis along the lines of attachment of levator ani, are composed of white fibrous connective tissue with some involuntary muscle fibres and are pierced in their upper part by the ureters.
2. The ***uterosacral ligaments***, which pass backwards from the posterolateral aspect of the cervix at the level of the isthmus and from the lateral vaginal fornices deep to the uterosacral folds of peritoneum in the lateral boundaries of the pouch of Douglas, are attached to the periosteum in front of the sacro-iliac joints and the lateral part of the third piece of the sacrum.
3. The ***pubocervical ligament*** extends forwards from the cardinal ligament to the pubis on either side of the bladder, for which it acts as a sling.

These three ligaments act as supports to the cervix of the uterus and the vault of the vagina, in conjunction with the important elastic muscular foundation provided by levator ani. In prolapse, these ligaments lengthen (in *procidentia* – complete uterine prolapse – they may be 6 in. (15 cm) long) and any repair operation must include their reconstitution.

Two other pairs of ligaments take attachments from the uterus as follows:

1. The **broad ligament** is a fold of peritoneum connecting the lateral margin of the uterus with the side wall of the pelvis on each side. The uterus and its broad ligaments, therefore, form a partition across the pelvic floor dividing off an anterior compartment, containing the bladder (the *uterovesical pouch*), from a posterior compartment, containing the rectum (the pouch of Douglas or *recto-uterine pouch*).

   The broad ligament contains or carries (Figs 2.65 and 2.67):
   - The Fallopian (uterine) tube in its free edge
   - The ovary, attached by the mesovarium to its posterior aspect
   - The round ligament
   - The ovarian ligament, crossing from the ovary to the uterine cornu (*see* 'Ovary', page 85)
   - The uterine vessels and branches of the ovarian vessels
   - Lymphatics and nerve fibres

   The ureter passes forwards to the bladder deep to this ligament and lateral to and immediately above the lateral fornix of the vagina.
2. The **round ligament** – a fibromuscular cord – passes from the lateral angle of the uterus in the anterior layer of the broad ligament to the internal inguinal ring; thence it traverses the inguinal canal to the labium majus. Taken together with the ovarian ligament, it is equivalent to the male gubernaculum testis and can be thought of as the pathway along which the female gonad might have descended, but in fact did not, to the labium majus (the female homologue of the scrotum). Compare this process with descent of the testis (page 72).

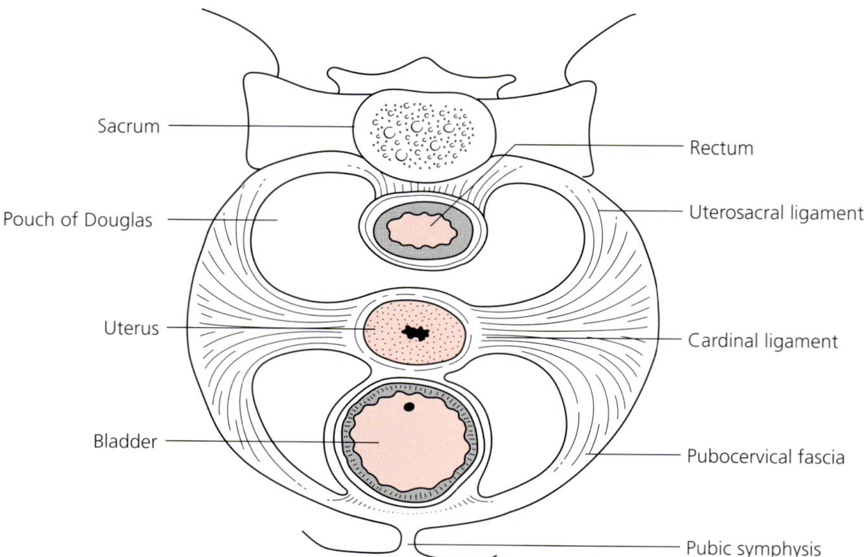

Figure 2.68 The pelvic ligaments seen from above.

Vaginal examination

The relations of the vagina to the other pelvic organs must be constantly borne in mind when carrying out a vaginal examination.

Inspection (by means of a speculum) enables the vaginal walls and cervix to be examined and a biopsy or cytological smear to be taken. Inspection of the introitus while straining detects prolapse and the presence of stress incontinence.

- **Anteriorly:** The urethra, bladder and symphysis pubis are felt.
- **Posteriorly:** The rectum (invasion of the vagina by a rectal neoplasm must always be sought after in this disease). Collections of fluid, malignant deposits, prolapsed uterine tubes and ovaries or coils of distended bowel may be felt in the pouch of Douglas.
- **Laterally:** The ovary and tube, and the side wall of the pelvis. Rarely, a stone in the ureter may be felt through the lateral fornix. The strength of the perineal muscles can be assessed by asking the patient to tighten up her perineum.
- **Apex:** The cervix is felt projecting back from the anterior wall of the vagina. In the normal anteverted uterus the anterior lip of the cervix presents; in retroversion, either the cervical os or the posterior lip are first to be felt.

Pathological cervical conditions – for example, neoplasm – can be felt, as can the softening of the cervix in pregnancy and its dilatation during labour.

Bimanual examination assesses the pelvic size and position of the uterus, enlargements of ovary or uterine tubes and the presence of other pelvic masses.

The obstetrician can assess the pelvic size in both the transverse and anteroposterior diameter. Particularly important is the distance from the lower border of the symphysis pubis to the sacral promontory, which is termed the *diagonal conjugate*. If the pelvis is of normal size, the examiner's fingers should fail to reach the promontory of the sacrum. If it is readily palpable, pelvic narrowing is present (*see* 'Obstetrical pelvic measurements', page 77).

Embryology of the Fallopian tubes, uterus and vagina (Fig. 2.69)

The *paramesonephric* (or *Müllerian*) *ducts* develop, one on each side, adjacent to the *mesonephric* (*Wolffian*) *ducts* in the posterior abdominal wall – they are mesodermal in origin. All these four tubes lie close together caudally, projecting into the anterior (urogenital) compartment of the cloaca.

One system disappears in the male, the other in the female, each leaving behind congenital remnants of some interest to the clinician.

In the male, the paramesonephric duct disappears, apart from the appendix testis and the prostatic utricle. In the female, the mesonephric system (which in the male develops into the vas deferens and epididymal ducts) persists as remnants in the broad ligament termed the *epoöphoron, paroöphoron* and *ducts of Gärtner*.

The paramesonephric ducts in the female form the Fallopian tubes cranially. More caudally, they come together and fuse in the midline (dragging, as they do so, a peritoneal fold from the side wall of the pelvis which becomes the broad ligament). The median structure so formed differentiates into the epithelium of the uterine body (endometrium), cervical canal and upper one-third of the vagina, which are first solid and later become canalized. The rest of the vaginal epithelium develops by canalization of the solid sinuvaginal node at the back of the urogenital sinus. This accounts for the differences in lymphatic drainage of the upper and lower vagina (Fig. 2.66). The muscle of the Fallopian tubes, uterine body, cervix and vagina develops from surrounding mesoderm, so that remnants of the mesonephric duct system of the female are found in the myometrium, cervix and vaginal wall.

Developmental abnormalities of this system can easily be deduced. All stages of division of the original double tube may persist from a bicornuate uterus to a complete reduplication of the uterus and vagina. Alternatively, there may be absence, hypoplasia or atresia of the duct system on one or both sides.

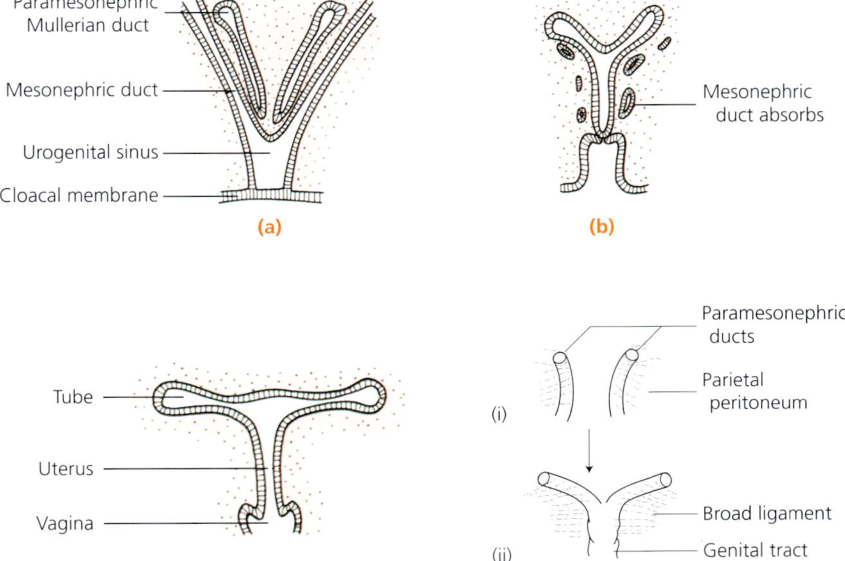

Figure 2.69 Development of the Fallopian tubes, uterus and vagina from the paramesonephric (Müllerian) ducts and the urogenital sinus (after Hollinshead) **(a–c)**, and formation of the broad ligament **(d)**.

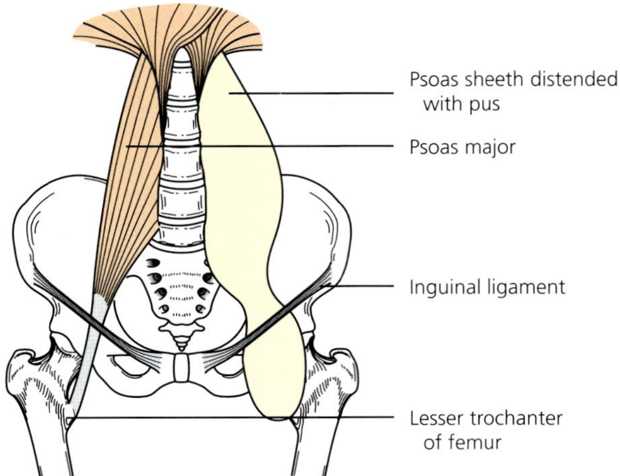

Figure 2.70 Psoas sheath and psoas abscess. On the right side is a normal psoas sheath; on the left side it is shown distended with pus, which tracks under the inguinal ligament to present in the groin.

Failure of canalization of the originally solid caudal end of the duct results, after puberty, in the accumulation of menstrual blood above the obstruction. First the vagina may distend with blood, then the uterus and then the tubes (haematocolpos, haematometra and haematosalpinx, respectively).

Posterior abdominal wall

The *bed of the posterior abdominal wall* is made up of three bony and four muscular structures. *The bones are* as follows*:*

- The bodies of the lumbar vertebrae
- The sacrum
- The wings of the ilium

The muscles are as follows*:*

- The diaphragm – posterior part
- The quadratus lumborum
- The psoas major
- The iliacus

The diaphragm has been considered in the section on the thorax (*see* page 9).

The psoas must be dealt with in more detail because of the involvement of its sheath in the formation of a psoas abscess.

The *psoas major* arises from the transverse processes of all the lumbar vertebrae and from the sides of the bodies and the intervening discs of the T12 to L5 vertebrae. It passes downwards and laterally at the margin of the brim of the pelvis, narrowing down to a tendon which crosses the front of the hip joint beneath the inguinal ligament to be inserted, with iliacus, into the lesser trochanter of the femur (Fig. 2.70).

The psoas major, together with iliacus, flexes the hip on the trunk, or, alternatively, the trunk on the hips (e.g. in sitting up from the lying position). *Psoas minor*, absent in 40% of subjects, lies on psoas major. It has a common origin with psoas major from T12 and L1 vertebrae and attaches to the iliopubic eminence.

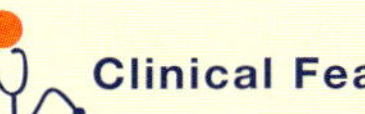

Clinical Features

1 The femoral artery lies on the psoas tendon in the groin, and it is this firm posterior relation of the femoral artery at the groin which enables it here to be identified and compressed easily by the finger.

2 The psoas is enclosed in the psoas sheath, which is a compartment of the lumbar fascia. Pus from a tuberculous infection of the lumbar vertebrae is limited in its anterior spread by the anterior longitudinal vertebral ligament, and therefore passes laterally into its sheath (***psoas abscess***), which may also be entered by pus tracking down from the posterior mediastinum in disease of the thoracic vertebrae. Pus may then spread under the inguinal ligament into the femoral triangle, where it produces a soft swelling (Fig. 2.70). Occasionally, in completely neglected cases, pus tracks along the femoral vessels, along the subsartorial canal and eventually appears in the popliteal fossa.

The retroperitoneal organs are: the pancreas, kidneys and ureters (which have already been considered), the suprarenals, the aorta and inferior vena cava and their main branches, the para-aortic lymph nodes and the lumbar sympathetic chain.

Suprarenal glands (Fig. 2.41)

The suprarenal glands cap the upper poles of the kidneys and lie against the crura of the diaphragm. The left is related anteriorly to the stomach across the lesser sac; the right lies behind the right lobe of the liver and tucks medially behind the inferior vena cava.

Blood supply

Each gland, although weighing only 3–4 g, has the following three arteries supplying it:

1. A direct branch from the aorta
2. A branch from the phrenic artery
3. A branch from the renal artery

The single main vein drains from the hilum of the gland into the nearest available vessel – the inferior vena cava on the right, the renal vein on the left. The stubby right suprarenal vein, coming directly from the inferior vena cava, presents the most dangerous feature in performing an adrenalectomy – the tiro should always choose the easier left side and leave the right to his chief.

Structures

The suprarenal gland comprises a cortex and medulla, which represent two developmentally and functionally independent endocrine glands within the same anatomical structure. The medulla is derived from the neural crest (neuroectoderm), whose cells also give rise to the sympathetic ganglia. The cortex, on the other hand, is derived from the mesoderm. The suprarenal medulla receives preganglionic sympathetic fibres from the greater splanchnic nerve and secretes adrenaline (epinephrine) and noradrenaline (norepinephrine). The cortex secretes the adrenocortical hormones.

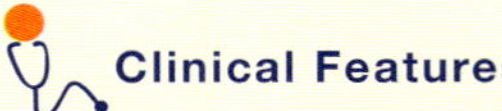

A tumour arising from adrenal medulla is called *pheochromocytoma*. It releases an excess amount of catecholamines in blood leading to paroxysmal palpitation, perspiration, pallor headache and hypertension.

Abdominal aorta (Fig. 2.71)

The abdominal aorta is the continuation of descending thoracic aorta. It enters the abdomen via the aortic hiatus in the diaphragm at the level of the 12th thoracic vertebra and ends at the level of L4 in. the supracristal (transcristal) plane (Fig. 2.2). It lies throughout this course against the vertebral bodies and is easily palpable in the midline. The normal abdominal aorta measures approximately 0.5 in. (1–1.5 cm) in diameter. In the elderly it is frequently thickened and dilated. An early aneurysmal dilatation is considered to be present if the diameter reaches 1.5 in. (4 cm).

Anteriorly, from above down, it is related to the pancreas (separating it from the stomach), the third part of the duodenum and coils of small intestine. It is crossed by the left renal vein. A large tumour of pancreas or stomach, a mass of enlarged para-aortic nodes or a large ovarian cyst may transmit the pulsations of the aorta and be mistaken for an aneurysm.

Branches

The branches of the aorta are as follows

1. **Three anterior unpaired branches** passing to the viscera:
   a. The *coeliac axis* – giving off the
      - Hepatic artery
      - Splenic artery
      - Left gastric artery

   b. The *superior mesenteric artery*
   c. The *inferior mesenteric artery*
2. **Three lateral paired branches** passing to viscera:
   a. The *suprarenal artery*
   b. The *renal artery*
   c. The *testicular or ovarian artery*
3. **Five lateral paired branches** to the parietes:
   a. The *inferior phrenic artery*
   b. Four *lumbar* branches
4. **Terminal branches**:
   a. The *common iliacs*
   b. The *median sacral artery*

The ***common iliac arteries*** pass, one on each side, downwards and outwards to bifurcate into the internal and external iliacs in front of the sacro-iliac joint, at the level of the sacral promontory. They give no other branches.

At the bifurcation, the common iliac artery is crossed superficially by the ureter – a convenient site to identify this latter structure in pelvic operations.

The ***external iliac artery*** runs along the brim of the pelvis on the medial side of psoas major. The artery passes below the inguinal ligament to form the femoral artery, giving off, immediately before its termination, the *inferior epigastric artery*, which demarcates the medial edge of the internal inguinal ring (Fig. 2.5) and also the *deep circumflex iliac artery*.

The ***internal iliac artery*** passes backwards and downwards into the pelvis, sandwiched between the ureter anteriorly and the internal iliac vein posteriorly. At the upper border of the

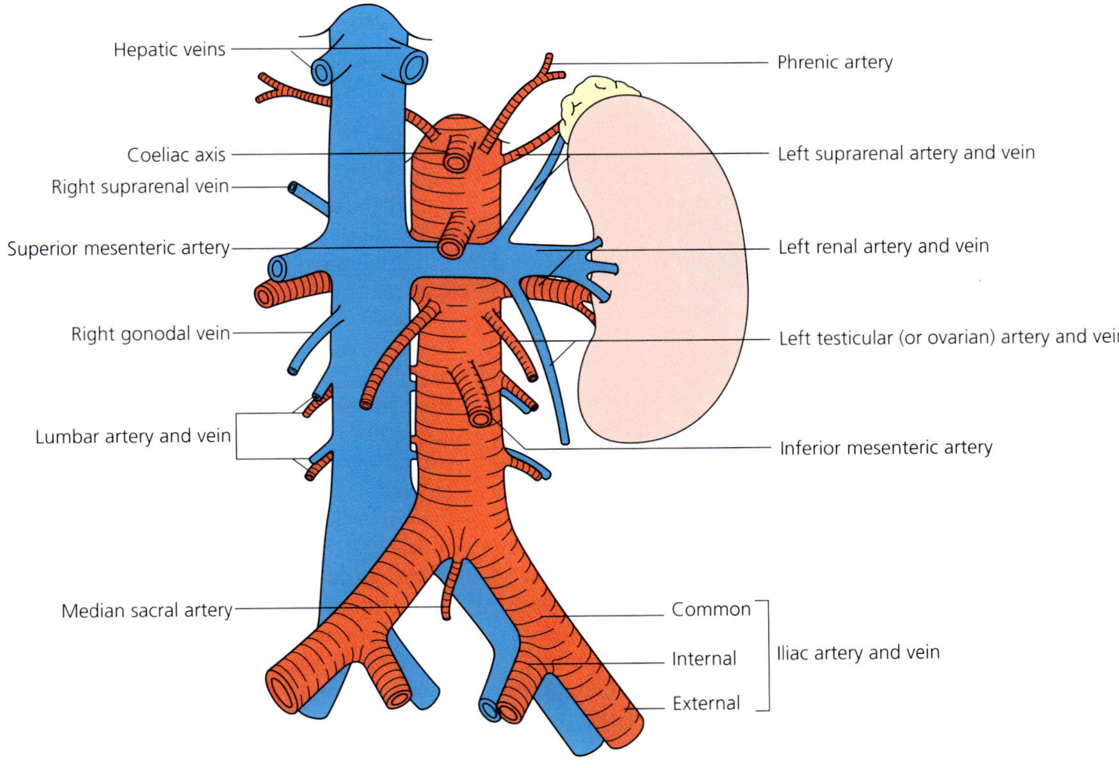

Figure 2.71 The abdominal aorta, the inferior vena cava and their main branches.

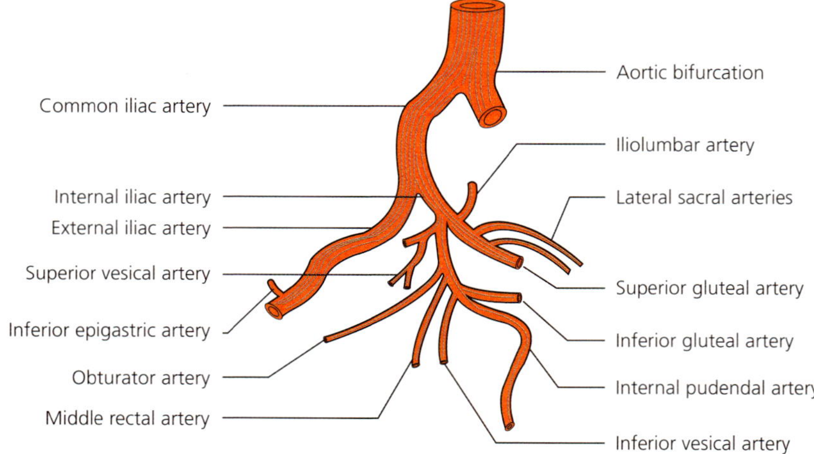

Figure 2.72 The aortic bifurcation and the right internal iliac artery. The internal iliac artery divides into anterior and posterior divisions. The latter gives rise to the superior gluteal artery, whereas the former gives off all the visceral branches. (Although the branches of the internal iliac artery are fairly constant, the arrangement of these branches is variable.) Hatching indicates arteries present only in the female.

greater sciatic notch it divides into an anterior and posterior division, which give off numerous branches to supply the pelvic organs, perineum, buttock and sacral canal (Fig. 2.72). These are as follows:

1. *Parietal branches* to the inner and outer walls of the pelvis, sacrum and sacral canal, the perineum and the buttock:
   a. Iliolumbar
   b. Lateral sacral
   c. Obturator
   d. Superior gluteal
   e. Inferior gluteal
   f. Internal pudendal
2. *Visceral branches* to the pelvic organs:
   a. Superior vesical
   b. Inferior vesical (vaginal in the female)
   c. Middle rectal

In addition, in the female, the uterine artery, which arises above the vaginal.

These arteries are accompanied by their corresponding veins, which drain to the internal iliac vein

Inferior vena cava (Fig. 2.71)

The inferior vena cava commences at L5 by the junction of the common iliac veins *behind* the right common iliac artery (unlike the usual arrangement of a vein being superficial to its corresponding artery). It lies to the right of the aorta as it ascends until separated from it by the right crus of the diaphragm when the aorta pierces this muscle. The inferior vena cava itself passes through the diaphragm at T8 (Fig. 1.12), traverses the pericardium and drains into the right atrium.

As the inferior vena cava ascends, it is related anteriorly to coils of small intestine, the third part of the duodenum, the head of the pancreas with the common bile duct and the first part of the duodenum. It then passes behind the foramen of Winslow, in front of which lies the portal vein, separating it from the common bile duct and hepatic artery. Finally, the inferior vena cava lies in a deep groove in the liver before piercing the diaphragm. Within the liver it receives the right and left hepatic veins. Occasionally, these veins fuse into a single trunk that opens directly into the inferior vena cava; on other occasions, the central hepatic vein (which usually enters the left hepatic near its termination) drains directly into the inferior vena cava (Fig. 2.34). These variations are now of importance because of the possibility of carrying out resection of one or other lobe of the liver.

Lumbar sympathetic chain

The lumbar part of the sympathetic trunk commences deep to the medial arcuate ligament of the diaphragm as a continuation of the thoracic sympathetic chain (*see* Fig. 6.39). On each side it lies against the bodies of the lumbar vertebrae, overlapped, on the right side, by the inferior vena cava and, on the left, by the aorta.

The lumbar arteries lie deep to the chain but the lumbar veins may cross superficial to it and are of importance because they may be damaged in performing a sympathectomy.

Below, the lumbar trunk passes deep to the iliac vessels to continue as the sacral trunk in front of the sacrum. Inferiorly, the chains converge and unite in front of the coccyx as the small ganglion impar.

Usually the lumbar trunk carries four ganglia, although sometimes these are condensed to three. All four send grey rami communicantes to the lumbar spinal nerves; in addition, the upper two ganglia receive white rami.

Branches from the chain pass to plexuses around the abdominal aorta and its branches, which also receive fibres from the splanchnic nerves and the vagus. Other branches pass in front of the common iliac vessels as the hypogastric plexus ('presacral nerves') to supply the pelvic viscera via plexuses of nerves distributed along the branches of the internal iliac artery.

The parasympathetic supply to the pelvic viscera arises from the anterior primary rami of S2, S3 and S4 and is distributed with the pelvic plexuses (*see* page 237).

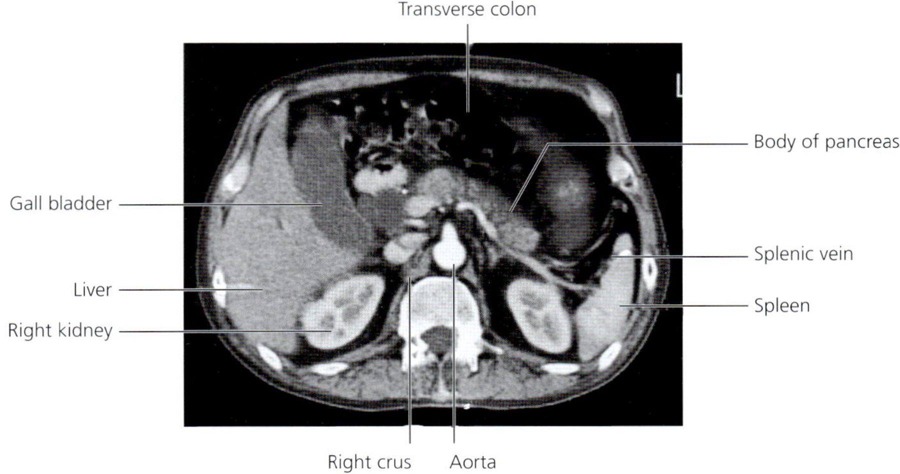

Figure 2.73 CT scan at the level of the 1st lumbar vertebra. This demonstrates the liver, gall bladder, aorta with the commencement of the superior mesenteric artery, the inferior vena cava, the crura of the diaphragm, the kidneys, the pancreas and the spleen. The splenic vein can be seen as it passes to the splenic hilum posterior to the body of the pancreas. The vena cava lies on the right crus. The vessels have been enhanced by an intravenous injection of contrast.

Computed axial tomography

Computed axial tomography (CT scanning) has revealed a fresh dimension to the importance of topographical anatomy. It is now necessary for clinicians to possess a detailed knowledge of the cross-sectional relationships of the body in health so that pathological abnormalities can be appreciated. Figures 2.73 and 2.74 demonstrate CT scan cuts of the abdomen at the levels of the 1st and 2nd lumbar vertebral bodies, respectively. Clinical students should take every opportunity of studying normal scans with the help of a skilled radiologist.

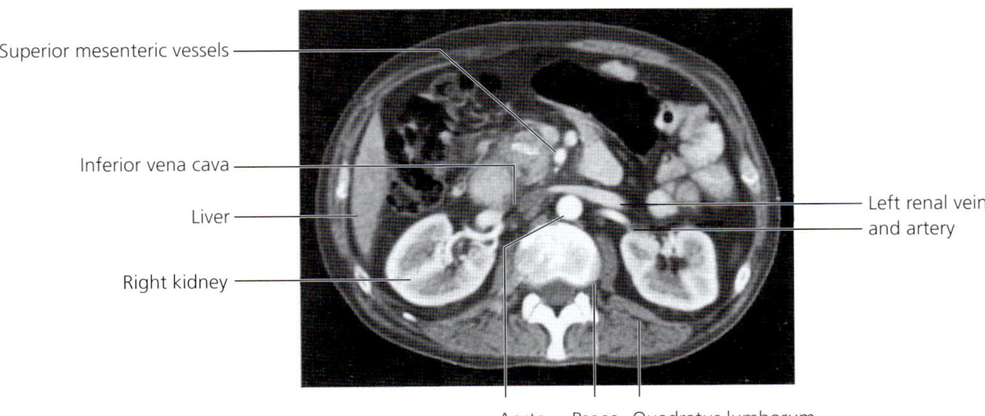

Figure 2.74 CT scan at the level of the 2nd lumbar vertebra demonstrating the kidneys, aorta, inferior vena cava, the liver, renal and superior mesenteric vessels, and the muscles of the abdominal wall. The blood vessels, again, have been enhanced by an intravenous injection of contrast.

Part III

The upper limb

Surface anatomy and surface markings of the upper limb

Much of the anatomy of the limbs can be revised on oneself; otherwise, choose a thin colleague.

Bones and joints (*see* Figs 3.6 and 3.8–3.11)

The subcutaneous border of the *clavicle* can be palpated along its entire length; the supraclavicular nerves crossing it can be rolled against the bone.

The *acromion process* forms a sharp bony edge at the lateral extremity of the *scapular spine*. It lies immediately above the smooth bulge of the *deltoid muscle*, which itself covers the *greater tubercle of the humerus*. Less easily identified is the *coracoid process* of the scapula, lying immediately below the clavicle at the junction of the middle and outer thirds, and covered by the anterior fibres of the deltoid.

The medial border of the scapula can be both seen and felt. Abduction of the arm is a complex affair made up of abduction at the shoulder joint, depression at the sternoclavicular joint and rotation of the scapula; the last two are readily confirmed on self-palpation.

With the shoulder abducted, the *head of the humerus* can be felt in the axilla; note its movement with rotation of the arm.

At the elbow, the three bony landmarks are the *olecranon process* and the *medial* and *lateral epicondyles*. A supracondylar fracture lies above these points, which, therefore, remain in their triangular relationship to each other; in dislocation of the elbow, however, the olecranon comes more or less in line with the epicondyles (Fig. 3.1).

Note a hollow in the posterolateral aspect of the extended elbow distal to the lateral epicondyle; this lies over the *head of the radius*, which can be felt to rotate during pronation and supination.

The posterior border of the *ulna* is completely subcutaneous and crossed by no named vessels or nerve; it can, therefore, be exposed surgically from end to end without danger.

At the wrist, the *styloid processes* of the radius and ulna can be felt; the former extends more distally. The radial styloid process lies in the floor of the 'anatomical snuffbox', while the ulnar styloid process can be felt (and usually seen) on the dorsal aspect of the *head* of the ulna. The *dorsal tubercle of Lister* is palpable on the posterior aspect of the distal end of the radius.

In the palm of the hand, palpate the *pisiform* at the base of the hypothenar eminence. *Flexor carpi ulnaris* is inserted into it, and when this tendon is relaxed by flexing the wrist the pisiform can be moved a little from side to side. The *hook of the hamate* can be felt by deep palpation just distal to the pisiform. The *scaphoid* is felt at the base of the thenar eminence and also within the anatomical snuffbox, where there is characteristic tenderness when this bone is fractured. In a thin subject, the pisiform and the tubercle of the scaphoid can be seen as bulges when the wrist is extended.

Muscles and tendons

The anterior fold of the axilla is formed by the *pectoralis major*, and its posterior fold by the *teres major* and *latissimus dorsi*. The digitations of *serratus anterior* can be seen in a muscular subject on the medial axillary wall.

In the upper arm the *deltoid* forms the smooth contour of the shoulder. The *biceps* and *brachialis* constitute the bulk of the anterior aspect of the arm, and the *triceps* its posterior aspect. The tendon of biceps is easily felt, and often seen, at the elbow when this is flexed to a right angle. Immediately medial to this, palpate the pulse of the brachial artery. Firm pressure immediately medial to this will, in turn, produce paraesthesiae in the hand as the median nerve is palpated (*see* Fig. 3.23).

When the forearm is flexed against resistance, the *brachioradialis* presents prominently along its radial border.

At the wrist (Figs 3.2 and 3.4) it is convenient to commence at the radial pulse. The tendon medial to this is that of the *flexor carpi radialis*, then *palmaris longus* (which may be absent), then the cluster of tendons of *flexor digitorum superficialis*. The tendon of *flexor carpi ulnaris* lies most medially, inserting into the pisiform; the ulnar pulse can be felt just to the radial side of this tendon.

On the dorsal aspect of the wrist (Figs 3.3 and 3.4) the anatomical snuffbox is bordered by the tendons of *abductor pollicis longus* and *extensor pollicis brevis* laterally and that of *extensor pollicis longus* medially (i.e. towards the ulnar

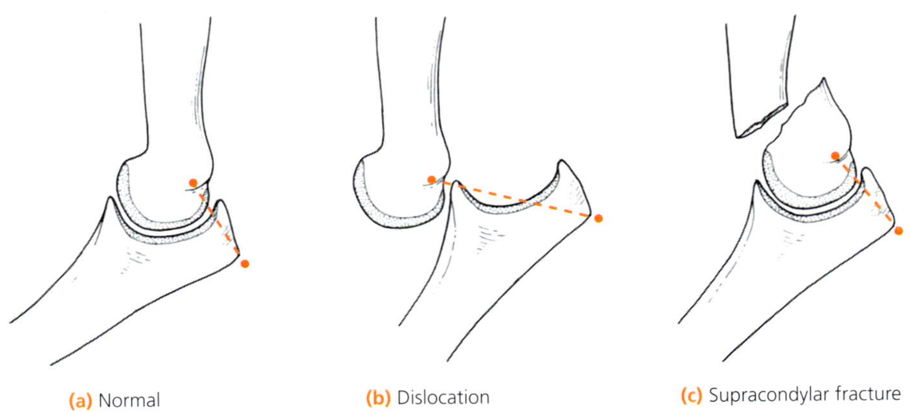

Figure 3.1 The relationship of the medial and lateral epicondyles to the olecranon process **(a)** is disturbed in a dislocation of the elbow **(b)** but maintained in a supracondylar fracture **(c)**.

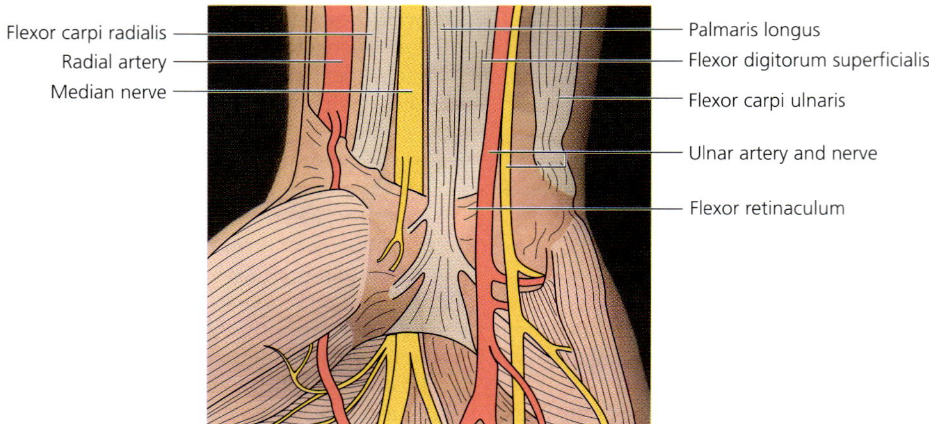

Figure 3.2 The structures on the anterior aspect of the right wrist.

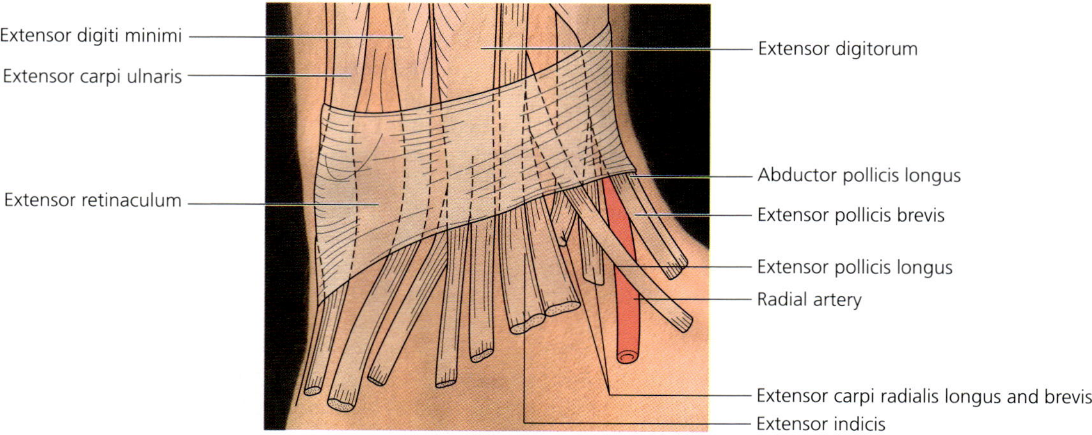

Figure 3.3 The structures on the posterior aspect of the right wrist.

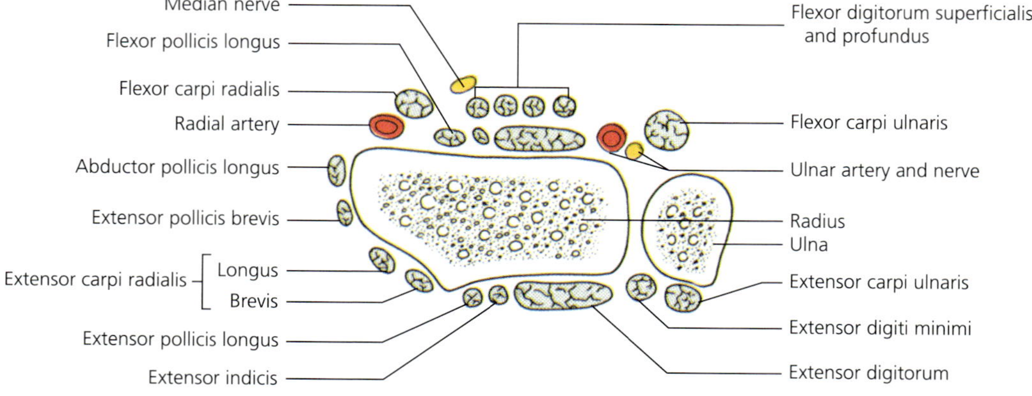

Figure 3.4 Section immediately above the wrist joint.

border) – the last can be traced to the base of the terminal phalanx of the extended thumb. The tendons of extensor digitorum are seen in the extended hand passing over the dorsal aspects of the proximal phalanges of the fingers.

Vessels

Arteries

The arteries of upper limb comprise the axillary, brachial, radial and ulnar arteries. The axillary artery is the continuation of subclavian artery at the outer border of the 1st rib.

Feel the pulsations of the *subclavian artery* against the 1st rib, the *brachial artery* against the humerus, the *radial* and *ulnar* arteries at the wrist and the *radial artery* again in the anatomical snuffbox.

The **brachial artery** bifurcates into its **radial and ulnar branches** at the level of the neck of the radius and the line of the radial artery then corresponds to the slight groove which can be seen along the ulnar border of the tensed brachioradialis.

Veins

The veins of the upper limb (Fig. 3.5) comprise the *deep venae comitantes*, which accompany all the main arteries, usually in pairs, and the much more important superficial veins – more important both in size and in practical value because of their use for venepuncture and transfusion.

These superficial veins can be seen as a dorsal venous network on the back of the hand that drains into a lateral *cephalic* and medial *basilic* vein.

The **cephalic vein** at its origin lies fairly constantly in the superficial fascia just posterior to the radial styloid; even if not visible it can be cut down upon confidently at this site. It then runs up the anterior aspect of the forearm to lie in a groove along the lateral border of the biceps and then, after piercing the deep fascia, in

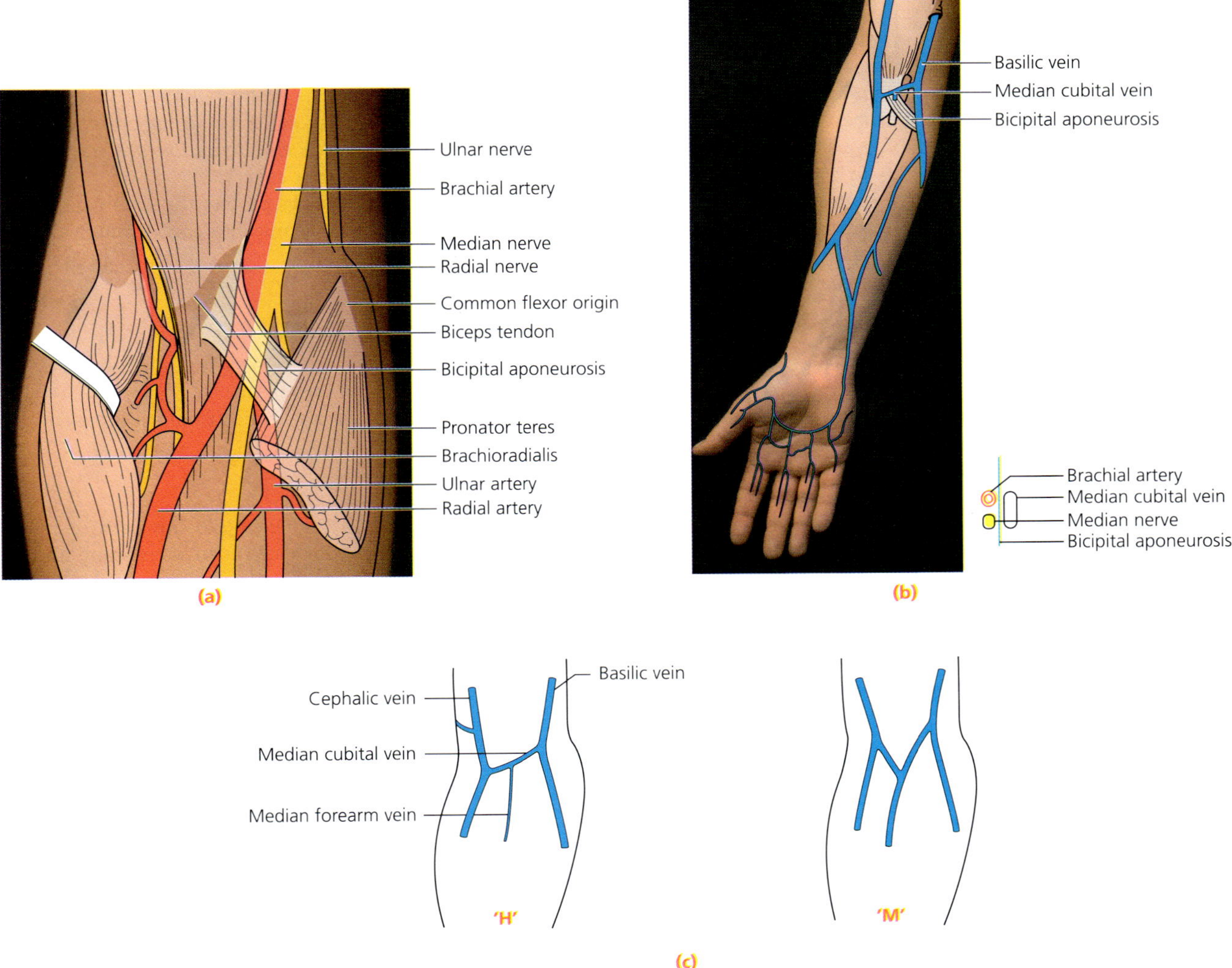

Figure 3.5 (a) The cubital fossa with the bicipital aponeurosis in detail. (b) The superficial veins of the upper limb. (Note the bicipital aponeurosis situated between the median cubital vein and brachial artery*.) (c) Two common arrangements in the formation of the median cubital vein.

the groove between pectoralis major and the deltoid, where again it can readily be exposed for an emergency cut-down. It finally penetrates the clavipectoral fascia to enter the axillary vein.

The **basilic vein** runs along the posteromedial aspect of the forearm, passes on to the anterior aspect just below the elbow and pierces the deep fascia at about the middle of the upper arm. At the edge of the posterior axillary fold it is joined by the venae comitantes of the brachial artery to form the axillary vein.

Linking the cephalic and basilic veins just distal to the front of the elbow is the **median cubital vein**, usually the most prominent superficial vein in the body and visible or palpable when all others are hidden in fat or collapsed in shock. It usually runs upwards and medially from the cephalic to the basilic vein, giving a rather drunken 'H'-shaped appearance, and receiving a median forearm vein. A frequent variant is for the median forearm vein to bifurcate just distal to the fossa – one branch passing to the cephalic, the other to the basilic vein – giving an 'M'-shaped pattern, which replaces the median cubital vein. Since this area is so often used in venepuncture, you will soon be familiar with these two appearances (Fig. 3.5(b) and (c)). It was the antecubital vein that was favoured for the operation of bleeding, or phlebotomy, in days gone by; the underlying brachial artery was protected from the barber–surgeon's knife by the *bicipital aponeurosis*, a condensation of deep fascia passing across from the biceps tendon, which was, therefore, termed the 'grâce à Dieu' (praise be to God) fascia.

In more modern times one tries to avoid using this vein for injection of intravenous barbiturates and other irritant drugs because of the slight risk of entering the brachial artery and also because of the danger of piercing a superficially placed abnormal ulnar artery in occasional instances of high brachial bifurcation.

Nerves

A number of nerves in the upper limb can be palpated, particularly in a thin subject; these are the *supraclavicular nerves*, as they pass over the clavicle, the cords of the *brachial plexus* against the humeral head (with the arm abducted), the *median nerve* in the mid-upper arm, crossing over the brachial artery, the *ulnar nerve* in the groove of the medial epicondyle and the *superficial radial nerve* as it passes over the tendon of extensor pollicis longus at the wrist.

The median nerve lies first lateral then medial to the brachial artery, crossing it at the mid-upper arm, usually superficially but occasionally deeply. This close relationship is of historical interest: Nelson (Lord (Viscount) Horatio Nelson (1758–1805) was one of England's greatest heroes; he was the most inspiring leader ever to command the British Navy) had his median nerve accidentally incorporated in the ligature around the artery when his arm was amputated above the elbow.

Useful surface markings of other, impalpable, nerves may be listed as follows:

1. The *axillary nerve* is related closely to the surgical neck of the humerus 2 in. (5 cm) below the acromion process.
2. The *radial nerve* crosses the posterior aspect of the humeral shaft at its mid-point.
3. The *posterior interosseous branch* of the radial nerve is located by Henry's method as it winds round the radius. Place three fingers along the lateral aspect of the upper end of the radius; the uppermost finger lies on the radial head (feel it rotate on pronation and supination), and the lowermost lies over the nerve.
4. The *median nerve* (Figs 3.2 and 3.4) in the forearm lies, as its name suggests, in the median plane; its area of distribution in the hand is thus anaesthetized if local anaesthetic is injected exactly in the midline at the wrist.
5. The *ulnar nerve* at the wrist lies immediately medial to the ulnar pulse (Figs 3.2 and 3.4). In the hand, it passes on the radial side of the pisiform and then lies on the hook of the hamate. If you press with your fingernail just lateral to the pisiform bone, you will experience tingling in your ulnar two fingers.

Bones and joints of the upper limb

Scapula (Fig. 3.6)

The scapula is a flat triangular bone on the upper part of the back of chest. This triangular bone bears three prominent features: the *glenoid fossa* laterally (which is the scapula's contribution to the shoulder joint), the *spine* on its posterior aspect, projecting laterally as the *acromion process*, and the *coracoid process* on its anterior aspect.

Its strong muscular coverings protect the scapula and only rarely is it fractured, and then only as a consequence of direct and severe violence.

Clavicle (Fig. 3.6)

The clavicle is a curbed long bone lying horizontally at the junction neck and front of the chest.

This long bone has a number of unusual features. They are as follows:

1. It has no medullary cavity.
2. It is the first to ossify in the foetus (5th–6th week).
3. Although a long bone, it develops in membrane and not in cartilage.
4. It is the most commonly fractured long bone in the body.

The clavicle is made up of a medial two-thirds, which is circular in section and convex anteriorly, and a lateral one-third, which is flattened in section and convex posteriorly.

Medially it articulates with the manubrium at the *sternoclavicular joint*, which contains a cartilaginous disc (an important, and often overlooked, structure). It is a ball-and-socket joint that moves reciprocally with the movements of the shoulder joint, around its fulcrum – the costoclavicular ligament. Put a finger on the medial end of your clavicle; raise your shoulder – the sternoclavicular joint is depressed; retract your shoulder – the sternoclavicular joint protracts, and so on. The patient may complain of a 'painful stiff shoulder' when he actually has arthritis of the sternoclavicular joint.

Laterally it articulates with the acromion at the *acromioclavicular joint* (the joint containing an incomplete articular disc) and, in addition, is attached to the coracoid process by the tough coracoclavicular ligament.

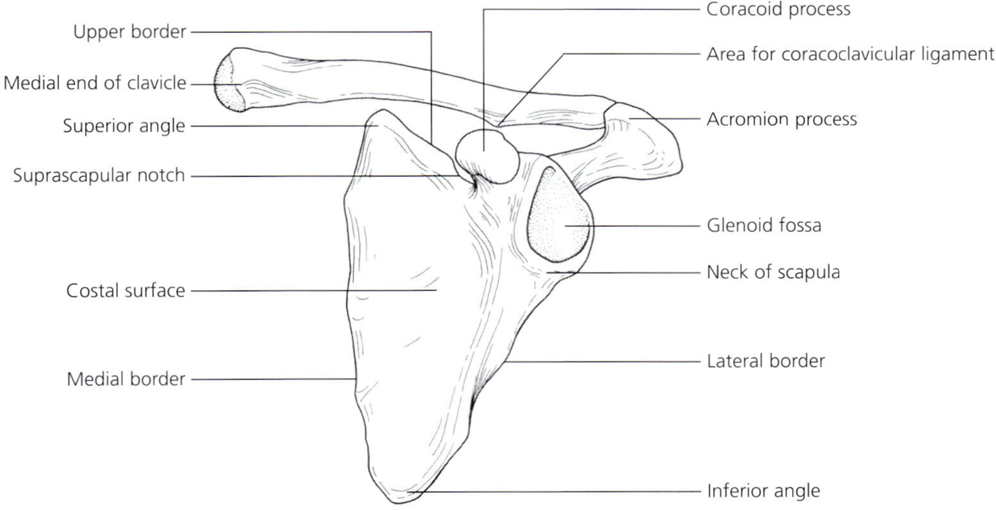

Figure 3.6 The left scapula and clavicle (anterior aspect).

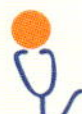

Clinical Features

The clavicle has three functions as mentioned below:

1 To transmit forces from the upper limb to the axial skeleton;
2 To act as a strut holding the arm free from the trunk, to hang supported principally by trapezius;
3 To provide attachment for muscles.

The weakest point along the clavicle is the junction of the middle and outer third. Transmission of forces to the axial skeleton in falls on the shoulder or hand may prove greater than the strength of the bone at this site, and this indirect force is the usual cause of fracture.

When fracture occurs, the trapezius is unable to support the weight of the arm so that the characteristic picture of the patient with a fractured clavicle is that of a man supporting his sagging upper limb with his opposite hand. The lateral fragment is not only depressed but also drawn medially by the shoulder adductors, principally teres major, latissimus dorsi and pectoralis major (Fig. 3.7).

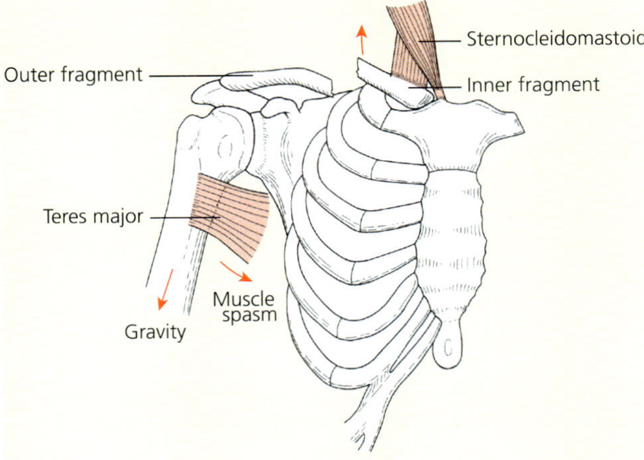

Figure 3.7 The deformity of a fractured clavicle – downward displacement and adduction of the outer fragment by gravity and muscle spasm, respectively; slight elevation of the inner fragment by the sternocleidomastoid.

The third part of the subclavian vessels and the trunks of the brachial plexus pass behind the middle third of the shaft of the clavicle, separated only by the thin subclavius muscle. Fractures of the clavicle are common, yet associated injury of the underlying subclavian vessels (except in penetrating gunshot wounds) is extremely rare because of the protection offered by this functionally insignificant slip of a muscle. Rarely, these vessels (protected by the subclavius) are torn by the fragments of a fractured clavicle; this was the cause of death of Sir Robert Peel (Prime Minister of the United Kingdom 1834–1835, and again 1841–1846) following a fall from his horse.

The sternal end of the clavicle has important posterior relations; behind the sternoclavicular joints lie the common carotid artery on the left and the bifurcation of the brachiocephalic artery on the right. The internal jugular vein lies a little more laterally on either side. These vessels are separated from bone by the strap muscles – the sternohyoid and sternothyroid.

Humerus (Fig. 3.8)

The humerus is the long bone of the arm. The upper end of the humerus consists of a *head* (one-third of a sphere) facing medially, upwards and backwards, separated from the *greater* and *lesser tubercles* by the *anatomical neck*. The tubercles, in turn, are separated from each other by the *bicipital groove (intertubercular sulcus)* along which emerges the long head of biceps from the shoulder joint.

Where the upper end and the shaft of the humerus meet there is the narrow *surgical neck* against which lie the axillary nerve and circumflex humeral vessels. The shaft itself is circular in section above and flattened in its lower part. The posterior aspect of the shaft bears the faint *spiral groove* demarcating the origins of the medial and lateral heads of the triceps between which wind the radial nerve and the accompanying profunda brachii vessels.

The lower end of the humerus bears the rounded *capitulum* laterally, for articulation with the radial head, and the spool-shaped *trochlea* medially, articulating with the trochlear notch of the ulna.

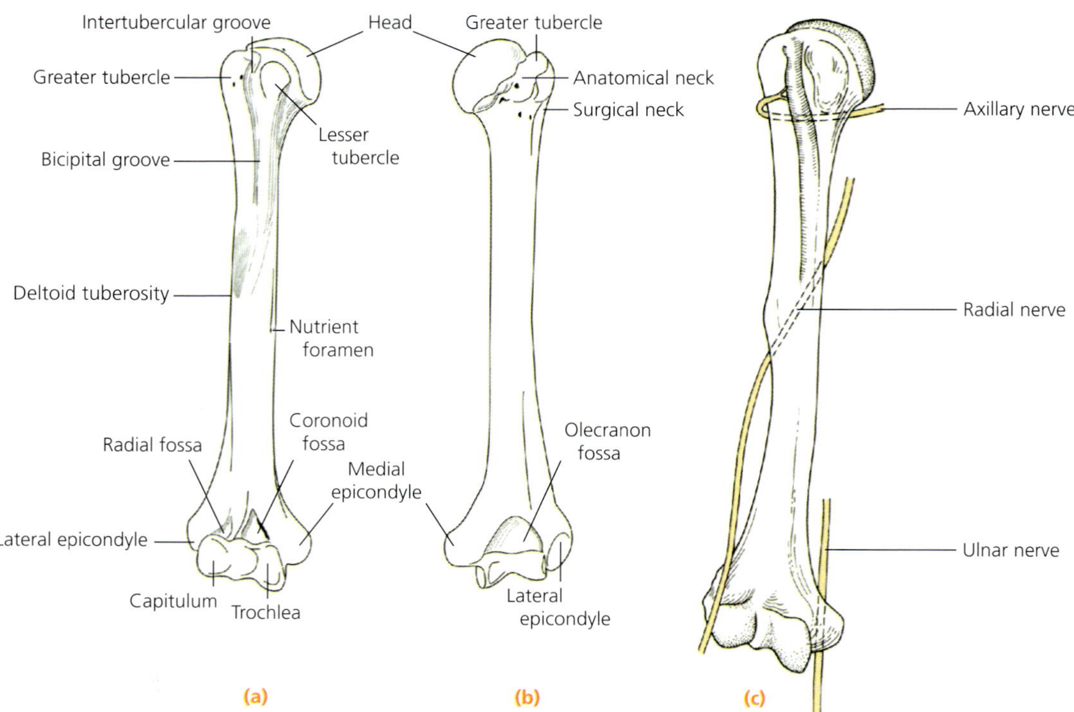

Figure 3.8 The (a) anterior and (b) posterior views of the right humerus. (c) The humerus with its three major related nerves – axillary, radial and ulnar – all of which are in danger of injury in humeral fractures.

The *medial* and *lateral epicondyles,* on either side, are extracapsular; the medial is the larger of the two, extends more distally and bears a groove on its posterior aspect for the *ulnar nerve.*

Three important nerves thus come into close contact with the humerus – the axillary, the radial and the ulnar; they may be damaged, respectively, in fractures of the humeral neck, midshaft and lower end (Fig. 3.8).

It is an important practical point to note that the lower end of the humerus is angulated forwards 45° on the shaft. This is easily confirmed by examining a lateral radiograph of the elbow, when it will be seen that a vertical line continued downwards along the front of the shaft bisects the capitulum. Any decrease of this angulation indicates backward displacement of the distal end of the humerus and is good radiographic evidence of a supracondylar fracture.

Radius and ulna (Fig. 3.9)

The radius is a long, lateral bone of the forearm. It consists of the *head, neck, shaft* (with its *radial tuberosity*) and expanded distal end. The ulna is a long, medial bone of the forearm. It consists of an upper end, a shaft and a lower end. Its upper expanded end comprises *olecranon, trochlear fossa, coronoid process* (with its *radial notch* for articulation with the radial head), *shaft* and small distal *head,* which articulates with the medial side of the distal end of the radius at the inferior radio-ulnar joint.

In pronation and supination, the head of the radius rotates against the radial notch of the ulna, the shaft of the radius swings round the relatively fixed ulnar shaft (the two bones being connected by a fibrous interosseous membrane/ligament) and the distal end of the radius rotates against the head of the ulna. This axis of rotation passes from the radial head proximally to the ulnar head distally.

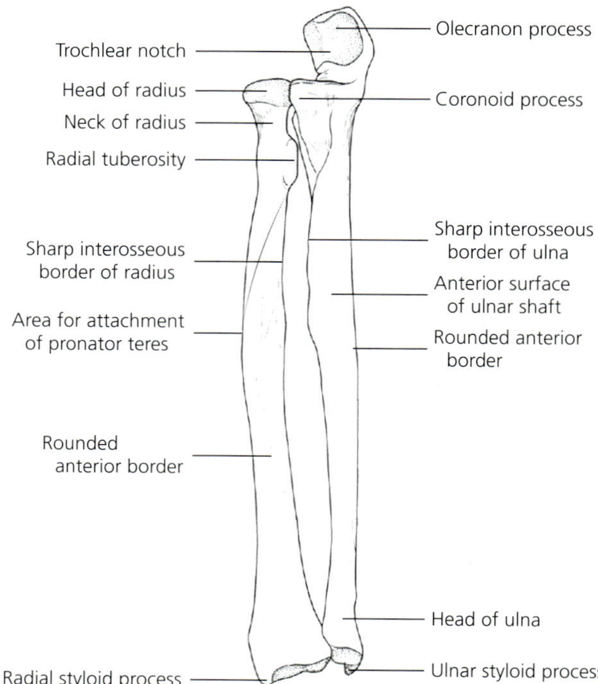

Figure 3.9 The right radius and ulna – anterior aspect.

Clinical Features

1 The pronator teres is inserted midway along the radial shaft. If the radius is fractured proximal to this, the proximal fragment is supinated (by the action of the biceps) and the distal fragment is pronated by pronator teres. The fracture must, therefore, be splinted with the forearm supinated so that the distal fragment is aligned with the supinated proximal end. If the fracture is distal to the midshaft, the actions of biceps and the pronator muscles more or less balance and the fracture is, therefore, immobilized with the forearm in the neutral position (Fig. 3.10).

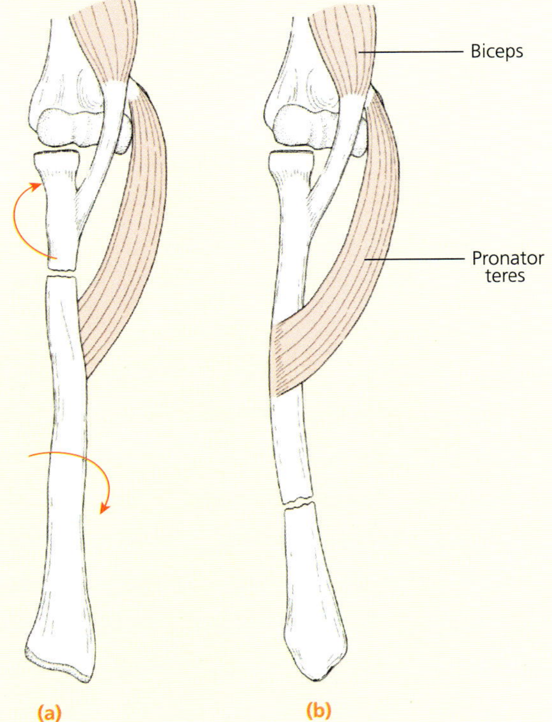

Figure 3.10 The important role of pronator teres in radial fractures. **(a)** In proximal fractures, above the insertion of pronator teres, the distal fragment is pronated. Such a fracture must be splinted in the supinated position. **(b)** When the fracture is distal to the insertion of pronator teres, the action of this muscle on the proximal fragment is cancelled by the supinator action of biceps. This fracture is, therefore, held reduced in the neutral position, midway between pronation and supination.

2 The force of a fall on the hand produces different effects in different age groups: in a child it may cause a posterior displacement of the distal radial epiphysis; in the young adult the shafts of the radius and ulna may fracture, or the scaphoid may fracture (*see* page 102); in the elderly the most likely result will be a *Colles' fracture*. In the last injury, the radius fractures approximately 1 in. (2.5 cm) proximal to the wrist joint; the distal fragment is displaced posteriorly and usually becomes impacted. The shortening which results brings the styloid processes of the radius and ulna more or less in line with each other.

Another forearm injury resulting from a fall on the outstretched hand is fracture of the head of the radius, due to its being crushed against the capitulum of the humerus.

(*Continued ...*)

(*... continued*)

3 The olecranon process may be fractured by direct violence but more often it is avulsed by forcible contraction of the triceps, which is inserted into its upper aspect. In these circumstances the bone ends are widely displaced and operative repair, to reconstruct the integrity of the elbow joint, becomes essential.

4 A subcutaneous bursa is constantly present over the olecranon and is likely to become inflamed when exposed to repeated trauma. Students and coal miners share this hazard so that olecranon bursitis goes by the nicknames of '**student's elbow**' and '**miner's elbow**'. Although I have seen many miners with this lesion, I have yet to see a medical student thus disabled.

Bones of the hand (Fig. 3.11)

Bones of hand comprises the carpals, metacarpals and phalanges. The carpal bones together form the corpus (anatomical wrist).The *carpus* is made up of two rows, each containing four bones. In the proximal row, from the lateral to the medial side, are the *scaphoid*, *lunate* and *triquetral*, the last bearing the *pisiform* on its anterior surface, into which sesamoid bone the flexor carpi ulnaris tendon is inserted.

In the distal row, from the lateral to the medial side, are the *trapezium*, *trapezoid*, *capitate* and *hamate*.

The carpus as a whole is arched transversely, the palmar aspect being concave. This is maintained by the following:

1. The shapes of the individual bones, which are broader posteriorly than anteriorly (except for the lunate, which is broader anteriorly)
2. The tough *flexor retinaculum* passing from the scaphoid and the ridge of the trapezium laterally to the pisiform and the hook of the hamate medially (Fig. 3.12)
3. Distal to the carpal bones lie the five metacarpals, slender bones apart from the first – that of the thumb, which is stout and set at right angles to the palm of the hand. In front of

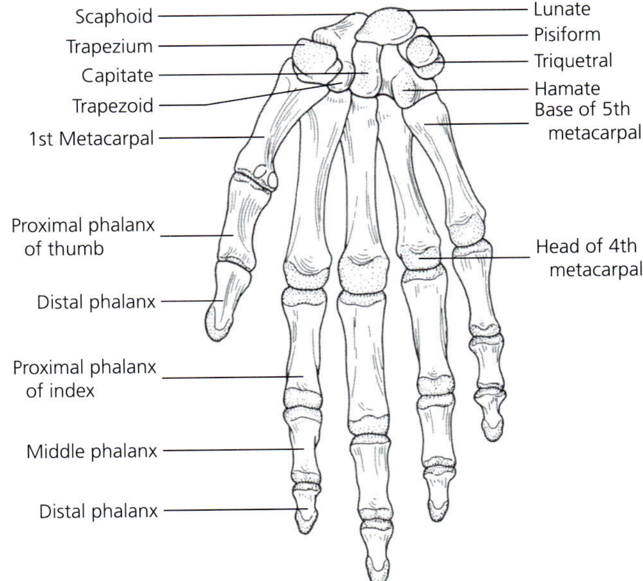

Figure 3.11 The right carpus, metacarpus and phalanges (anterior aspect).

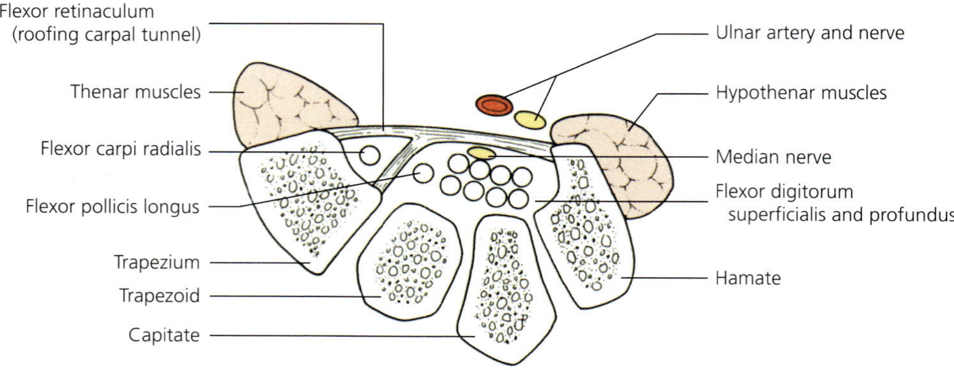

Figure 3.12 Transverse section through the distal carpus (right side viewed from the distal end), showing the attachments of the flexor retinaculum. Note the separate osseofascial compartment for the tendon of flexor carpi radialis. Note also that, at this level, the tendon of flexor carpi ulnaris has 'disappeared'. It attaches to the pisiform, in the proximal row of carpal bones.

the head of this metacarpal are two tiny sesamoid bones (in the insertions of the heads of flexor pollicis brevis), which are easily visible on a plain radiograph of the hand. Distally, the metacarpals articulate with the phalanges, of which there are two in the thumb and three in each of the other four fingers (Fig. 3.11). The important articulations between these small bones of the hand are considered on page 107

Clinical Features

1 A fall on the hand may dislocate the rest of the carpal arch backwards from the lunate which, as commented on above, is wide-based anteriorly (perilunate dislocation of the carpus). The dislocated carpus may then reduce spontaneously, only to push the lunate forwards and tilt it over so that its distal articular surface faces forwards (dislocation of the lunate).

2 The scaphoid may be fractured by a fall on the palm with the hand abducted, in which position the scaphoid lies directly facing the radius.

The blood supply of the scaphoid in one-third of cases enters distally along its waist so that, if the fracture is proximal, the blood supply to this small proximal fragment may be completely cut off with resultant avascular necrosis of this portion of bone (Fig. 3.13).

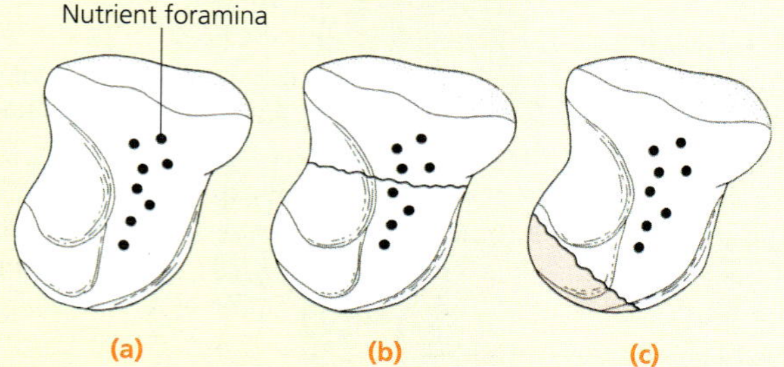

Figure 3.13 Blood supply of the scaphoid. **(a)** Blood vessels enter the bone principally in its distal half. **(b)** A fracture through the waist of the scaphoid – vessels to the proximal fragment are preserved. **(c)** A fracture near the proximal pole of the scaphoid – in this case there are no vessels supplying the proximal fragment and aseptic necrosis of bone is, therefore, inevitable.

(Continued ...)

(... continued)

3 *'The carpal tunnel syndrome'*. The flexor retinaculum forms the roof of a tunnel, the floor and walls of which are made up of the concavity of the carpus. Packed within this tunnel are the long flexor tendons of the fingers and thumb together with the median nerve (Fig. 3.11). Any lesion diminishing the size of the compartment – for example, an old fracture or arthritic change – may result in compression of the median nerve, resulting in paraesthesiae, numbness and motor weakness in its distribution. Since the superficial palmar branch of the median nerve is given off proximal to the retinaculum, there is usually no sensory impairment in the palm.

It is interesting that this syndrome also often occurs, especially in elderly women, without any very obvious cause, although symptoms are relieved by dividing the retinaculum longitudinally.

Shoulder joint (Figs 3.14 and 3.15)

The shoulder joint (glenohumeral joint) is a typical synovial joint of the ball-and-socket type, between the relatively large *head of humerus* and the relatively small and shallow *glenoid fossa,* although the latter is deepened somewhat by the cartilaginous ring of the *labrum glenoidale.*

The joint *capsule* is lax and is attached around the epiphyseal lines of both the glenoid and the humeral head. However, it does extend down on to the diaphysis on the medial aspect of the neck of the humerus, so that an osteomyelitis of the upper end of the humeral shaft may involve the joint by direct spread.

The capsule is lined on the inside by synovial membrane, which is prolonged along the tendon of the long head of the biceps as this traverses the joint. The synovium also communicates with the *subscapular bursa* beneath the tendon of subscapularis.

The stability of the shoulder joint depends almost entirely on the strength of the surrounding muscles, which may be grouped into the following:

1. The closely related short muscles of the 'rotator cuff' (*see* the following section)

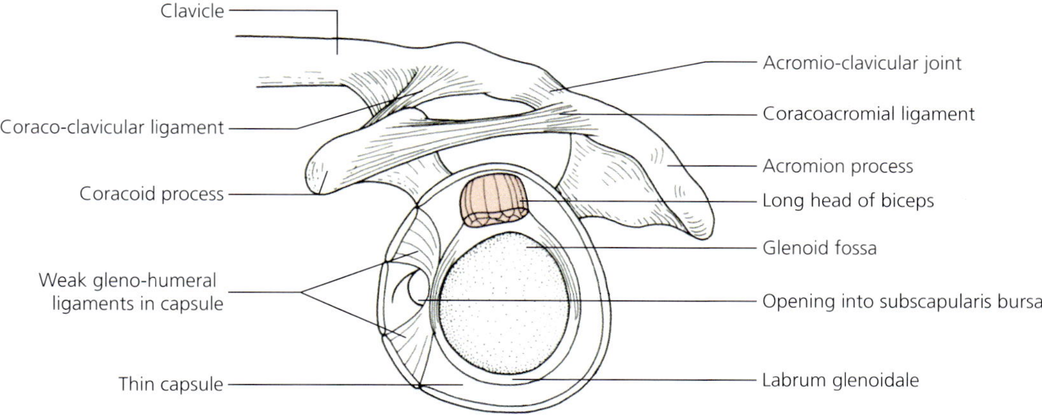

Figure 3.14 The left shoulder joint (viewed from the lateral aspect) – its ligaments are shown after removal of the humerus.

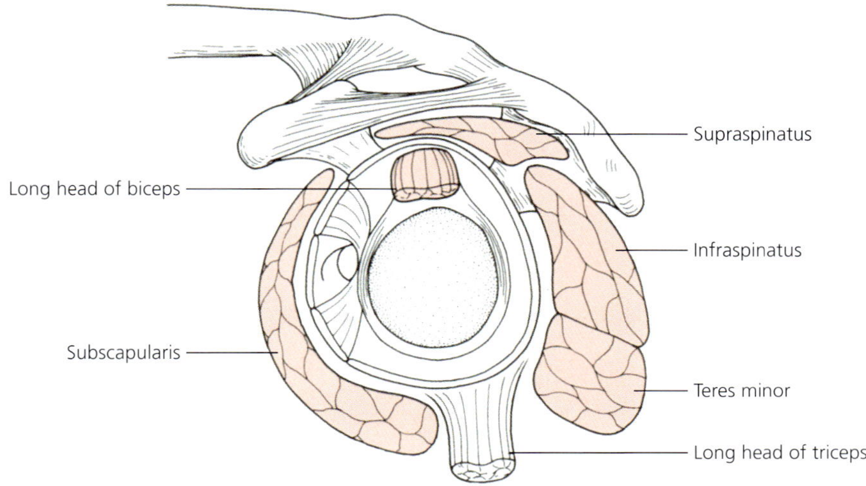

Figure 3.15 The shoulder joint – the same view as in Fig. 3.14, but now with the addition of the surrounding muscles.

2. The long head of biceps brachii, arising from the supraglenoid tubercle and crossing over the head of the humerus, thus lying actually within the joint, although enclosed in a tube of synovium
3. The more distantly related long muscles of the shoulder: the deltoid, long head of triceps, pectoralis major, latissimus dorsi and teres major

Movements of the shoulder girdle

The movements of the shoulder joint itself cannot be divorced from those of the whole shoulder girdle. Even if the shoulder joint is fused, a wide range of movement is still possible by elevation, depression, rotation and protraction of the scapula, leverage occurring at the sternoclavicular joint, the pivot being the costoclavicular ligament.

Abduction of the shoulder is initiated by the supraspinatus; the deltoid can then abduct to 90°. Further movement to 180° (elevation) is brought about by rotation of the scapula upwards by the trapezius and serratus anterior. Shoulder and shoulder girdle movements combine into one smooth action. As soon as abduction commences at the shoulder joint, so rotation of the scapula begins. Test this on yourself or on a colleague by palpating the lower pole of the scapula. This will be felt to swing outwards on initiation of shoulder abduction. Movements of the scapula occur with reciprocal movements at the sternoclavicular joint. Place a finger on this joint; elevate the shoulder and the joint will be felt to depress; swing the shoulder forwards and it will be felt to move backwards, and so on.

Rotator cuff' (Figs 3.15 and 3.16) is the name given to the sheath of tendons of the short muscles of the shoulder which covers and blends with all but the inferior aspect of that joint. The muscles are the supraspinatus, infraspinatus and teres minor, which are inserted from above down into the humeral greater tubercle, and the subscapularis, which is inserted into the lesser tubercle. All originate from the scapula.

Of these muscles, the supraspinatus is of the greatest practical importance. It passes over the apex of the shoulder beneath the acromion process and coracoacromial ligament, from which it is separated by the *subacromial bursa*. This bursa is continued beneath the deltoid as the *subdeltoid bursa* forming, together, the largest bursa in the body.

The supraspinatus initiates the abduction of the humerus on the scapula; if the tendon is torn as a result of injury, active

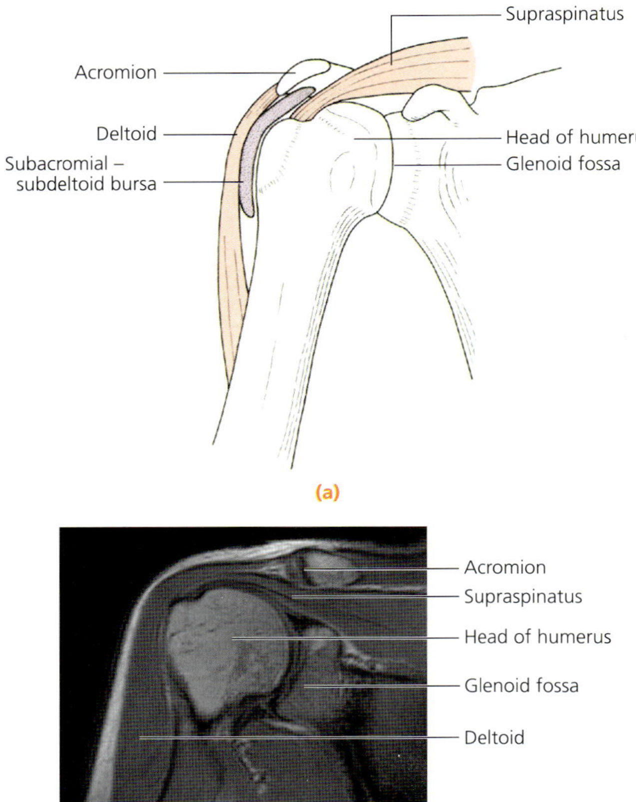

Figure 3.16 **(a)** Supraspinatus and the subacromial–subdeltoid bursa. Note that the supraspinatus tendon lies close against the acromion – if this tendon is inflamed, there is a painful arc of movement as the shoulder is abducted from 60° to 120°, because, in this range, the inflamed tendon impinges against the acromion. **(b)** Magnetic resonance imaging of the shoulder showing the detailed anatomy revealed by this technique.

initiation of abduction becomes impossible and the patient has to develop the trick movement of tilting his body towards the injured side so that gravity passively swings the arm from his trunk. Once this occurs, the deltoid and the scapular rotators can then come into play.

Inflammation of the supraspinatus tendon ('*supraspinatus tendinitis*') is characterized by a painful arc of shoulder movement between 60° and 120°; in this range, the tendon impinges against the overlying acromion and the coracoacromial ligament. The investigation of soft-tissue lesions around the shoulder has been greatly facilitated by magnetic resonance imaging (MRI), which reveals the anatomical structures in exquisite detail (Fig. 3.16(b)).

Principal muscles acting on the shoulder joint

Abductors
- supraspinatus (initiates)
- deltoid

Adductors
- pectoralis major
- latissimus dorsi
- subscapularis

Flexors
- biceps brachii
- pectoralis major
- coracobrachialis
- deltoid (anterior fibres)

Extensors
- triceps brachii
- teres major
- latissimus dorsi
- deltoid (posterior fibres)

Medial rotators
- pectoralis major
- latissimus dorsi
- teres major
- deltoid (anterior fibres)
- subscapularis

Lateral rotators
- infraspinatus
- teres minor
- deltoid (posterior fibres)

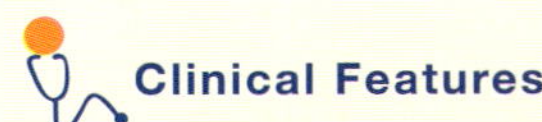

Clinical Features

Dislocation of the shoulder

The wide range of movement possible at the shoulder is achieved only at the cost of stability, and for this reason it is the most commonly dislocated major joint. Its inferior aspect is completely unprotected by muscles and it is here that, in violent abduction, the humeral head may slip away from the glenoid to lie in the subglenoid region, whence it usually passes anteriorly into a subcoracoid position (Fig. 3.17).

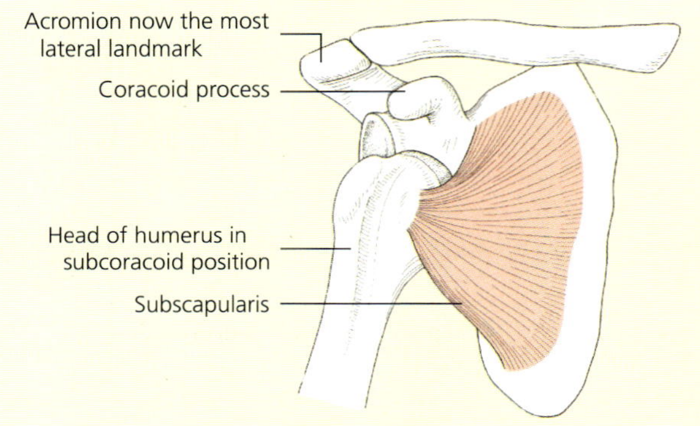

Figure 3.17 The deformity of shoulder dislocation. The dislocated head of the humerus is held adducted by the shoulder girdle muscles and internally rotated by subscapularis.

The axillary nerve, lying in relation to the surgical neck of the humerus, may be torn in this injury. Assess this in the patient before reducing the dislocation by testing for loss of cutaneous sensation over the deltoid.

The head of the humerus is drawn medially by the powerful adductors of the shoulder; its greater tubercle, therefore, no longer remains the most lateral bony projection of the shoulder region, being replaced for this honour by the acromion process. The normal bulge of the deltoid over the greater tubercle is lost; instead, there is the characteristic flattening of this muscle.

In reducing the dislocation by *Kocher's method* the elbow is flexed and the forearm rotated outwards; this stretches the subscapularis, which is holding the humeral head internally rotated. The elbow is then swung medially across the trunk, thus levering the head of the humerus laterally so that it slips back into place.

In the *Hippocratic method*, the foot is used as a fulcrum in the axilla, traction and adduction being applied to the forearm; in this way, the humeral head is levered outwards into its normal position.

Elbow joint (Figs 3.18 and 3.19)

The elbow joint is generally described as a synovial joint of hinge variety. This joint, although has a single synovial cavity, is made up of three distinct articulations, which are:

1. The *humero-ulnar*, between the trochlea of the humerus and the trochlear notch of the ulna (a hinge joint)
2. The *humeroradial*, between the capitulum and the upper concave surface of the radial head (a ball-and-socket joint)
3. The *superior radio-ulnar*, between the head of the radius and the radial notch of the ulna, the head being held in place by the tough annular ligament (a pivot joint)

The *capsule* of the elbow joint is closely applied around this complex articular arrangement; the non-articular medial and lateral epicondyles are extracapsular. The capsule is thin and loose anteriorly and posteriorly to allow flexion and extension, whereas it is strongly thickened on either side, being reinforced by the *medial* and *lateral collateral* ligaments. The lateral ligament is attached distally to the *annular ligament* around the radial head. In order to allow rotation of the radius, the lower margin of the annular ligament is free and, beneath it, the synovium of the elbow bulges downwards onto the neck of the radius.

Two sets of movements take place at the elbow as mentioned below:

1. Flexion and extension at the humero-ulnar and humeroradial joints
2. Pronation and supination at the proximal radio-ulnar (in conjunction with associated movements of the distal radio-ulnar joint)

Muscles acting on the elbow

Flexors	*Extensors*
biceps brachii	triceps brachii
brachialis	anconeus
brachioradialis	
the forearm flexor muscles	

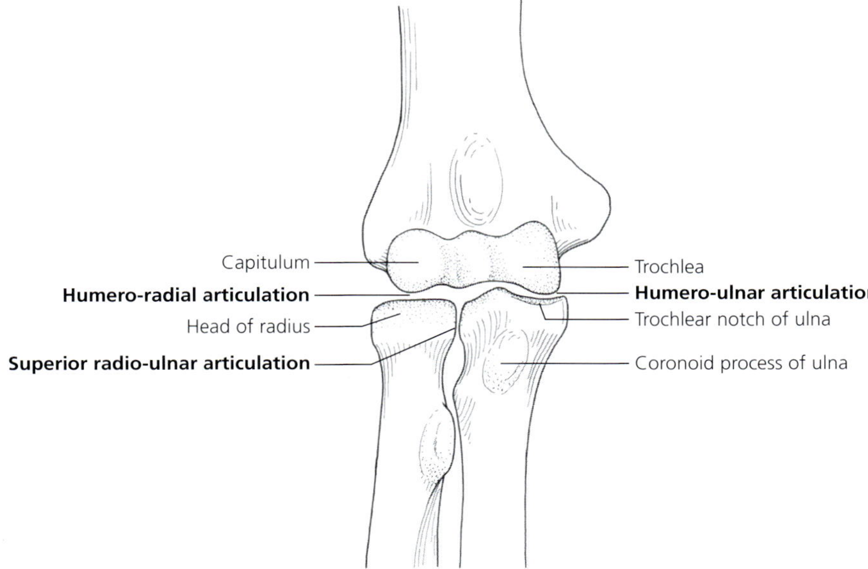

Figure 3.18 The bony components of the elbow joint (right side; anterior aspect). Note the three sets of articular surfaces.

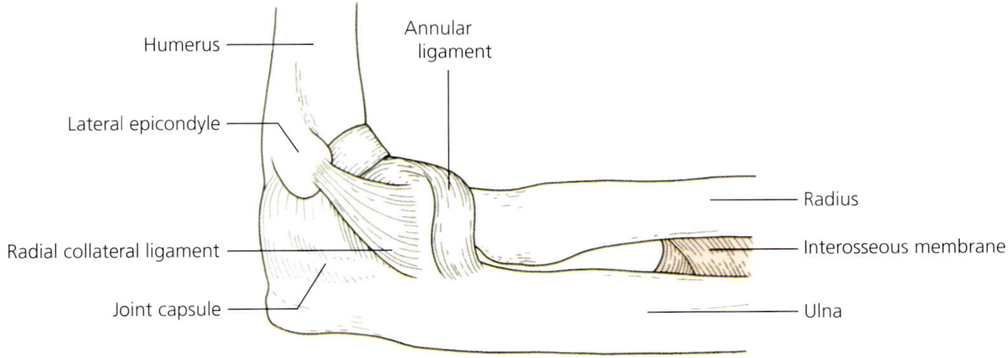

Figure 3.19 The joint capsule of the right elbow – lateral aspect.

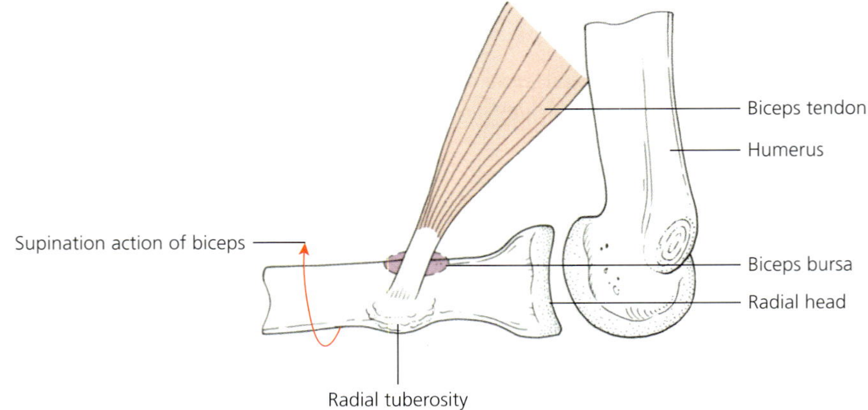

Figure 3.20 The supination action of biceps (right elbow viewed from the medial side with the ulna removed).

Pronators	*Supinators*
pronator teres	biceps
pronator quadratus	supinator

The supinator action of the biceps is due to its insertion on to the *posterior* aspect of the tuberosity of the radius. When the biceps contracts, not only is the forearm flexed, but the radius 'unwinds' as its tuberosity is rotated anteriorly, i.e. the forearm supinates (Fig. 3.20). Biceps is a powerful muscle; hence, supination is more powerful than pronation – try it on yourself. Screwdrivers and cork screws are made for right-handed people to screw in using this supination action.

Wrist joint (Fig. 3.21)

The wrist joint is a synovial joint of ellipsoid variety. The articular disc of the inferior radio-ulnar joint covers the head of the ulna and is attached to the base of the ulnar styloid process. This disc, together with the distal end of the radius, forms the proximal face of the wrist joint, the distal surface being the proximal articular surfaces of the scaphoid, lunate and triquetral.

The wrist joint allows flexion, extension, abduction, adduction and circumduction, the last being a combination of the previous four. Flexion and extension are increased by

Clinical Features

1 The elbow joint is safely approached by a vertical posterior incision that divides the triceps expansion.
2 As the capsule is relatively weak anteriorly and posteriorly it will be distended at these sites by an effusion, particularly posteriorly, since the anterior aspect is covered by muscles and dense deep fascia. Aspiration of such an effusion is readily performed posteriorly on one or other side of the olecranon.
3 The annular ligament is funnel-shaped in adults, but its sides are vertical in young children. A sudden jerk on the arm of a child under the age of 8 years may subluxate the radial head through this ligament ('*pulled elbow*'). Reduction is easily effected by firm supination of the elbow, which 'screws' the radial head back into place.
4 *Posterior dislocation of the elbow* may occur as a result of the indirect violence of a fall on the hand. Occasionally, the coronoid process of the ulna is fractured in this injury, being snapped off against the trochlea of the humerus. Characteristically, the triangular relationship between the olecranon and the two humeral epicondyles is lost (Fig. 3.1). Reduction is effected by traction to overcome the protective spasm of the muscles acting on the joint, together with flexion of the elbow, which levers the humero-ulnar joint back into place.

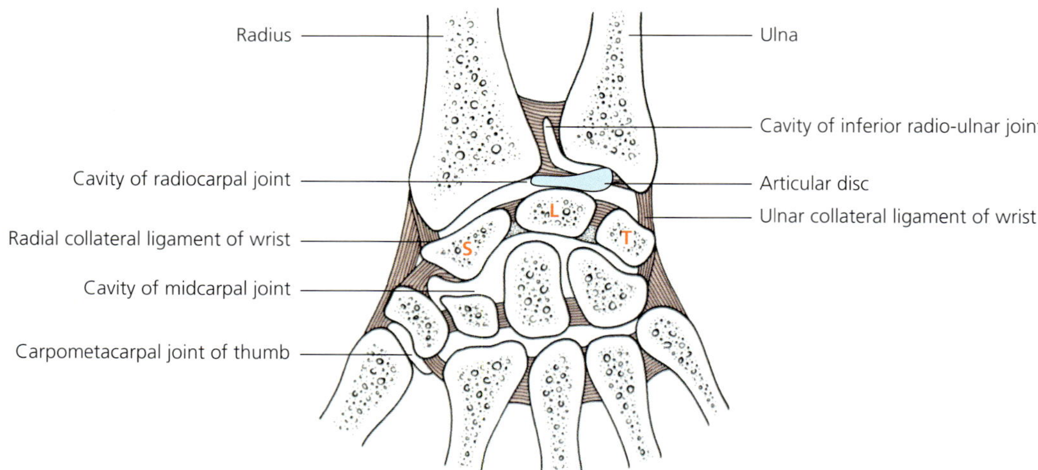

Figure 3.21 The wrist, carpal and carpometacarpal joints in section. S: scaphoid; L: lunate; T: triquetral.

associated sliding movements of the intercarpal joints; although the range of flexion at the wrist is actually less than that of extension, these associated movements make it apparently greater.

Because of the greater distal projection of the radial styloid, the range of abduction at the wrist is considerably less than that of adduction.

Muscles acting on the wrist

Flexors: All the long muscles crossing the anterior aspect of the wrist joint

Extensors: All the long muscles crossing the posterior aspect of the joint

Adductors: Flexor carpi ulnaris acting in concord with extensor carpi ulnaris

Abductors: Flexor carpi radialis and extensores carpi radialis longus and brevis together with the long abductor and short extensor of the thumb

Joints of the hand (Fig. 3.21)

The intercarpal joints between the individual carpal bones are a plane type of synovial joints. They allow gliding movements to occur that increase the range of extension and, more particularly, flexion permitted at the wrist joint.

The *carpometacarpal joint of the thumb* is a synovial joint of a saddle variety. It permits flexion and extension (in a plane parallel to the palm of the hand), abduction and adduction (in a plane at a right angle to the palm) and opposition, in which the thumb is brought across in contact with the 5th finger. This joint's range contrasts with the limited movements of the other carpometacarpal joints, which allow a few degrees of gliding movement of the 2nd and 3rd metacarpals and a small range of flexion and extension of the 4th and 5th metacarpals.

The opposite state of affairs holds at the *metacarpophalangeal joints*; only a 60° range of flexion and extension is possible at the metacarpophalangeal joint of the thumb, whereas a 90° range of flexion and extension, together with abduction, adduction and circumduction, is possible at the four other metacarpophalangeal joints, which are condyloid in shape.

Note that, when the metacarpophalangeal joints of the fingers are flexed, abduction and adduction become impossible. This is because each metacarpal head, although rounded at its distal extremity, is flattened anteriorly; when the base of the proximal phalanx moves onto this flattened surface, side movements become impossible. Moreover, the collateral ligaments on either side of the metacarpophalangeal joints become taut in flexion and thus prevent abduction and adduction.

The metacarpophalangeal joints of the fingers, but not the thumb, are linked by the tough *deep transverse ligaments*, which prevent any spreading of the palm when a firm grip is taken.

All the *interphalangeal joints* have pulley-shaped opposing surfaces and are, therefore, hinge joints, allowing flexion and extension only. At all the metacarpophalangeal and interphalangeal joints the ligamentous arrangements are the same.

1. **Posteriorly:** The joint capsule is replaced by the expansion of the extensor tendon of the digit concerned.
2. **Anteriorly:** The capsule is formed by a dense plate of fibrocartilage. This *palmar ligament* is the response to the friction of the adjacent flexor tendons.
3. **On either side:** The joints are reinforced by the *collateral ligaments*, which are lax in extension and taut in flexion of the joint.

The *carpometacarpal joint of the thumb* may be regarded as the most important joint in the human upper limb. It allows the unique movement, only possible in man, of opposition of the tip of the thumb to one or other of the other fingers – for example, in holding a pen or a scalpel. A fracture of the base of the 1st metacarpal (*Bennett's fracture*) is, therefore, a dangerous injury. Unless anatomical reduction is achieved by pinning the fragments at open operation, osteoarthritic change will take place in the deformed joint with consequent painful limitation of this important movement.

Muscles acting on the hand

The **long flexors of the fingers** are as follows:

1. *Flexor digitorum profundus*, inserted into the bases of the four distal phalanges
2. *Flexor digitorum superficialis*, inserted into the sides of the bases of the four middle phalanges

The profundus tendon pierces that of superficialis over the proximal phalanx.

The profundus flexes the distal interphalangeal joint, superficialis the proximal interphalangeal joint; acting together they flex the fingers and the wrist (Fig. 3.22).

The **long extensors of the fingers** are as follows:

- *Extensor digitorum longus*, reinforced by
- *Extensor indicis*
- Extensor digiti minimi

which join the appropriate tendons of extensor digitorum longus on their edial sides

The tendons of extensor digitorum terminate in each finger by an aponeurotic extensor expansion that covers the dorsum of the proximal phalanx and the sides of its base. It then attaches by a central slip into the base of the middle phalanx and by two lateral slips to the distal phalanx (Fig. 3.22).

The margins of the extensor expansion are reinforced by the tendons of the intrinsic muscles of the fingers in the following ways:

1. The *dorsal* and *palmar interossei* arising from the sides and the fronts of the metacarpals, respectively
2. The *lumbricals*, which arise from the four profundus tendons and run on the radial side of the metacarpophalangeal joints to join the extensor expansion

These intrinsic muscles, arising from the palmar aspect of the hand and inserting along the dorsal aspects of the fingers, have a unique action in that they *flex* the metacarpophalangeal joints and *extend* the interphalangeal joints.

The interossei, together with *abductor digiti minimi*, are responsible for abduction (dorsal interossei) and adduction (ventral interossei) of the fingers. A weak abduction movement accompanies the action of extensor digitorum and the long flexors adduct the fingers in the movement of full flexion. However, if these movements of extension and flexion are eliminated by laying the hand flat on the table, abduction and adduction become purely the actions of the intrinsic muscles.

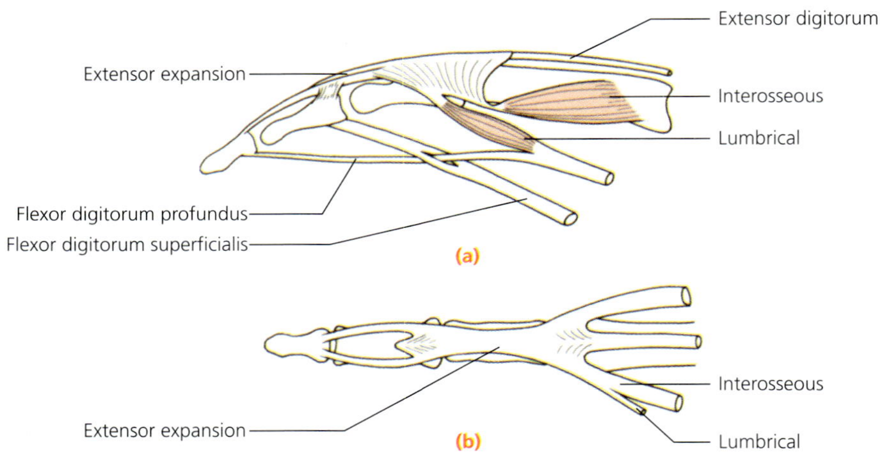

Figure 3.22 The tendons of a finger. **(a)** Lateral view. **(b)** Dorsal (posterior) view.

A card gripped between the fingers in this position of the hand is kept there entirely by intrinsic muscle action.

The 5th finger receives two further intrinsic muscles, *opponens digiti minimi* and *flexor digiti minimi*, from the *hypothenar eminence.*

The **eight muscles acting on the thumb** may be divided into the long (proceeding from the forearm) and the short or intrinsic muscles as mentioned below:

- **Long muscles**
  Flexor pollicis longus – inserted into the distal phalanx
  Extensor pollicis longus – inserted into the distal phalanx
  Extensor pollicis brevis – inserted into the proximal phalanx
  Abductor pollicis longus – inserted into the metacarpal
- **Short muscles**
  Adductor pollicis, *Flexor pollicis brevis*, *Abductor pollicis brevis* – inserted into the base of the proximal phalanx
  Opponens pollicis – along the metacarpal

The flexors and extensors of the wrist play an important synergic role in movements of the hand. Notice how weak the grip becomes when the wrist is fully flexed; it must be held firmly in the extended or neutral position by balanced muscle action in order to allow the long flexors of the fingers and thumb to work at their full stretch and, therefore, at their maximum efficiency.

Three important zones of the upper limb

The three important zones of the upper limb comprise axilla, cubital fossa and carpal tunnel.

Axilla

The axilla (*see* Figs 3.28 and 3.32) is a zone of transition between the neck and the upper limb. It is in the shape of an irregular and somewhat tilted pyramid.

The anterior wall of the axilla is two layers thick. The superficial layer is made up of pectoralis major, while the deep layer is made up of pectoralis minor and subclavius and the clavipectoral fascia that stretches between the two muscles, enclosing both.

The posterior wall is considerably longer, and, from above downwards, it is made up successively of subscapularis, teres major and latissimus dorsi.

The medial wall of the axilla is made up of the lateral aspects of the upper four intercostal spaces, covered by digitations of serratus anterior, while its lateral wall is the medial aspect of the upper part of the arm.

The base of the axillary pyramid is the deep fascia, which stretches from the lateral aspect of the chest wall to the medial aspect of the arm. Termed the axillary fascia, it is attached to the lower edges of both pectoralis major and latissimus dorsi.

The apex of the axilla is truncated and is, in fact, the gap between the middle third of the clavicle and the outer edge of the 1st rib. This gap, known as the cervico-axillary opening, transmits the subclavian artery and brachial plexus from the neck into the axilla, and the axillary vein from the axilla into the neck. The cervico-axillary opening is also traversed by numerous lymphatic channels.

The *contents* of the axilla are the axillary artery and its branches, the axillary vein and its tributaries, the cords of the brachial plexus and their branches, axillary lymph nodes, and the intercostobrachial nerve. All these structures are contained in the axillary fat, which is usually quite substantial.

The organization of the brachial plexus and the course of the axillary artery will be described later (*see* pages 110 and 109, respectively).

Cubital fossa

The cubital fossa (Fig. 3.23) is a zone of transition between the arm and forearm. Situated in front of the elbow joint, the cubital fossa is a triangular intermuscular space.

Boundaries

Its boundaries are as follows:

- **Proximally:** An imaginary line running between the medial and lateral epicondyles of the humerus (this is the base of the triangle)

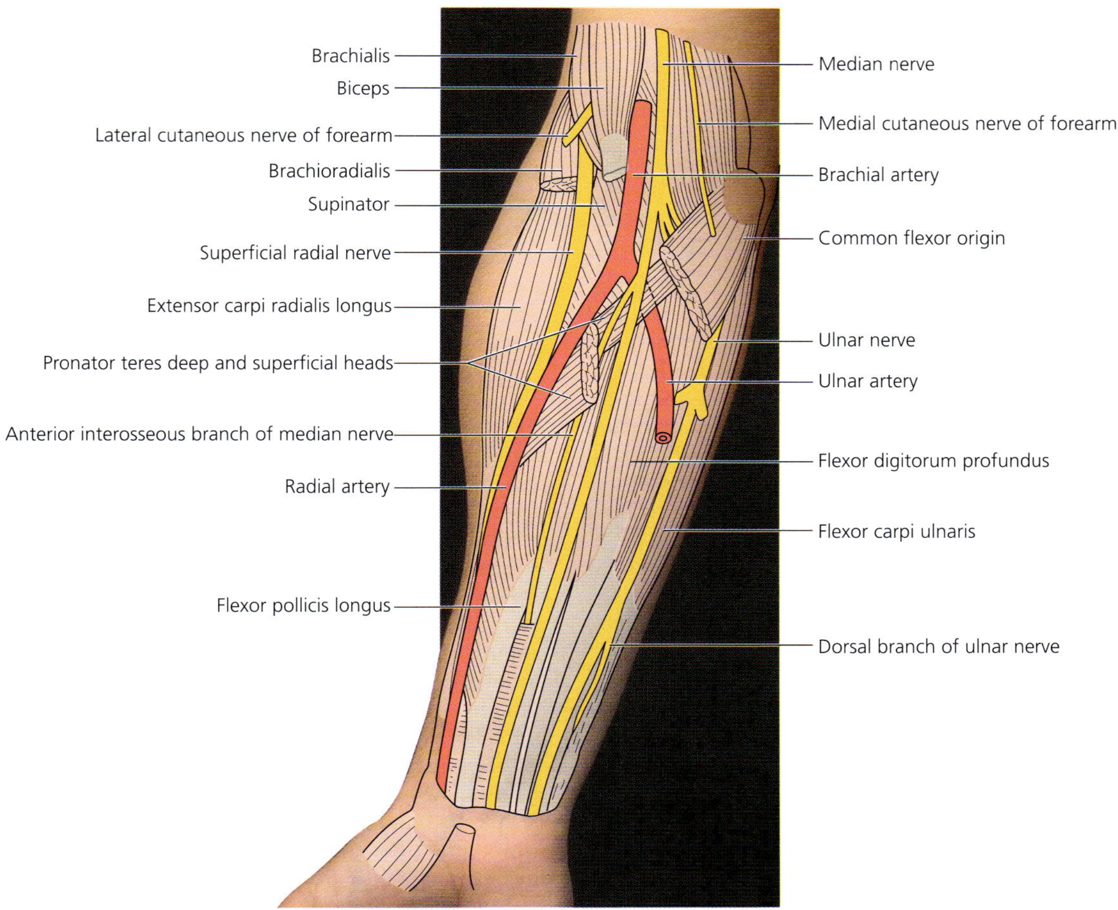

Figure 3.23 Dissection of the right forearm (anterior aspect) to show the principal vessels and nerves. The superficial forearm muscles of the common flexor origin have been removed, apart from pronator teres, which has been partly divided.

- **Laterally:** The brachioradialis muscle
- **Medially:** The pronator teres muscle running obliquely from the medial epicondyle of humerus to the lateral aspect of the radial shaft (Fig. 3.10). The apex of the cubital fossa is, self-evidently, the point where the brachioradialis crosses pronator teres

The *roof* of the cubital fossa is the overlying deep fascia, which is partially reinforced by an extension from the biceps brachii tendon known as the bicipital aponeurosis.

The *floor* of the fossa is the brachialis muscle, behind which is the capsule of the elbow joint.

Contents

The contents of the fossa are, from medial to lateral, the median nerve, the brachial artery flanked by its venae comitantes and the tendon of biceps brachii. If the brachioradialis muscle is undermined and retracted radially, the radial nerve can be brought into view. Of these contents, the brachial artery and the tendon of biceps brachii are readily palpable.

In the distal part of the cubital fossa, the brachial artery divides into its two terminal branches – the radial and ulnar arteries (the latter usually being the larger one).

The contents of the cubital fossa (particularly the brachial artery and median nerve) are vulnerable in supracondylar fractures of the humerus (Fig. 3.1).

Carpal tunnel

The carpal tunnel (Figs 3.2, 3.11 and 3.12) is an osseofibrous space, bounded dorsally by the concave palmar surface of the articulated carpus.

The ventral boundary (i.e. *roof*) of the carpal tunnel is the flexor retinaculum (also known as the transverse carpal ligament).

The flexor retinaculum is a quadrangular sheet of dense fibrous tissue that attaches by its four corners to four carpal bones as follows.

On the radial side it is attached, proximally, to the tubercle of the scaphoid and, distally, to a ridge on the ventral surface of the trapezium. On the ulnar side, it is attached proximally to the pisiform and, distally, to the hook of the hamate. These four bony points are readily palpable in most individuals, enabling the clinician to surface-mark the flexor retinaculum and carpal tunnel with precision.

As has been noted (Fig. 3.12) the carpal tunnel is traversed longitudinally by the four tendons of flexor digitorum superficialis, the four tendons of flexor digitorum profundus, the tendon of flexor pollicis longus and the tendon of flexor carpi radialis (which runs in its own fibrous compartment within the carpal tunnel). Running within the carpal tunnel, adhering to the deep surface of the flexor retinaculum, is the median nerve. *Carpal tunnel syndrome* (described on page 102) denotes a sustained, symptomatic compression of the median nerve in the carpal tunnel. It is by far the most common of all entrapment neuropathies in human pathology.

Arteries of the upper limb

Axillary artery

The axillary artery (*see* Fig. 3.28) commences at the lateral border of the 1st rib, as a continuation of the subclavian, and ends at the lower border of the axilla (i.e. the lower border of teres major) to become the brachial artery. It is divided into three parts by the overlying pectoralis minor muscle and, apart from its very distal extremity, it lies covered by pectoralis major.

Above pectoralis minor, the brachial plexus lies above and behind the artery, but, distal to this, the cords of the plexus take up their positions around the artery according to their names, i.e. lateral, medial and posterior.

The branches of the axillary artery supply the chest wall and shoulder; conveniently; the 1st, 2nd and 3rd parts give off the following one, two and three branches, respectively:

1st Part: 1, Superior thoracic artery

2nd Part: 1, Acromiothoracic trunk
2, Lateral thoracic artery

3rd Part: 1, Subscapular artery
2, Anterior circumflex humeral artery
3, Posterior circumflex humeral artery

All but the circumflex humeral vessels are encountered in the axillary dissection of a radical mastectomy.

Brachial artery

The brachial artery continues on from the axillary artery at the lower border of the teres major and ends at the level of the neck of the radius by dividing into the radial and ulnar arteries. It is superficial (immediately below the deep fascia) along its whole course, except where it is crossed, at the level of the middle of the humerus, by the median nerve, which passes superficially from its lateral to medial side; occasionally, the nerve crosses deep to the artery. Fairly frequently the artery divides into its two terminal branches in the upper arm.

The named branches of the artery are as follows:

- The *profunda* brachii artery (accompanying the radial nerve)
- The *superior ulnar collateral* arteries (accompanying the ulnar nerve)
- The *nutrient* artery (to the humerus)
- The *inferior ulnar collateral* artery

Radial artery

The radial artery (Fig. 3.23) commences at the level of the radial neck by lying on the tendon of biceps. In its upper half it lies overlapped by brachioradialis, the surface marking of the artery being the groove which can be seen on the medial side of this tensed muscle in the muscular subject. Distally in the forearm the artery lies superficially between brachioradialis and flexor carpi radialis, and it is between these two tendons that it is palpated at the wrist (Fig. 3.2).

In the middle third of the forearm the radial nerve lies along the lateral side of the artery; the nerve may here be incorporated in a carelessly placed ligature.

Distal to the radial pulse, the artery gives off a branch to assist in forming the superficial palmar arch. It then passes deep to the tendons of abductor pollicis longus and extensor pollicis brevis to enter the anatomical snuffbox (in which it can be felt), pierces the 1st dorsal interosseous muscle and adductor pollicis, between the 1st and 2nd metacarpals, and goes on to form the deep palmar arch with the deep branch of the ulnar artery.

Ulnar artery

The ulnar artery (Fig. 3.23) is the larger of the two terminal branches of the brachial artery. From its commencement it passes beneath the muscles arising from the common flexor origin, lies upon flexor digitorum profundus and is overlapped by flexor carpi ulnaris. The median nerve crosses superficially to the ulnar artery, separated from it by only part of one muscle, the deep head of pronator teres.

In the distal half of the forearm the artery becomes superficial between the tendons of flexor carpi ulnaris and flexor digitorum sublimis; it then crosses the flexor retinaculum to form the superficial palmar arch with the superficial branch of the radial artery.

The ulnar nerve accompanies the artery on its medial side in the distal two-thirds of its course in the forearm and across the flexor retinaculum (Fig. 3.2).

Note that there is a rich anastomosis of arteries around all major joints. Apart from remembering this fact, the clinical student need not commit to memory the numerous named branches involved.

Brachial plexus

The brachial plexus is of great practical importance to the surgeon. It may be damaged in open, closed or obstetrical injuries, be pressed upon by a cervical rib or be involved in tumour. It is encountered, and hence put in danger, in operations upon the root of the neck.

Formation

The plexus is formed as follows (Fig. 3.24):

1. Five *roots*, derived from the anterior primary rami of C5, C6, C7, C8 and T1, link up into:
2. Three *trunks*, formed by the union of
   - C5 and C6 (upper trunk)
   - C7 alone (middle trunk)
   - C8 and T1 (lower trunk)

   These split into:
3. Six *divisions*, formed by each trunk dividing into an anterior and posterior division, which link up again into:
4. Three *cords*
   - A lateral, from the fused anterior divisions of the upper and middle trunks
   - A medial, from the anterior division of the lower trunk
   - A posterior, from the union of all three posterior divisions

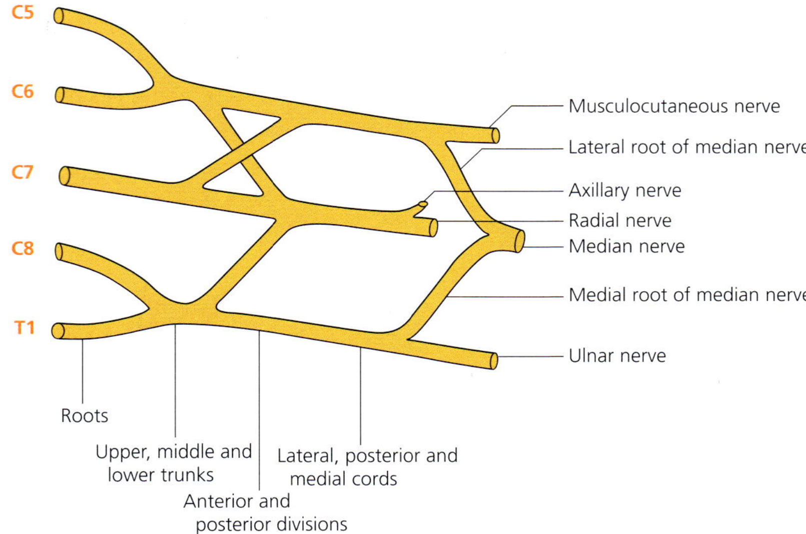

Figure 3.24 Scheme of the brachial plexus formation.

The *roots* lie between the anterior and middle scalene muscles. The *trunks* lie deep to the fascial floor of the posterior triangle of the neck. The *divisions* lie behind the clavicle. The *cords* lie in the axilla.

Branches

The cords continue distally to form the following main nerve trunks of the upper limb, thus:

1. The lateral cord continues as the *musculocutaneous nerve*
2. The medial cord, as the *ulnar nerve*
3. The posterior cord, as the *radial nerve* and the *axillary nerve*
4. A cross-communication between the lateral and medial cords forms the *median nerve*

For reference purposes, the derivatives of the various components of the brachial plexus are given below (Fig. 3.25):

- *From the roots*
  - Nerve to rhomboids
  - Nerve to subclavius
  - Nerve to serratus anterior (C5, C6, C7)

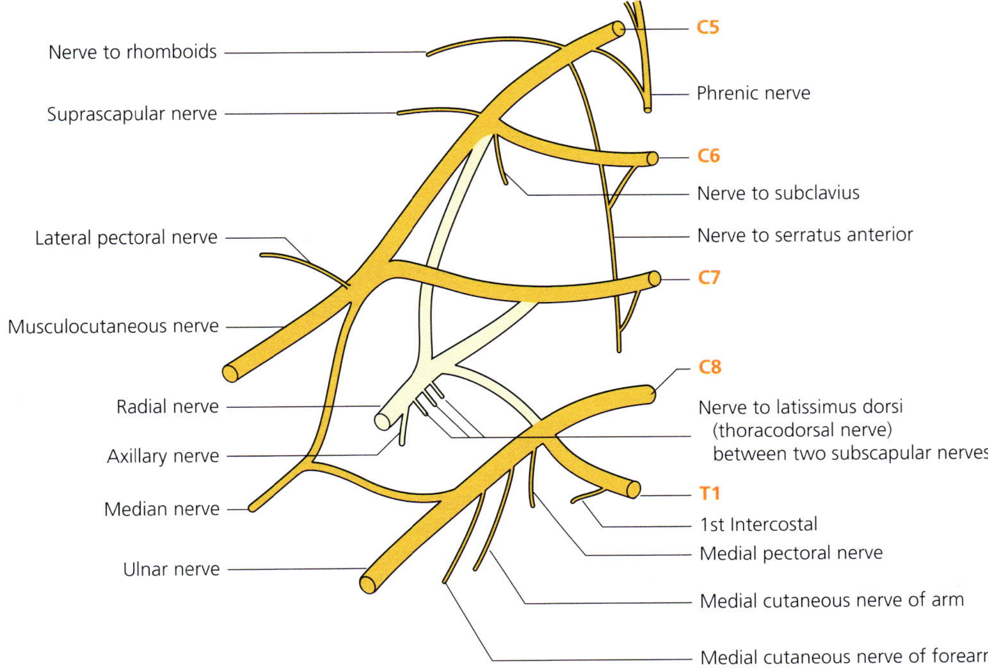

Figure 3.25 The branches of the brachial plexus. The lightly coloured areas show the posterior divisions.

- *From the trunk*
  - Suprascapular nerve – from the upper trunk (supplies supraspinatus and infraspinatus)
- *From the lateral cord*
  - Musculocutaneous nerve
  - Lateral pectoral nerve
  - Lateral root of the median nerve
- *From the medial cord*
  - Medial pectoral nerve
  - Medial cutaneous nerves of the arm and forearm
  - Ulnar nerve
  - Medial root of the median nerve
- *From the posterior cord*
  - Subscapular nerves
  - Nerve to latissimus dorsi (thoracodorsal nerve)
  - Axillary nerve
  - Radial nerve

Note that the posterior cord supplies the skin and muscles of the posterior aspect of the limb, whereas the anteriorly placed lateral and medial cords supply the anterior compartment structures.

Segmental cutaneous supply of the upper limb (Fig. 3.26)

In spite of this complex interlacing of the nerve roots in the brachial plexus, the skin of the upper limb, as with the skin of the rest of the body, has a perfectly regular segmental nerve supply.

This is derived from C4 to T2 and is arranged approximately as follows:

- **C4:** Supplies skin over the shoulder tip
- **C5:** Radial side of the upper arm
- **C6:** Radial side of the forearm
- **C7:** The skin of the hand
- **C8:** Ulnar side of the forearm
- **T1:** Ulnar side of the upper arm
- **T2:** Skin of the axilla (via its intercostobrachial branch)

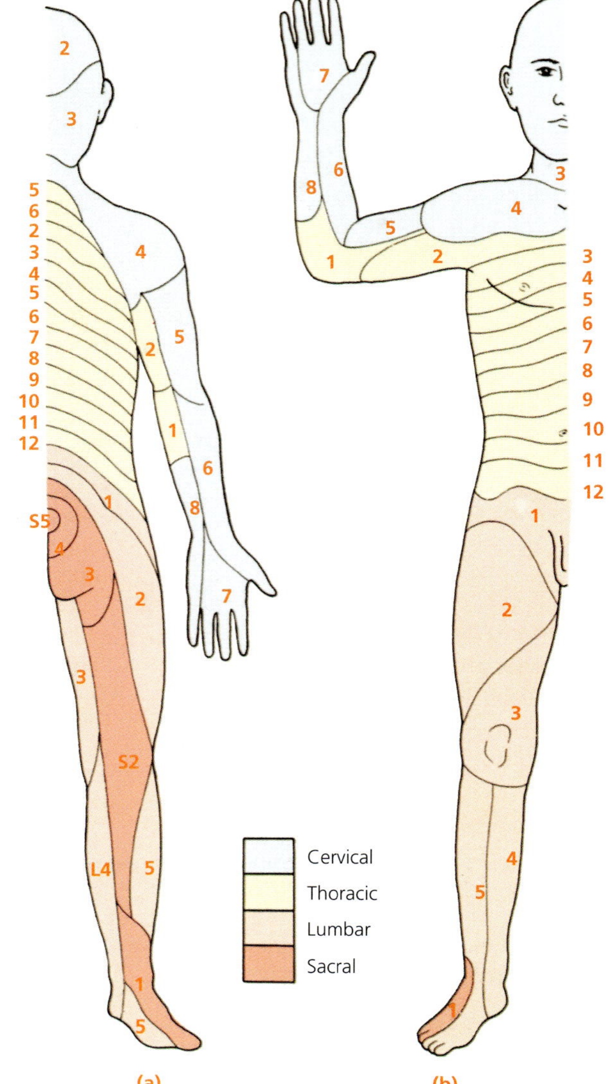

Figure 3.26 The segmental cutaneous innervation of the body. (a) Posterior aspect. (b) Anterior aspect.

Course and distribution of the principal nerves of the upper limb

The nerves of the upper limb are derived from the brachial plexus. The principal nerves of the upper limb are: axillary, radial, musculocutaneous, ulnar and median.

Axillary nerve

The axillary (circumflex) nerve (C5, C6) arises from the posterior cord of the plexus and winds round the surgical neck of the humerus in company with the posterior circumflex humeral vessels (Figs 3.8 and 3.27). Its branches are as follows:

- **Muscular:** To deltoid and teres minor; the nerve to teres minor possesses pseudoganglion
- **Cutaneous:** To a palm-sized area of skin over the deltoid

The axillary nerve may be injured in fractures of the humeral neck or in dislocations of the shoulder. This will be followed by weakness of shoulder abduction, wasting of the deltoid and a small patch of anaesthesia over this muscle.

Radial nerve

The radial nerve (C5, C6, C7, C8, T1) is the main branch of the posterior cord. Lying first behind the axillary artery, it then passes backwards between the long and medial heads of the triceps to lie in the spiral groove on the back of the humerus between the medial and lateral heads of triceps (Fig. 3.27). The profunda branch of the brachial artery and its venae comitantes accompany the nerve in this part of its course (Fig. 3.8).

At the lower third of the humerus, the radial nerve pierces the lateral intermuscular septum to re-enter the anterior compartment of the arm between brachialis and brachioradialis (a convenient site for surgical exposure; Fig. 3.23). At the level of the lateral epicondyle its important *posterior*

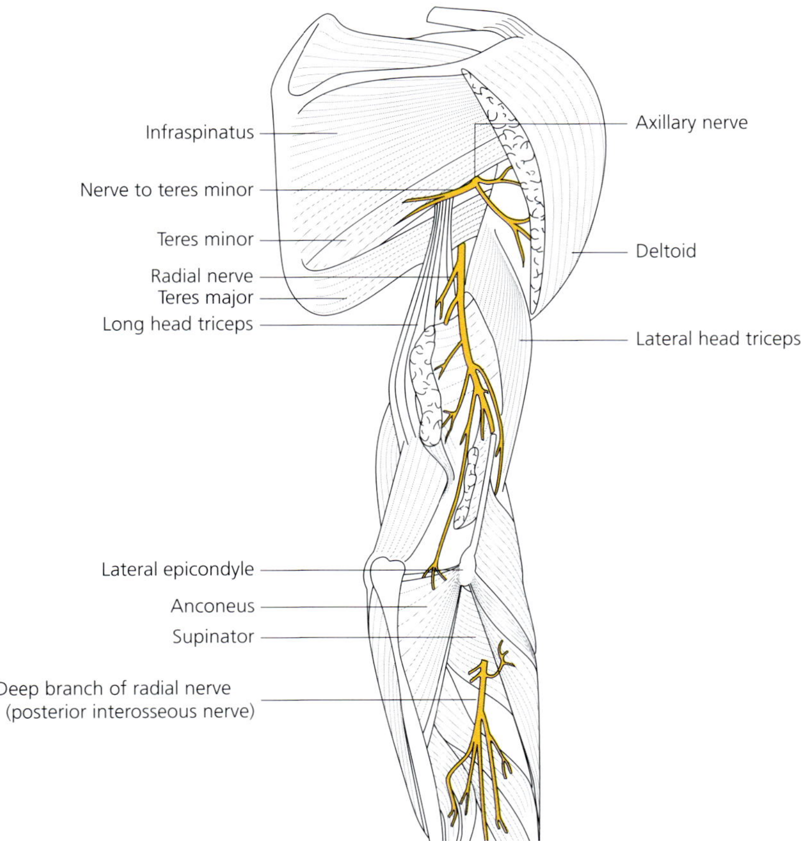

Figure 3.27 The distribution of the radial nerve (right upper limb, dorsal aspect).

interosseous nerve is given off, which winds round the radius within the supinator muscle then sprays out to be distributed to the extensor muscles of the forearm.

The radial nerve itself continues as the superficial radial nerve, lying deep to brachioradialis (Fig. 3.23). Above the wrist, it emerges posteriorly from beneath this muscle to end by dividing into cutaneous nerves to the posterior aspects of the radial 3½ digits. Run a fingertip over the extended tendons of extensor pollicis longus (Fig. 3.3) just distal to the wrist joint. The nerve will be felt as a thin cord flicking over the tendon.

The radial nerve is the nerve of supply to the extensor aspect of the upper limb. The main trunk itself innervates: triceps, anconeus, brachioradialis and extensor carpi radialis longus. It also gives a twig to the lateral part of brachialis.

The posterior interosseous branch of the radial nerve supplies all the remaining extensor muscles of the forearm, including supinator and abductor pollicis longus.

Cutaneous branches are distributed to the back of the arm, forearm and radial side of the dorsum of the hand. So great is the overlap from adjacent nerves, however, that division of the radial nerve results, surprisingly, in only a small area of anaesthesia over the dorsum of the hand, in the web between the thumb and index finger (*see* Fig. 3.33(a)).

Musculocutaneous nerve

The musculocutaneous nerve (C5, C6, C7) continues on from the lateral cord of the plexus. It pierces coracobrachialis then runs between biceps and brachialis (supplying all these three muscles) to innervate, by its terminal cutaneous branch, now termed the lateral cutaneous nerve of the forearm, the skin of the lateral forearm.

Ulnar nerve

The ulnar nerve (C7, C8, T1; Fig. 3.28) is formed from the medial cord of the plexus. It lies medial to the axillary and brachial artery as far as the middle of the humerus, then pierces the medial intermuscular septum (in company with the superior ulnar collateral artery) to descend on the anterior face of triceps. It passes behind the medial epicondyle (where it can readily be rolled against the bone), to enter the forearm (Fig. 3.8). Here, it descends beneath flexor carpi ulnaris until this muscle thins out into its tendon, leaving the nerve to lie superficially on its radial side. In the distal two-thirds of the forearm the nerve is accompanied by the ulnar artery, which lies on the nerve's radial side. Approximately 2 in. (5 cm) above the wrist, a dorsal cutaneous branch passes deep to flexor carpi ulnaris to supply the dorsal aspects of the ulnar 1½ fingers and the dorsal aspect or the ulnar side of the hand (Fig. 3.29).

The ulnar nerve crosses the flexor retinaculum superficially (Figs 3.2 and 3.4) to break up into a superficial terminal branch, supplying the ulnar 1½ fingers, and a deep terminal branch that supplies the hypothenar muscles and the intrinsic muscles of the hand.

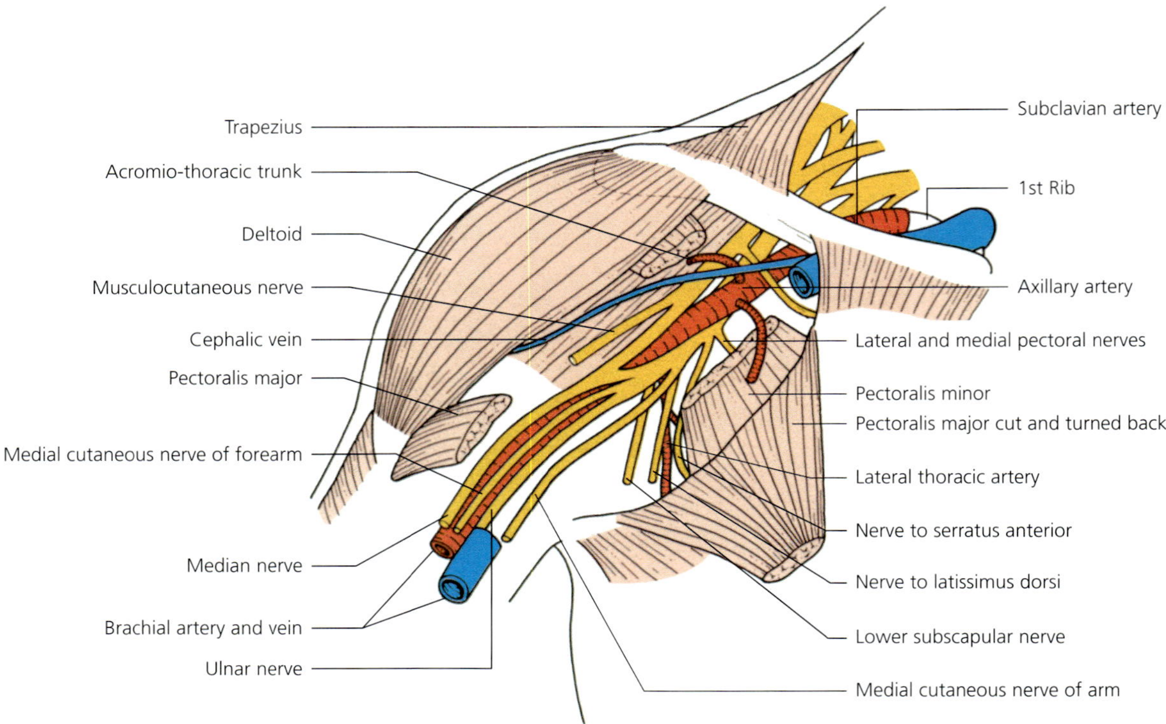

Figure 3.28 Dissection of the right axilla and upper arm to show the course of the major nerves.

Its branches are as follows:

- **Muscular:** To flexor carpi ulnaris, medial half of flexor digitorum profundus, the hypothenar muscles, the interossei, 3rd and 4th lumbricals and adductor pollicis (i.e. it supplies all the intrinsic muscles of the hand apart from those of the thenar eminence and the 1st and 2nd lumbricals, which are innervated by the median nerve)
- **Cutaneous:** To the ulnar side of both aspects of the hand and both surfaces of the ulnar 1½ fingers

Median nerve

The median nerve (C6, C7, C8, T1; Fig. 3.28) arises by the junction of a branch from the medial and another from the lateral cord of the plexus, which unite anterior to the third part of the axillary artery. Continuing along the lateral aspect of the brachial artery, the nerve then crosses superficially (occasionally deep) to the artery at the mid-humerus to lie on its medial side. The nerve enters the forearm between the heads of pronator teres, the deeper of which separates it from the ulnar artery (Fig. 3.23). Here, the nerve gives off its *anterior interosseous branch* (which supplies flexor pollicis longus, flexor digitorum profundus to the index and middle fingers, and pronator quadratus), and then lies on the deep aspect of flexor digitorum superficialis, to which it adheres.

At the wrist, the median nerve becomes superficial on the ulnar side of flexor carpi radialis, exactly in the midline (Fig. 3.2). Here, it gives off a *palmar cutaneous branch*, which supplies the skin of the mid-palm. It then passes deep to the flexor retinaculum, giving off an important branch to the thenar muscles beyond the distal skin crease, twigs to the radial two lumbricals and cutaneous branches to the palmar aspects of the radial 3½ digits.

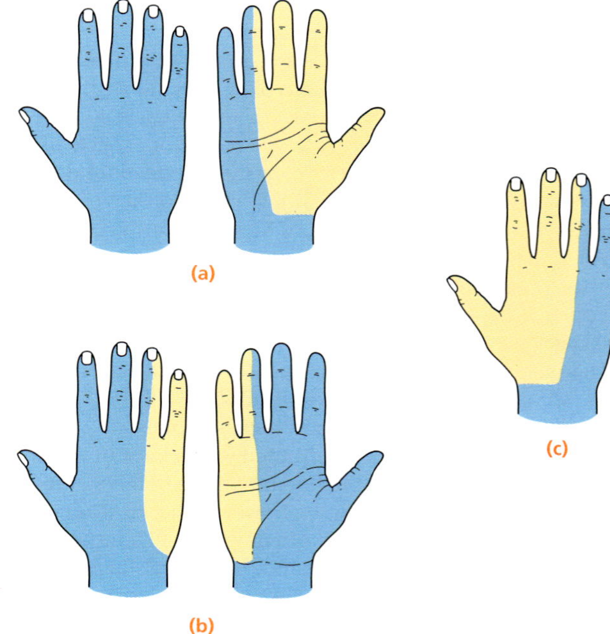

Figure 3.29 The usual cutaneous distribution (shown in yellow) of the **(a)** median, **(b)** ulnar and **(c)** radial nerves in the hand (considerable variations and overlap occur).

Within the carpal tunnel, deep to the flexor retinaculum, the nerve may be compressed – *the carpal tunnel syndrome* (*see* page 102).

Its branches are as follows:

- **Muscular:** To all the muscles of the flexor aspects of the forearm, apart from the flexor carpi ulnaris and the ulnar half of flexor digitorum profundus, and to the thenar eminence muscles and the radial two lumbricals
- **Cutaneous:** To the skin of the radial side of the palm, the palmar aspect and a variable degree of the dorsal aspect of the radial 3½ digits

Note that there is considerable variation in the exact cutaneous distribution of the nerves in the hand; for example, the ulnar nerve may encroach on median territory and supply the whole of the 4th and 5th digits (Fig. 3.29).

Compartments of the upper limb

In each of the limbs, the skeletal muscles are collectively ensleeved in a layer of deep fascia. From the inner surface of this stocking-like deep fascial envelope, fibrous septa project inwards and attach to the bone(s) lying within a given segment of the limb, thereby separating the muscles of that limb segment into functional groups. Thus, the muscles within each segment of the upper and lower limbs may be pictured as being located in discrete, osseofascial compartments (*see* Fig. 3.30). As a general rule, each compartment possesses its own complement of neurovascular structures, with the nerve being responsible for the motor innervation of all the muscles of the compartment.

Compartments in the segments of the upper limb

The arm contains two compartments as mentioned below:

1. Anterior (flexor) compartment containing biceps brachii, brachialis and coracobrachialis, all innervated by the musculocutaneous nerve
2. Posterior (extensor) compartment containing triceps brachii, innervated by the radial nerve

The forearm contains two compartments – the anterior (flexor) compartment and the posterior (extensor) compartment, which are separated from each other by the radius, ulna and interosseous membrane.

1. The muscles of the anterior compartment of the forearm are arranged in two groups:
   - A superficial group comprising pronator teres, flexor carpi radialis, palmaris longus, flexor digitorum superficialis and flexor carpi ulnaris
   - A deep group comprising flexor pollicis longus, flexor digitorum profundus and pronator quadratus

   In the superficial group, all but flexor carpi ulnaris are innervated by the median nerve. Flexor carpi ulnaris is innervated by the ulnar nerve. In the deep group, the median nerve innervates flexor pollicis longus, pronator quadratus and the radial half of flexor digitorum profundus. The medial half of flexor digitorum profundus is innervated by the ulnar nerve.
2. The muscles of the posterior compartment of the forearm (comprising the radial and ulnar extensors of the wrist, the long and short extensors of the thumb, the long abductor of the thumb, the extensors of the digits and supinator) are innervated by the radial nerve (chiefly through the posterior interosseous nerve)

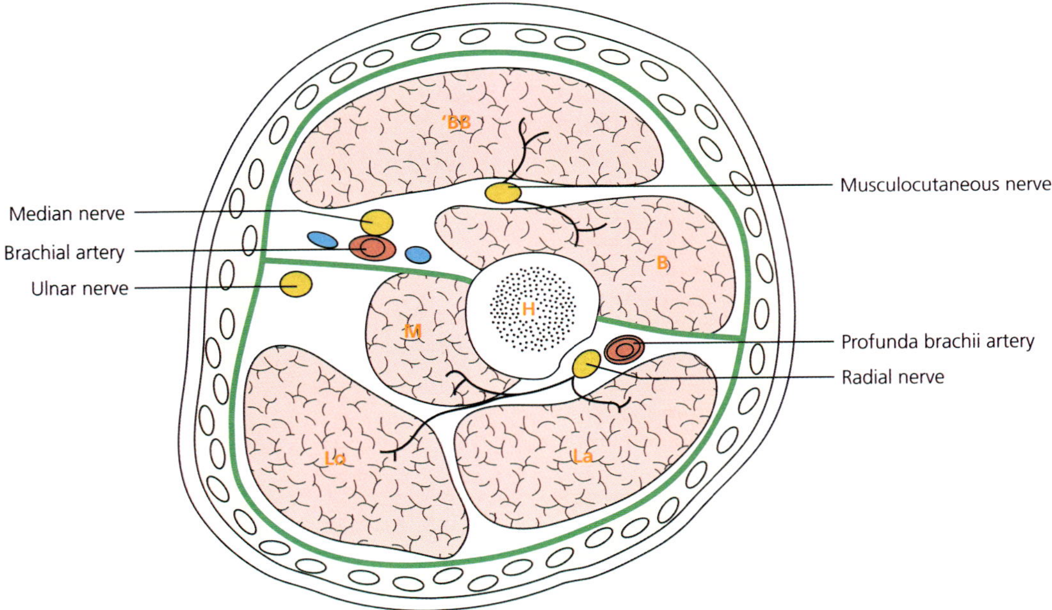

Figure 3.30 Cross sectional representation of the right mid-arm. BB: biceps brachii; B: brachialis; H: humerus; M: medial head of triceps; Lo: long head of triceps; La: lateral head of triceps.

Compartment syndrome

The fascial boundaries which limit the osseofascial compartments are inelastic sheets. Any condition that leads to an increase in the volume of the compartmental contents is, therefore, likely to result in a rise in intracompartmental pressure. Such conditions include haemorrhage following closed fractures, muscle swelling caused by trauma or unaccustomed overuse and local infection. If unrelieved, the increased pressure leads to compression of the vessels in the compartment and secondary ischaemic damage to the nerves and muscles of the compartment. This phenomenon is known as *compartment syndrome*.

Compartment syndrome is a surgical emergency and is treated by performing a *fasciotomy*; this is a procedure in which a generous incision is made in the deep fascia overlying the compartment in order to decompress the compartment.

Female breast

The breast or mammary gland is a modified sweat gland in the superficial fascia of the pectoral region. The female breast overlies the 2nd–6th rib; two-thirds of it rests on pectoralis major, one-third on serratus anterior, while its lower medial edge just overlaps the upper part of the rectus sheath.

Structure

The breast is made up of 15–20 lobules of glandular tissue embedded in fat; the latter accounts for its smooth contour and most of its bulk. These lobules are separated by fibrous septa running from the subcutaneous tissues to the fascia of the chest wall (the *ligaments of Cooper*).

Each lobule drains by its lactiferous duct onto the *nipple*, which is surrounded by the pigmented *areola*. This area is lubricated by the *areolar glands of Montgomery*; these are large, modified sebaceous glands that may form sebaceous cysts, which may, in turn, become infected.

The male breast is rudimentary, comprising small ducts without alveoli and supported by fibrous tissue and fat. Insignificant it may be, but it is still prone to the major diseases that affect the female organ.

Blood supply

Arteries

The blood supply to the breast is provided by the following vessels:

1. From the axillary artery, principally via its lateral thoracic and acromiothoracic branches
2. From the internal thoracic (hence its former name – the internal mammary artery) via its perforating branches; these pierce the 1st–4th intercostal spaces, then traverse pectoralis major to reach the breast along its medial edge. The 1st and 2nd perforators are the largest of these branches
3. From the intercostal arteries via their lateral perforating branches; a relatively unimportant source

Veins

The venous drainage takes place by the following veins: axillary, internal thoracic and posterior intercostal.

Lymphatic drainage

This is of considerable importance in the spread of malignant tumours of the breast.

The lymph drainage of the breast, as with any other organ, follows the pathway of its blood supply and, therefore, travels in the following directions:

1. Along the tributaries of the axillary vessels to axillary lymph nodes; this accounts for approximately 75% of the total lymphatic drainage of the breast
2. Along the tributaries of the internal thoracic vessels, piercing pectoralis major to traverse each intercostal space to lymph nodes along the internal thoracic chain (internal mammary nodes); these also receive lymphatics penetrating along the lateral perforating branches of the intercostal vessels

Although the lymph vessels lying between the lobules of the breast freely communicate, there is a tendency for the lateral part of the breast to drain towards the axilla and the medial part to the internal thoracic chain (Fig. 3.31).

A subareolar plexus of lymphatics below the nipple (the *plexus of Sappey*) and another deep plexus on the pectoral fascia have, in the past, been considered to be the central points to which, respectively, the superficial and deep parts of the breast drain before communicating with the main efferent lymphatics. These plexuses appear, however, to be relatively unimportant; the vessels from these plexuses, in the main, pass directly to the regional lymph nodes.

The *axillary lymph nodes* (some 20–30 in number) drain not only the lymphatics of the breast, but also those of the pectoral region, upper abdominal wall and the upper limb, and are arranged in five groups as mentioned below (Fig. 3.32):

1. **Anterior:** Lying deep to pectoralis major along the lower border of pectoralis minor

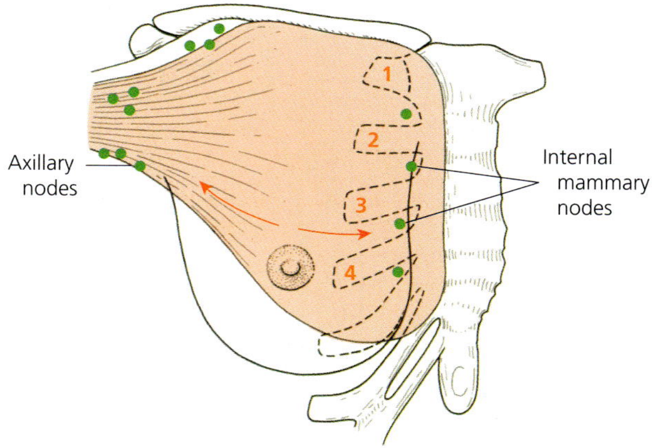

Figure 3.31 The principal pathways of lymphatic drainage of the breast. These follow the venous drainage of the breast – to the axilla and to the internal mammary (internal thoracic) chain.

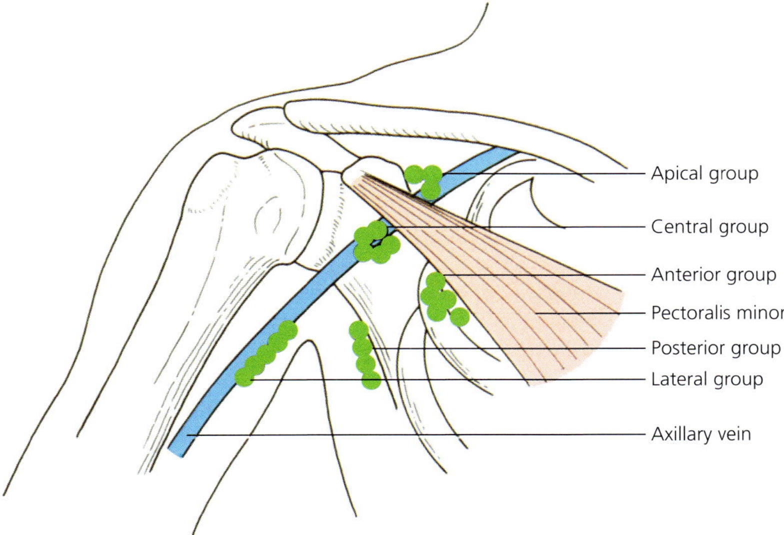

Figure 3.32 The lymph nodes of the axilla.

2. **Posterior:** Along the subscapular vessels
3. **Lateral:** Along the axillary vein
4. **Central:** In the axillary fat
5. **Apical (through which all the other axillary nodes drain):** Immediately behind the clavicle at the apex of the axilla above pectoralis minor and along the medial side of the axillary vein.

Clinicians and pathologists often define metastatic axillary node spread simply into the following three levels:

- **Level I:** Nodes lateral to pectoralis minor
- **Level II:** Nodes deep to pectoralis minor
- **Level III:** Nodes medial to pectoralis minor

From the apical nodes emerges the subclavian lymph trunk. On the right, this either drains directly into the subclavian vein or else joins the right jugular trunk; on the left, it usually drains directly into the thoracic duct.

The parasternal *internal thoracic (internal mammary) nodes,* lying along the internal thoracic vessels, drain to the mediastinal nodes and thence to the thoracic duct on the left and to the right thoracic duct on the right. Inferiorly, they communicate distantly with the groin nodes via lymphatics which accompany the superior and inferior epigastric vessels.

Lymphatic spread of a neoplastic growth of the breast may occur further afield when these normal pathways have become interrupted by malignant deposits, surgery or radiotherapy. Secondaries may then be found in the lymphatics of the opposite breast or in the opposite axillary lymph nodes, the groin lymph nodes (via lymph vessels in the trunk wall), the cervical nodes (as a result of retrograde extension from the blocked thoracic duct or jugular trunk) or in peritoneal lymphatics, spreading there in a retrograde manner from the lower internal thoracic nodes; this is in addition, of course, to spread via the bloodstream.

Development

The breast develops from milk line which appears on the chest wall by the invagination of the surface ectoderm. It extends

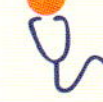

Clinical Features

1 Developmental abnormalities are not uncommon. The nipple may fail to evert, and it is important to find out from the patient whether or not an inverted nipple is a recent event or has been present since birth. Supernumerary nipples (*polythelia*) or even breasts (*polymastia*) may occur along a vertical 'milk line' – a reminder of the line of mammary glands in more primitive mammals; on the other hand, the breast on one or both sides may be small or even absent (amastia).

2 An abscess of the breast should be opened by a radial incision to avoid cutting across a number of lactiferous ducts. Such an abscess may rupture from one fascial compartment into its neighbours, and it is important at operation to break down any loculi which thus form in order to provide ample drainage.

3 Dimpling of the skin over a carcinoma of the breast results from malignant infiltration and fibrous contraction of Cooper's ligaments – as these pass from breast to skin, their shortening results in tethering of the skin to the underlying tumour. This may also occur, however, in chronic infection, after trauma and, very rarely, in fibroadenosis, so that skin fixation to a breast lump is not necessarily diagnostic of malignancy.

4 Retraction of the nipple, if of recent origin, is suggestive of involvement of the milk ducts in the fibrous contraction of a scirrhous tumour.

5 The excision of a breast carcinoma by *radical mastectomy* involves the removal of a wide area of skin around the tumour, all the breast tissue, the pectoralis major (through which the lymphatics pass to the internal mammary chain), the pectoralis minor (which lies as a gateway to the axilla), and the whole axillary contents of fatty tissue and contained lymph nodes. This excision also removes the bulk of the lymphatics from the arm that pass along the anterior and medial aspects of the axillary vein. A few lymph vessels from the upper limb pass above the axillary vein and are, therefore, saved.

between the two limb buds in the pectoral region. It forms a series of branching ducts. Shortly before birth, this site of invagination everts to form the nipple. At puberty, alveoli sprout from the ducts and considerable fatty infiltration of the breast tissue takes place. With pregnancy there is tremendous development of the alveoli which, in lactation, secrete the fatty droplets of milk. At the menopause the gland tissue atrophies.

Most surgeons today perform less extensive surgery for breast cancer; for example, a *simple mastectomy*, in which the breast alone is removed, or an *extended simple mastectomy*, which combines this with clearance of the axillary fat and its contained nodes. Comparable results are obtained by excision of the lump, followed by radiotherapy to the breast and to the nodal areas of the axilla and the internal thoracic chain.

Oedema of the arm after mastectomy usually occurs only if further damage is done to this precarious lymph drainage by infection, malignant infiltration or heavy irradiation, or if additional strain is put on the evacuation of fluid from the limb by ligation or thrombosis of the axillary vein.

Anatomy of upper limb deformities

The deformities of the upper limb commonly occur due to nerve injuries, Volkmann's ischaemic contracture and Dupuytren's contracture.

Deformities due to the nerve injuries

Many deformities of the upper limb, resulting from nerve injuries, are readily interpreted anatomically. Now is a good time to revise all the palpable nerves in the upper limb (page 98).

Brachial plexus injuries

Brachial plexus injuries may occur from traction on the arm during birth. The force of downward traction falls upon roots C5 and C6, resulting in paralysis of the deltoid and short muscles of the shoulder, and of brachialis and biceps, both of which flex the elbow. In addition, biceps is also the powerful supinator of the forearm (Fig. 3.20). The arm, therefore, hangs limply by the side with the forearm pronated and the palm facing backwards, like a porter hinting for a tip (**Erb–Duchenne paralysis**). The sensory loss in this lesion affects the lateral aspect of the upper arm and the radial side of the forearm (C5 and C6; Fig. 3.26). In adults, this lesion is seen in violent falls on the side of the head and shoulder, forcing the two apart and thus putting a tearing strain on the upper roots of the plexus.

Upward traction on the arm (e.g. in a forcible breech delivery) may tear the lowest root, T1, which is the segmental supply of the intrinsic hand muscles. The hand assumes a clawed appearance because of the unopposed action of the long flexors and extensors of the fingers; the extensors, inserting into the bases of the proximal phalanges, extend the metacarpophalangeal joints while the flexor profundus and sublimis, inserting into the distal and middle phalanges, flex the interphalangeal joints (**Klumpke's paralysis**). The sensory loss in this injury is along the medial aspect of the arm (T1; Fig. 3.26). There is often an associated *Horner's syndrome* (ptosis and constriction of the pupil), due to traction on the cervical sympathetic chain.

A mass of malignant supraclavicular lymph nodes or the direct invasion of a pulmonary carcinoma (*Pancoast's syndrome*) may produce a similar neurological picture by involvement of the lowest root of the plexus.

Not infrequently, the lower trunk of the plexus (C8, T1) is pressed upon by a cervical rib, or by the fibrous strand running from the extremity of such a rib, resulting in paraesthesiae along the ulnar border of the arm and weakness and wasting of the small muscles of the hand.

Radial nerve injuries

The *radial nerve* may be injured in the axilla by the pressure of a crutch ('crutch palsy') or may be compressed when a drunkard falls into an intoxicated sleep with the arm hanging over the back of a chair ('**Saturday night palsy**'). Fractures of the humeral shaft may damage the main radial nerve, whereas its posterior interosseous branch, to the extensor muscles of the forearm, may be injured in fractures or dislocations of the radial head. An ill-placed incision to expose the head of the radius taken more than three fingers' breadth below the head will divide the nerve as it lies in the supinator muscle.

Damage to the main trunk of the radial nerve results in a **wrist drop** owing to paralysis of all the wrist extensors (Fig. 3.33). Damage to the posterior interosseous nerve, however, leaves extensor carpi radialis longus intact, as it is supplied from the radial nerve above its division; this muscle alone is sufficiently powerful to maintain extension of the wrist.

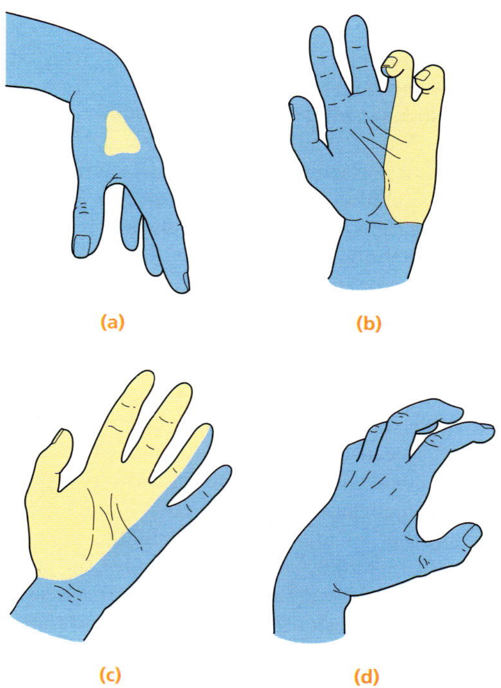

Figure 3.33 Deformities of the hand. (a) Radial palsy – wrist drop. (b) Ulnar nerve palsy – 'main en griffe' or claw hand. (c) Median nerve palsy – 'monkey's hand'. (d) Volkmann's contracture – another claw hand deformity. The yellow areas represent the usual distribution of anaesthesia.

The disability produced by a wrist drop is inability to grip firmly, since, unless the flexor muscles are stretched by extending the wrist, they act at a mechanical disadvantage. Try yourself to grip strongly with the wrist flexed and realize how, by operative fusion of the wrist joint in extension, the weakness produced by a radial nerve paralysis would be overcome.

Nerve overlap means that division of the radial nerve produces only a small area of anaesthesia of the dorsum of the hand between the 1st and 2nd metacarpals (Fig. 3.33(a)).

Ulnar nerve injuries

The *ulnar nerve*, in its vulnerable position behind the medial epicondyle of the humerus, may be damaged in fractures or dislocations of the elbow; it is also frequently divided in lacerations of the wrist. In the latter case, all the intrinsic muscles of the fingers (apart from the radial two lumbricals) are paralysed so that the hand assumes the clawed position already described under Klumpke's palsy (Fig. 3.33(d)). The clawing is slightly less intense in the 2nd and 3rd digits because of their intact lumbricals, supplied by the median nerve. In late cases, wasting of the interossei is readily seen on inspecting the dorsum of the hand.

If the nerve is injured at the elbow, the flexor digitorum profundus to the 4th and 5th fingers is paralysed so that the clawing of these two fingers is less intense than in division at the wrist. Paralysis of the flexor carpi ulnaris results in a tendency to radial deviation of the wrist.

Division of the ulnar nerve leaves a surprisingly efficient hand. The long flexors enable a good grip to be taken; the thumb, apart from loss of adductor pollicis, is intact and sensation over the palm of the hand is largely maintained. Indeed, it may be difficult to determine clinically with certainty that the nerve is injured; a reliable test is loss of ability to adduct and abduct the fingers with the hand laid flat, palm downwards on the table; this eliminates 'trick' movements of adduction and abduction of the fingers brought about as part of their flexion and extension, respectively.

A high division of the ulnar nerve, anywhere above the level of a hand's breadth above the wrist, will be followed by sensory loss over the ulnar side of the hand and the ulnar 1½ fingers on both the palmar and dorsal aspects (Fig. 3.29). However, if the nerve is divided at, or just above, the wrist, which is the common site for this to occur, the sensory loss is confined to the *palmar* aspect of the ulnar side of the hand and the ulnar 1½ fingers, with sparing of the dorsum of the hand. This is because the dorsal branch of the ulnar nerve, which supplies this area, is given off about a hand's breadth above the level of the wrist (Fig. 3.23) and is, therefore, spared from injury.

Median nerve injuries

The *median nerve* is occasionally damaged in supracondylar fractures, but it is in greatest danger in lacerations of the wrist.

If divided at the wrist, only the thenar muscles (excluding adductor pollicis) and the radial two lumbricals are paralysed and wasting of the thenar muscles occurs. The best clinical test for this is to ask the patient, with his hand resting palm upwards on the table, to touch a pencil held above the thumb. Failure to be able to do this (abduction) is diagnostic of paralysis of abductor pollicis brevis. It might be thought that such a lesion is relatively trivial since the only motor defect is loss of accurate opposition movement of the thumb to other fingers. In point of fact, this injury is a serious disability because of the loss of sensation over the thumb, adjacent 2½ fingers and the radial two-thirds of the palm of the hand, which prevents the accurate and delicate adjustments the hand makes in response to tactile stimuli (Fig. 3.33).

If the median nerve is divided at the elbow, there is serious muscle impairment. Pronation of the forearm is lost and is replaced by a trick movement of rotation of the upper arm. Wrist flexion is weak and accompanied by ulnar deviation, since this now depends on the flexor carpi ulnaris and the ulnar half of flexor digitorum profundus.

Deformity due to Volkmann's ischaemic contracture

The *Volkmann's contracture* of the hand follows ischaemia and subsequent fibrosis and contraction of the long flexor and extensor muscles of the forearm (Fig. 3.33(d)).

The deformities are readily explained as follows:

1. Since the flexors of the wrist are bulkier than the extensors, their fibrous contraction is greater and the wrist is, therefore, flexed.
2. The long extensors of the fingers are inserted into the proximal phalanges; their contracture extends the metacarpophalangeal joints.
3. The long flexors are inserted into the distal and middle phalanges and, therefore, flex the interphalangeal joints.

There is, therefore, flexion at the wrist, extension at the metacarpophalangeal and flexion at the interphalangeal joints.

If the wrist is passively further flexed by the examiner, the tight flexor tendons are somewhat relaxed and, therefore, the fingers become a little less clawed.

Deformity due to Dupuytren's contracture

The *Dupuytren's contracture* results from a fibrous contraction of the palmar aponeurosis, particularly of the 4th and 5th fingers.

The palmar aponeurosis is merely part of the deep fascial sheath of the upper limb; it passes from the palm along either side of each finger, blends with the fibrous flexor sheath of the fingers and is attached to the sides of the proximal and middle phalanges. Contracture of this fascia results in a longitudinal thickening in the palm together with flexion of the metacarpophalangeal and proximal interphalangeal joints. However, the distal interphalangeal joints are not involved and, in fact, in an advanced case, are actually *extended* by the distal phalanx being pushed backwards against the palm of the hand.

Spaces of the hand

The spaces of the hand are of practical significance because they may become infected and, in consequence, become distended with pus. The important spaces are as follows:

1. The superficial pulp spaces of the fingers
2. The synovial tendon sheaths of the 2nd, 3rd and 4th fingers

3. The ulnar bursa
4. The radial bursa
5. The mid-palmar space
6. The thenar space

Superficial pulp space of the fingers (Fig. 3.34)

The tips of the fingers and thumb are composed entirely of subcutaneous fat broken up and packed between fibrous septa, which pass from the skin down to the periosteum of the terminal phalanx. The tight packing of this compartment is responsible for the severe pain of a 'septic finger' – there is little room for the expansion of inflamed and oedematous tissues.

The blood vessels to the shaft of the distal phalanx must traverse this space and may become thrombosed in a severe pulp infection with resulting necrosis of the diaphysis of the bone. The base of the distal phalanx receives its blood supply more proximally from a branch of the digital artery in the middle segment of the finger and, therefore, survives. At each of the skin creases of the fingers, the skin is bound down to the underlying flexor sheath so that the pulp over each phalanx is in a separate compartment cut off from its neighbours. Infection may, however, track from one space to another along the neurovascular digital bundles.

Over the palm of the hand there is very little subcutaneous tissue, the skin adhering to the underlying palmar aponeurosis; in contrast, the skin of the dorsum of the fingers and hand is loose and fluid can, therefore, readily collect beneath it. Unless this is remembered, the marked dorsal oedema which may accompany sepsis of the palmar aspect of the fingers or hand may result in the primary site of the infection being overlooked.

Ulnar and radial bursae and the synovial tendon sheaths of the fingers (Fig. 3.35)

The flexor tendons traverse a fibro-osseous tunnel in each digit. This tunnel is made up posteriorly by the metacarpal head, the phalanges and the fronts of the intervening joints. The anterior fibrous part consists of condensed deep fascia attached to the sharp anterolateral margin of each phalanx and is termed the *fibrous flexor sheath*. This is particularly tough over the phalanges but loose over the front of each joint; it, therefore, holds the flexor tendons in place without 'bow-stringing' during flexion of the fingers, but does not impede movement of the joints.

Distally, the fibrous sheath ends at the insertion of the profundus tendon (or flexor pollicis longus tendon in the case of the thumb) at the base of the distal phalanx.

These fibrous sheaths are lined by synovial membrane, which is reflected around each tendon. The tendons of the 2nd, 3rd and 4th fingers have synovial sheaths which are closed off proximally at the metacarpal head, but the synovial sheaths of the thumb and little finger extend proximally into the palm.

That of the long flexor tendon of the thumb extends through the palm, deep to the flexor retinaculum, to approximately 1 in. (2.5 cm) proximal to the wrist and is termed the *radial bursa*. The synovial sheath of the 5th finger continues as the *ulnar bursa*, an expanded synovial sheath which encloses all the finger tendons in the palm and which also extends proximally below the flexor retinaculum for 1 in. (2.5 cm) above the wrist. In approximately 50% of cases the radial and ulnar bursae communicate. These synovial sheaths either may become infected directly – for example, following the entry of a splinter – or may be secondarily involved from a neglected pulp-space infection. Infections of the 2nd, 3rd and 4th sheaths are confined to the finger concerned, but sepsis in the 1st and 5th sheaths may spread proximally into the palm through the radial and ulnar bursa, respectively, and may pass from one bursa to the other via the frequent cross-communication between the two.

Since these bursae both extend proximally beyond the wrist, infection may, on occasion, spread into the forearm.

Palmar spaces

Two spaces deep in the palm of the hand may rarely become distended with pus; these are the mid-palmar and thenar spaces (Fig. 3.36).

The *mid-palmar space* lies behind the flexor tendons and ulnar bursa in the palm and in front of the 3rd, 4th and 5th metacarpals with their attached interossei. The 1st and 2nd metacarpals are curtained off from this space by the adductor pollicis, which arises from the shaft of the 3rd metacarpal and passes as a triangular sheet to the base of the proximal phalanx of the thumb.

The *thenar space* is the space superficial to the 2nd and 3rd metacarpals and the adductor pollicis. It is separated from the mid-palmar space by a fibrous partition.

Infection of these two spaces sometimes results from penetrating wounds or may be due to secondary involvement from a long-neglected tendon sheath infection. Nowadays, they are fortunately extremely rare, thanks to antibiotic treatment and the early surgical drainage of pus collections.

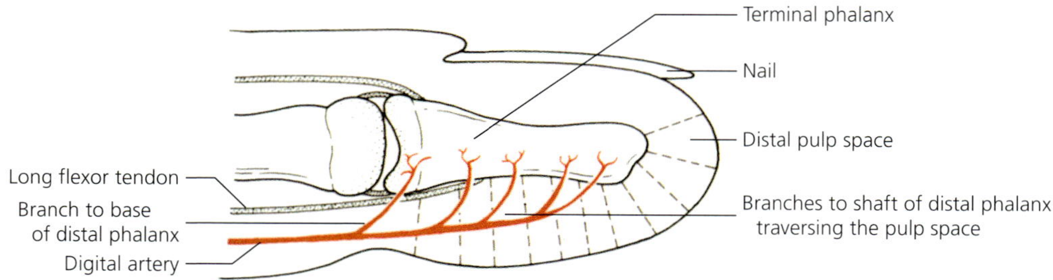

Figure 3.34 The distal pulp space of the finger; note the distribution of the arterial supply to the distal phalanx.

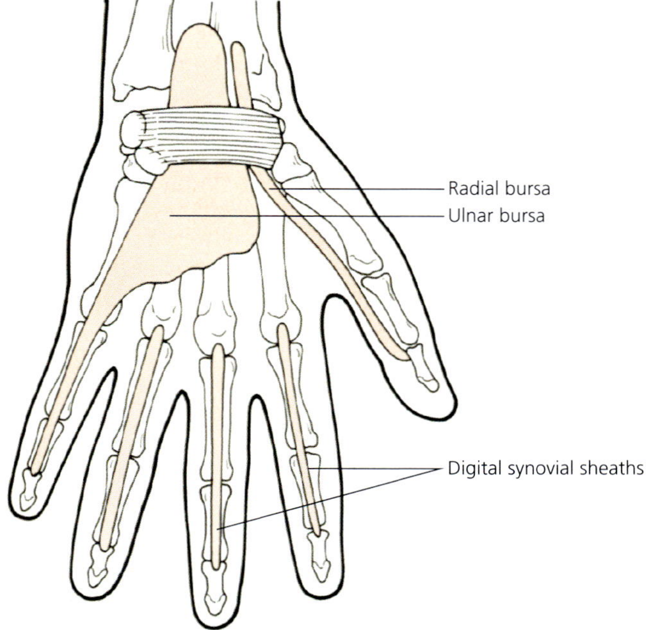

Figure 3.35 The synovial sheaths of the flexor tendons of the hand (left) – the radial and ulnar bursae track proximally deep to the flexor retinaculum and provide a potential pathway of infection into the forearm. In many cases, these bursae communicate.

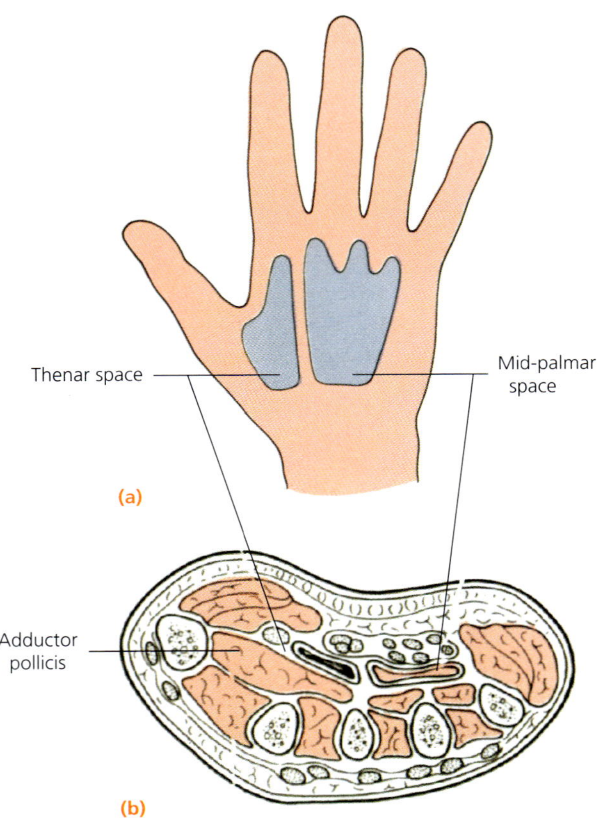

Figure 3.36 The mid-palmar and thenar spaces (left hand): **(a)** projected onto the surface of the hand and **(b)** in transverse section (viewed from the proximal aspect).

Part IV

The lower limb

Surface anatomy and surface markings of the lower limb

Anatomically the upper and lower limbs are comparable to each other as regards the arrangement of the bones, joints, main muscle groups, vessels and nerves. However, compared with the complex movements of the upper limb, designed to place the hand in a multiplicity of positions, together with the intricate and multiple functions of the hand, fingers and thumb, the functions of the lower limb are simple indeed – first, to act as a rigid column in the standing position and, second, to turn into a lever system when the subject walks or runs.

Bones and joints

The tip of the *anterior superior spine of the ilium* is easily felt and may be visible in the thin subject. The *greater trochanter* of the femur lies a hand's breadth below the iliac crest; it is best palpated with the hip passively abducted so that the overlying hip abductors (tensor fasciae latae and gluteus medius and minimus) are relaxed. In the very thin patient, the greater trochanter may be seen as a prominent bulge and its overlying skin is a common site for a pressure sore to form in such a case.

The *ischial tuberosity* is covered by gluteus maximus when one stands. In the sitting position, however, the muscle slips away laterally so that weight is taken directly on the bone. To palpate this bony point, therefore, feel for it uncovered by gluteus maximus in the flexed position of the hip.

At the knee, the *patella* forms a prominent landmark. When quadriceps femoris is relaxed, this bone is freely mobile from side to side; note that this is so when you stand erect. The *condyles* of the femur and tibia, the *head of the fibula* and the joint line of the knee are all readily palpable; less so is the *adductor tubercle* of the femur, best identified by running the fingers down the medial side of the thigh until they are halted by it, the first bony prominence so to be encountered.

The *tibia* can be felt along the entire length of its anterior subcutaneous border from the *tibial tuberosity* above, which marks the insertion of the quadriceps tendon, to the *medial malleolus* at the ankle. The subcutaneous surface of the tibia, which can be felt immediately medial to its subcutaneous border, is crossed by only two structures – the long saphenous vein, which is readily visible immediately in front of the medial malleolus of the tibia, and the adjacent saphenous nerve. The head of the fibula, as noted above, is easily palpable; note that it lies below and towards the posterior part of the lateral tibial condyle. Distal to its neck, the fibula 'disappears' as it dives into the muscle mass of the peroneal muscles, becoming subcutaneous distally. The *fibula* is subcutaneous for its terminal 3 in. (7 cm) above the *lateral malleolus*, which extends more distally than the stumpier *medial malleolus* of the tibia.

Immediately in front of the malleoli can be felt a block of bone which is the *head of the talus*. Feel it move up and down in dorsiflexion and plantarflexion of the ankle.

The *tuberosity of the navicular* stands out as a bony prominence 1 in. (2.5 cm) in front of the medial malleolus; it is the principal point of insertion of tibialis posterior. The base of the 5th metatarsal is easily felt on the lateral side of the foot and is the site of insertion of peroneus brevis.

If the *calcaneus* (*os calcis*) is carefully palpated, the *peroneal tubercle* can be felt 1 in. (2.5 cm) below the tip of the lateral malleolus and the *sustentaculum tali* 1 in. (2.5 cm) below the medial malleolus; these represent pulleys for peroneus longus and for flexor hallucis longus, respectively.

Bursae of the lower limb

A number of these bony prominences are associated with overlying bursae, which may become distended and inflamed: the one over the ischial tuberosity may enlarge with too much sitting ('**weaver's bottom**'); that in front of the patella is affected by prolonged kneeling forwards, as in scrubbing floors or hewing coal ('**housemaid's knee**', the 'beat knee' of north-country miners, or prepatellar bursitis); whereas the bursa over the ligamentum patellae is involved by years of kneeling in a more erect position – as in praying ('**clergyman's knee**' or infrapatellar bursitis). Young women who wear fashionable but tight shoes are prone to bursitis over the insertion of the Achilles tendon (calcaneal tendon or tendo calcaneus) into the calcaneus and may also develop bursae over the navicular tuberosity and dorsal aspects of the phalanges.

A '**bunion**' is a thickened bursa on the inner aspect of the 1st metatarsal head, usually associated with hallux valgus deformity. Note that the bursae that may develop (and become inflamed) over the calcaneus, navicular, the phalanges and the head of the 1st metatarsal are called *adventitial* bursae. They are not found in normal anatomy but occur only under the pathological conditions described. This is in contrast to the pre- and infrapatellar bursae, which are normal anatomical structures and which may become distended with fluid as a result of repeated trauma.

Measurements in the lower limb

Measurement is an important part of the clinical examination of the lower limb. Unfortunately, students find difficulty in carrying this out accurately and still greater difficulty in explaining the results they obtain, yet this is nothing more or less than a simple exercise in applied anatomy.

First note the differences between *real* and *apparent* shortening of the lower limbs. Real shortening is due to actual loss of bone length; for example, when a femoral fracture has united with a good deal of overriding of the two fragments. Apparent shortening is due to a *fixed* deformity of the limb (Fig. 4.1). Stand up and flex your knee and hip on one side, imagine these are both ankylosed at 90° and note that, although there is no loss of tissue in this limb, it is apparently some 2 ft. (60 cm) shorter than its partner.

If there is a fixed pelvic tilt or fixed joint deformity in one limb, there may be this apparent difference between the lengths of the two limbs. By experimenting on yourself you will find that adduction apparently shortens the limb, whereas it is apparently lengthened in abduction.

To measure the real length of the limbs (Fig. 4.2), overcome any disparity due to fixed deformity by putting both limbs into exactly the same position; where there is no joint fixation, this means that the patient lies with his pelvis 'square', his limbs abducted symmetrically and both limbs lying flat on the couch. If, however, one hip is in 60° of fixed flexion, for example, the other hip must first be put into this identical position. The length of each limb is then measured from

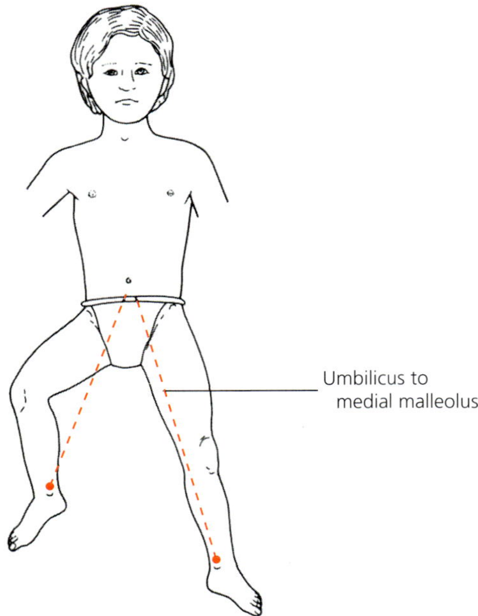

Figure 4.1 Apparent shortening – one limb may be apparently shorter than the other because of fixed deformity; the legs in this illustration are actually equal in length but the right is *apparently* considerably shorter because of a gross flexion contracture at the hip. Apparent shortening is measured by comparing the distance from the umbilicus to the medial malleolus on each side.

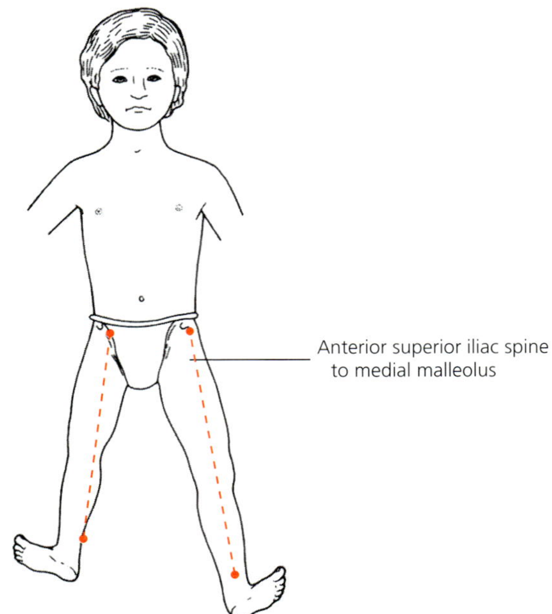

Figure 4.2 Measuring real shortening – the patient lies with the pelvis 'square' and the legs placed symmetrically. Measurement is made from the anterior superior spine to the medial malleolus on each side.

the anterior superior iliac spine to the medial malleolus. In order to obtain identical points on each side, slide the finger upwards along Poupart's inguinal ligament and mark the bony point first encountered by the finger. Similarly, slide the finger upwards from just distal to the malleolus to determine the apex of this landmark on each side.

To determine apparent shortening, the patient lies with his legs parallel (as they would be when he stands erect) and the distance from umbilicus to each medial malleolus is measured (Fig. 4.1).

Now suppose we find 4 in. (10 cm) of apparent shortening and 2 in. (5 cm) of real shortening of the limb; we interpret this as meaning that 2 in. (5 cm) of the shortening is due to true loss of limb length and another 2 in. (5 cm) is due to fixed postural deformity.

If the apparent shortening is *less* than the real, this can only mean that the hip has ankylosed in the abducted, and hence apparently elongated, position.

Note this important point: one reason why the orthopaedic surgeon immobilizes a tuberculous hip in the abducted position is that, when the hip becomes ankylosed, shortening due to actual destruction at the hip (i.e. true shortening) will be compensated, to a considerable extent, by the apparent lengthening produced by the fixed abduction.

Having established that there is real shortening present, the examiner must then determine whether this is at the hip, the femur or the tibia, or at a combination of these sites.

At the hip

Place the thumb on the anterior superior spine and the index finger on the greater trochanter on each side; a glance is sufficient to tell if there is any difference between the two sides.

Measuring *Nelaton's line* and *Bryant's triangle* is seldom undertaken in clinical practice these days. Nevertheless, some examiners remain partial to asking questions about them (Fig. 4.3).

Nelaton's line joins the anterior superior iliac spine to the ischial tuberosity and should normally lie above the greater trochanter; if the line passes through or below the trochanter, there is shortening at the head or neck of the femur.

Bryant's triangle might better be called '*Bryant's* T' because it is not necessary to construct all of its three sides. With the patient supine, a perpendicular is dropped from each anterior

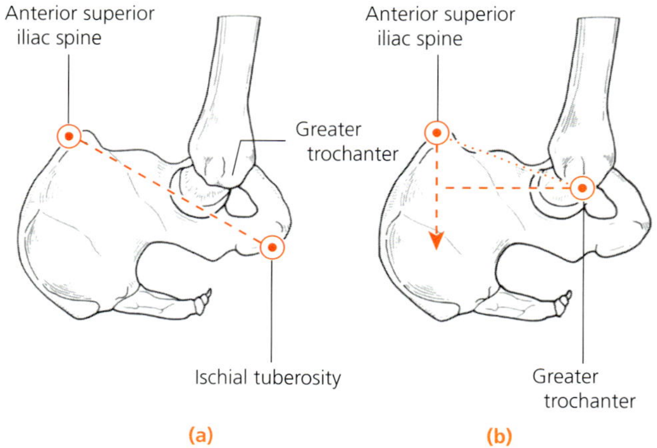

Figure 4.3 (a) Nelaton's line joins the anterior superior iliac spine to the ischial *tuberosity* – normally this passes above the greater trochanter. (b) Bryant's triangle – in the supine subject, drop a vertical from each superior spine; compare the perpendicular distance from this line to the greater trochanter on either side. (There is no need to complete the third side of the triangle.)

superior spine and the distance between this line and the greater trochanter compared on each side. (The third side of the triangle, joining the trochanter to the anterior spine, need never be completed.)

At the femur

Measure the distance from the anterior superior spine (if hip disease has been excluded) or from the greater trochanter to the line of the knee joint (not to the patella, whose height can be varied by contraction of the quadriceps).

At the tibia

Compare the distance from the line of the knee joint to the medial malleolus on each side.

Muscles and tendons

Quadriceps femoris forms the prominent muscle mass on the anterior aspect of the thigh; its insertion into the medial aspect of the patella can be seen to extend more distally than on the lateral side. In the well-developed subject, *sartorius* can be defined when the hip is flexed and externally rotated against resistance. It extends from the anterior superior iliac spine to the medial side of the upper end of the tibia and, as the lateral border of the *femoral triangle*, it is an important landmark.

Gluteus maximus forms the bulk of the buttock and can be felt to contract in extension of the hip.

Gluteus medius and *minimus* and the *adductors* can be felt to tighten, respectively, in resisted abduction and adduction of the hip.

Define the tendons around the knee with this joint comfortably flexed in the sitting position:

- **Laterally:** The *biceps* tendon passes to the head of the fibula, the *iliotibial tract* lies approximately 0.5 in. (1.25 cm) in front of this tendon and passes to the lateral condyle of the tibia.
- **Medially:** The bulge which one feels is the *semimembranosus insertion* on which two tendons, *gracilis*, medially and more anteriorly, and *semitendinosus*, laterally and more posteriorly, are readily palpable.

Between the tendons of biceps and semitendinosus can be felt the heads of origin of *gastrocnemius*. This muscle, with soleus, forms the bulk of the posterior bulge of the calf; the two end distally in the *Achilles tendon* (calcaneal tendon).

At the front of the ankle (Fig. 4.4) the tendon of *tibialis anterior* lies most medially, passing to its insertion at the base of the 1st metatarsal and the medial cuneiform. More laterally, the tendons of *extensor hallucis longus* and *extensor digitorum longus* are readily visible in the dorsiflexed foot. *Peroneus longus* and *brevis* tendons pass behind the lateral malleolus. Behind the medial malleolus, from the medial to the lateral

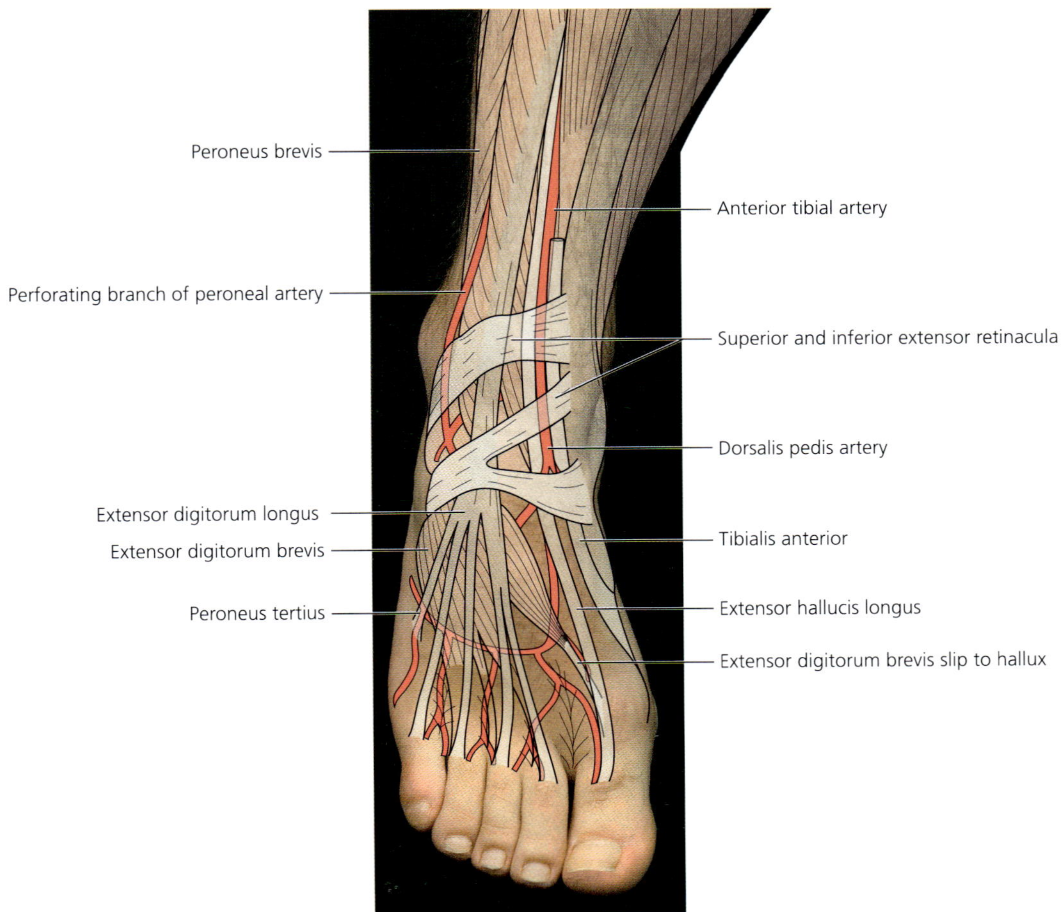

Figure 4.4 The structures passing over the dorsum of the ankle (right ankle, anterior aspect).

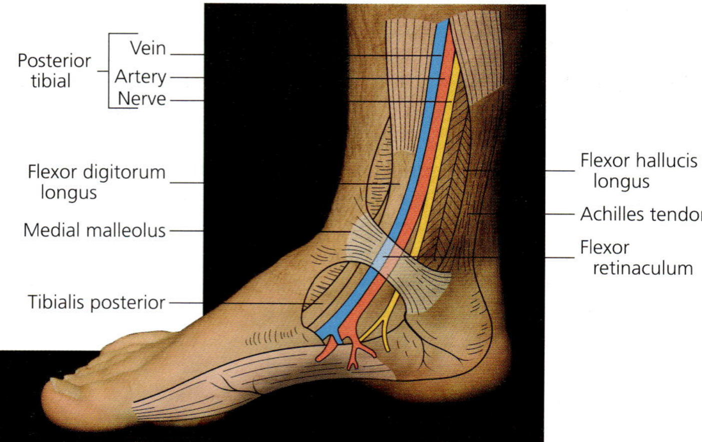

Figure 4.5 The structures passing behind the medial malleolus (right ankle, medial aspect).

side, pass the tendons of *tibialis posterior* and *flexor digitorum longus*, the *posterior tibial artery* with its venae comitantes, the *tibial nerve* and, finally, *flexor hallucis longus* (Fig. 4.5).

Vessels

The *femoral artery* (Fig. 4.6) can be felt pulsating at the mid-inguinal point, half-way between the anterior superior iliac spine and the pubic symphysis. The upper two-thirds of a line joining this point to the adductor tubercle, with the hip somewhat flexed, abducted and externally rotated, accurately defines the surface marking of this vessel. A finger on the femoral pulse lies directly over the head of the femur, immediately lateral to the femoral vein (and the termination of the great saphenous vein) and a finger's breadth medial to the femoral nerve.

The *pulse of popliteal artery* is often not easy to detect. It is most readily felt with the patient prone, his knee flexed and his muscles relaxed by resting the leg on the examiner's arm. The pulse is sought by firm pressure downwards against the popliteal fossa of the femur.

The *pulse of dorsalis pedis artery* (Fig. 4.4) is felt between the tendons of extensor hallucis longus and extensor digitorum longus on the dorsum of the foot – it is absent in approximately 2% of normal subjects. The *posterior tibial artery* (Fig. 4.5) may be felt a finger's breadth below and behind the medial malleolus. In approximately 1% of healthy subjects this artery is replaced by the *peroneal (fibular) artery*.

The absence of one or both pulses at the ankle is not, therefore, in itself diagnostic of vascular disease.

The *small (or short) saphenous vein* commences as a continuation of the veins on the lateral side of the dorsum of the foot, runs proximally *behind* the lateral malleolus, and terminates by draining into the popliteal vein behind the knee. The *great (or long) saphenous vein* arises from the medial side of the dorsal network of veins, passes upwards *in front* of the medial malleolus, with the saphenous nerve anterior to it, to enter the femoral vein in the groin, 1 in. (2.5 cm) below the inguinal ligament and immediately medial to the femoral pulse.

These veins are readily studied in any patient with extensive varicose veins and are usually visible, in their lower part, in the thin normal subject on standing. (The word 'saphenous' is derived from the Greek for 'clear'.)

From the practical point of view, the position of the long saphenous vein immediately in front of the medial malleolus is perhaps the most important single anatomical relationship; no matter how collapsed or obese, or how young and tiny the patient, the vein can be relied upon to be available at this site when urgently required for transfusion purposes (Fig. 4.7).

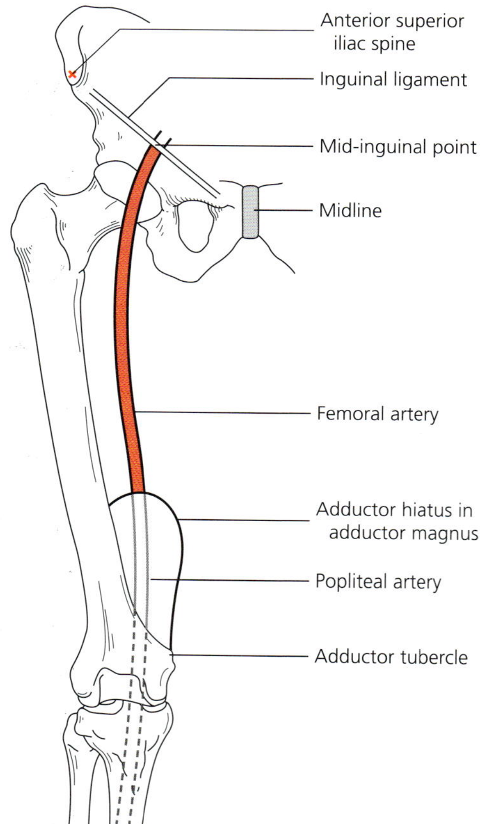

Figure 4.6 The surface markings of the femoral artery; the upper two-thirds of a line joining the mid-inguinal point (halfway between the anterior superior iliac spine and the symphysis pubis) to the adductor tubercle.

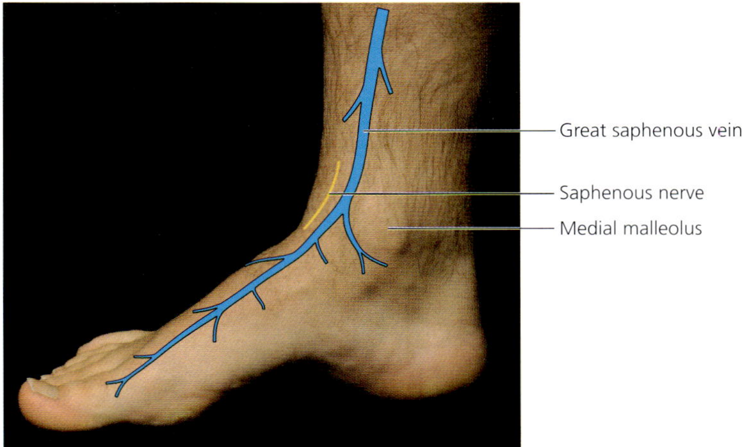

Figure 4.7 The relationship of the great (long) saphenous vein to the medial malleolus (right ankle).

Nerves

Only one nerve is easily felt in the lower limb; this is the *common peroneal (fibular) nerve*, which can be rolled against the bone as it winds round the neck of the fibula (Fig. 4.8). Not unnaturally, it may be injured at this site in adduction injuries to the knee or compressed by a tight plaster cast or firm bandage, with a resultant foot drop and inversion (talipes equinovarus; *see* page 154).

The *femoral nerve* emerges from under the inguinal ligament 0.5 in. (1.25 cm) lateral to the femoral pulse. After a course of approximately 2 in. (5 cm) the nerve breaks up into its terminal branches.

The surface markings of the *sciatic nerve* (Fig. 4.9) can be represented by a line which commences at a point midway between the posterior superior iliac spine (identified by the overlying easily visible sacral dimple) and the ischial tuberosity, curves outwards and downwards through a point midway between the greater trochanter and ischial tuberosity and then continues vertically downwards in the midline of the posterior aspect of the thigh. The nerve ends at a variable point above the popliteal fossa by dividing into the *tibial* and *common peroneal nerves*, respectively.

It would seem inconceivable that a nerve with such constant and well-defined landmarks could be damaged by intramuscular injections, yet this has happened so frequently that it has seriously been proposed that this site should be prohibited. The explanation is, we believe, a psychological one. The standard advice is to use the upper outer quadrant of the buttock for these injections, and when the full anatomical extent of the buttock – extending upwards to the iliac crest and outwards to the greater trochanter – is implied, perfectly sound and safe advice this is. Many health-care professionals, however, have an entirely different mental picture of the buttock; a much smaller and more aesthetic affair comprising merely the hillock of the natus. An injection into the upper outer quadrant of this diminutive structure lies in the immediate vicinityof the sciatic nerve!

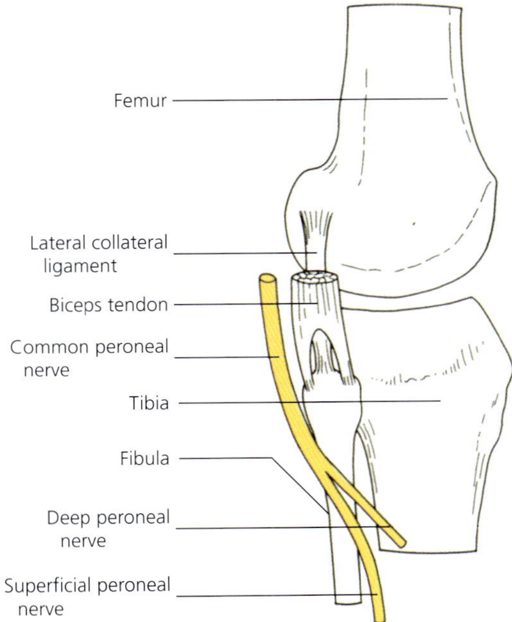

Figure 4.8 The close relationship of the common peroneal nerve to the neck of the fibula; at this site it may be compressed by a tight bandage or plaster cast (right knee, lateral aspect).

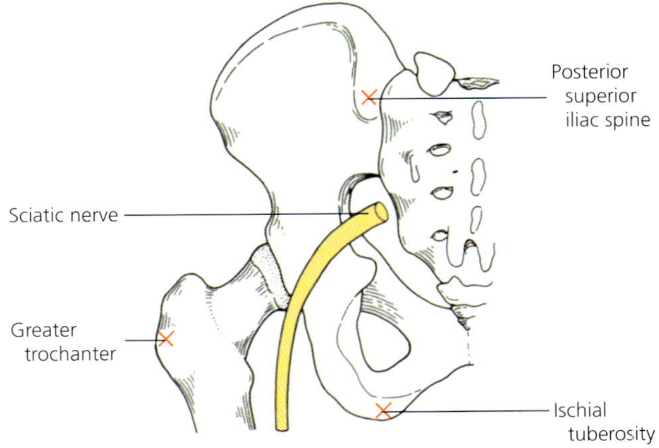

Figure 4.9 The surface markings of the sciatic nerve (left gluteal region). Join the midpoint between the ischial tuberosity and posterior superior iliac spine to the midpoint between the ischial tuberosity and the greater trochanter by a curved line; continue this line vertically down the leg – it represents the course of the sciatic nerve.

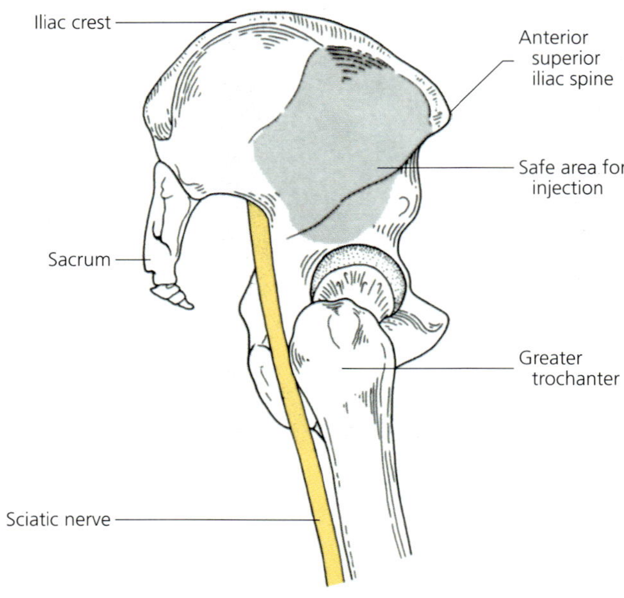

Figure 4.10 The 'safe area' for injections in the buttock.

A better surface marking for the 'safe area' of buttock injections can be defined as that area which lies under the outstretched hand when the thumb and thenar eminence are placed along the iliac crest with the tip of the thumb touching the anterior superior iliac spine (Fig. 4.10).

Bones and joints of the lower limb

The bones of the lower limb comprise os innominatum/hip bone, femur, patella, fibula and bones of the foot.

Os innominatum

See 'Bony and ligamentous pelvis', pages 73–75.

Femur (Figs 4.11 and 4.12)

The femur or the thigh bone is the longest and the strongest bone in the body. It is 18 in. (45 cm) in length, a measurement it shares with the vas deferens, the spinal cord and the thoracic duct and which is also the distance from the teeth to the cardia of the stomach.

The femoral *head* is two-thirds of a sphere and faces upwards, medially and forwards. It is covered with articular hyaline cartilage except for its central *fovea,* where the ligamentum teres is attached.

The *neck* is 2 in. (5 cm) long and is set at an angle of 135° to the shaft. In the female, with her wider pelvis, the angle is smaller.

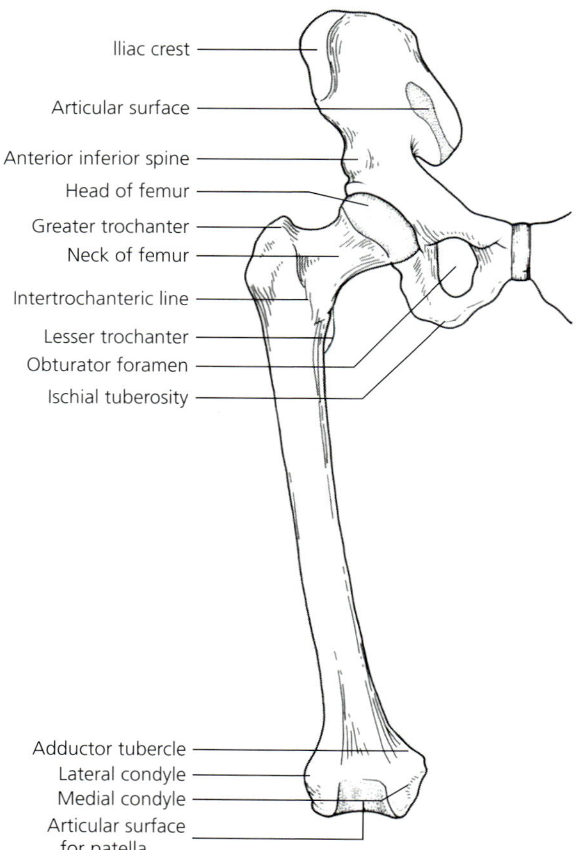

Figure 4.11 The anterior aspect of the right femur.

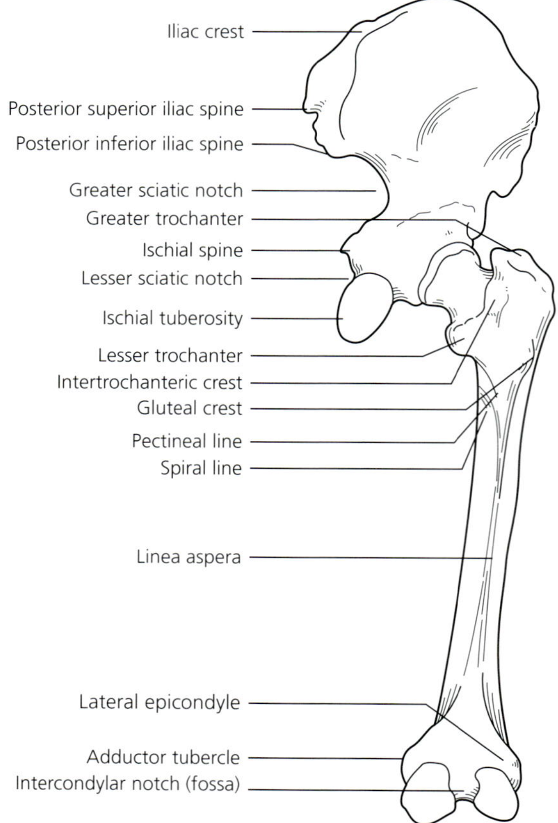

Figure 4.12 The posterior aspect of the right femur.

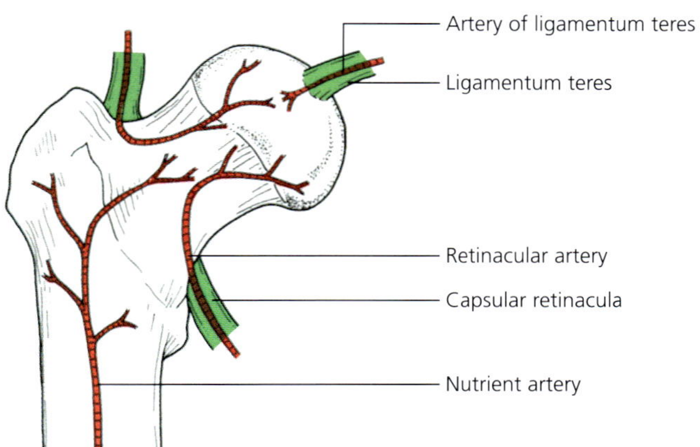

Figure 4.13 The sources of blood supply to the femoral head – along the ligamentum teres, through the diaphysis and via the retinacula.

The junction between the neck and the shaft is marked anteriorly by the *trochanteric line*, laterally by the *greater trochanter*, medially and somewhat posteriorly by the *lesser trochanter* and posteriorly by the prominent *trochanteric crest*, which unites the two trochanters.

The blood supply to the femoral head is derived from vessels travelling up from the diaphysis along the cancellous bone, from vessels in the hip capsule, where this is reflected onto the neck in longitudinal bands or retinacula, and from the artery in the ligamentum teres; this third source is negligible in adults, but essential in children, when the femoral head is separated from the neck by the cartilage of the epiphyseal line (Fig. 4.13).

The femoral *shaft* is roughly circular in section at its middle but is flattened posteriorly at each extremity. Posteriorly also it is marked by a strong crest, the *linea aspera*. Inferiorly,this crest splits into the medial and lateral *supracondylar lines*, leaving a flat *popliteal surface* between them. The medial supracondylar line ends distally in the *adductor tubercle*.

The lower end of the femur bears the prominent *condyles*, which are separated by a deep *intercondylar notch* (fossa) posteriorly but which blend anteriorly to form an articular surface for the patella. The lateral condyle is the more prominent of the two and acts as a buttress to assist in preventing lateral displacement of the patella.

Clinical Features

1 The upper end of the femur is a common site for fracture in the elderly. The neck may break immediately beneath the head (*subcapital*), near its midpoint (*cervical*) or adjacent to the trochanters (*basal*), or the fracture line may pass between, along or just below the trochanters (Fig. 4.14).

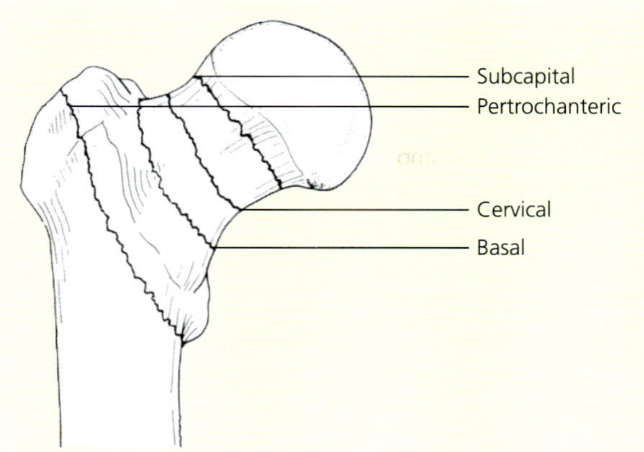

Figure 4.14 The head and neck of the femur, showing the terminology of the common fracture sites.

Fractures of the femoral neck will interrupt completely the blood supply from the diaphysis and, should the retinacula also be torn, avascular necrosis of the head will be inevitable. The nearer the fracture to the femoral head, the more tenuous the retinacular blood supply and the more likely it is to be disrupted.

Avascular necrosis of the femoral head in children is seen in Perthes' disease and in severe slipped femoral epiphysis; both resulting from thrombosis of the artery of the ligamentum teres.

In contrast, pertrochanteric fractures, being outside the joint capsule, leave the retinacula undisturbed; avascular necrosis, therefore, does not follow such injuries (Fig. 4.15).

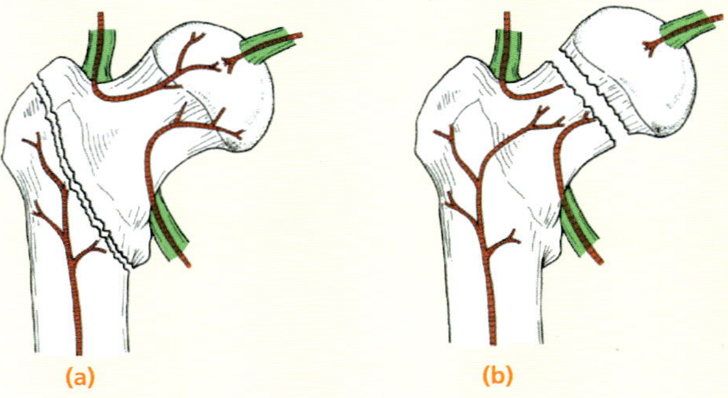

Figure 4.15 (a) A pertrochanteric fracture does not damage the retinacular blood supply – aseptic bone necrosis does not occur. **(b)** A subcapital fracture cuts off most of the retinacular supply to the head – aseptic bone necrosis is common. Note that the blood supply via the ligamentum teres is negligible in adult life.

There is a curious age pattern of hip injuries: children may sustain greenstick fractures of the femoral neck; schoolboys may displace the epiphysis of the femoral head; in adult life the hip dislocates; and in old age fracture of the neck of the femur again becomes the usual lesion.

2 Fractures of the femoral shaft are accompanied by considerable shortening as a result of the longitudinal contraction of the extremely strong surrounding muscles.

The proximal segment is flexed by iliacus and psoas and abducted by gluteus medius and minimus, whereas the distal

(Continued ...)

(... *continued*)

segment is pulled medially by the adductor muscles. Reduction requires powerful traction, to overcome the shortening, and then manipulation of the distal fragment into line with the proximal segment; the limb must therefore be abducted and also pushed forwards by using a large pad behind the knee.

Fractures of the lower end of the shaft, immediately above the condyles, are relatively rare; fortunately so, because they can be extremely difficult to treat since the small distal fragment is tilted backwards by gastrocnemius, the only muscle which is attached to it. The sharp proximal edge of this distal fragment may also tear the popliteal artery, which lies directly behind it (Fig. 4.16).

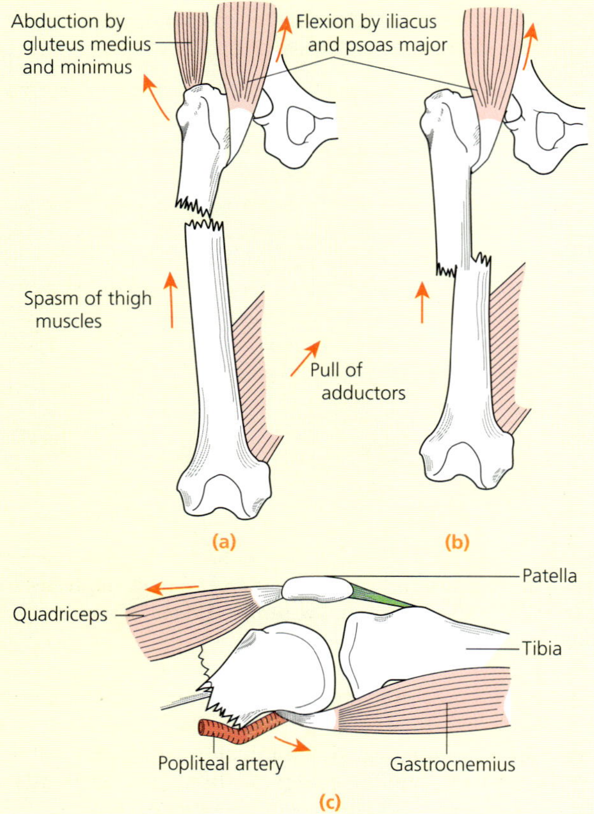

Figure 4.16 The deformities of femoral shaft fractures. **(a)** Fracture of the proximal shaft – the proximal fragment is flexed by iliacus and psoas and abducted by gluteus medius and minimus. **(b)** Fracture of the mid-shaft – flexion of the proximal fragment by iliacus and psoas. **(c)** Fracture of the distal shaft – the distal fragment is angulated backwards by gastrocnemius; the popliteal artery may be torn in this injury. (In all these fractures overriding of the bone ends is produced by muscle spasm.)

3 The angle subtended by the femoral neck to the shaft may be decreased, producing a *coxa vara* deformity. This may result from adduction fractures, slipped femoral epiphysis or bone-softening diseases. *Coxa valga*, in which the angle is increased, is much rarer but occurs in impacted abduction fractures. Note, that the angle measures less in females due to wider pelvis; however, that in children the normal angle between the neck and shaft is approximately 160°.

Patella

The patella is a sesamoid bone, the largest in the body, in the expansion of the quadriceps tendon. The tendon continues from the apex of the bone as the ligamentum patellae.

The posterior surface of the patella is covered with cartilage and articulates with the two femoral condyles by means of a larger lateral and smaller medial facet.

Clinical Features

1 Lateral dislocation of the patella is resisted by the prominent, anteriorly projecting articular surface of the lateral femoral condyle and by the medial pull of the lowermost fibres of vastus medialis, which insert almost horizontally along the medial margin of the patella. If the lateral condyle of the femur is underdeveloped, or if there is a considerable *genu valgum* (knock-knee deformity), recurrent dislocations of the patella may occur (Fig. 4.17).

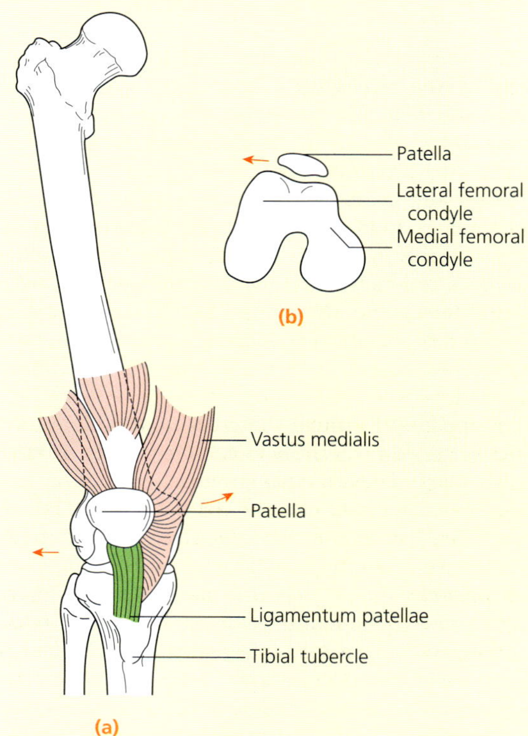

Figure 4.17 Factors in the stability of the patella: **(a)** the medial pull of vastus medialis and **(b)** the high patellar articular surface of the lateral femoral condyle. These resist the tendency for lateral displacement of the patella, which results from the valgus angulation between the femur and the tibia.

2 A direct blow on the patella may split or shatter it but the fragments are not avulsed because the quadriceps expansion remains intact.

The patella may also be fractured transversely by violent contraction of the quadriceps – for example, in trying to stop a backwards fall. In this case, the tear extends outwards into the quadriceps expansion, allowing the upper bone fragment to be pulled proximally; there may be a gap of over 2 in. (5 cm) between

(*Continued ...*)

(... *continued*)

the bone ends. Reduction is impossible by closed manipulation and operative repair of the extensor expansion is imperative.

Occasionally, this same mechanism of sudden forcible quadriceps contraction tears the quadriceps expansion above the patella, ruptures the ligamentum patellae or avulses the tibial tubercle.

It is interesting that, following complete excision of the patella for a comminuted fracture, knee function and movement may return to near-100% efficiency; it is difficult, then, to ascribe any particular function to this bone other than protection of the soft tissues of the knee joint anteriorly.

Tibia (Fig. 4.18)

The tibia is a larger medial bone of the leg. Its upper end is expanded into the *medial* and *lateral condyles*, the former having the greater surface area of the two. Between the condyles on the upper surface of the tibia (tibial plateau) is the *intercondylar area*, which bears, at its waist, the *intercondylar eminence*, projecting upwards slightly on either side as the *medial* and *lateral intercondylar tubercles*.

The *tuberosity* of the tibia is at the upper end of the anterior border of the shaft and gives attachment to the ligamentum patellae.

The anterior aspect of this tuberosity is subcutaneous, only excepting the infrapatellar bursa immediately in front of it.

The shaft of the tibia is triangular in cross-section, its anterior border and anteromedial surface being subcutaneous throughout their whole extent. The subcutaneous surface is crossed only by the easily visible *great saphenous vein*, accompanied by the *saphenous nerve*, immediately in front of the medial malleolus (Fig. 4.7).

The posterior surface of the shaft bears a prominent oblique line at its upper end termed the *soleal line*, which not only marks the tibial origin of the soleus but also delimits an area above, into which is inserted the popliteus.

The lower end of the tibia is expanded and quadrilateral in section, bearing an additional surface, the *fibular notch*, for the lower tibiofibular joint.

The *medial malleolus* projects from the medial extremity of the bone and is grooved posteriorly by the *tendon of tibialis posterior*.

The inferior surface of the lower end of the tibia is smooth, cartilage-covered and forms, with the malleoli, the upper articular surface of the ankle joint.

Clinical Features

1 The upper end of the tibial shaft is one of the most common sites for *acute osteomyelitis*. Fortunately, the capsule of the knee joint is attached closely around the articular surfaces so that the upper extremity of the tibial diaphysis is extracapsular; involvement of the knee joint therefore occurs only in the late and neglected case.

2 The shaft of the tibia is subcutaneous and unprotected anteromedially throughout its course and is particularly slender in its lower third. It is not surprising that the tibia is the commonest long bone to be fractured and to suffer compound injury.

3 The extensive subcutaneous surface of the tibia makes it a delightfully accessible donor site for bone grafts.

Fibula (Fig. 4.18)

The fibula is a smaller lateral bone of the leg. It serves three functions as mentioned below:

1. Provides origin to muscles
2. Forms a part of the ankle joint
3. Provides a pulley for the tendons of peroneus longus and brevis

It comprises the *head* with a *styloid process* (into which is inserted the tendon of biceps), the *neck* (around which passes the common peroneal nerve; Fig. 4.8), the *shaft* and the *lower end* or *lateral malleolus*. The last bears a roughened surface on its medial aspect for the lower tibiofibular joint, below which is the articular facet for the talus. A groove on the posterior aspect of the malleolus lodges the tendons of peroneus longus and brevis.

A note on growing ends and nutrient foramina in the long bones

The shaft of every long bone bears one or more *nutrient foramina* which are obliquely placed; this obliquity is the result of unequal growth at the upper and lower epiphyses. The artery is obviously dragged in the direction of more rapid growth and the direction of slope of entry of the nutrient foramen therefore points *away* from the more rapid growing end of the bone.

The *direction of growth of the long bones* can be remembered by a little jingle, which runs:

'From the knee, I flee
To the elbow, I grow.'

With one exception, the epiphysis of the growing end of a long bone is the first to appear and last to fuse with its diaphysis; the exception is the epiphysis of the upper end of the fibula which, although at the growing end, appears *after* the distal epiphysis and fuses after the latter has blended with the shaft.

The site of the growing end is of considerable practical significance; for example, if a child has to undergo an above-elbow amputation, the humeral upper epiphyseal line continues to grow and the elongating bone may well push its way through the stump end, requiring reamputation.

Bones of the foot

These are best considered as a functional unit and are therefore dealt with together under 'the arches of the foot' (*see* pages 141–142).

Hip joint (Figs 4.19 and 4.20)

The hip joint is a synovial joint of the ball and socket variety. It is the largest joint in the body. To the surgeon, the examiner and, therefore, the student it is also the most important.

It is a perfect example of a ball-and-socket joint. Its articular surfaces are the femoral head and the horseshoe-shaped articular surface of the acetabulum, which is deepened by the fibrocartilaginous *labrum acetabulare*. The non-articular lower part of the acetabulum, the *acetabular notch*, is closed off below by the *transverse acetabular ligament*. From this

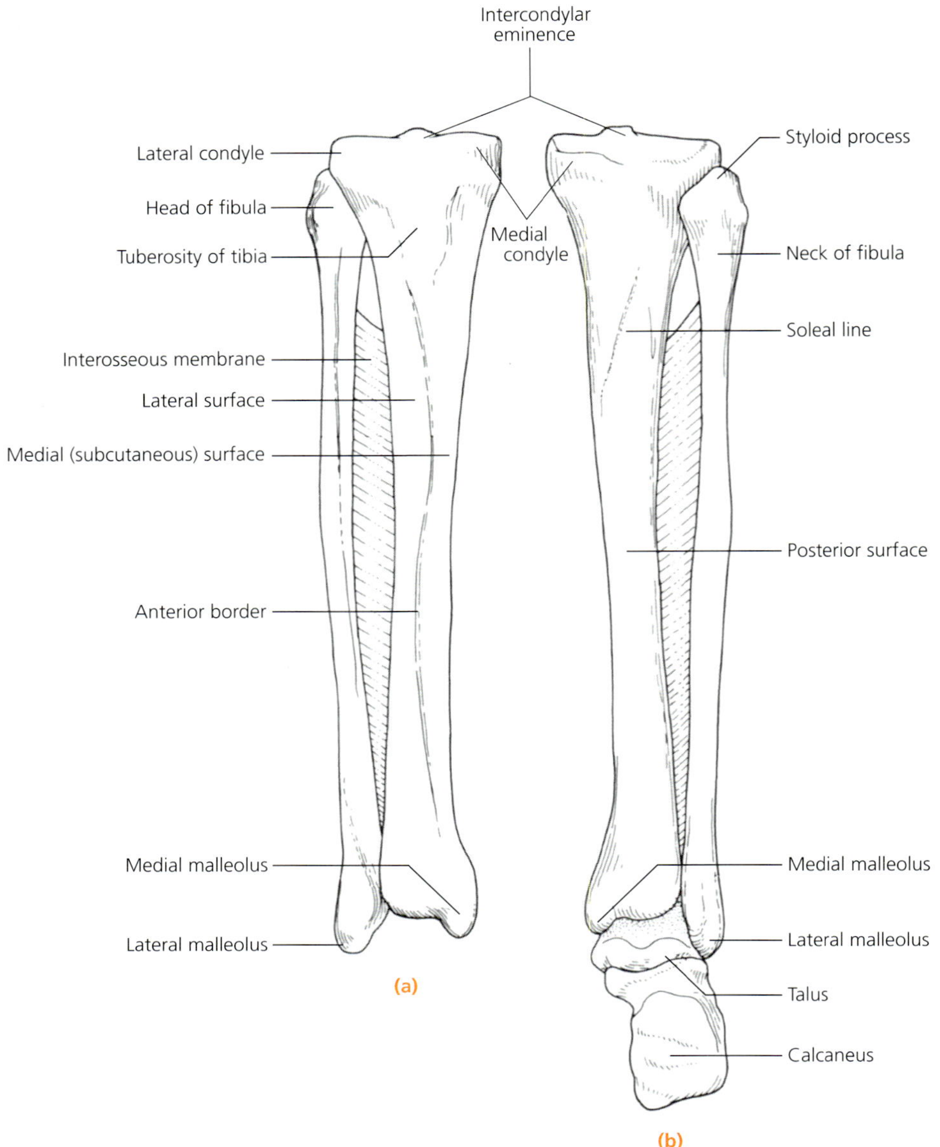

Figure 4.18 The tibia and fibula of the right side. **(a)** Anterior aspect. **(b)** Posterior aspect.

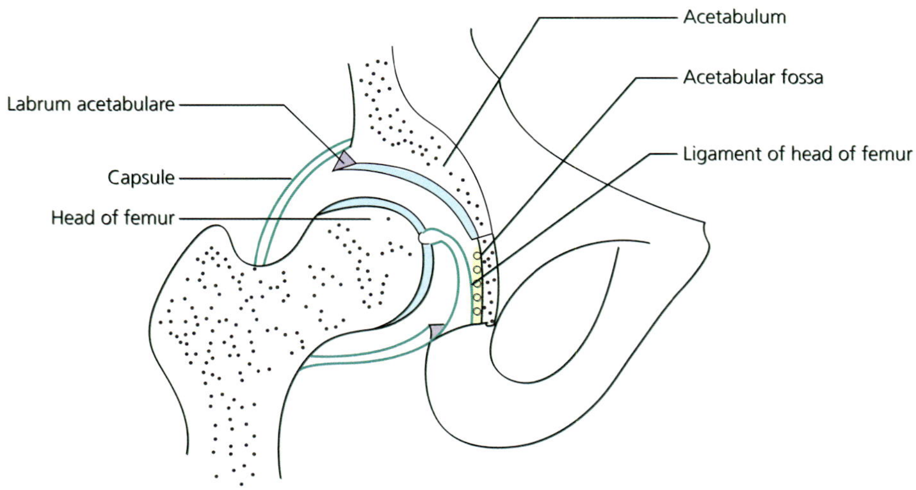

Figure 4.19 The articular surfaces of the hip joint as seen in the coronal section.

notch is given off the *ligamentum teres*, passing to the fovea on the femoral head (Fig. 4.19).

The *capsule* of the hip is attached proximally to the margins of the acetabulum and to the transverse acetabular ligament. Distally, it is attached along the trochanteric line, the bases of the greater and lesser trochanters and, posteriorly, to the femoral neck approximately 0.5 in. (1.25 cm) from the trochanteric crest. From this distal attachment, capsular fibres are reflected onto the femoral neck as *retinacula* and provide one pathway for the blood supply to the femoral head (*see* 'Femur', Fig. 4.13).

Note that *acute osteomyelitis* of the upper femoral metaphysis will involve the neck, which is intracapsular and which will therefore rapidly produce a secondary *pyogenic arthritis of the hip joint*.

Three ligaments reinforce the capsule are follows:

1. The *iliofemoral* (Y-shaped ligament of Bigelow), which arises from the anterior inferior iliac spine, bifurcates and is inserted at each end of the trochanteric line (Fig. 4.20).
2. The *pubofemoral* arising from the iliopubic junction to blend with the medial aspect of the capsule.
3. The *ischiofemoral* arising from the ischium to be inserted into the base of the greater trochanter.

Of these, the iliofemoral is by far the strongest and resists hyperextension strains on the hip. In posterior dislocation it usually remains intact.

The *synovium* of the hip covers the non-articular surfaces of the joint and occasionally bulges out anteriorly through an

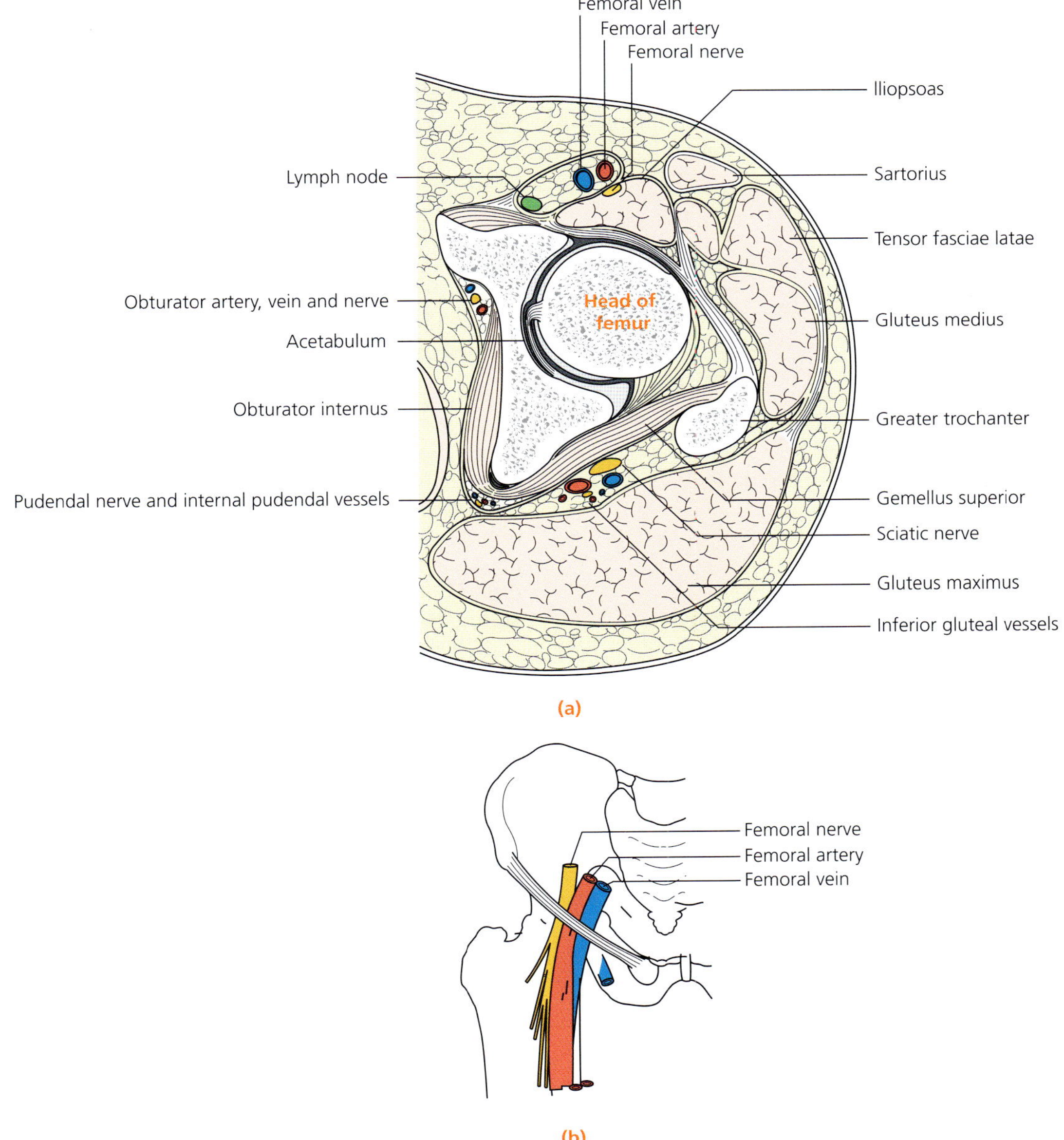

Figure 4.20 (a) The immediate relations of the hip joint (in diagrammatic horizontal section; right hip, viewed from proximal aspect). **(b)** Scout diagram indicating the level of the section.

opening in the capsule between iliofemoral and ischiofemoral ligaments to form a bursa beneath the psoas tendon (also called psoas bursa) where this crosses the front of the joint.

Movements

The hip is capable of a wide range of movements – flexion, extension, abduction, adduction, medial and lateral rotation and circumduction.

The principal muscles acting on the joint are as follows:

- **Flexors:** Iliacus and psoas major assisted by rectus femoris, sartorius, pectineus
- **Extensors:** Gluteus maximus, the hamstrings
- **Adductors:** Adductor longus, brevis and magnus assisted by gracilis and pectineus
- **Abductors:** Gluteus medius and minimus, tensor fasciae latae
- **Lateral rotators:** Principally gluteus maximus assisted by the obturators, gemelli and quadratus femoris
- **Medial rotators:** Tensor fasciae latae and anterior fibres of gluteus medius and minimus. Medial rotation is therefore a much weaker movement than lateral rotation

Relations (Figs 4.20 and 4.21)

The hip joint is surrounded by the following muscles:

- **Anteriorly:** Iliacus, psoas major and pectineus, together with the femoral artery vein and nerve
- **Laterally:** Tensor fasciae latae, gluteus medius and minimus
- **Posteriorly:** The tendons of piriformis, obturator internus with the gemelli, quadratus femoris, the sciatic nerve and, more superficially, gluteus maximus
- **Superiorly:** The reflected head of rectus femoris lying in contact with the joint capsule
- **Inferiorly:** The obturator externus, passing back to be inserted into the trochanteric fossa

Surgical exposure of the hip joint therefore inevitably involves considerable and deep dissection.

The *lateral approach* comprises splitting down through the fibres of tensor fasciae latae, gluteus medius and minimus on to the femoral neck. Further access may be obtained by detaching the greater trochanter with the gluteal insertions.

The *anterior approach* passes between gluteus medius and minimus laterally and sartorius medially, then dividing the reflected head of rectus femoris to expose the anterior aspect of the hip joint. More room may be obtained by detaching these glutei from the external aspect of the ilium.

The *posterior approach* is through an angled incision commencing at the posterior superior iliac spine, passing to the greater trochanter and then dropping vertically downwards from this point. Gluteus maximus is split in the line of its fibres and then incised along its tendinous insertion. Deep to gluteus maximus, the short lateral rotators are divided a few centimetres medial to their attachments on the greater trochanter. The medial stumps of the divided short lateral rotators are retracted medially to protect the sciatic nerve. An excellent view of the posterior aspect of the hip joint is thus obtained.

Nerve supply

Hilton's law states that the nerves crossing a joint supply the muscles acting on it, the skin over the joint and the joint itself. The hip is no exception and receives fibres from the *femoral, sciatic and obturator nerves*. It is important to note that these nerves also supply the knee joint and, for this reason, it is not uncommon for a patient, particularly a child, to complain bitterly of pain in the knee and for the cause of the mischief, the diseased hip, to be overlooked.

Dislocation of the hip (Fig. 4.22)

The hip is usually dislocated backwards and this is produced by a force applied along the femoral shaft with the hip in the flexed position (e.g. the knee striking against the opposite seat when a train runs into the buffers). If the hip is also in the adducted position, the head of the femur is unsupported posteriorly by the acetabulum and dislocation can occur without an associated acetabular fracture. If the hip is abducted, dislocation must be accompanied by a fracture of the posterior acetabular lip.

The sciatic nerve, a close posterior relation of the hip, is in danger of damage in these injuries, as will be appreciated by a glance at Fig. 4.9.

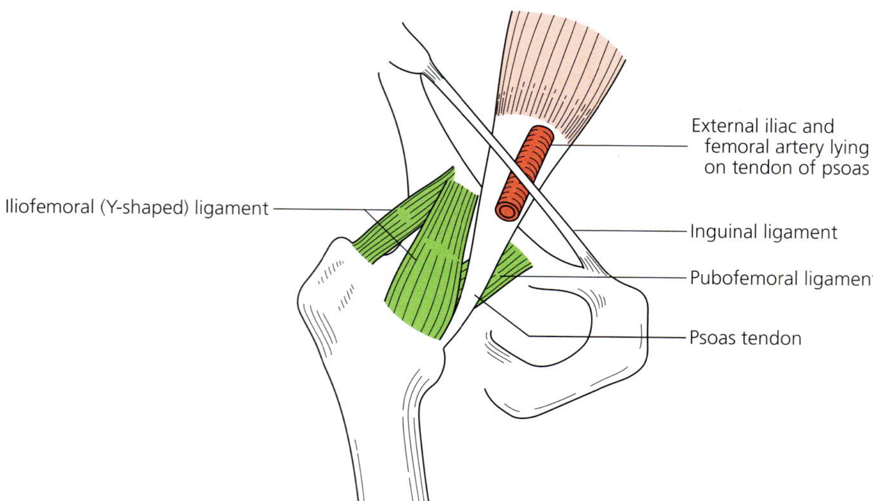

Figure 4.21 The anterior aspect of the right hip. Note that the psoas tendon and the femoral artery are intimate anterior relations of the joint.

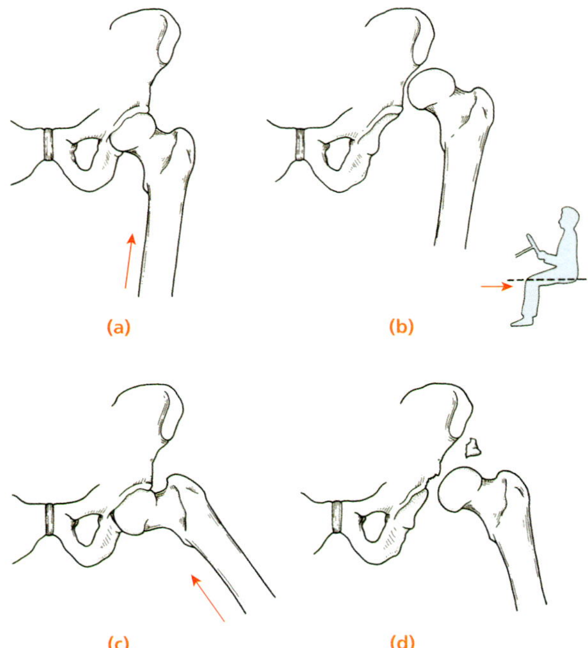

Figure 4.22 Dislocation of the hip. If the hip is forced into posterior dislocation while adducted **(a)**, there is no associated fracture of the posterior acetabular lip **(b)**. Dislocation in the abducted position **(c)** can occur only with a concomitant acetabular fracture **(d)**. (The inset figure indicates the plane of these diagrams.)

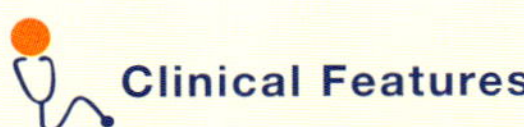

Trendelenburg's test

The stability of the hip in the standing position depends on two factors: the strength of the surrounding muscles and the integrity of the lever system of the femoral neck and head within the intact hip joint. When standing on one leg, the abductors of the hip on this side (gluteus medius and minimus and tensor fasciae latae) come into powerful action to maintain fixation at the hip joint, so much so that the pelvis actually rises slightly on the opposite side. If, however, there is any defect in these muscles or lever mechanism of the hip joint, the weight of the body in these circumstances forces the pelvis to tilt downwards on the opposite side.

This positive Trendelenburg test is seen if the hip abductors are paralysed (e.g. poliomyelitis), if there is an old unreduced or congenital dislocation of the hip, if the head of the femur has been destroyed by disease or removed operatively (pseudarthrosis), if there is an un-united fracture of the femoral neck or if there is a very severe degree of coxa vara.

The test may be said to indicate '*a defect in the osseomuscular stability of the hip joint*'.

A patient with any of the conditions enumerated above walks with a characteristic '*dipping gait*'.

Reduction of a dislocated hip is quite simple providing that a deep anaesthetic is used to relax the surrounding muscles; the hip is flexed, rotated into the neutral position and lifted back into the acetabulum. Occasionally, forcible abduction of the hip will dislocate the hip forwards. Violent force along the shaft (e.g. a fall from a height) may thrust the femoral head through the floor of the acetabulum, producing a central dislocation of the hip.

Knee joint (Figs 4.23, 4.24 and 4.25)

The knee joint is the largest and most complicated joint in the body. It is a modified hinge joint, made up of the articulations between the femoral and tibial condyles and between the patella and the patellar surface of the femur (Fig. 4.25). Primitively, there were three joint cavities, now merged into one: one between medial condyle of the femoral and tibia (medial tibiofemoral articulation), one between lateral condyle of the femur and tibia (lateral tibiofemoral articulation) and one between patella and femur (patellofemoral articulation).

The *capsule* is attached to the margins of these articular surfaces but communicates above with the *suprapatellar bursa* (between the lower femoral shaft and the quadriceps), posteriorly with the bursa under the medial head of gastrocnemius and often, through it, with the bursa under semimembranosus. It may also communicate with the bursa under the lateral head of gastrocnemius. The capsule is also perforated posteriorly by popliteus, which emerges from it in much the same way that the long head of biceps bursts out of the shoulder joint.

The capsule of the knee joint is reinforced on each side by the *medial* and *lateral collateral ligaments*, the latter passing to the head of the fibula and lying free from the capsule.

Anteriorly, the capsule is considerably strengthened by the *ligamentum patellae*, and, on each side of the patella, by the *medial* and *lateral patellar retinacula*, which are expansions from vastus medialis and lateralis, respectively.

Posteriorly, the tough *oblique ligament* arises as an expansion from the insertion of semimembranosus and blends with the joint capsule.

Internal structures (Figs 4.24 and 4.25)

Within the joint are a number of important structures. The *cruciate ligaments* are extremely strong connections between the tibia and femur. They arise from the anterior and posterior intercondylar areas of the superior aspect of the tibia, taking their names from their tibial origins, and pass obliquely upwards to attach to the intercondylar notch of the femur.

The anterior cruciate ligament resists forward displacement of the tibia on the femur and becomes taut in hyperextension

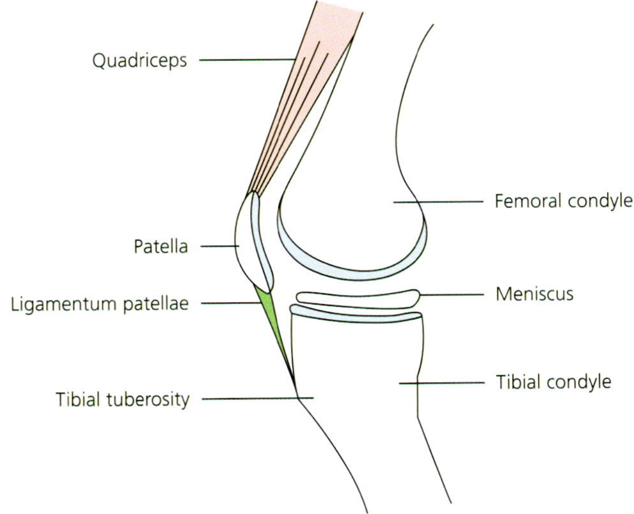

Figure 4.23 Knee joint, lateral view.

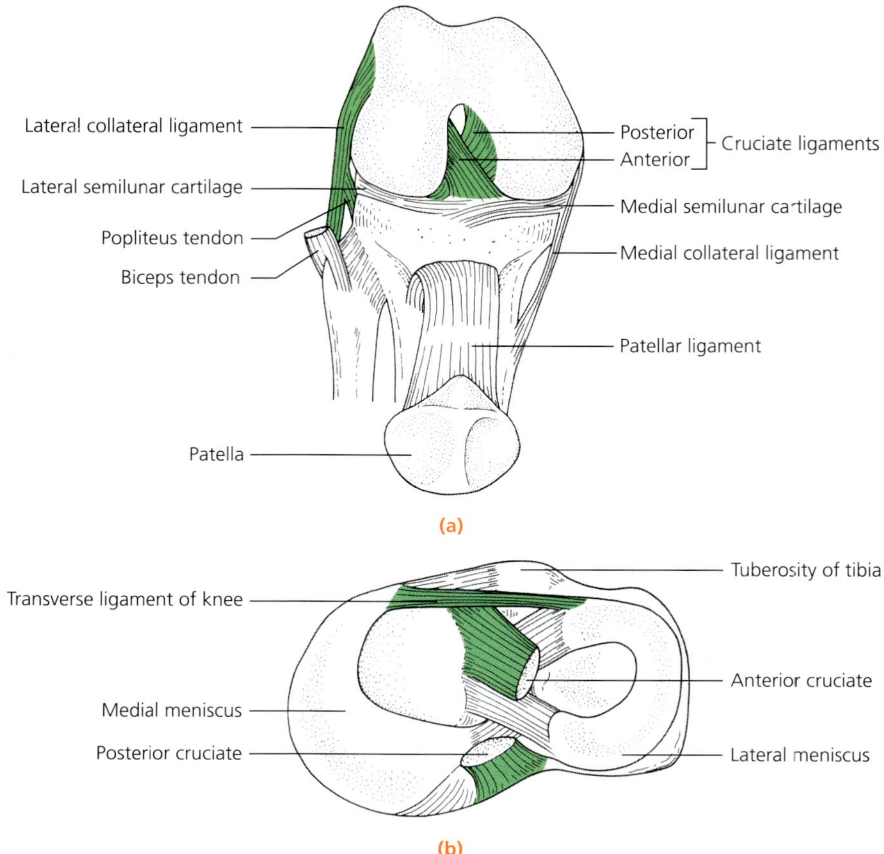

Figure 4.24 **(a)** The right knee – anterior view; the knee is flexed and the patella has been turned downwards. **(b)** The right knee in transverse section.

of the knee; it also resists rotation. The posterior cruciate ligament resists backward displacement of the tibia and becomes taut in hyperflexion.

The *semilunar cartilages (menisci)* are crescent-shaped and are triangular in cross-section, the medial being larger and less curved than the lateral. They are attached by their extremities to the tibial intercondylar area and by their periphery to the capsule of the joint, although the lateral cartilage is only loosely adherent and the popliteus tendon intervenes between it and the lateral collateral ligament.

They deepen, although to only a negligible extent, the articulations between the tibial and femoral condyles and probably act as shock absorbers. If both menisci are removed, the knee can regain complete functional efficiency, although it is interesting that, following surgery, a rim of fibrocartilage regenerates from the connective tissue margin of the excised menisci.

An *infrapatellar pad of fat* fills the space between the ligamentum patellae and the femoral intercondylar notch. The synovium covering this pad projects into the joint as two folds termed the *alar folds*.

Movements of the knee

The principal knee movements are flexion and extension, but note on yourself that some degree of rotation of the knee is possible when this joint is in the flexed position. In full extension, i.e. in the standing position, the knee is quite rigid because the medial condyle of the tibia, being rather larger

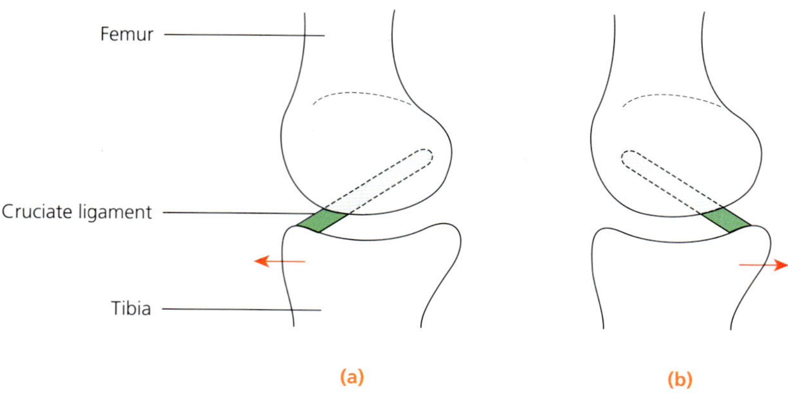

Figure 4.25 The actions of the cruciate ligaments. **(a)** Anterior cruciate ligament – resists forward movement of tibia on femur. **(b)** Posterior cruciate ligament – resists backward movement of tibia on femur

than the lateral condyle, rides forwards on the medial femoral condyle, thus '*screwing*' the joint firmly together. The first step in flexion of the fully extended knee is '*unscrewing*' or internal rotation. This is brought about by *popliteus*, which arises from the lateral side of the lateral condyle of the femur, emerges from the joint capsule posteriorly and is inserted into the back of the upper end of the tibia.

The principal muscles acting on the knee are as follows:

- **Extensor:** Quadriceps femoris
- **Flexors:** Hamstrings assisted by gracilis, gastrocnemius and sartorius
- **Medial rotator:** Popliteus ('unscrews the knee')

Tibiofibular joints

The tibia and fibula are connected by the following:

1. The *superior tibiofibular joint*, a synovial joint of plane variety between the head of the fibula and the lateral condyle of the tibia
2. The *interosseous membrane*, which is crossed by the anterior tibial vessels above and pierced by the perforating branch of the peroneal artery below
3. The *inferior tibiofibular joint*, a fibrous joint, the only one in the limbs, between the triangular areas of each bone immediately above the ankle joint. It represents, in fact, the reinforced distal end of the fibrous tissue of the tibiofibular interosseous membrane

Clinical Features

1 The stability of the knee depends upon the strength of its surrounding muscles and of its ligaments. Of the two, the muscles are by far the more important. Providing quadriceps femoris is powerfully developed, the knee will function satisfactorily even in the face of considerable ligamentous damage. Conversely, the most skilful surgical repair of torn ligaments is doomed to failure unless the muscles are functioning strongly; without their support, reconstructed ligaments will merely stretch once more.

2 When considering soft-tissue injuries of the knee joint, think of three the Cs that may be damaged – the Collateral ligaments, the Cruciates and the Cartilages.

The *collateral ligaments* are taut in full extension of the knee and are, therefore, liable to injury only in this position. The medial ligament may be partly or completely torn when a violent abduction strain is applied, whereas an adduction force may damage the lateral ligament. If one or other collateral ligament is completely torn, the extended knee can be rocked away from the affected side.

The *cruciate ligaments* may both be torn (along with the collateral ligaments) in severe abduction or adduction injuries. The anterior cruciate, which is taut in extension, may be torn by violent hyperextension of the knee or in anterior dislocation of the tibia on the femur. Since it resists rotation, it may also be torn in a violent twisting injury to the knee. The posterior cruciate tears in a posterior dislocation (Fig. 4.24).

If both the cruciate ligaments are torn, unnatural anteroposterior mobility of the knee can be demonstrated.

(Continued ...)

(... continued)

If there is only increased forward mobility, the anterior cruciate ligament has been divided or is lax. Increased backward mobility implies a lesion of the posterior cruciate.

The *semilunar cartilages* can tear only when the knee is flexed and is thus able to rotate. If you place a finger on either side of the ligamentum patellae on the joint line and then rotate your flexed knee first internally and then externally, you will note how the lateral and medial cartilages are respectively sucked into the knee joint. If the flexed knee is forcibly abducted and externally rotated, the medial cartilage will be drawn between, and then split by, the grinding surfaces of the medial condyles of the femur and tibia. This occurs when a footballer twists his flexed knee while running or when a miner topples over in the crouched position while hewing coal in a narrow seam. A severe adduction and internal rotation strain may similarly tear the lateral cartilage, but this injury is less common.

The knee 'locks' in this type of injury because the torn and displaced segment of cartilage lodges between the condyles and prevents full extension of the knee.

Ankle joint (Fig. 4.26)

The ankle joint (talocrural joint) is a hinge joint between a mortice formed by the malleoli and lower end of the tibia and the body of the talus.

The *capsule* of the joint fits closely around its articular surfaces, and, as in every hinge joint, it is weak anteriorly and posteriorly but reinforced laterally and medially by *collateral ligaments*.

The *medial collateral ligament* (or deltoid ligament) is the stronger of the two. It radiates from its attachment to the tip of the medial malleolus to attach, from before backwards, to the tuberosity of the navicular, the spring ligament, the sustentaculum tali and the medial tuberosity of the talus (Fig. 4.26(b)). The *lateral collateral ligament* is a complex of three bands (or ligaments) which radiate from the fibular malleolus. These are the anterior talofibular band, running forwards to the neck of the talus, the calcaneofibular, passing downwards and backwards to the calcaneus, and the posterior talofibular, passing backwards to the talus (Fig. 4.26(c)). At the first glance, the direction of the anterior talofibular ligament seems all wrong! However, put your foot, or the bones of an articulated skeleton, into the plantar-flexed position and invert it – you will note that now this ligament will come directly into the line of strain.

Movements of the ankle

The ankle joint is capable of being flexed and extended (plantar- and dorsiflexion).

The body of the talus is slightly wider anteriorly and, in full extension (i.e. dorsiflexion), becomes firmly wedged between the malleoli. Conversely, in flexion (i.e. plantarflexion), there is slight laxity at the joint and some degree of side-to-side tilting is possible; test this fact on yourself.

The principal muscles acting on the ankle are as follows:

- **Dorsiflexors:** Tibialis anterior assisted by extensor digitorum longus, extensor hallucis longus and peroneus tertius
- **Plantarflexors:** Gastrocnemius and soleus assisted by tibialis posterior, flexor hallucis longus and flexor digitorum longus

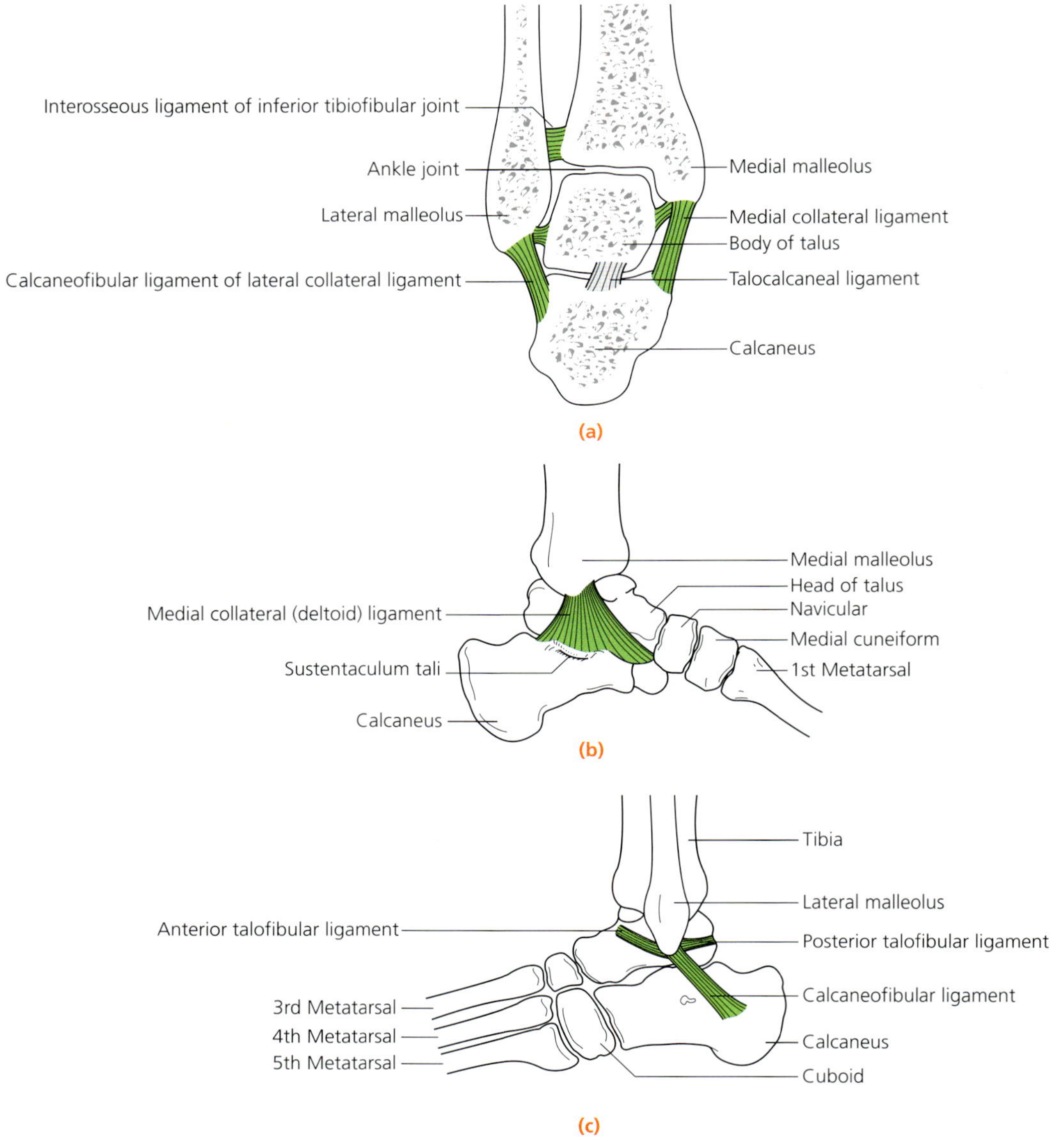

Figure 4.26 The left ankle. **(a)** In coronal section (viewed from behind). **(b)** Medial aspect. **(c)** Lateral aspect.

Joints of the foot

The *inversion* and *eversion* of the foot take place at the *talocalcaneal articulations* and at the *midtarsal joints* between the calcaneus and the cuboid and between the talus and the navicular (Fig. 4.27). Of these, the talocalcaneal joint is far the more important. Test this on yourself – hold your calcaneus between your finger and thumb; inversion and eversion of the foot are prevented.

Loss of these rotatory movements of the foot, for example after injury or due to arthritis, results in quite severe disability

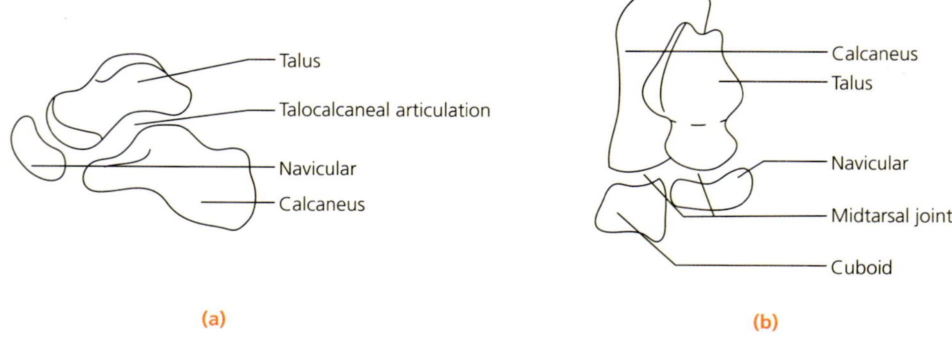

Figure 4.27 Joints of the foot. **(a)** Talocalcaneal articulation. **(b)** Mid-tarsal joint.

because the foot cannot adapt itself to walking on uneven, rough or sloping ground.

Inversion is brought about by tibialis anterior and tibialis posterior assisted by the long extensor and flexor tendons of the hallux; *eversion* is the duty of peroneus longus and brevis (assisted by peroneus tertius which is a member of the extensor muscles).

The other tarsal joints allow slight gliding movements only, and, individually, are not of clinical importance. The arrangement of the metatarsophalangeal and interphalangeal joints is on the same basic plan as in the upper limb.

Clinical Features

1 The collateral ligaments of the ankle can be sprained or completely torn by forcible abduction or adduction, the lateral ligament being far the more frequently affected. This is because, first, the medial collateral ligament is more powerful than the lateral and, second, and you can test this on yourself, you are more likely to twist your ankle into forcible inversion than eversion. The first part of the lateral collateral ligament to come under strain is the anterior talofibular ligament, and it is this strand that tears in partial rupture of the lateral ligament. If the ligament is completely disrupted the talus can be tilted in its mortice; this is difficult to demonstrate clinically and is best confirmed by taking an anteroposterior radiograph of the ankle while forcibly inverting the foot.

(Continued ...)

(... continued)

2 The most usual ankle fracture is that produced by an abduction–external rotation injury; the patient catches his foot in a rabbit hole, his body and his tibia internally rotate while the foot is rigidly held. First, there is a torsional spinal fracture of the lateral malleolus, then avulsion of the medial collateral ligament, with or without avulsion of a flake of the medial malleolus, and, finally, as the tibia is carried forwards, the posterior margin of the lower end of the tibia shears off against the talus. These stages are termed *1st, 2nd* and *3rd degree Pott's fractures*. Notice that, with widening of the joint, there is forward dislocation of the tibia on the talus, producing characteristic prominence of the heel in this injury.

Arches of the foot (Fig. 4.28)

On standing, the heel and the metatarsal heads are the principal weight-bearing points, but a moment's study of wet footprints on the bathroom floor will show that the lateral margin of the foot and the tips of the phalanges also touch the ground.

The bones of the foot are arranged in the form of *two longitudinal arches*. The *medial arch* comprises calcaneus, talus, navicular, the three cuneiforms and the three medial metatarsals; the apex of this arch is the talus. The *lateral arch*, which is lower, comprises the calcaneus, cuboid and the lateral two metatarsals.

The foot plays a double role; it functions as a rigid support for the weight of the body in the standing position, and as a mobile springboard during walking and running.

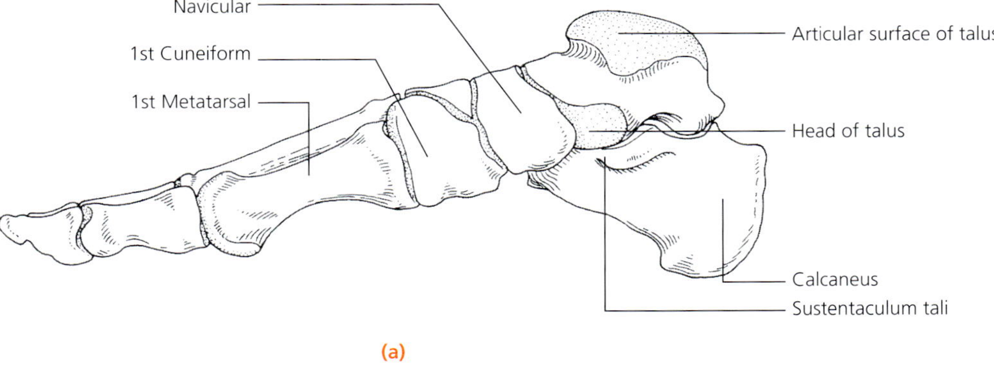

(a)

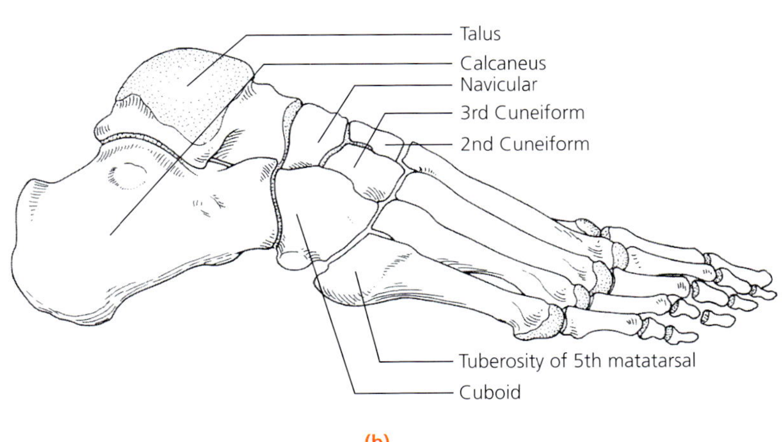

(b)

Figure 4.28 The longitudinal arches of the right foot. **(a)** Medial view. **(b)** Lateral view.

When one stands, the arches sink somewhat under the body's weight, the individual bones lock together, the ligaments linking them are at maximum tension and the foot becomes an immobile pedestal. When one walks, the weight is released from the arches, which unlock and become a mobile lever system in the spring-like actions of locomotion.

The arches are maintained by the following:

1. The shape of the interlocking bones
2. The ligaments of the foot
3. Muscle action

The ligaments concerned are the following (Fig. 4.29):

1. The dorsal, plantar and interosseous ligaments between the small bones of the forefoot
2. The *spring ligament*, which passes from the *sustentaculum tali* of the calcaneus forwards to the *tuberosity of the navicular* and which supports the inferior aspect of the head of the talus
3. The *short plantar ligament*, which stretches from the plantar surface of the calcaneus to the cuboid
4. The *long plantar ligament*, which arises from the posterior tuberosity on the plantar surface of the calcaneus, covers the short plantar ligament, forms a tunnel for the peroneus longus tendon with the cuboid, and is inserted into the bases of the 2nd, 3rd and 4th metatarsals

These ligaments are reinforced in their action by the *plantar aponeurosis*, which is the condensed deep fascia of the sole of the foot. This arises from the plantar aspect of the calcaneus (medial process of the calcaneal tubercle) and is attached to the deep transverse ligaments linking the heads of the metatarsals; it also continues forwards into each toe to form the fibrous flexor sheaths, in a similar arrangement to that of the palmar fascia of the hand. Indeed, like the palmar fascia, it may be subject to Dupuytren's contracture (page 119).

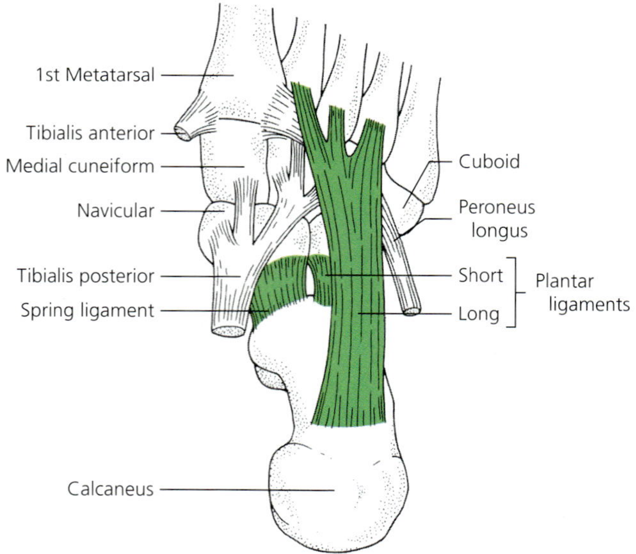

Figure 4.29 Plantar aspect of the left foot to show the attachments of the important ligaments and long tendons. (The head of the talus is hidden, deep to the spring ligament.)

The principal muscles concerned in the mechanism of the arches of the foot are peroneus longus, tibialis anterior and posterior, flexor hallucis longus and the intrinsic muscles of the foot.

Peroneus longus tendon passes obliquely across the sole in a groove on the cuboid bone and is inserted into the lateral side of the base of the 1st metatarsal and the medial cuneiform. Into the medial aspect of these two bones is inserted the tendon of *tibialis anterior* so that these muscles form, in effect, a stirrup between them that supports the arches of the foot.

The medial arch is further reinforced by flexor hallucis longus, whose tendon passes under the sustentaculum tali of the calcaneus, and by *tibialis posterior*, two-thirds of whose fibres are inserted into the tuberosity of the navicular and support the spring ligament.

The longitudinally running intrinsic muscles of the foot also act as ties to the longitudinal arches.

Anatomy of walking

In the process of walking, the heel is raised from the ground, the metatarsophalangeal joints flex to give a 'push-off' movement; the foot then leaves the ground completely and is dorsiflexed to clear the toes.

Just before the toes of one foot leave the ground, the heel of the other makes contact.

Forward progression is produced partly by the 'push-off' of the toes, partly by powerful plantarflexion of the ankle and partly by the forward swing of the hips accentuated by swinging movements of the pelvis. Paraplegics can be taught to walk purely by this pelvic swing action, even though paralysed from the waist downwards.

When one foot is off the ground, dropping of the pelvis to the unsupported side is prevented by the hip abductors (gluteus medius and minimus and tensor fasciae latae). Their paralysis is one cause of a 'dipping gait' and of a positive Trendelenburg sign (*see* page 137).

Three important zones of the lower limb

The three important zones of the lower limb comprise the femoral triangle, adductor canal and popliteal fossa.

Femoral triangle (Fig. 4.30)

The femoral triangle (Scarpa's triangle) is a triangular depression on the front of thigh below the inguinal ligament.

This triangle is bounded by the following:

- **Superiorly:** By the inguinal ligament
- **Medially:** By the medial border of adductor longus
- **Laterally:** By the medial border of sartorius

Its *floor* consists of iliacus, the tendon of psoas, pectineus and adductor longus.

The *roof* is formed by the superficial fascia, containing the superficial inguinal lymph nodes and the great saphenous vein with its tributaries, and the deep fascia (fascia

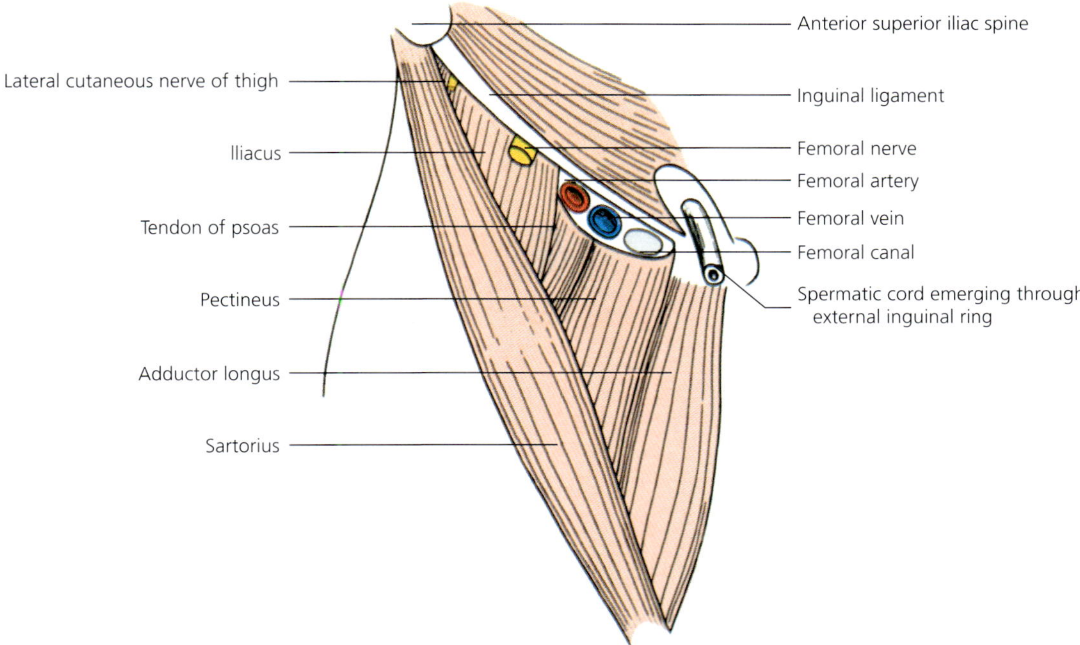

Figure 4.30 The right femoral triangle and its contents.

lata), which is pierced by the great saphenous vein at the saphenous opening.

The *contents* of the triangle are the femoral vein, artery and nerve together with the deep inguinal nodes.

Some of these structures must now be considered in greater detail.

Fascia lata

The deep fascia of the thigh, or fascia lata, extends downwards to ensheath the whole lower limb except over the subcutaneous surface of the tibia (to whose margins it adheres), and at the saphenous opening. Above, it is attached all around to the root of the lower limb – that is to say, to the inguinal ligament, pubis, ischium, sacrotuberous ligament, sacrum and coccyx and the iliac crest. The fascia of the thigh is particularly dense laterally (the *iliotibial tract*), where it receives tensor fasciae latae, and posteriorly, where the greater part of gluteus maximus is inserted into it. The iliotibial tract, when tensed by its attached muscles, assists in the stabilization of the hip and the extended knee when standing.

The fact that a considerable part of the largest muscle of the lower limb, gluteus maximus, inserts into it shows the importance of this tract. Note that when you stand for a long period of time, for example in the operating theatre, you shift from one leg to the other and maintain the leg you are standing on by tension of the iliotibial tract.

The tough lateral fascia of the thigh is an excellent source of this material for hernia and dural repairs.

Femoral sheath and femoral canal (Fig. 4.31)

The femoral artery and vein enter the femoral triangle from beneath the inguinal ligament within a fascial tube termed the *femoral sheath*. This is derived from the extraperitoneal intra-abdominal fascia, its anterior wall arising from the transversalis fascia and its posterior wall from the fascia iliaca, the fascia covering the iliacus.

The medial part of the femoral sheath contains a small, almost vertically placed, gap, the *femoral canal*, which is approximately 0.5 in. (1.25 cm) in length and which just admits the tip of the little finger. The greater width of the female pelvis means that the canal is somewhat larger in the female and femoral herniae are, consequently, commoner in this sex.

The **boundaries of the femoral canal** are as follows:

- **Anteriorly:** The inguinal ligament
- **Medially:** The sharp free edge of the pectineal part of the inguinal ligament, termed the *lacunar ligament (Gimbernat's ligament)*
- **Laterally:** The femoral vein
- **Posteriorly:** The pectineal ligament (of Astley Cooper), which is the thickened periosteum along the pectineal border of the superior pubic ramus and which continues medially with the pectineal part of the inguinal ligament

The canal contains a plug of fat and a constant lymph node – the *node of the femoral canal* or *Cloquet's gland*.

The canal has two functions: first, as a dead space for expansion of the distended femoral vein and, second, as a lymphatic pathway from the lower limb to the external iliac nodes.

Femoral hernia

The great importance of the femoral canal is, of course, that it is a potential point of weakness in the abdominal wall through which may develop a femoral hernia. Unlike the indirect inguinal hernia, this is never due to a congenital sac and, although cases do occur rarely in children, it is never found in the newborn.

As the hernia sac enlarges, it emerges through the saphenous opening then turns upwards along the pathway presented

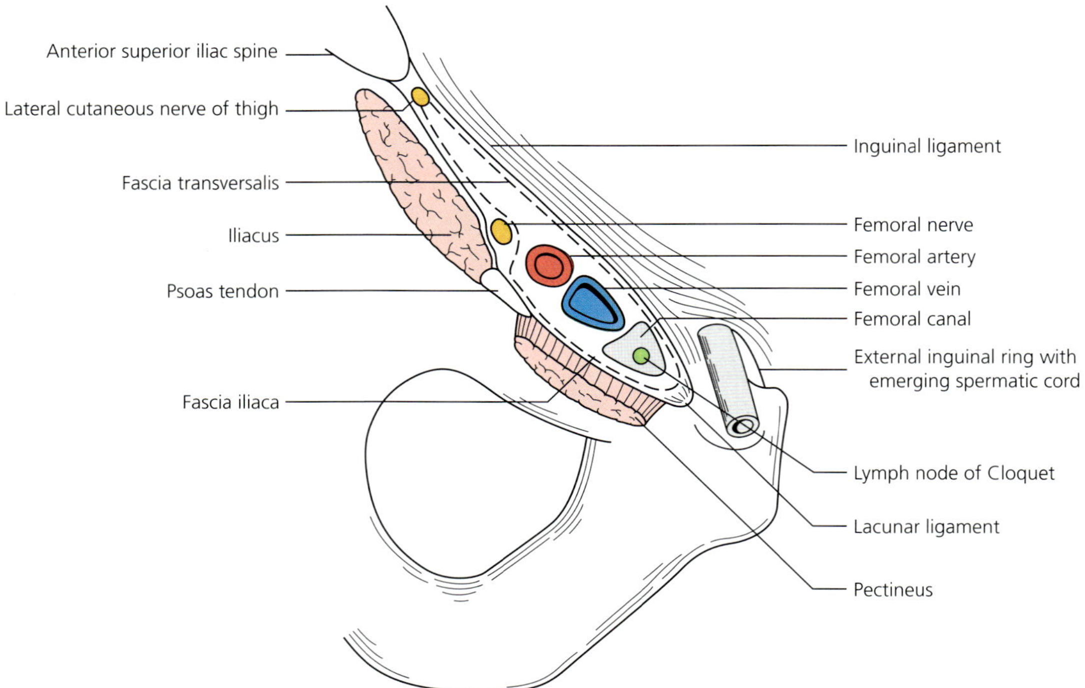

Figure 4.31 The femoral canal and its surrounds (right inguinal region).

by the superficial epigastric and superficial circumflex iliac vessels so that it may come to project above the inguinal ligament. There should not, however, be any difficulty in differentiating between an irreducible femoral and inguinal hernia; the neck of the former must always lie below and lateral to the pubic tubercle, whereas the sac of the latter extends above and medial to this landmark (Fig. 4.32).

The neck of the femoral canal is narrow and bears a particular sharp medial border; for this reason, irreducibility and strangulation occur more commonly at this site than at any other. In order to enlarge the opening of the canal at operation on a strangulated case, this sharp edge of Gimbernat's lacunar ligament may require incision; there is a slight risk of damage to the abnormal obturator artery in this manoeuvre and

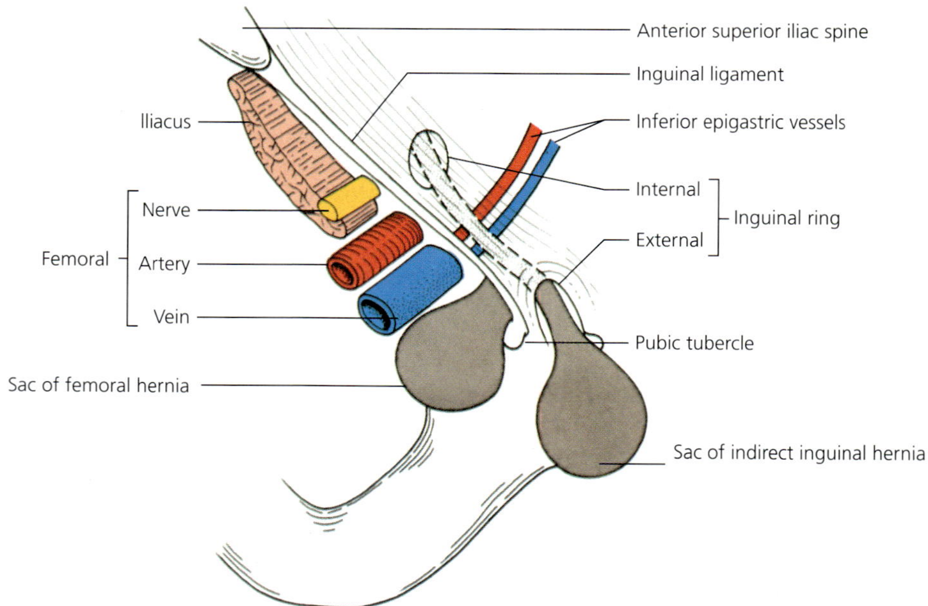

Figure 4.32 The relationship of an indirect inguinal and a femoral hernia to the pubic tubercle; the inguinal hernia emerges above and medial to the tubercle, the femoral hernia lies below and lateral to it (right inguinal region).

it is safer to enlarge the opening by making several small nicks into the ligament. The safe alternative is to divide the inguinal ligament, which can then be repaired.

Note that normally there is an anastomosis between the pubic branch of the inferior epigastric artery and the pubic branch of the obturator artery. Occasionally, the obturator artery is entirely replaced by this branch from the inferior epigastric – the *abnormal obturator artery*. This aberrant vessel usually passes laterally to the femoral canal and is out of harm's way; more rarely, it passes behind Gimbernat's ligament and it is then in surgical danger.

Lymph nodes of the groin and the lymphatic drainage of the lower limb

The lymph nodes of the groin are arranged in a superficial and a deep group. The *superficial nodes* lie in two chains, a *longitudinal chain* along the great saphenous vein, receiving the bulk of the superficial lymph drainage of the lower limb, and a *horizontal chain*, just distal to the inguinal ligament. These horizontal nodes receive lymphatics from the skin and superficial tissues of the following:

1. The lower trunk and back, below the level of the umbilicus
2. The buttock
3. The perineum, scrotum and penis (or lower vagina and vulva) and the anal canal below its mucocutaneous junction

In addition, some lymphatics drain via the round ligament to these nodes from the fundus of the uterus.

(All these sites, as well as the whole leg, must be examined carefully when a patient presents with an *inguinal lymphadenopathy*.)

The two groups of superficial nodes drain through the saphenous opening in the fascia lata into the *deep nodes* lying medial to the femoral vein, which also receive the lymph drainage from the tissues of the lower limb beneath the deep fascia. In addition, a small area of skin over the heel and lateral side of the foot drains by lymphatics along the small saphenous vein to nodes in the popliteal fossa and then along the femoral vessels directly to the deep nodes at the groin.

The deep groin nodes drain to the external iliac nodes by lymphatics that travel partly in front of the femoral artery and vein and partly through the femoral canal.

Clinical Features

1 Minor sepsis and abrasions of the leg are so common that it is usual to find that the inguinal nodes are palpable in perfectly healthy people.

2 Secondary involvement of the inguinal nodes by malignant deposits may be dealt with by *block dissection of the groin*. This involves removal of the superficial and deep fascial roof of the femoral triangle, the saphenous vein and its tributaries and the fatty and lymphatic contents of the triangle, leaving only the femoral artery, vein and nerve. The inguinal ligament is detached so that, in addition, an extraperitoneal removal of the external iliac nodes can be carried out.

(*Continued ...*)

(*... continued*)

3 In making a differential diagnosis of a lump in the femoral triangle, think of each anatomical structure and of the pathological conditions to which it may give rise, thus:
- **Skin and soft tissues:** Lipoma, sebaceous cyst, sarcoma
- **Artery:** Aneurysm of the femoral artery
- **Vein:** Varix of the great saphenous vein
- **Nerve:** Neuroma of the femoral nerve or its branches
- **Femoral canal:** Femoral hernia
- **Psoas sheath:** Psoas abscess
- **Lymph nodes:** Any of the causes of lymphadenopathy

Adductor canal (of Hunter) or subsartorial canal (Fig. 4.33)

The adductor canal is an intermuscular space on the medial side of the middle one-third of the thigh.

This canal leads on from the apex of the femoral triangle and ends at the hiatus of the adductor magnus.

Boundaries

Its **boundaries** are as follows:

- **Posteriorly:** Adductor longus and magnus
- **Anterolaterally:** Vastus medialis
- **Anteromedially:** The sartorius, which lies on a fascial sheet forming the roof of the canal

Contents

The **contents** of the canal are the femoral artery, the femoral vein (which lies behind the artery), the saphenous nerve and, in its upper part, the nerve to vastus medialis from the femoral nerve.

John Hunter described the exposure and ligation of the femoral artery in this canal for *aneurysm of the popliteal artery*; this method has the advantage that the artery at this site is healthy and will not tear when tied, as may happen if ligation is attempted immediately above the aneurysm.

Popliteal fossa (Fig. 4.34)

The popliteal fossa is a diamond-shaped (rhomoid-shaped) hollow behind the knee joint. It is the distal continuation of the adductor canal. This 'fossa' is, in fact, a closely packed compartment which becomes the rhomboid-shaped space of anatomical diagrams only when opened up at operation or by dissection.

Boundaries

Its boundaries are as follows:

- **Superolaterally:** Biceps femoris tendon
- **Superomedially:** Semimembranosus reinforced by semitendinosus
- **Inferomedially and inferolaterally:** The medial and lateral heads of gastrocnemius, respectively

The *roof* of the fossa is deep fascia, which is pierced by the small saphenous vein as this enters the popliteal vein.

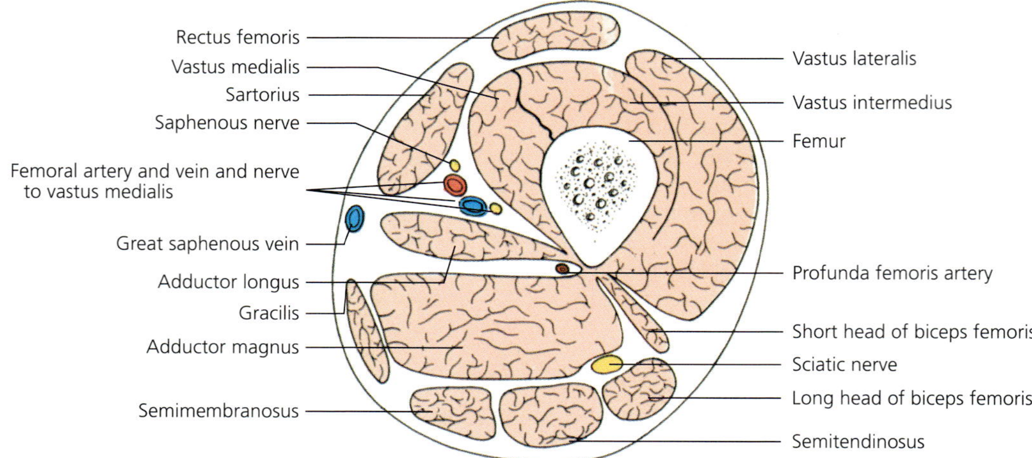

Figure 4.33 Cross-section through the right thigh in the region of the adductor, or subsartorial, canal of Hunter (viewed from the proximal aspect).

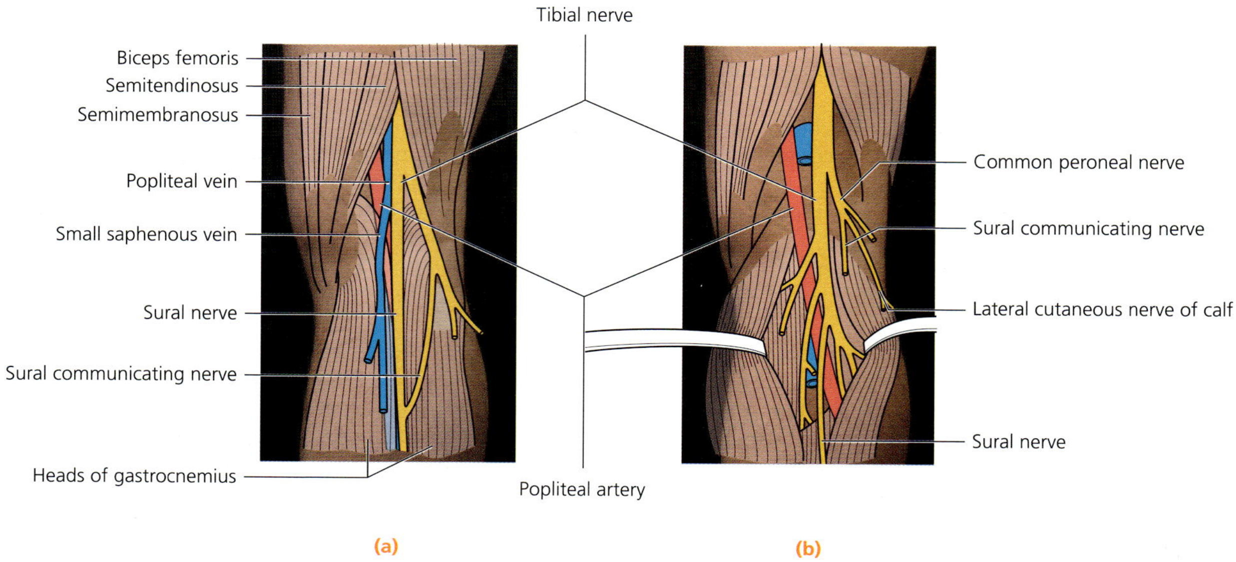

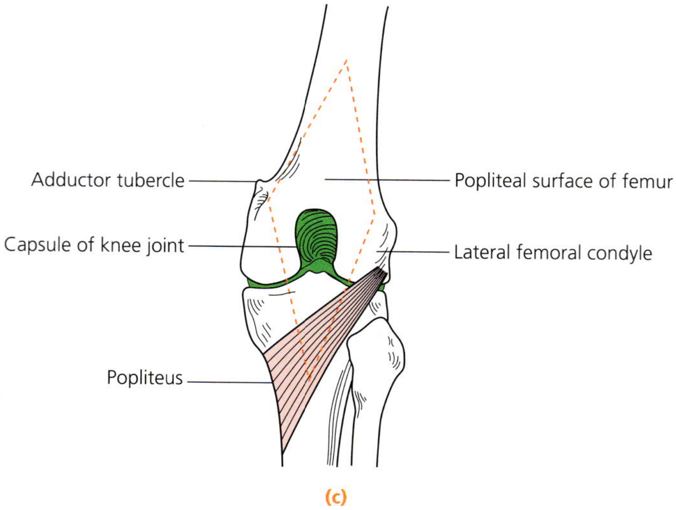

Figure 4.34 The right popliteal fossa. **(a)** Superficial dissection. **(b)** Deep dissection. **(c)** Floor.

Its *floor*, from above down, is formed by the following:

- The popliteal surface of the femur
- The posterior aspect of the knee joint
- The popliteus muscle covering the upper posterior surface of the tibia

Contents

From without in, the popliteal fossa contains nerves, vein and artery.

The *common peroneal nerve* passes out of the fossa along the medial border of the biceps tendon; the *tibial nerve* is first lateral to the popliteal vessels and then crosses superficial to these vessels to lie on their medial side.

The *popliteal vein* lies immediately superficial to the artery; the *popliteal artery* itself lies deepest of all in the fossa.

As well as these important structures, the fossa contains fat, popliteal lymph nodes and a variable number of thin-walled sacs termed bursae.

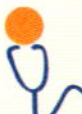

Clinical Features

The popliteal fossa is another good example of the value of thinking anatomically when considering the differential diagnosis of a mass situated in a particular anatomical area.

When examining a lump in the popliteal region, let the following possibilities pass through your mind:

- **Skin and soft tissues:** Sebaceous cyst, lipoma, sarcoma
- **Vein:** Varicosities of the short saphenous vein in the roof of the fossa
- **Artery:** Popliteal aneurysm
- **Lymph nodes:** Infection secondary to suppuration in the foot
- **Knee joint:** Joint effusion
- **Tendons:** Enlarged bursae, especially those beneath semimembranosus (e.g. Baker's cyst) and the heads of gastrocnemius
- **Bones:** A tumour of the lower end of the femur or upper end of the tibia

Arteries of the lower limb

The main arteries of the lower limb comprise femoral, popliteal, posterior tibial and anterior tibial.

Femoral artery

The femoral artery is the distal continuation of the external iliac artery beyond the inguinal ligament. It traverses the femoral triangle and the adductor canal of Hunter, then terminates a hand's breadth above the adductor tubercle by passing through the hiatus in adductor magnus to become the popliteal artery (Fig. 4.6).

Throughout its course, the femoral artery is accompanied by its vein, which lies first on the medial side of the artery and then passes posteriorly to it at the apex of the femoral triangle.

Branches

In the groin, the femoral artery gives off the following arteries:

1. The superficial circumflex iliac artery
2. The superficial epigastric artery
3. The superficial external pudendal artery
4. The deep external pudendal artery

The first three of these vessels are encountered in the groin incision for repair of an inguinal hernia. Their corresponding veins drain into the great saphenous vein (Fig. 4.36).

The *profunda femoris artery* arises posterolaterally from the femoral artery 2 in. (5 cm) distal to the inguinal ligament. It is conventional to call the femoral artery above this branch the *common femoral*, and, below it, the *superficial femoral artery*.

The profunda femoris artery passes deep to adductor longus and gives off *medial* and *lateral circumflex branches* and four *perforating branches*. These are important both as the source of blood supply to the great muscles of the thigh and as collateral channels that link the rich arterial anastomoses around the hip and the knee.

Popliteal artery

The popliteal artery continues on from the femoral artery at the adductor hiatus and terminates at the lower border of the popliteus muscle. It lies deep within the popliteal fossa (*see* below), being covered superficially by the popliteal vein and, more superficially still, crossed by the tibial nerve.

The popliteal artery gives off muscular branches, geniculate branches (to the knee joint) and terminal branches – the anterior and posterior tibial arteries.

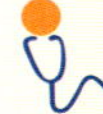

Clinical Features

1 Recapitulate the surface markings of the femoral artery – the upper two-thirds of a line connecting the mid-inguinal point with the adductor tubercle, the hip being held somewhat flexed and externally rotated (Fig. 4.6).

The femoral artery in the upper 4 in. (10 cm) of its course lies in the femoral triangle, where it is relatively superficial and, in consequence, easily injured. A laceration of the femoral artery at this site is an occupational hazard of butchers and bullfighters.

2 The femoral artery at the groin is readily punctured by a hypodermic needle and is the most convenient site from which to obtain arterial blood samples. Arteriography of the peripheral leg vessels is also easily performed at this point. A Seldinger catheter can be passed proximally through a femoral artery puncture in order to carry out aortography or selective renal, coeliac and mesenteric angiography.

3 Arteriosclerotic changes, with consequent thrombotic arterial occlusion, frequently commence at the lower end of the femoral artery, perhaps as a result of compression of the diseased vessel by the margins of the hiatus in adductor magnus. Collateral circulation is maintained via anastomoses between the branches of profunda femoris and the popliteal artery. If arteriography demonstrates a patent arterial tree distal to the block, it is possible to bypass the occluded segment by means of a graft between the common femoral and popliteal arteries.

Clinical Features

1 *Aneurysm of the popliteal artery*, once common, is now rare. Its frequency in former days was associated with the repeated traumata of horse-riding and the wearing of high riding-boots.

Pressure of the aneurysm on the adjacent vein may cause venous thrombosis and peripheral oedema; pressure on the tibial nerve may cause severe pain in the leg.

2 The popliteal artery is exposed by deep dissection in the midline within the popliteal fossa, care being taken not to injure the more superficial vein and nerve. It can also be exposed by a medial approach, which divides the insertion of adductor magnus and partially detaches the origin of the medial head of gastrocnemius from the femur.

Posterior tibial artery

The posterior tibial artery is the larger of the two terminal branches of the popliteal artery. From its origin, at the lower border of the popliteus, it descends deep to soleus, where it can be exposed by splitting gastrocnemius and soleus in the midline, then becomes superficial in the lower third of the leg and passes behind the medial malleolus between the tendons of flexor digitorum longus and flexor hallucis longus. It is accompanied by its corresponding vein and by the tibial nerve (Fig. 4.35).

Below the ankle, the posterior tibial artery divides into the *medial* and *lateral plantar arteries*, which constitute the principal blood supply to the foot.

As well as branches to muscles and skin and a large nutrient branch to the tibia, the posterior tibial artery gives off the *peroneal artery* approximately 1.5 in. (4 cm) from its origin. The peroneal artery runs down the posterior aspect of the fibula, close to the medial margin of the bone, supplying adjacent muscles and giving a nutrient branch to the fibula. Above the ankle it gives off its *perforating branch*, which pierces the interosseous membrane, descends over the lateral malleolus and anastomoses with the arteries of the dorsum of the foot.

Anterior tibial artery

The anterior tibial artery arises at the bifurcation of the popliteal artery. It passes forwards into anterior compart of the leg between the tibia and fibula, over the upper margin of the interosseous membrane and descends on the anterior surface of this structure flanked by venae comitantes.

At first deeply buried, it becomes superficial just above the ankle between the tendons of extensor hallucis longus and tibialis anterior, being crossed superficially by the former immediately proximal to the line of the ankle joint.

The artery continues over the dorsum of the foot as the *dorsalis pedis* (where its pulse may be palpated); this gives off the *arcuate artery*, which, in turn, supplies cutaneous branches to the dorsal aspects of the toes. Dorsalis pedis itself plunges between the 1st and 2nd metatarsals to join the lateral plantar artery in the formation of the *plantar arch*, from which branches run forwards to supply the plantar aspects of the toes.

Veins of the lower limb

The veins of the lower limb are divided into the deep and superficial groups according to their relationship to the investing deep fascia of the leg. The *deep veins* accompany the corresponding major arteries. The *superficial veins* are the *great* and *small* (or *long* and *short*) *saphenous veins* and their tributaries (Fig. 4.36).

The ***small (short) saphenous vein*** commences at the ankle behind the lateral malleolus where it drains the lateral side of the dorsal venous plexus of the foot. It courses over the back of the calf, perforates the deep fascia over the popliteal fossa and terminates in the popliteal vein. One or more branches run upwards and medially from it to join the great saphenous vein. The small saphenous vein is accompanied by the sural nerve – a sensory branch of the tibial nerve (Fig. 4.34(a)), which may be damaged when operating on varices of this vein.

The ***great (long) saphenous vein*** commences on the medial side of the dorsum of the foot. It drains the medial part of the venous plexus on the dorsum of the foot and passes upwards immediately in front of the medial malleolus (Fig. 4.7); here, branches of the saphenous nerve lie in front of and behind the vein. The vein then ascends over the posterior parts of the medial condyles of the tibia and femur to the groin, where it pierces the deep fascia at the saphenous opening 1 in. (2.5 cm) below the inguinal ligament,

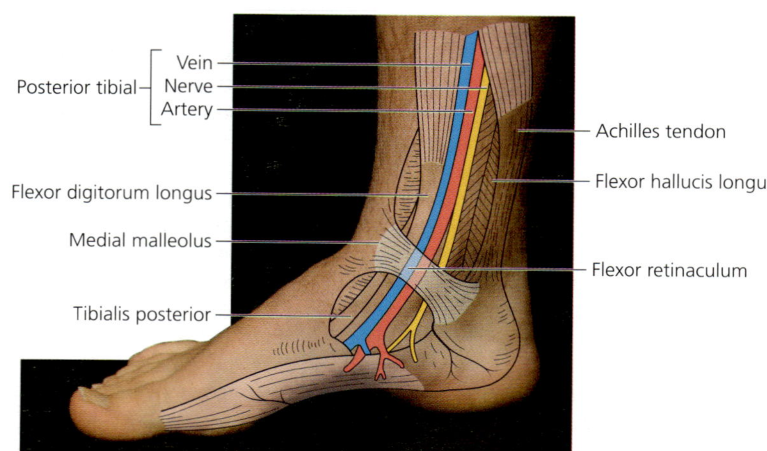

Figure 4.35 The relations of the posterior tibial artery as it passes behind the medial malleolus (right ankle region).

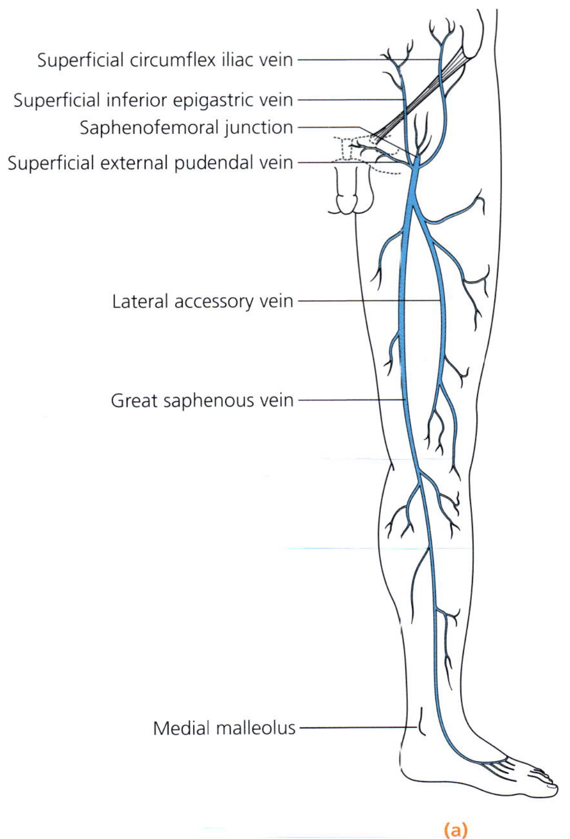

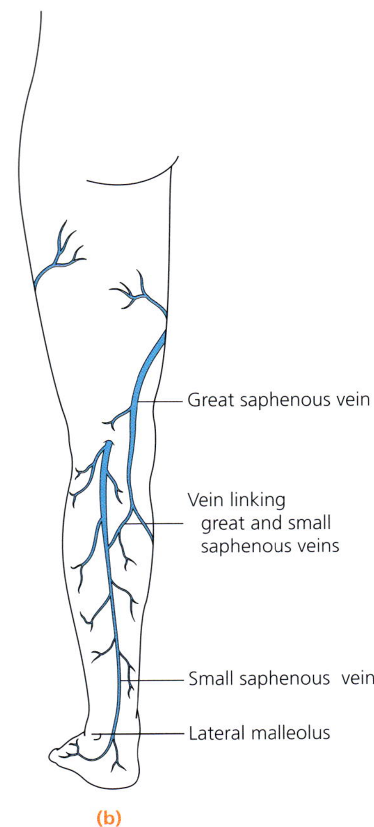

Figure 4.36 The superficial veins of the left lower limb. **(a)** Anteromedial. **(b)** Posterior view.

to enter the femoral vein immediately medial to the femoral pulse.

The great saphenous vein is joined by one or more branches from the small saphenous vein and by the *lateral accessory vein*, which usually enters the main vein at the mid-thigh, although it may not do so until the saphenous opening is reached.

At the groin a number of tributaries from the lower abdominal wall, thigh and scrotum enter the great saphenous vein; these tributaries are variable in number and arrangement but usually comprise the following (Fig. 4.36):

1. The superficial epigastric vein
2. The superficial circumflex iliac vein
3. The superficial external pudendal vein

The superficial epigastric vein communicates with the lateral thoracic tributary of the axillary vein via the *thoraco-epigastric vein*. This dilates (and may become readily visible coursing over the trunk) following obstruction of the inferior vena cava. The great saphenous vein communicates with the deep venous system not only at the groin but also at a number of points along its course through *perforating veins*; one is usually present a hand's breadth above the knee, another a hand's breadth below.

The skin of the medial aspect of the leg is drained to the deep veins by two or three *direct perforating veins* that pierce the deep fascia behind the great saphenous vein.

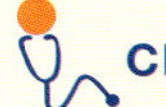

Clinical Features

1 We have already noted (under 'The surface anatomy and surface markings of the lower limb') the great importance of the constant position of the great saphenous vein lying immediately in front of the medial malleolus (Fig. 4.7). Knowledge that a vein *must* be present at this site, even if not visible in an obese or collapsed patient, may be life-saving when urgent transfusion is required. Occasionally, the immediately adjacent saphenous nerve is caught up by a ligature during this procedure – the patient, if conscious, will complain bitterly of pain if this is done.

2 The saphenous veins frequently become dilated, incompetent and varicose. Usually this is idiopathic but may result from the increased venous pressure caused by more proximal venous obstruction (a pelvic tumour or the pregnant uterus, for example) or may be secondary to obstruction of the deep venous pathway of the leg by thrombosis.

3 Stagnation of blood in the skin of the lower limb may result from venous thrombosis or valve incompetence; the skin, in consequence, is poorly nourished and easily breaks down into a *varicose ulcer* if subjected to even minor trauma. This is especially liable to occur over the subcutaneous anteromedial surface of the tibia where the cutaneous blood supply is least generous.

4 In operating upon varicose veins it is important that all tributaries of the groin are ligated as well as the main saphenous trunk; if one tributary escapes, it in turn becomes dilated and

(Continued ...)

(... continued)

produces recurrence of the varices. The proximal termination of the great saphenous vein at the groin is found by palpating the femoral pulse. The femoral vein lies a finger's breadth medial to this pulse, so that a vertical or transverse incision at this site will come down upon the great saphenous vein as it lies in the superficial fascia immediately before it plunges through the hiatus in the deep fascia to join the femoral vein. The great saphenous vein is distinguished from the femoral vein in that (a) it lies in the superficial fascia, whereas the femoral vein lies deep to the deep facia, and (b) the great saphenous vein bears a number of tributaries, whereas the femoral vein receives only the great saphenous vein. There is really no excuse for the occasional disaster of the femoral vein being injured in varicose vein surgery.

Course and distribution of the principal nerves of the lower limb

The nerves of the lower limb are derived from the lumbar and sacral plexuses.

Lumbar plexus (Fig. 4.37)

The lumbar plexus is formed from the anterior primary rami of L1–L4 in the substance of the psoas major.

The branches of the plexus traverse psoas major and emerge from its lateral border. There are two exceptions: the obturator nerve appears at the medial border of psoas tendon, and the genitofemoral nerve emerges on the anterior aspect of the muscle.

The principal branches of the plexus are the femoral nerve and the obturator nerve.

The *femoral nerve* (L2–L4) passes through the substance of psoas then under the inguinal ligament a finger's breadth lateral to the femoral artery, to break up into its terminal branches after a course in the lower limb of only some 2 in. (5 cm).

Its branches are the following:

- **Muscular:** To the anterior compartment of the thigh (quadriceps, sartorius and pectineus)
- **Cutaneous:** The medial and intermediate cutaneous nerves of the thigh and the saphenous nerve, which traverses the adductor canal to supply the skin of the medial side of the leg, ankle and foot to the great toe
- **Articular:** To the hip and knee joints

The femoral nerve supplies the skin of the medial and anterior aspects of the thigh via its medial and intermediate cutaneous branches, but the lateral aspect is supplied by the *lateral cutaneous nerve of the thigh* (L2–L3). This arises directly from the lumbar plexus and enters the thigh usually by passing deep to the inguinal ligament. Occasionally, the nerve pierces the ligament and may then be pressed upon by it with resultant pain and anaesthesia over the upper outer thigh (*meralgia paraesthetica*). This is relieved by dividing the deeper fasciculus of the inguinal ligament where the nerve passes over it.

The *obturator nerve* (L2–L4) emerges from the medial aspect of the psoas and runs downwards and forwards, deep to the internal iliac vessels, to reach the superior part of the obturator foramen. This the nerve traverses, in company with the obturator vessels, to enter the thigh.

Its branches are the following:

- **Muscular:** To obturator externus, the adductor muscles and gracilis
- **Cutaneous:** To an area of skin over the medial aspect of the thigh
- **Articular:** To the hip and knee joints

Sacral plexus (Fig. 4.38)

This plexus originates from the anterior primary rami of L4–L5, S1–S4.

Note that L4 is shared by both plexuses, a branch from it joining L5 to form the *lumbosacral trunk*, which carries its important contribution to the sacral plexus.

The sacral nerves emerge from the anterior sacral foramina and unite in front of piriformis, where they are joined by the lumbosacral trunk.

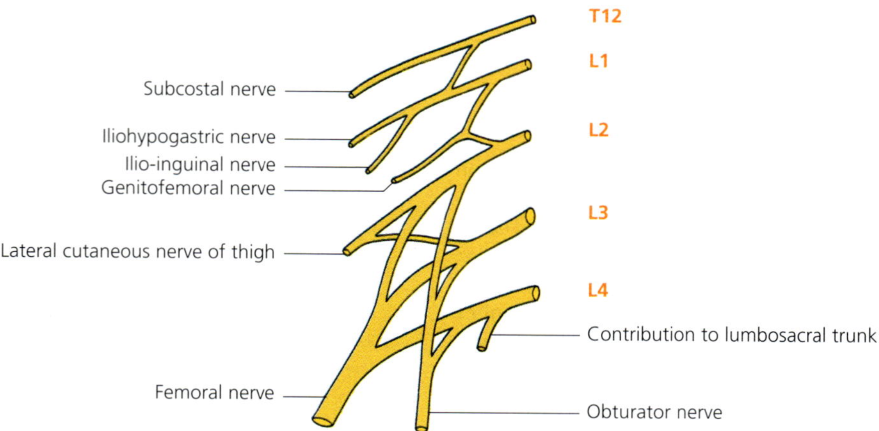

Figure 4.37 Plan of the lumbar plexus (muscular branches have been omitted for clarity).

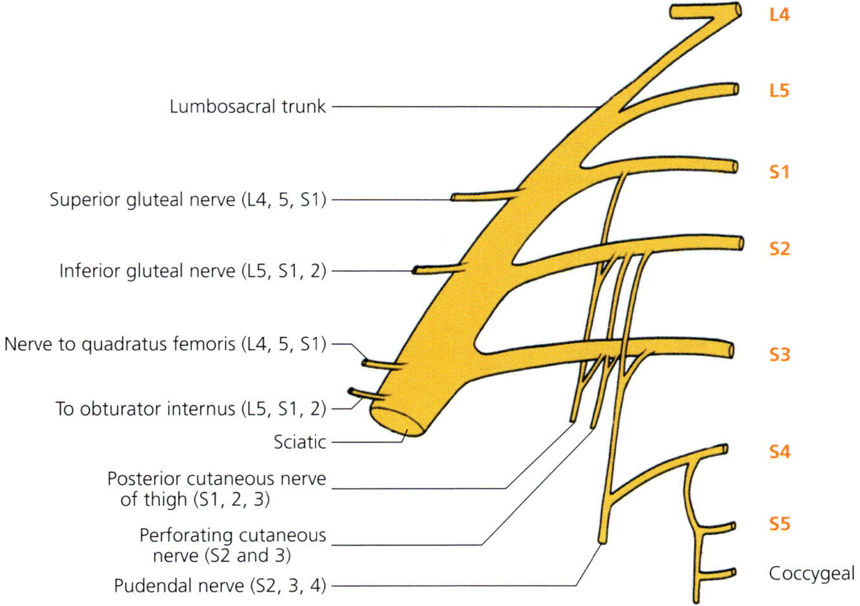

Figure 4.38 Plan of the sacral plexus.

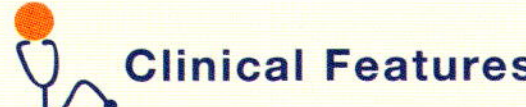

Clinical Features

1. Spasm of the adductor muscles of the thigh in spastic paraplegia can be relieved by division of the obturator nerve (*obturator neurectomy*). This can be performed through a midline lower abdominal incision exposing the nerve trunk extraperitoneally on each side as it passes towards the obturator foramen.
2. Rarely, an *obturator hernia* develops through the canal where the obturator nerve and vessels traverse the membrane covering the obturator foramen. Pressure of a strangulated obturator hernia upon the nerve causes referred pain in its area of cutaneous distribution, so that intestinal obstruction associated with pain along the medial side of the thigh should suggest this diagnosis.
3. The femoral and obturator nerves, as well as the sciatic nerve and its branches, supply sensory fibres to both the hip and the knee; it is not uncommon for hip disease to present disguised as pain in the knee.

Branches from the plexus supply the following:

- The pelvic muscles
- The muscles of the hip
- The skin of the buttock and the back of the thigh

The plexus itself terminates as the pudendal nerve and the sciatic nerve.

The *pudendal nerve* (S2–S4) provides the principal innervation of the perineum. It has a complex course, passing from the pelvis, briefly through the gluteal region, along the side-wall of the ischiorectal fossa and through the deep perineal pouch to end by supplying the skin of the external genitalia (Fig. 4.39).

It arises as the lower main division of the sacral plexus, although it is dwarfed by the giant sciatic nerve. It leaves the pelvis through the greater foramen below the piriformis muscle. It crosses the dorsum of the ischial spine and immediately disappears through the lesser sciatic foramen into the perineum. The nerve now traverses the lateral wall of the ischio-anal fossa in company with the internal pudendal vessels, and lies within a distinct fascial compartment on the medial aspect of obturator internus termed the pudendal canal (Alcock's canal; Fig. 2.59). Within the canal it first gives off the *inferior rectal nerve*, which crosses the fossa to innervate the external anal sphincter and the perianal skin, and then divides into the perineal nerve and the dorsal nerve of the penis (or clitoris).

The *perineal nerve* is the larger of the two. It bifurcates almost at once; its deeper branch supplies the sphincter urethrae and the other muscles of the anterior perineum (the ischiocavernosus, bulbospongiosus and the superficial and deep transverse perinei). Its more superficial branch innervates the skin of the posterior aspect of the scrotum or vulva.

The *dorsal nerve of the penis* (or *clitoris*) traverses the deep perineal pouch, pierces the perineal membrane and then penetrates the suspensory ligament of the penis to supply the dorsal aspect of this structure.

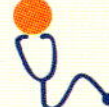

Clinical Features

In obstetric practice the pudendal nerve can be blocked with local anaesthetic prior to forceps delivery by inserting a long needle through the vaginal wall and, guided by a finger, to the ischial spine, which can be palpated per vaginam. Alternatively, the needle can be introduced just medial to the ischial tuberosity to a depth of 1 in. (2.5 cm). When the procedure is carried out bilaterally, there is loss of the anal reflex (which is a useful test that a successful block has been achieved), relaxation of the pelvic floor muscles and loss of sensation to the vulva and lower one-third of the vagina (Fig. 2.59(b)).

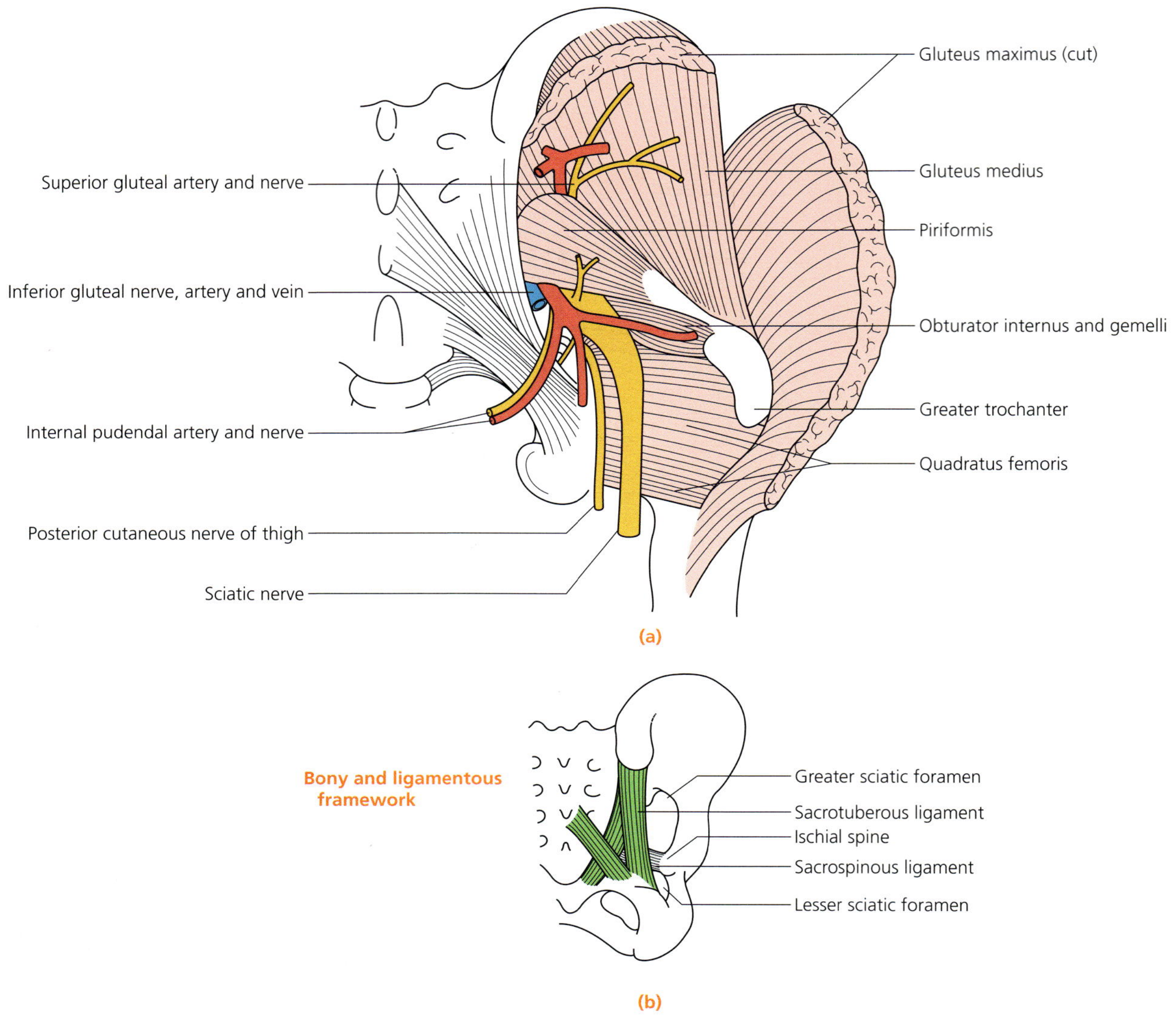

Gluteus maximus (cut)
Superior gluteal artery and nerve
Gluteus medius
Piriformis
Inferior gluteal nerve, artery and vein
Obturator internus and gemelli
Greater trochanter
Internal pudendal artery and nerve
Quadratus femoris
Posterior cutaneous nerve of thigh
Sciatic nerve

(a)

Bony and ligamentous framework
Greater sciatic foramen
Sacrotuberous ligament
Ischial spine
Sacrospinous ligament
Lesser sciatic foramen

(b)

Figure 4.39 The sciatic foramina (right side). **(a)** Contents and related muscles. **(b)** Boundaries and ligamentous framework.

Sciatic nerve

The sciatic nerve (L4, L5, S1–S3) is the largest nerve in the body (Fig. 4.40). It is broad and flat at its origin, although peripherally it becomes rounded.

The nerve emerges from the greater sciatic foramen distal to piriformis and under cover of gluteus maximus, crosses the posterior surface of the ischium, crosses obturator internus, with its gemelli, quadratus femoris and descends on adductor magnus (Figs 4.39 and 4.40). Here, it lies deep to the hamstrings and is crossed only by the long head of biceps.

The sciatic nerve terminates by dividing into the *tibial* and *common peroneal nerves* (Fig. 4.34). The level of this division is variable – usually it is at the mid-thigh, but the two nerves may be separate even at their origins from the sacral plexus.

Branches

The trunk of the sciatic nerve supplies the hamstring muscles (biceps, semimembranosus, semitendinosus) and also the adductor magnus, the latter being innervated also by the obturator nerve.

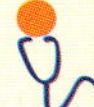

Clinical Features

1 The sciatic nerve may be wounded in penetrating injuries or in posterior dislocation of the hip associated with fracture of the posterior lip of the acetabulum, to which the nerve is closely related (Fig. 4.22).

Damage to the sciatic nerve is followed by paralysis of the hamstrings and all the muscles of the leg and foot (supplied by its distributing branches); there is loss of all movements in the lower limb below the knee joint with foot drop deformity. Sensory loss is complete below the knee, except for an area along the medial side of the leg, over the medial malleolus and down to the hallux, which is innervated by the saphenous branch of the femoral nerve.

2 The sciatic nerve is accompanied by a companion artery (derived from the inferior gluteal artery), which bleeds quite sharply when the nerve is divided during an above-knee amputation. The artery must be neatly isolated and tied without any nerve fibres being incorporated in the ligature, since this would be followed by severe pain in the stump.

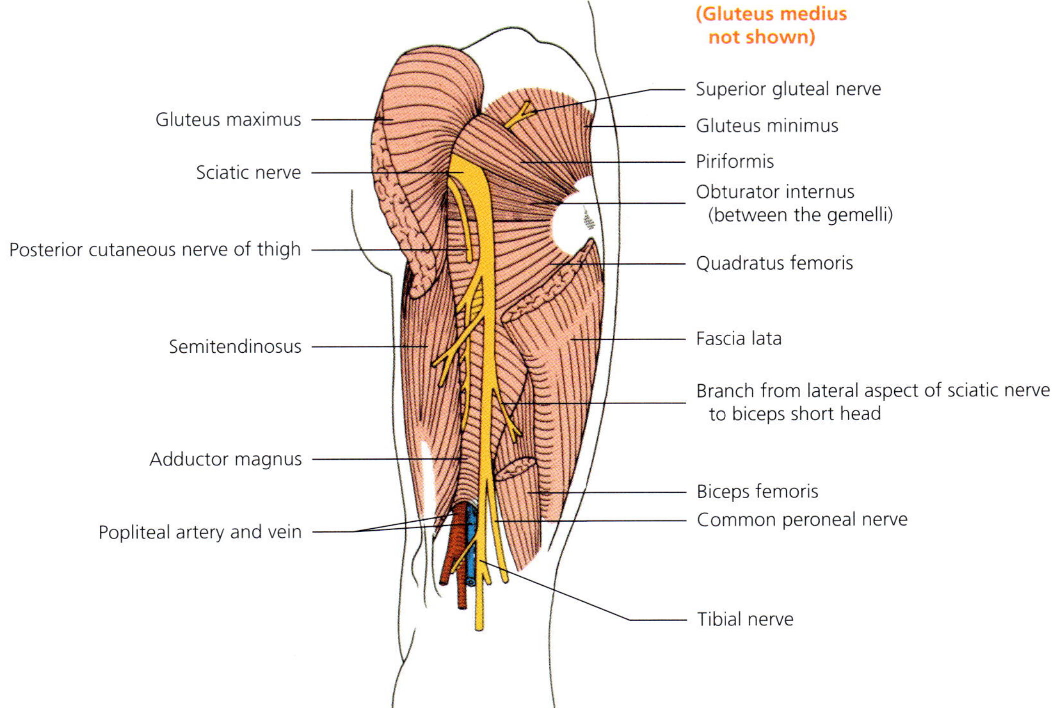

Figure 4.40 Dissection of the sciatic nerve in the thigh and popliteal fossa (right side). Note that gluteus medius has been removed to show the otherwise completely hidden gluteus minimus.

All the muscle branches apart from the one to the short head of biceps arise on the medial side of the nerve; its lateral border is therefore the side of relative safety in its operative exposure.

Tibial nerve (Fig. 4.34(a) and (b))

The tibial nerve (L4, L5, S1–S3) is the larger of the two terminal branches of the sciatic nerve; it traverses the popliteal fossa superficial to the popliteal vein and artery, which it crosses from the lateral to the medial side.

Branches

The branches of tibial nerve are as under:

1. *In the popliteal fossa*:
   - **Muscular:** To gastrocnemius, soleus and popliteus
   - **Cutaneous:** The *sural nerve*, which descends over the back of the calf, behind the lateral malleolus to the 5th toe; it receives a communicating branch from the common peroneal nerve and supplies the lateral side of the leg, foot and 5th toe
   - **Articular:** To the knee joint

   It then descends deep to soleus, in company with the posterior tibial vessels, passes on their lateral side behind the medial malleolus to end by dividing into the *medial* and *lateral plantar* nerves.
2. *In the leg* – the tibial nerve supplies flexor hallucis longus, flexor digitorum longus and tibialis posterior. Its terminal plantar branches supply the intrinsic muscles and skin of the sole of the foot; the medial plantar nerve having an equivalent distribution to that of the median nerve in the hand, the lateral plantar nerve being comparable to the ulnar nerve.

Common peroneal (fibular) nerve

The common peroneal nerve (L4, L5, S1, S2) is the smaller of the terminal branches of the sciatic nerve. It enters the upper part of the popliteal fossa, passes along the medial border of the biceps tendon, then curves around the neck of the fibula where it lies in the substance of peroneus longus and divides into its terminal branches, the *deep peroneal* and *superficial peroneal nerves* (Fig. 4.8).

Branches

While still in the popliteal fossa, the common peroneal nerve gives off the *lateral cutaneous nerve of the calf*, a *peroneal (sural) communicating branch* and twigs to the knee joint, but has no muscular branches.

Deep peroneal (fibular) nerve

The deep peroneal nerve pierces extensor digitorum longus, then descends, in company with the anterior tibial vessels, over the interosseous membrane and then over the ankle joint. Medially lies tibialis anterior, whereas laterally lies first extensor digitorum longus, then extensor hallucis longus. Its branches are as follows:

- **Muscular:** To the muscles of the anterior compartment of the leg – extensor digitorum longus, extensor hallucis longus, tibialis anterior, peroneus tertius – and extensor digitorum brevis
- **Cutaneous:** To a small area of skin in the web between the 1st and 2nd toes

Superficial peroneal (fibular) nerve

The superficial peroneal nerve runs in the lateral compartment of the leg. Its branches are as follows:

- **Muscular:** To the lateral compartment muscles (peroneus longus and brevis)
- **Cutaneous:** To the skin of the distal two-thirds of the lateral aspect of the leg and to the dorsum of the foot (apart from the small area between the 1st and 2nd toes supplied by the deep peroneal nerve)

Segmental cutaneous supply of the lower limb (Fig. 4.41)

The arrangement of root segments supplying the lower limb is as follows:

- **L1, L2 and L3:** Supply the anterior aspect of the thigh from above down
- **L4:** Supplies the anteromedial aspect of the leg
- **L5:** Supplies the anterolateral aspect of the leg but also extends onto the medial side of the foot
- **S1:** Supplies the lateral side of the foot and the sole
- **S2:** Supplies the posterior surface of the leg and thigh
- **S3 and S4:** Supply the buttocks and perianal region

A little aid to memory is that 5 supplies the 1st toe and 1 supplies the 5th.

Note that, although S3 supplies the posterior part of the scrotum (or vulva), L1 supplies the anterior part of these structures via the ilio-inguinal nerve.

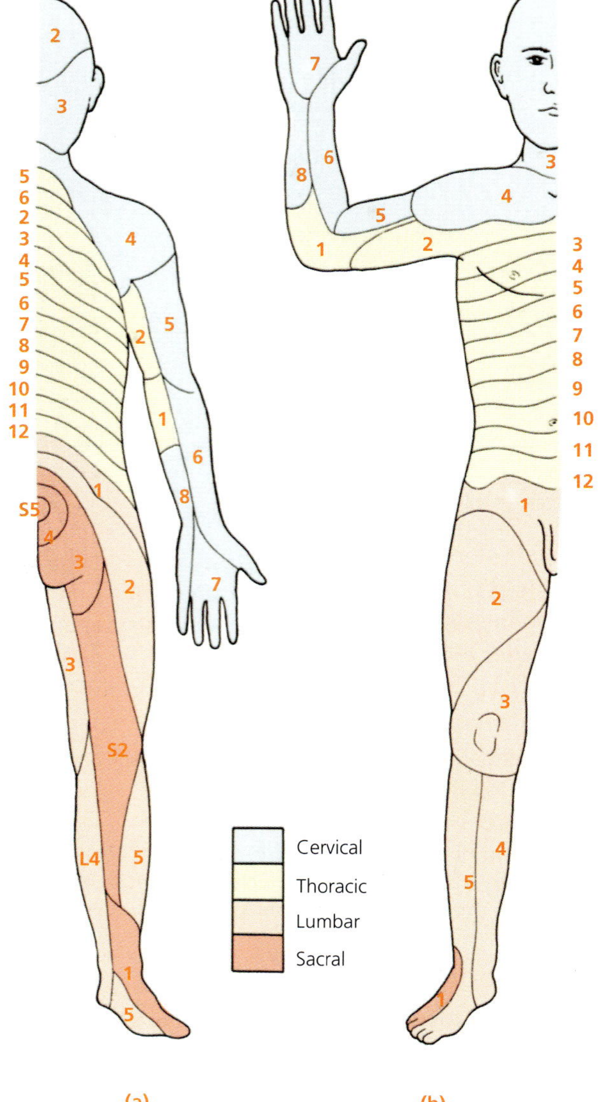

Figure 4.41 The segmental cutaneous nerve supply of the skin. **(a)** Posterior aspect. **(b)** Anterior aspect.

Compartments of the lower limb

In each of the limbs, the skeletal muscles are collectively ensleeved in a layer of deep fascia. From the inner surface of this stocking-like deep fascial envelope, fibrous septa project inwards and attach to the bone(s) lying within a given segment of the limb, thereby separating the muscles of that limb segment into functional groups. Thus, the muscles within each segment of the upper and lower limbs may be pictured as being located in discrete, osseofascial compartments (Fig. 4.42). As a general rule, each compartment possesses its own complement of neurovascular structures, with the nerve being responsible for the motor innervation of all the muscles of the compartment.

Clinical Features

The common peroneal nerve is in a particularly vulnerable position as it winds around the neck of the fibula. It may be damaged at this site by the pressure of a tight bandage or plaster cast or may be torn in severe adduction injuries to the knee. Damage to this nerve is followed by foot drop (due to paralysis of the ankle and foot extensors) and inversion of the foot (due to paralysis of the peroneal muscles with unopposed action of the foot flexors and invertors). This deformity is termed *talipes equinovarus* (*talipes* refers to the foot; *equino*, the foot is held plantar flexed, as in the horse; and *varus* means the foot is adducted, i.e. internally rotated). There is also anaesthesia over the anterior and lateral aspects of the leg and foot, although the medial side escapes since this is innervated by the saphenous branch of the femoral nerve.

Compartments in the segments of the lower limb

Thigh

The thigh contains two distinct and physically separate compartments as mentioned below:

1. The *anterior (extensor) compartment* comprising quadriceps femoris and sartorius. The nerve of this compartment is the femoral nerve.

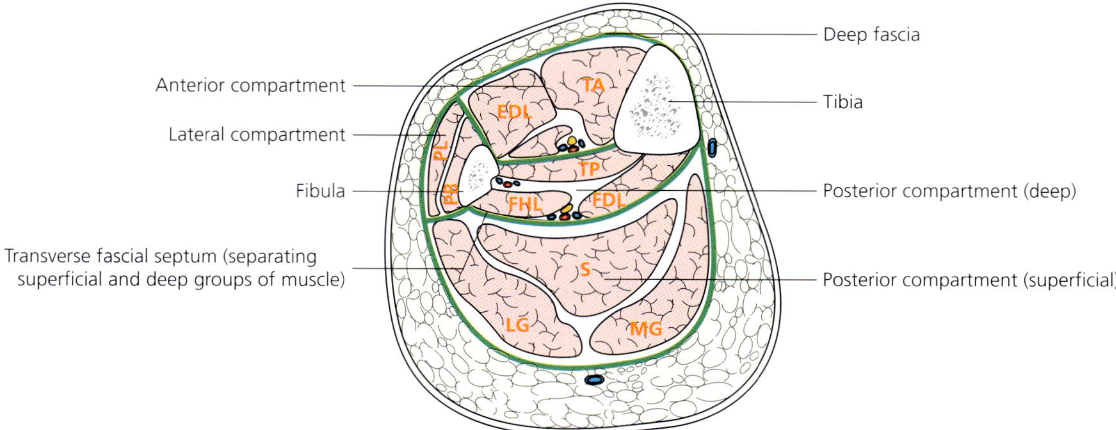

Figure 4.42 Cross-sectional representation of the compartments of the right leg. EDL, extensor digitorum longus; FDL, flexor digitorum longus; FHL, flexor hallucis longus; LG, lateral head of gastrocnemius; MG, medial head of gastrocnemius; PB, peroneus brevis; PL, peroneus longus; S, soleus; TA, tibialis anterior; TP, tibialis posterior.

2. The *posterior compartment* contains two groups of muscles that are functionally distinct – the hamstrings, which are innervated by the sciatic nerve, and the adductors, which are innervated by the obturator nerve.

Leg

A very definite fascial separation into anterior (extensor), posterior (flexor) and lateral (evertor) compartments exists in the leg (Fig. 4.42). Furthermore, the posterior compartment is divided by a fascial layer into superficial and deep subdivisions. Thus, the leg contains four distinct compartments. The anterior compartment contains tibialis anterior, extensor digitorum longus, extensor hallucis longus and peroneus tertius, all of which are innervated by the deep peroneal nerve and supplied by the anterior tibial artery. The lateral compartment contains the peroneus longus and brevis muscles, which are innervated by the superficial peroneal nerve. The superficial group of posterior compartment muscles comprises gastrocnemius, soleus and plantaris, whereas the deep group is made up of flexor digitorum longus, flexor hallucis longus, tibialis posterior and popliteus. All the muscles of the posterior compartment (superficial and deep groups) are innervated by the tibial nerve. (In the view of some authorities, the posterior compartment of the leg has three, rather than two, subdivisions. According to this view, tibialis posterior occupies a compartment of its own.)

Compartment syndrome

The fascial boundaries that limit the osseofascial compartments are inelastic sheets. Any condition that leads to an increase in the volume of the compartmental contents is therefore likely to result in a rise in intracompartmental pressure. Such conditions include haemorrhage following closed fractures, muscle swelling caused by trauma or unaccustomed overuse, and local infection. If unrelieved, the increased pressure leads to compression of the vessels in the compartment and secondary ischaemic damage to the nerves and muscles of the compartment. This phenomenon is known as *compartment syndrome*, and involves, most commonly, the compartments of the leg (especially, the anterior compartment of leg).

Compartment syndrome is a surgical emergency and is treated by performing a fasciotomy; a procedure in which a generous incision is made in the deep fascia overlying the compartment in order to decompress the compartment.

Part V

The head and neck

Surface anatomy of the neck

Introduction

The differential diagnosis of lumps in the neck and the effective clinical and surgical management of pathological lesions in the neck require a sound knowledge of the surgical anatomy of the head and neck. From a practical perspective, it is helpful to picture the neck as being made up of the following two parts:

1. *A posterior portion*, comprising the cervical vertebral column, the cervical segment of the spinal cord and the postvertebral musculature.
2. *An anterior portion,* which includes the prevertebral musculature draped in prevertebral fascia, in front of which lies the centrally located visceral compartment; this portion includes also the right and left carotid sheaths, the submandibular glands and the anterior cervical musculature.

In the midline, from above down, the following can be felt (Fig. 5.1):

1. The *hyoid bone* at the level of C3
2. The notch of the *thyroid cartilage* at the level of C4
3. The *cricothyroid* ligament important in cricothyroid puncture
4. The *cricoid cartilage* terminating in the trachea at the level of C6
5. The rings of the *trachea*, over the 2nd and 3rd of which lies the *isthmus of the thyroid gland* (*sometimes palpable*)
6. *The suprasternal notch*

Note that the lower border of the cricoid is an important level in the neck; it corresponds not only to the level of the 6th cervical vertebra but also to the following:

1. The junction of the larynx with the trachea
2. The junction of the pharynx with the oesophagus
3. The level at which the inferior thyroid artery enters and the middle thyroid vein leaves the thyroid gland
4. The level at which the vertebral artery enters the transverse foramen in the 6th cervical vertebra
5. The level at which the superior belly of the omohyoid crosses the carotid sheath
6. The level of the middle cervical sympathetic ganglion
7. The site at which the carotid artery can be compressed against the transverse process of C6 (the carotid tubercle)

By pressing the jaw laterally against the resistance of one's hand, the opposite *sternocleidomastoid* is tensed. This muscle helps define the posterior triangle of the neck, bounded by sternocleidomastoid, trapezius and the clavicle, and the anterior triangle, defined by sternocleidomastoid, the mandible and the midline (Fig. 5.2).

Violently clench the jaws; the platysma then comes into view as a sheet of muscle, passing from the mandible down over the clavicles, lying in the superficial fascia of the neck. The *external jugular vein* lies immediately deep to the platysma, crosses the sternocleidomastoid into the posterior triangle, perforates the deep fascia just above the clavicle and enters the subclavian vein. It is readily visible in a thin subject on straining and is seen from the audience when a singer hits a sustained high note or when an orthopaedic surgeon attempts to reduce a difficult fracture!

The *common carotid artery* pulse can be felt by pressing backwards against the prominent anterior tubercle of the transverse process of C6. The line of the carotid sheath can be marked out by a line joining a point midway between the tip of the mastoid process and the angle of the jaw to the sternoclavicular joint. Along this line, the common carotid bifurcates into the *external* and *internal carotid arteries* at the level of the upper border of the thyroid cartilage; at this level, the vessels lie within the carotid sheath just beneath the investing layer of the deep cervical fascia, where their pulsation is palpable and sometimes visible.

Fascial compartments of the neck (Fig. 5.3)

A thorough appreciation of the topographical arrangement of the fascial and muscular planes in the anterior aspect of the neck is fundamental to accuracy in the clinical diagnosis of

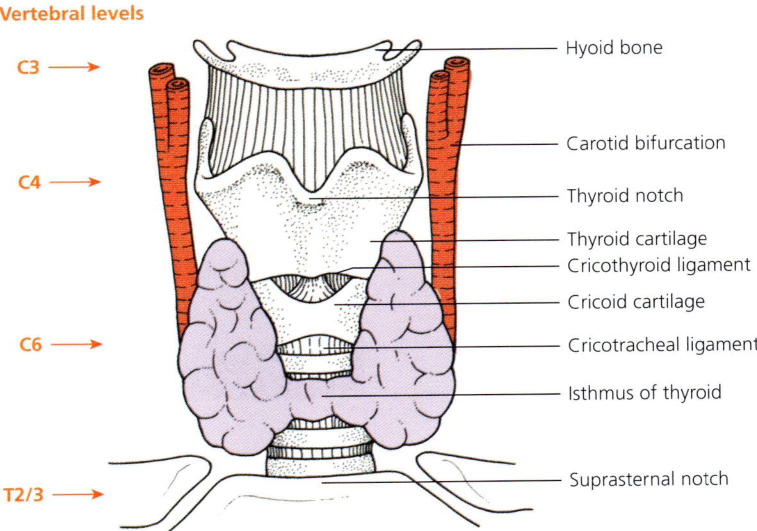

Figure 5.1 Structures palpable on the anterior aspect of the neck, together with their corresponding vertebral levels.

Digastric (anterior belly)
Digastric triangle
Carotid triangle
Muscular triangle
Anterior triangle
Omohyoid
Digastric (posterior belly)
Trapezius
Sternocleidomastoid
Posterior triangle

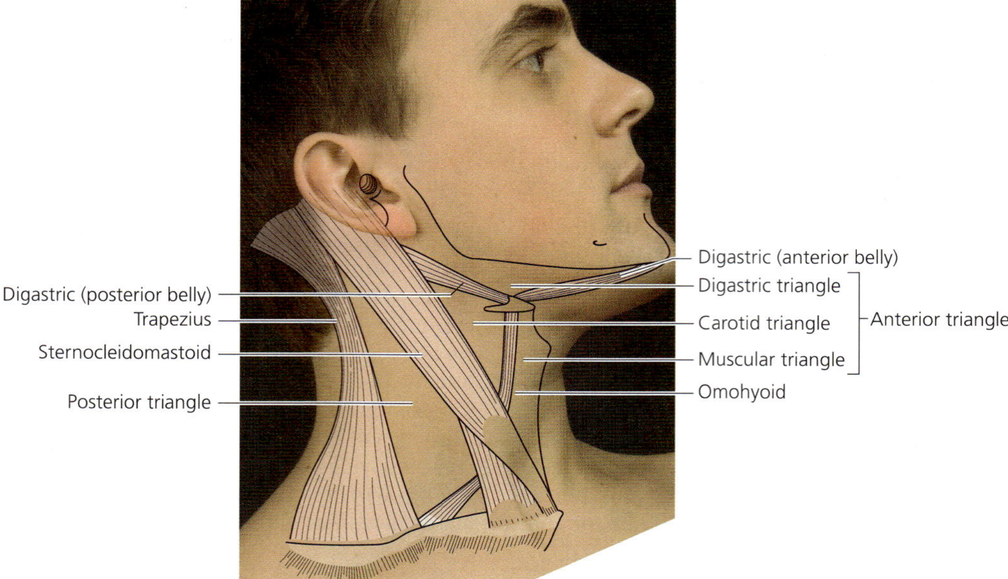

Figure 5.2 Triangles of the neck.

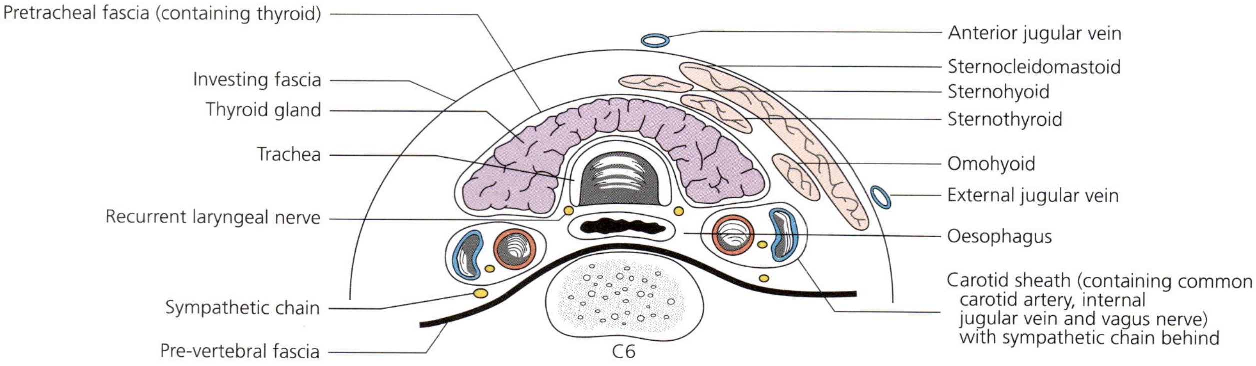

Pretracheal fascia (containing thyroid)
Investing fascia
Thyroid gland
Trachea
Recurrent laryngeal nerve
Sympathetic chain
Pre-vertebral fascia
C6
Anterior jugular vein
Sternocleidomastoid
Sternohyoid
Sternothyroid
Omohyoid
External jugular vein
Oesophagus
Carotid sheath (containing common carotid artery, internal jugular vein and vagus nerve) with sympathetic chain behind

(a)

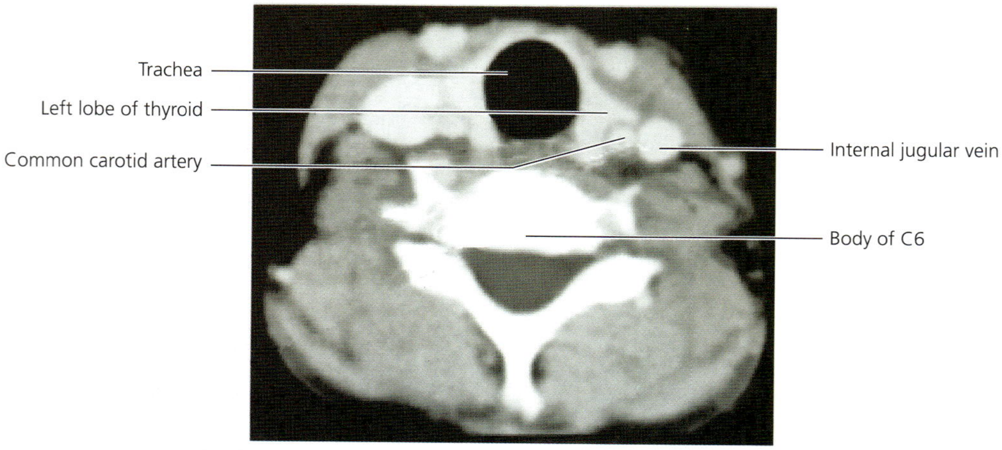

Trachea
Left lobe of thyroid
Common carotid artery
Internal jugular vein
Body of C6

(b)

Figure 5.3 **(a)** Transverse section of the neck through C6, showing the fascial planes and also the contents of the pretracheal fascia (or 'visceral compartment of the neck'). **(b)** Computed tomography (CT) scan through the C6 level; compare this with (a).

neck lumps, besides being an essential prerequisite to safety and precision in neck surgery.

Tissue planes and fascial layers in the anterior part of the neck

Deep to the skin of the neck is the superficial fascia or *panniculus adiposus*, which is essentially a layer of subcutaneous fat, more or less homogeneous. The degree of adiposity in this layer varies between individuals; it also varies, to some extent, between the anterior and posterior aspects of the neck in the same individual, being generally somewhat thinner in the front of the neck than in the back. Lying immediately deep to the subcutaneous fat, on either side of the anterior midline, is the *platysma*, a relatively thin but wide sheet of muscle. The platysma is a feature of the anterolateral part of the neck and does not extend to the back of the neck. Above the level of the hyoid, the medial borders of the right and left platysma muscles are contiguous, whereas, below the hyoid level, they are separated from each other by an interval of 1 in. (2.5 cm).

Deep fascia

The *deep fascia* of neck can be classified into four parts: investing layer of deep cervical fascia, pretracheal fascia, prevertebral fascia and carotid sheaths (right and left).

Immediately deep to the platysma is the **investing layer of deep cervical fascia**, the most superficial of the multiple layers of the deep cervical fascia. It invests the neck like a collar. Superiorly, its attachment may be traced circumferentially along the entire length of the lower border of the mandible, the mastoid processes and superior nuchal lines on either side and to the external occipital protuberance in the posterior midline. In the interval between the angle of the mandible and the mastoid process, the investing layer of deep cervical fascia encloses the parotid salivary gland as the *parotid fascia*.

Inferiorly, the circumferential attachment of the investing layer of deep cervical fascia is to the sternal notch (i.e. the notched, thick upper border of the manubrium sterni), and in continuity, on each side, to the upper surface of the clavicle, the acromion and the corresponding spine of the scapula and thus to the posterior midline. Traced laterally from the anterior midline, between its upper and lower attachments, the investing layer of deep cervical fascia meets, on each side, the medial border of the corresponding sternocleidomastoid muscle and splits to enclose the muscle. Thereafter, it continues posterolaterally as the fascial roof of the posterior triangle of the neck, and, upon reaching the anterior edge of the trapezius muscle, it splits to enclose the trapezius.

In its descent from the lower border of the mandible, the investing layer of deep cervical fascia is firmly adherent to the front of the hyoid body and to the lateral aspects of the greater horns of the hyoid. Thus, all the cervical viscera, major blood vessels and nerves of the neck and all the cervical muscles (with the sole exception of the platysma) come to lie within the sweep of the investing layer of deep cervical fascia.

The external jugular vein runs in the plane between the platysma and the underlying investing layer of deep fascia. It pierces the latter above the clavicle. If the vein is divided here, it is held open by the deep fascia that is attached to its margins, air is sucked into the vein lumen during inspiration and a fatal air embolism may ensue.

Lying immediately deep to the investing layer of deep cervical fascia and running longitudinally on either side of the anterior midline of the neck are the infrahyoid anterior cervical muscles, also known as the strap muscles. On each side of the vertical midline, the strap muscles are disposed in two planes. The superficial plane consists of the sternohyoid and omohyoid muscles lying side by side (sternohyoid medial to omohyoid), and the deep plane consists of the sternothyroid muscle, which extends vertically from the posterior surface of the manubrium sterni to the oblique line of the thyroid cartilage. Extending upwards from the oblique line of the thyroid cartilage to the greater horn of the hyoid is the thyrohyoid muscle, generally regarded as the upward continuation of the sternothyroid muscle.

The deepest layer of the deep cervical fascia is the **prevertebral fascia**, a relatively dense layer that covers the anterior aspects of the prevertebral musculature and the cervical vertebral column. The *prevertebral fascia* passes across the vertebrae and prevertebral muscles behind the oesophagus, the pharynx and the great vessels. Above, it is attached to the base of the skull. Laterally, the fascia covers the scalene muscles together with the phrenic nerve, as this lies on scalenus anterior, and the emerging brachial plexus and subclavian artery. These structures carry with them a sheath formed from the prevertebral fascia, which becomes the axillary sheath.

Inferiorly, the fascia blends with the anterior longitudinal ligament of the upper thoracic vertebrae in the posterior mediastinum.

Pus from a tuberculous cervical vertebra bulges behind this dense fascial layer and may form a midline swelling in the posterior wall of the pharynx. The abscess may then track laterally, deep to the prevertebral fascia, to a point behind the sternocleidomastoid. Rarely, pus has tracked down along the axillary sheath into the arm.

Deep to the strap muscles, and anterior to the prevertebral fascial layer, is the centrally located visceral compartment of the neck.

Lying lateral to the cervical visceral column, and in front of the prevertebral fascia, are the right and left **carotid sheaths**. Situated posteromedial to each carotid sheath and anterior to the prevertebral fascia is the ganglionated, cervical sympathetic chain.

The cervical visceral compartment flanked by the right and left carotid sheaths comprises, most posteriorly, the pharynx and its distal continuation – the oesophagus. The pharyngo-oesophageal junction, as has been noted, is typically at the level of the lower border of the cricoid cartilage (corresponding to the level of the lower border of the 6th cervical vertebra). Situated in front of the pharynx and oesophagus are, respectively, the larynx and trachea; the laryngotracheal junction being at the same horizontal level as the pharyngo-oesophageal junction. Lying astride the anterior aspect of the upper trachea is the thyroid isthmus, which on either side of the midline is confluent with the corresponding thyroid lobe. The entire thyroid gland is enveloped in a further layer of deep cervical fascia termed the ***pretracheal fascia***. The pretracheal fascia is itself firmly adherent to the front of the upper trachea behind the isthmus, and, elsewhere, to the sides of the cricoid and thyroid cartilages. Indeed, the encasement of the thyroid by the pretracheal fascia, and the attachment of the latter to the trachea and laryngeal cartilages, is the anatomical basis to the clinical observation that all thyroid swellings move upwards during the second phase of swallowing. During this phase of swallowing, the larynx and trachea ascend. The thyroid gland contained within the pretracheal fascia thus moves upwards obligatorily.

Inferiorly, the *pretracheal fascia* continues as a thin layer to fuse with the anterior surface of the fibrous pericardium.

The cervical lymph nodes may be broadly categorized into the following two sets:

1. Superficial cervical lymph nodes (i.e. those that are superficial to the investing layer of deep cervical fascia)
2. Deep cervical lymph nodes (i.e. those that are deep to the investing layer of deep cervical fascia)

Each of these categories is further subdivided into groups based on location and territory of drainage. The fascial planes of the neck are of considerable importance to the surgeon; they form convenient lines of cleavage through which he may separate the tissues in operative dissections and they may serve to delimit the spread of pus in neck infections.

(Some points of clinical significance concerning this fascia are to be found on page 161.)

Thyroid gland

The thyroid gland is the largest endocrine gland situated in the lower part of the front of the neck. It is made up of the following parts (Fig. 5.4):

1. The *isthmus* overlying the 2nd and 3rd rings of the trachea
2. The *lateral lobes* each extending from the side of the thyroid cartilage downwards to the 6th tracheal ring
3. An inconstant *pyramidal lobe* projecting upwards from the isthmus, usually on the left side, which represents a remnant of the embryological descent of the thyroid

Relations (Fig. 5.3)

The gland is enclosed in the *pretracheal fascia*, in turn covered by the strap muscles and overlapped by the sternocleidomastoids. The anterior jugular veins course over the isthmus. When the thyroid enlarges, the strap muscles stretch and adhere to the gland so that, at operation, they often appear to be thin layers of fascia.

On the deep aspect of the thyroid lie the larynx and trachea, with the pharynx and oesophagus behind and the carotid sheath on either side. Two nerves lie in close relationship to the gland; in the groove between the trachea and oesophagus lies the *recurrent laryngeal nerve*, and deep to the upper pole lies the *external branch* of the *superior laryngeal nerve* passing to the cricothyroid muscle.

Blood supply

Arterial supply

The following three arteries supply the thyroid gland (Fig. 5.4):

- The *superior thyroid artery* arises from the external carotid and passes to the upper pole
- The *inferior thyroid artery* arises from the thyrocervical trunk of the 1st part of the subclavian artery and passes behind the carotid sheath to the back of the gland
- The *thyroidea ima artery* is inconstant; when present, it arises from the aortic arch or the brachiocephalic artery

Venous drainage

The following three veins drain the thyroid gland (Fig. 5.4):

- The *superior thyroid vein* drains the upper pole to the internal jugular vein
- The *middle thyroid vein* drains from the lateral side of the gland to the internal jugular
- The *inferior thyroid veins* often several; drain the lower pole to the brachiocephalic veins

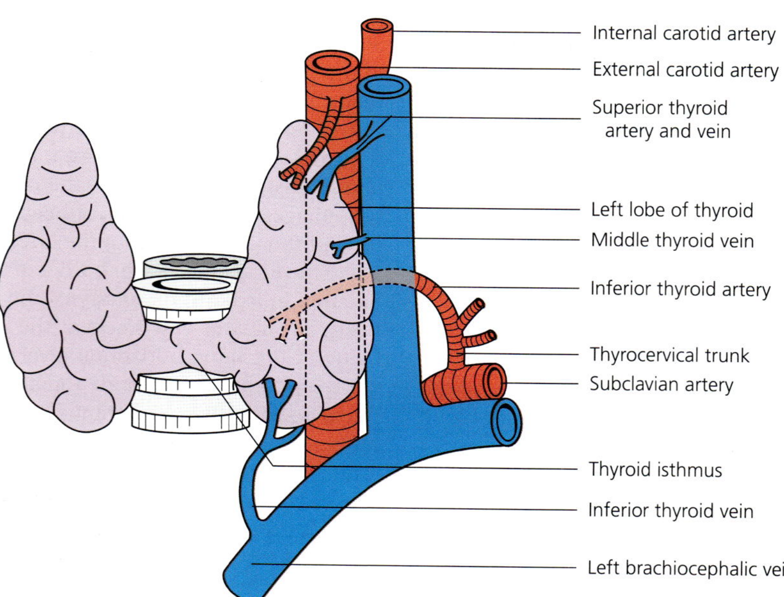

Figure 5.4 The thyroid and its blood vessels.

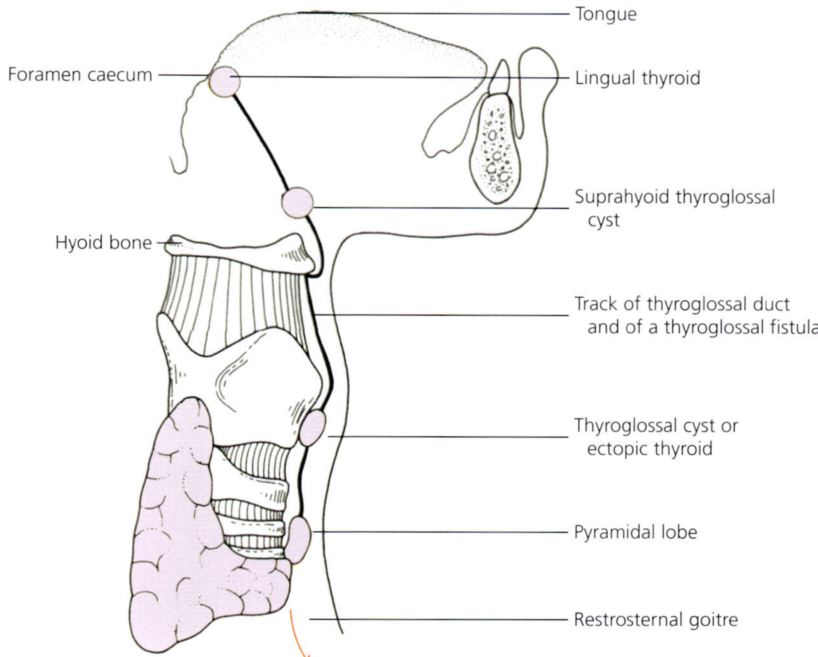

Figure 5.5 The descent of the thyroglossal duct, showing possible sites of ectopic thyroid tissue or thyroglossal cysts, and also the course of a thyroglossal fistula. (The arrow shows the further descent of the thyroid that may take place retrosternally into the superior mediastinum.)

As well as these named branches, numerous small vessels pass to the thyroid from the pharynx and trachea so that even when all the main vessels are tied, the gland still bleeds when cut across during a partial thyroidectomy.

Development

The thyroid develops from a bud that arises from the endodermal lining of the floor of the embryonic pharynx. It pushes out from the floor of the pharynx. This outgrowth is termed the thyroglossal duct, which descends to its definitive position in the neck. The lower end of the thyroglossal duct proliferates to become the thyroid gland, while the rest of the thyroglossal duct disintegrates and disappears. The origin of the thyroid is, however, commemorated by the *foramen caecum*, the midline punctum at the junction of the middle and posterior thirds of the tongue, and by the inconstant *pyramidal lobe* on the isthmus (Fig. 5.5).

Clinical Features

1 The embryological development of the thyroid accounts for the rare occurrence of the whole or a part of the gland remaining as a swelling at the tongue base (*lingual thyroid*) and for the much commoner occurrence of a *thyroglossal cyst* or *sinus* along the pathway of descent. Such a sinus can be dissected from the midline of the neck along the front of the hyoid (in such intimate contact with it that the centre of the hyoid must be excised during the dissection) then backwards through the muscles of the tongue to the foramen caecum (Fig. 5.5).

Descent of the thyroid may go beyond the normal position in the neck down into the superior mediastinum (*retro sternal goitre*).

(Continued ...)

(... continued)

2 A benign enlargement of the thyroid may compress or displace any of its close relations; the trachea and oesophagus may be narrowed, with resulting difficulty in breathing and swallowing, and the carotid may be displaced posteriorly. A carcinoma of the thyroid invades its neighbours rather than displacing them – eroding into trachea or oesophagus, surrounding the carotid sheath and occasionally causing severe haemorrhage therefrom. The recurrent laryngeal nerve and the cervical sympathetic chain may be involved, producing changes in the voice and Horner's syndrome, respectively.

3 We have already noted, in dealing with the fasciae of the neck, that the thyroid gland is enclosed in the *pretracheal fascia*. This thyroid capsule is much denser in front than behind and the enlarging gland therefore tends to push backwards, burying itself round the sides and even the back of the trachea and oesophagus. Because of the attachments of its fascial compartment, a large goitre will also extend downwards into the superior mediastinum ('plunging goitre').

Above, the pretracheal fascia blends with the larynx, accounting for the upward movement of the thyroid gland with each act of swallowing.

4 *Thyroidectomy* is carried out through a transverse 'collar' incision, two fingers' breadth above the suprasternal notch. This lies in the line of the natural skin folds of the neck. Skin flaps are reflected, together with platysma, and the investing fascia is opened longitudinally between the strap muscles and between the anterior jugular veins.

If more room is required in the case of a large goitre, the strap muscles are divided; this is carried out at their upper extremity because their nerve supply (the ansa hypoglossi) enters the lower part of the muscles and is hence preserved.

(Continued ...)

(... *continued*)

The pretracheal fascia is then divided, exposing the thyroid gland; unless this tissue plane deep to the fascia is found, dissection is a difficult and bloody procedure.

The thyroid is then mobilized and its vessels ligated *seriatim*. Both the external laryngeal and recurrent nerves are at risk during this procedure and must be carefully avoided. This is done by ligating the superior thyroid artery as close to the superior pole of gland as possible while inferior thyroid artery should be ligated as away from the lower pole as possible (for details *see* page 176). The relationship of recurrent laryngeal nerve to the thyroid gland is shown in Fig. 5.6.

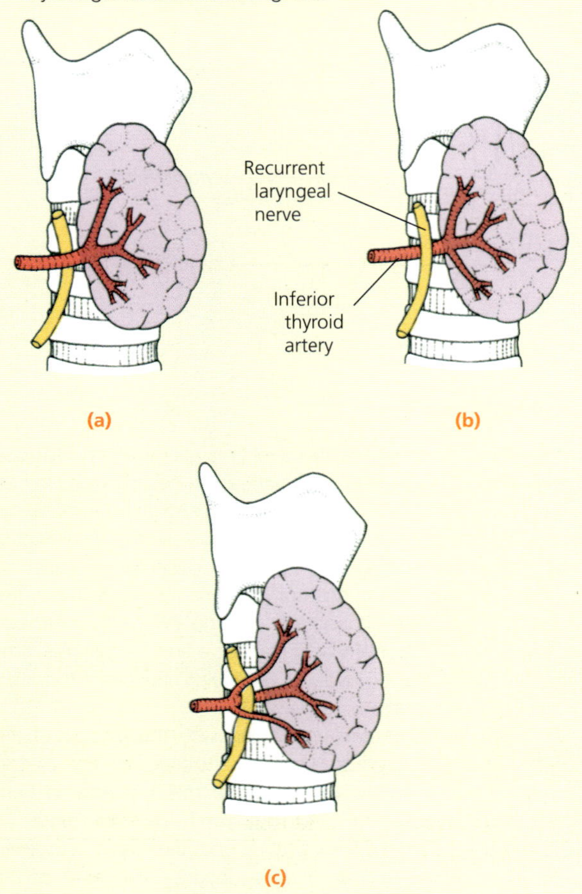

Figure 5.6 The relationship of the recurrent laryngeal nerve to the thyroid gland and the inferior thyroid artery. **(a)** The nerve is usually deep to the artery but may be **(b)** superficial to it or **(c)** pass through its branches. In these diagrams the lateral lobe of the thyroid is pulled forwards, as it would be in a thyroidectomy.

Parathyroid glands (Fig. 5.7)

The parathyroid glands are small endocrine glands (6 × 3 × 2 mm) situated along the posterior margin of the thyroid lobe.

These are usually four in number, a superior and inferior on either side; however, the numbers vary from two to six. Ninety per cent are in close relationship to the thyroid, 10% are aberrant, the latter most commonly being the inferior glands.

Each gland is about the size of a split pea and is of a yellowish-brown colour. The superior parathyroid is more constant in position than the inferior gland. It usually lies at the middle of the posterior border of the lobe of the thyroid above the level at which the inferior thyroid artery crosses the recurrent laryngeal nerve. The inferior parathyroid is most usually situated below the inferior artery near the lower pole of the thyroid gland. The next commonest site is within 0.5 in. (1.25 cm) of the lower pole of the thyroid gland. Aberrant inferior parathyroids may descend along the inferior thyroid veins in front of the trachea and may even track into the superior mediastinum in company with thymic tissues, for which there is an embryological explanation (*see* below). Less commonly, the inferior gland may lie behind and outside the fascial sheath of the thyroid and be found behind the oesophagus or even in the posterior mediastinum. Only on extremely rare occasions are the glands actually completely buried within thyroid tissue (Fig. 5.8).

Development

The superior parathyroids differentiate from the 4th pharyngeal (branchial) pouch. The inferior glands develop from the 3rd pharyngeal pouch in company with the thymus (Fig. 5.9; *see* Table 5.1, page 165). As the latter descends, the inferior parathyroids are dragged down with it.

It is thus easily understood that the inferior parathyroid may be dragged beyond the thyroid into the mediastinum and explains why, although very rarely, parathyroid tissue is found actually within the thymus.

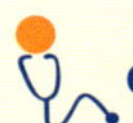

Clinical Features

1 These possible aberrant sites are, of course, of great importance when searching for a parathyroid adenoma in hyperparathyroidism.
2 The parathyroids are usually safe in subtotal thyroidectomy because the posterior rim of the thyroid is preserved in this operation. However, they may be inadvertently removed or damaged, with resultant tetany due to the lowered serum calcium.

Palate

The palate is an osseomuscular partition between nasopharynx and the nasal cavity above, and oropharynx and the buccal cavity below.
It comprises the following two parts:

1. The *hard palate*, which is vault-shaped and made up of the palatine plate of the maxilla and the horizontal plate of the palatine bone; it is bounded by the alveolar margin anteriorly and laterally, and merges posteriorly with the soft palate. It separates nasal and oral cavities.
2. The soft palate hanging as a curtain between the naso- and oropharynx; centrally, it bears the uvula on its free posterior edge; laterally, it blends into the palatoglossal and

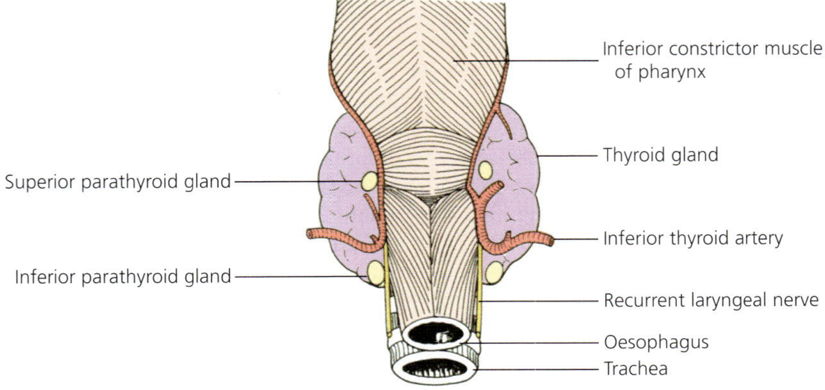

Figure 5.7 The normal sites of the parathyroid glands (posterior aspect).

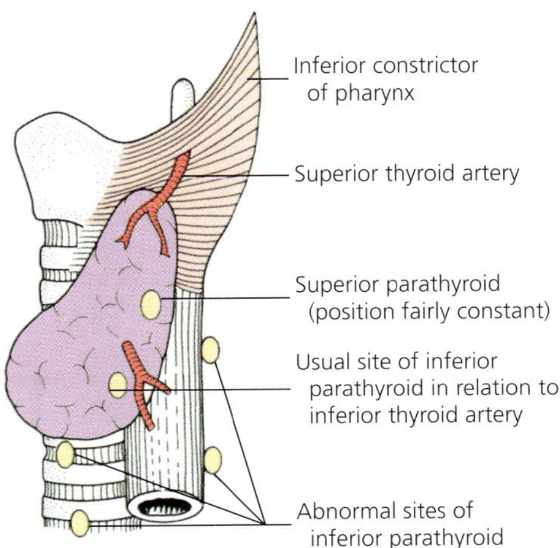

Figure 5.8 Normal and abnormal sites of the parathyroid glands (lateral view).

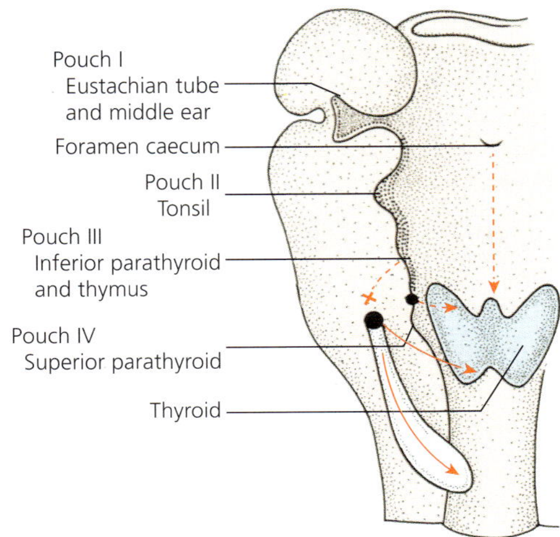

Figure 5.9 The derivatives of the branchial pouches. Note that the inferior parathyroid migrates downwards from the 3rd pouch, whereas the superior parathyroid (4th pouch) remains stationary.

Table 5.1 Derivatives of the branchial system (note the 5th arch disappears)

Arch	Nerve	Visceral	External cleft	Internal pouch	Floor	Cartilage	Muscle	Artery
I	V	Lower face	External auditory meatus	Eustachian tube, middle ear and mastoid antrum	Anterior 2/3 tongue	Meckel's, incus and malleus; sphenomandibular ligament	Muscles of mastication, anterior belly digastric, tensor palati, tensor tympani	Maxillary
II	VII	Grows down to cover remaining clefts to form skin of neck		Palatine tonsil	Contributes to anterior tongue; thyroid forms as outgrowth between I and II	Stapes, styloid process, stylohyoid ligament, upper body and lesser horn of hyoid	Muscles of facial expression, posterior belly digastric, stylohyoid, stapedius	Stapedial
III	IX			Thymus, inferior parathyroid	Posterior 1/3 tongue	Greater horn and lower part of body of hyoid	Stylopharyngeus	Common and internal carotids
IV	X (superior laryngeal)			Superior parathyroid		Thyroid cartilage	Muscles of pharynx, larynx and palate	Right, subclavian; left, aortic arch
VI	X (inferior laryngeal)				Outgrowth of lung buds	Cricoid cartilage		Pulmonary artery and ductus arteriosus

palatopharyngeal arches (respectively, the anterior and posterior pillars of the fauces). It separates the nasopharynx from the oropharynx.

The hard palate is made up of bone, periosteum and a squamous mucosa in which are embedded tiny accessory salivary glands.

The framework of the soft palate is formed by the aponeurosis of the tensor palati muscle, which adheres to the posterior border of the hard palate. To this fibrous sheet are attached the palatine muscles covered by a mucous membrane, which is squamous on its buccal aspect and ciliated columnar on its nasopharyngeal surface.

The sensory supply of the palate is largely from the maxillary division of V, but fibres of IX supply its most posterior part.

Motor innervation to the palatine muscles is from vagus (X) fibres in the pharyngeal plexus (with the qualification that the vagus derives these motor nerve fibres from XI, the cranial accessory nerve). The tensor palati is the exception to this rule and is supplied by the mandibular division of V.

In speaking, swallowing and blowing, the soft palate closes off the nasopharynx from the buccal cavity. If the palate is paralysed, as may occur in brainstem lesions or after diphtheria, the voice is impaired and fluids regurgitate through the nose on swallowing.

Development of the face, lips and palate with special reference to their congenital deformities (Fig. 5.10)

Around the primitive mouth, or stomodaeum, five processes develop as under:

1. The *frontonasal process*, which projects down from the cranium. Two olfactory pits develop in it and rupture into the pharynx to form the nostrils. Definitively, this process forms the nose, the nasal septum, nostrils, the philtrum of the upper lip (the small midline depression) and the premaxilla – the V-shaped anterior portion of the upper jaw which usually bears the four incisor teeth.
2. The *maxillary processes* on each side, which fuse with the frontonasal process and become the cheeks, upper lip (exclusive of the philtrum), upper jaw and palate (apart from the premaxilla).
3. The *mandibular processes*, which meet in the midline to form the lower jaw.

Abnormalities of this complex fusion process are numerous and constitute one of the commonest groups of congenital deformities. It is estimated that one child in 600 in England is born with some degree of either cleft lip or cleft palate (Fig. 5.11).

Frequently, these anomalies are associated with other congenital conditions such as spina bifida or syndactyly (fusion of fingers or toes). Indeed, it is good clinical practice to search a patient with any congenital defect for others.

The following anomalies are associated with defects of fusion of the face:

1. *Macrostoma* and *microstoma* are conditions in which either too little or too great a closure of the stomodaeum occurs.
2. *Cleft upper lip* (or 'hare lip') is only very rarely like the upper lip of a hare, i.e. a median cleft, although this may occur as a failure of development of the philtrum from the frontonasal process. Much more commonly, the cleft is on one or both sides of the philtrum, occurring as failure of fusion of the maxillary and frontonasal processes. The cleft may be a small defect in the lip or may extend into the nostril, split the alveolus or even extend along the side of the nose as far as the orbit. There may be an associated cleft palate.
3. *Cleft lower lip* occurs very rarely but may be associated with a cleft tongue and cleft mandible.
4. *Cleft palate* is a failure of fusion of the segments of the palate. The following stages may occur (Fig. 5.11):
   a. Bifid uvula, of no clinical importance
   b. Partial cleft, which may involve the soft palate only or the posterior part of the hard palate also
   c. Complete cleft, which may be unilateral, running the full length of the maxilla and then alongside one face of the premaxilla, or bilateral, in which the palate is cleft with an anterior V separating the premaxilla completely
5. *Inclusion dermoids* may form along the lines of fusion of the face. The most common of these is the *external angular dermoid* at the lateral extremity of the upper eyebrow. Occasionally, this dermoid extends through the skull to attach to the underlying dura.

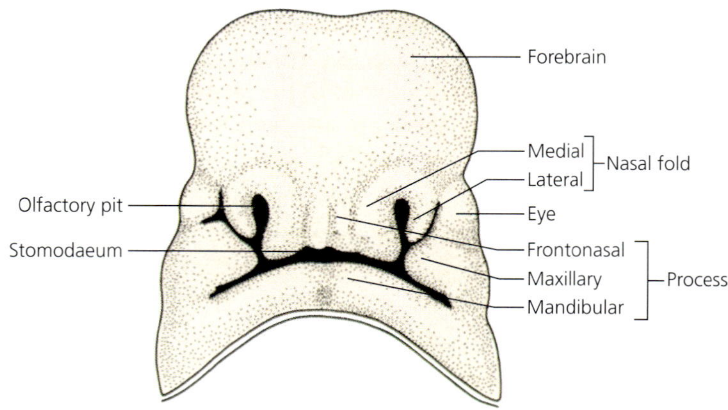

Figure 5.10 The ventral aspect of a foetal head showing the three processes, frontonasal, maxillary and mandibular, from which the face, nose and jaws are derived.

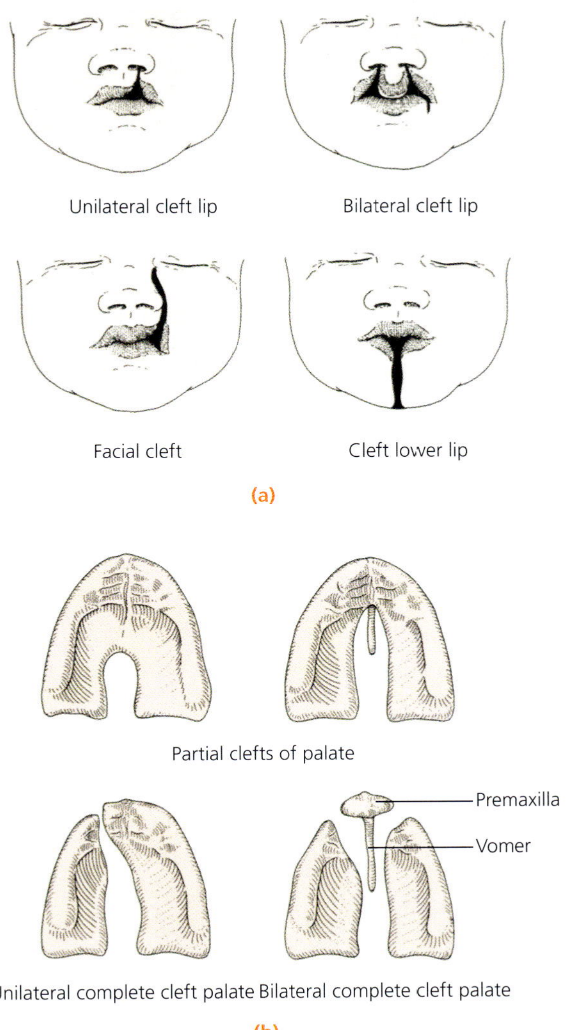

Figure 5.11 Types of **(a)** cleft lip and **(b)** cleft palate.

Tongue and floor of the mouth

Tongue

The tongue is a mobile muscular organ present in the oral cavity. It consists of a buccal and a pharyngeal portion separated by a V-shaped groove on its dorsal surface, the *sulcus terminalis*. At the apex of this groove is a shallow depression, the foramen caecum, marking the embryological origin of the thyroid (*see* page 164; Fig. 5.9). Immediately in front of the sulcus lies a row of large vallate papillae.

The under-aspect of the tongue bears the median *frenulum linguae*; the mucosa is thin on this surface and the lingual veins can thus be seen on either side of the frenulum. The lingual nerve and the lingual artery are medial to the vein but not visible. More laterally can be seen a fringed fold of mucous membrane termed the *plica fimbriata*. On either side of the base of the frenulum can be seen the orifice of the submandibular duct on its papilla. Inspect this in a mirror and note the discharge of saliva when you press on your submandibular gland just below the angle of the jaw.

Structure

The thick stratified squamous mucosa of the dorsum of the tongue bears papillae over the anterior two-thirds back as far as the sulcus terminalis. These papillae (particularly the vallate) bear the taste buds. The posterior one-third has no papillae but carries numerous lymphoid nodules which together form the **lingual tonsil.**

Small glands are scattered throughout the submucosa of the dorsum; these are predominantly serous anteriorly and mucous posteriorly.

The tongue is divided by a median vertical fibrous septum, as indicated on the dorsum by a shallow groove. On each side of this septum are the intrinsic and extrinsic muscles of the tongue (Fig. 5.12).

The **intrinsic muscles** are confined to the tongue. They are disposed in vertical, longitudinal and transverse bundles; they alter the shape of the tongue.

The **extrinsic muscles** move the tongue as a whole. They pass to the tongue from the symphysis of the mandible, the hyoid, styloid process and the soft palate, and are called the *genioglossus, hyoglossus, styloglossus* and *palatoglossus*, respectively. The functions of the individual extrinsic muscles can be deduced from their relative positions (Fig. 5.12). Genioglossus protrudes the tongue, styloglossus retracts it and hyoglossus depresses it. Palatoglossus is, in fact, a palatal muscle and helps to narrow the oropharynx in swallowing.

Blood supply

Blood is chiefly supplied from the lingual branch of the external carotid artery. There is little cross-circulation across the median raphe, which is, therefore, a relatively avascular plane.

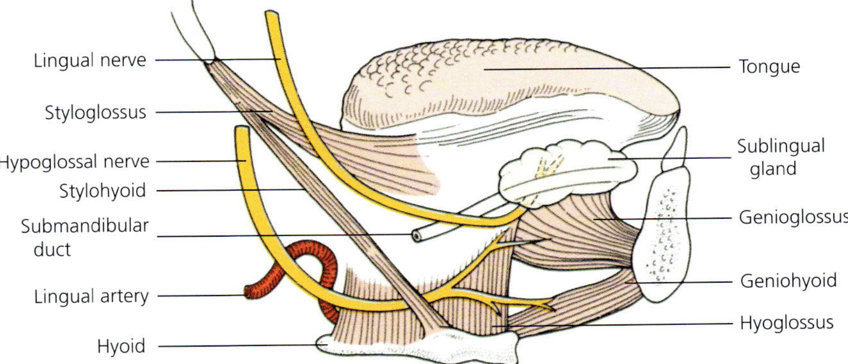

Figure 5.12 Lateral view of the tongue, its extrinsic muscles and its nerves.

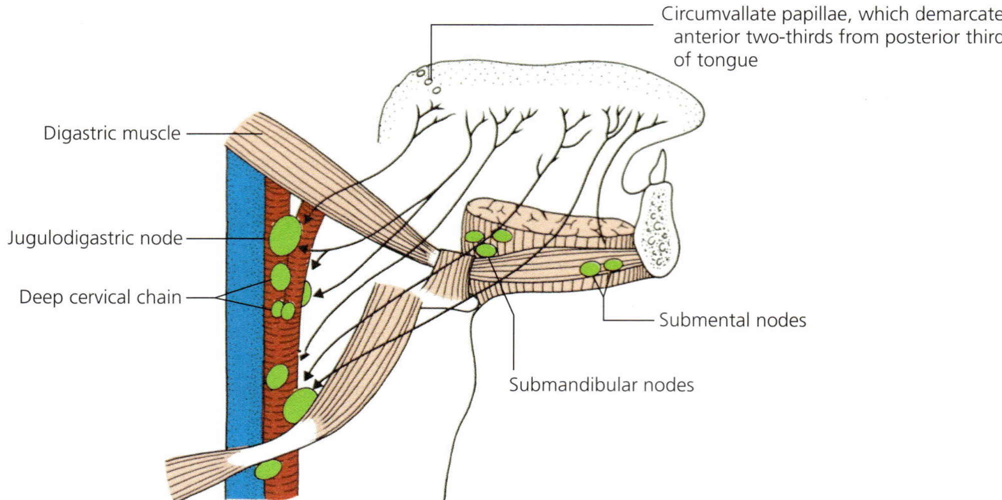

Figure 5.13 The lymph drainage of the tongue. Note two points. (i) The anterior part of the tongue tends to drain to the nodes farthest down the deep cervical chain, whereas the posterior part drains to the upper chain. (ii) The anterior two-thirds of the tongue drain unilaterally, the posterior one-third bilaterally.

Lymph drainage (Fig. 5.13)

The drainage zones of the mucosa of the tongue can be grouped into the following three:

1. The *tip* drains to the submental nodes
2. The *anterior two-thirds* drains to the submental and submandibular nodes and thence to the *lower* nodes of the deep cervical chain along the carotid sheath
3. The posterior one-third drains to the upper nodes of the deep cervical chain, and also to the deeply situated parapharyngeal and retropharyngeal nodes

There is a rich anastomosis across the midline between the lymphatics of the posterior one-third of the tongue so that a tumour on one side readily metastasizes to contralateral nodes. In contrast, there is little cross-communication in the anterior two-thirds, where growths more than 0.5 in. (1.25 cm) from the midline do not metastasize to the opposite side of the neck until late in the disease.

Nerve supply

The anterior two-thirds of the tongue receives its sensory supply from the *lingual nerve*, a branch of V, which also transmits the gustatory fibres of the *chorda tympani nerve*, a branch of VII.

Common sensation and taste to the posterior one-third, including the vallate papillae, are derived from *glossopharyngeal (IX) nerve*. A few fibres of the internal laryngeal branch of the *superior laryngeal nerve* (a branch of X) carry sensory fibres from the very posterior part of the tongue.

All the muscles of the tongue except palatoglossus are supplied by *hypoglossal (XII) nerve*; palatoglossus, a muscle of the soft palate, is innervated by the pharyngeal branch of vasoaccesory complex (i.e. cranial root of accessory nerve via vagus).

Development (Fig. 5.14)

The **tongue mucosa** develops from the following four swellings that appear in the floor of the primitive pharynx.

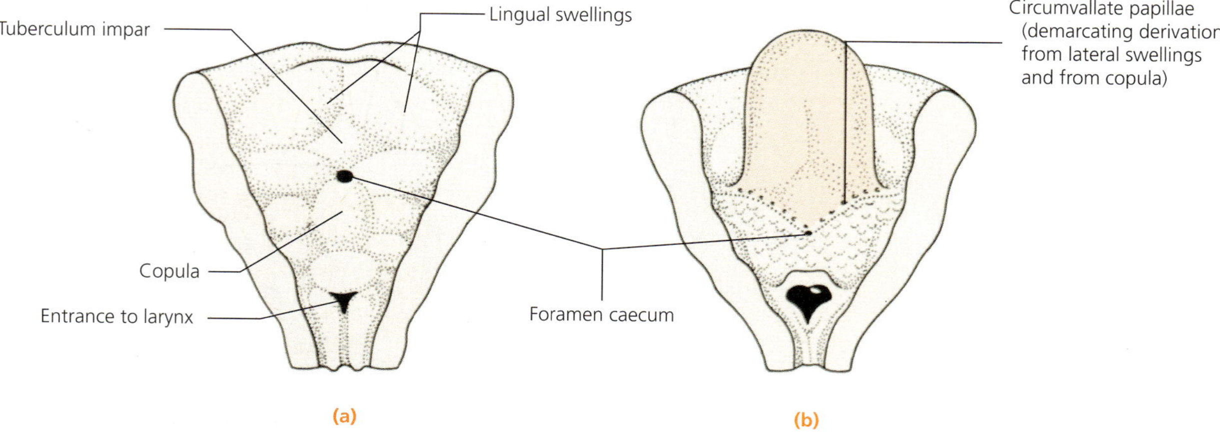

Figure 5.14 Stages in the development of the tongue.

A small nodule, the *tuberculum impar*, is the first evidence of the developing tongue in the floor of the primitive pharynx. This is soon covered over by the *lingual swellings*, one on each side, derived from the 1st branchial arch. These fuse in the midline to form the definitive anterior two-thirds of the tongue supplied by V and reinforced by the chorda tympani.

Posteriorly, this mass meets the *copula* (or *hypobranchial eminence*), a central swelling in the pharyngeal floor that represents the 2nd, 3rd and 4th arches and which forms the posterior one-third of the tongue (nerve supply IX and X).

The **tongue muscles** derive from the *occipital myotomes*, which migrate forwards dragging with them their nerve supply (XII, the hypoglossal nerve).

Clinical Features

1 Damage to the hypoglossal nerve is readily detected clinically by hemiatrophy of the ipsilateral side of the tongue and deviation of the projected organ towards the paralysed side.
2 If the unconscious or deeply anaesthetized patient is laid on his back, the posterior aspect of the tongue drops back to produce a laryngeal obstruction. This can be prevented either by lying the patient on his side with the head down ('the tonsil position'), when the tongue flops forwards with the weight of gravity, or by pushing the mandible forwards by pressure on the angle of the jaw on each side; this is effective because genioglossus, attached to the symphysis menti, drags the tongue forwards along with the lower jaw.
3 Although lymphatics pierce the floor of the mouth (i.e. the mylohyoid muscle) to reach the submental and submandibular lymph nodes, it is an interesting fact that these tissues are not affected by lymphatic spread of malignant cells (although they may be invaded by direct extension of growth). It seems that the nodes are involved by lymphatic emboli and not by a permeation of the lymphatic channels.
   The bilateral lymphatic spread of growths of the posterior one-third of the tongue is one factor contributing to the poor prognosis of tumours at this site.

Floor of the mouth

The floor of the mouth is formed principally by the mylohyoid muscles. These stretch as a diaphragm from their origin along the mylohyoid line on the medial aspect of the body of the mandible on each side, to their insertion along a median raphe and into the hyoid bone. Thus, together, the right and left mylohyoid muscles form a curved, sheet-like sling that supports the tongue (Fig. 5.15). The mylohyoid muscle is an important surgical landmark insofar as it constitutes the boundary between the neck and oral region.

On the lower aspect of this diaphragm, on each side, are the anterior belly of the digastric muscle, the superficial part of the submandibular gland and the submandibular lymph nodes, all covered by the investing layer of deep cervical fascia and platysma.

Lying above mylohyoid are the tongue muscles, as a central mass, with the sublingual salivary gland and the deep part of the submandibular gland and its duct lying beneath the mucosa of the mouth floor on either side.

Clinical Features

Ludwig's angina is a cellulitis of the floor of the mouth, usually originating from a carious molar tooth. The infection spreads above the mylohyoid; oedema forces the tongue upwards; and the mylohyoid itself is pushed downwards so that there is swelling both below the chin and within the mouth. There is considerable danger of spread of infection backwards with oedema of the glottis and asphyxia.

Drainage is carried out by a deep incision below the mandible that must divide the mylohyoid muscle.

Pharynx

The pharynx is a musculofascial tube, incomplete anteriorly, which extends from the base of the skull to the oesophagus and which acts as a common entrance to the respiratory and alimentary tracts.

From above downwards, it is made up of the following three portions (Fig. 5.16):

1. The *nasopharynx* lying behind the nasal fossae and above the soft palate
2. The *oropharynx* lying behind the anterior pillars of the fauces
3. The *laryngopharynx* lying behind the larynx

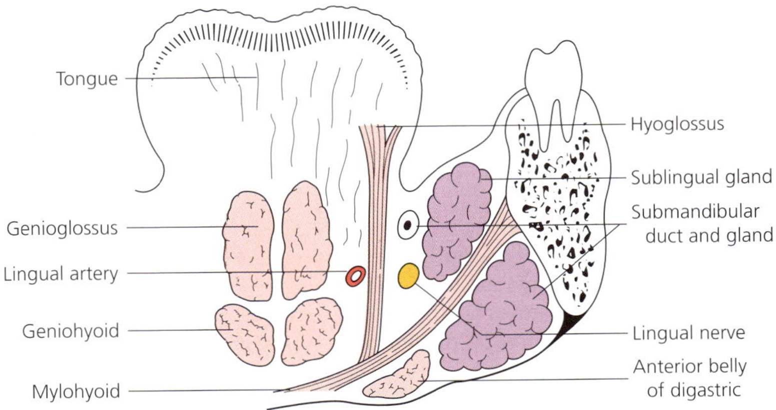

Figure 5.15 Coronal section of the floor of the mouth.

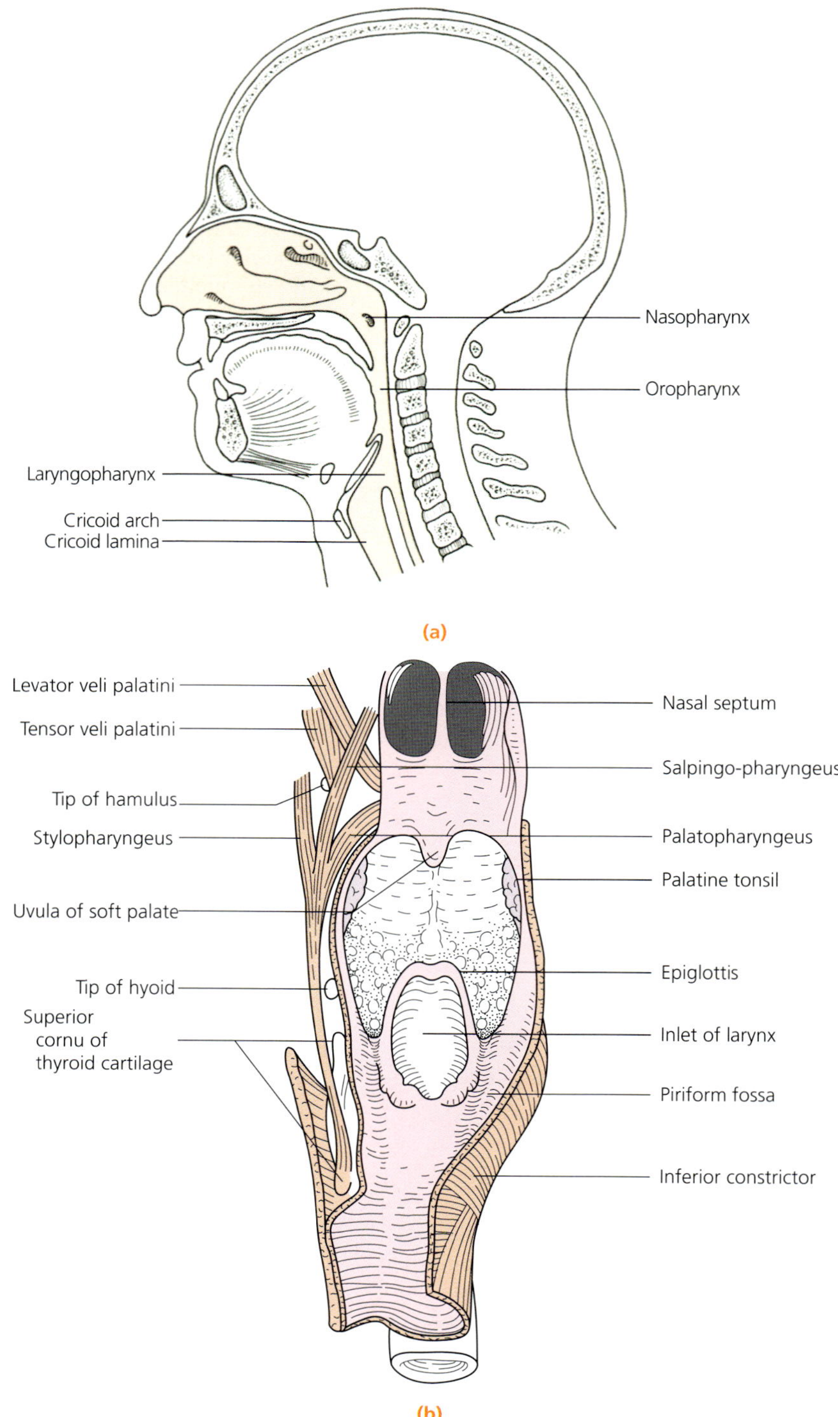

Figure 5.16 **(a)** Schematic sagittal section through the head and neck to show the subdivisions of the pharynx. **(b)** Interior of the pharynx viewed from behind after removing the posterior wall of the pharynx.

Nasopharynx

The nasopharynx lies above the soft palate, which cuts it off from the rest of the pharynx during deglutition and therefore prevents regurgitation of food through the nose.

Two important structures lie in this compartment.

The *nasopharyngeal tonsil* ('the *adenoids*') consists of a collection of lymphoid tissue beneath the epithelium of the roof and posterior wall of this region. It helps to form a continuous lymphoid ring with the palatine tonsils and the lymphoid nodules on the dorsum of the tongue (*Waldeyer's ring*).

The *orifice of the pharyngotympanic or auditory tube* (*Eustachian canal*) lies on the side-wall of the nasopharynx level with the floor of the nose. The posterior lip of this opening is prominent, due to the underlying cartilage of the Eustachian tube, and is termed the *Eustachian* or *pharyngeal cushion*, behind which lies the slit-like *pharyngeal recess*.

Clinical Features

1 The nasopharynx may be inspected indirectly by a mirror passed through the mouth (posterior rhinoscopy) or studied through a rhinoscope passed along the floor of the nose. Under anaesthesia, it can be palpated by a finger passed behind the soft palate.
2 The nasopharyngeal tonsils (adenoids) are prominent in children but usually undergo atrophy after puberty. When chronically inflamed they may all but fill the nasopharynx, causing mouth-breathing and also, by blocking the auditory tube, deafness and middle ear infection.
3 The Eustachian tube provides a ready pathway of sepsis from the pharynx to the middle ear and accounts for the frequency with which otitis media complicates infections of the throat.
4 The middle ear can be intubated through a catheter passed into the Eustachian tube. The catheter is passed along the nasal floor to the posterior wall of the nasopharynx. Its curved tip is then rotated laterally so that it lies in the pharyngeal recess; it is then withdrawn over the Eustachian cushion to slip into the orifice of the auditory tube.

Oropharynx

This part of the pharynx lies behind the mouth and tongue. Its anterior boundaries are the right and left palatoglossal arches (anterior pillars of the fauces) and it extends from the uvula of the soft palate above to the tip of the epiglottis below. Its most important contents are the palatine tonsils situated in the lateral wall on either side.

Waldeyer's ring

It is a ring of lymphatic tissues at the beginning of food and air passages. It is formed by palatine tonsils laterally, nasopharangeal tonsil posterosuperiorly, tubal tonsil posterolaterally and lingual tonsil anteriorly (Fig. 5.17).

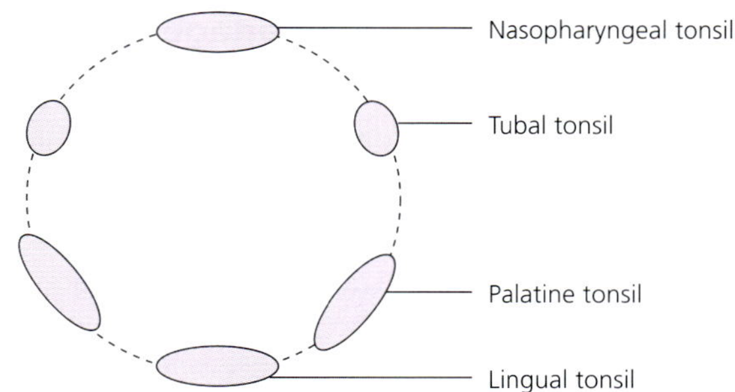

Figure 5.17 Schematic diagram of Waldeyer's ring.

Palatine tonsils

The palatine tonsil lies in the tonsillar fossa between the palatoglossal and palatopharyngeal arches (anterior and posterior pillars of the fauces, respectively). The anterior pillar, or palatoglossal arch, forms the boundary between the buccal cavity and the oropharynx; it fuses with the lateral wall of the tongue and contains the palatoglossus muscle. The posterior pillar, or palatopharyngeal arch, blends with the wall of the pharynx and contains the palatopharyngeus (Fig. 5.18).

The floor of the tonsillar fossa is formed by the superior constrictor of the pharynx separated from the tonsil by the *tonsillar capsule*, which is a thick condensation of the pharyngeal submucosa (the pharyngobasilar fascia). This capsule is itself separated from the superior constrictor by a film of loose areolar tissue.

The palatine tonsil consists of a collection of lymphoid tissue covered by a squamous epithelium, a unique histological combination which makes it easy to 'spot' in examinations. This epithelium is pitted by *crypts*, up to 20 in number, and often bears a deep *intratonsillar cleft* in its upper part.

The lymphoid material may extend up to the soft palate, down to the tongue or into the anterior faucial pillar. From late puberty onwards this lymphoid tissue undergoes progressive atrophy.

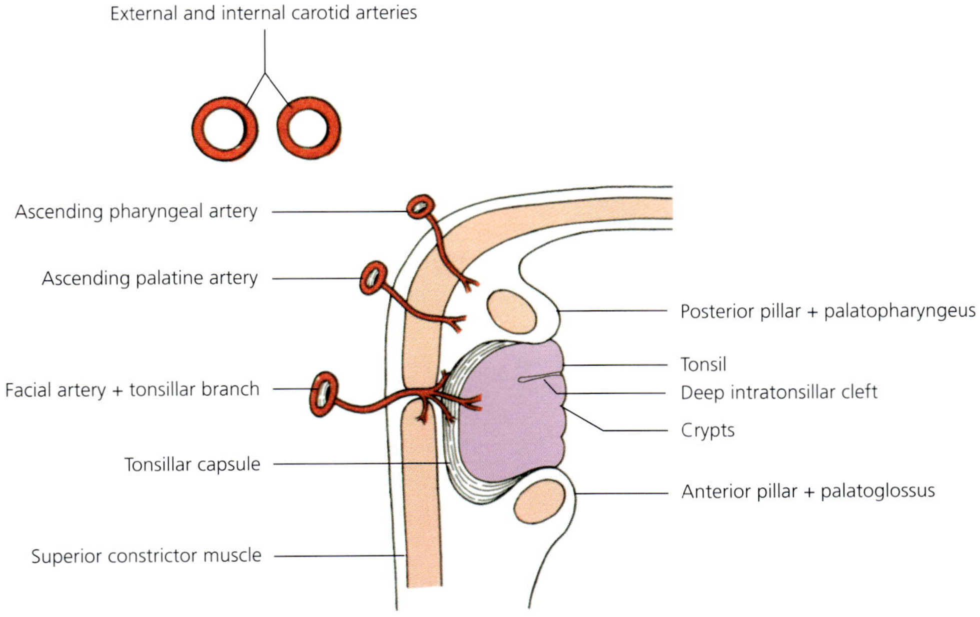

Figure 5.18 Diagram of the palatine tonsil and its relations – in horizontal section.

Blood supply, venous drainage and lymphatic drainage

Blood supply is principally from the tonsillar branch of the facial artery entering at the lower pole of the tonsil, although twigs are also derived from the lingual, ascending palatine and ascending pharyngeal arteries.

The venous drainage passes to the pharyngeal plexus. An important constant vein, the *paratonsillar vein*, descends from the soft palate across the lateral aspect of the tonsillar capsule. It is nearly always divided in tonsillectomy and may give rise to troublesome haemorrhage.

Lymph drainage is via lymphatics that pierce the superior constrictor muscle and pass to the nodes along the internal jugular vein, especially the *tonsillar or jugulodigastric node* at the angle of the jaw. Since this node is affected in tonsillitis it is the most common lymph node in the body to undergo pathological enlargement.

Embryologically, the tonsil derives from the 2nd pharyngeal (branchial) pouch (Fig. 5.9).

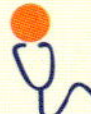

Clinical Features

1 *Tonsillectomy* may be carried out by dissection or by the guillotine method; both depend on removing the lymphoid tissue and underlying fascial capsule from the loose areolar tissue clothing the superior constrictor in the floor of the tonsillar fossa. In dissection, an incision is made in the mucosa of the anterior pillar immediately in front of the tonsil; the gland is then freed by blunt dissection until it remains attached only by its pedicle of vessels near its lower pole. This pedicle is then crushed and divided by means of a wire snare.

In the second method, the guillotine is applied so that the tonsil bulges through the ring in the instrument. The tonsil is then removed by closing the blade of the guillotine.

Unless there have been repeated infections, the superior constrictor lies separated from the palatine tonsil and its capsule by loose areolar tissue that prevents the pharyngeal wall being dragged into danger during tonsillectomy.

Similarly, the internal carotid artery, although only 1 in. (2.5 cm) behind the tonsil, is never injured in this operation since it lies safely freed from the pharynx by fatty tissue around the carotid sheath.

2 A *quinsy* is suppuration in the peritonsillar tissue secondary to tonsillitis. It is drained by an incision in the most prominent part of the abscess where softening can be felt.

Laryngopharynx

The laryngopharynx extends from the level of the tip of the epiglottis to the termination of the pharynx in the oesophagus at the level of C6.

The inlet of the larynx, defined by the epiglottis, aryepiglottic folds and the arytenoids, lies anteriorly. The larynx itself bulges into this part of the pharynx leaving a deep recess anterolaterally on either side, the *piriform fossa*, in which ingested sharp foreign bodies (for example, fish bones) may lodge.

The fossa is bounded medially by aryepiglottic fold and laterally by lamina of thyroid cartilage and thyrohyoid membrane.

Structure of the pharynx

The pharynx is made up of mucosa, containing mucus-secreting goblet cells, submucosa, muscle and a loose areolar sheath. The mucosa is a ciliated columnar epithelium in the nasopharynx, but elsewhere it is stratified and squamous. Beneath this, the submucosa is thick and fibrous (the *pharyngobasilar fascia*) and it is this layer which forms the capsule of the tonsil.

The three *pharyngeal constrictor muscles* (superior, middle and inferior) are arranged like flower pots (without bottoms) placed one inside the other, but are open in front at the entries of the nasal, buccal and laryngeal cavities.

Each constrictor muscle is attached anteriorly to the sidewall of these cavities and fans out to insert into a median raphe along the posterior aspect of the pharynx, extending from the base of the skull to the oesophagus (Fig. 5.19).

The three constrictors are so arranged that the inferior overlaps the middle, and which in turn overlaps the superior. Structures passing through the gaps in the pharyngeal wall are as follows:

1. A large gap between the upper border of superior constrictor and base of the skull (also called *sinus of Morgagni*) provides passage to the auditory tube, levator palati muscle and ascending palatine artery.
2. The gap between superior and inferior constrictors provide passage to stylopharyngeus muscle and glossopharyngeal nerve.
3. The gap between middle and inferior constrictors provides passage to internal laryngeal nerve and superior laryngeal vessels.
4. The gap between the lower border of inferior constrictor and oesophagus provides passage to recurrent laryngeal nerve and inferior laryngeal vessels.

Covering these muscles is a thin areolar layer continuous with that covering the buccinator and hence is termed the *buccopharyngeal fascia*.

Blood supply

The pharynx receives its arterial supply mainly from the superior thyroid and ascending pharyngeal branches of the external carotid.

A pharyngeal venous plexus lies in the areolar tissue that covers the pharynx and drains into the internal jugular vein.

Nerve supply

The pharyngeal branches of IX and X constitute the principal sensory and motor supply of the pharynx, respectively. The maxillary division of V supplies the sensory innervation of the nasopharynx.

Mechanism of deglutition

The act of swallowing not only conveys food down the oesophagus but also disposes of mucus loaded with dust

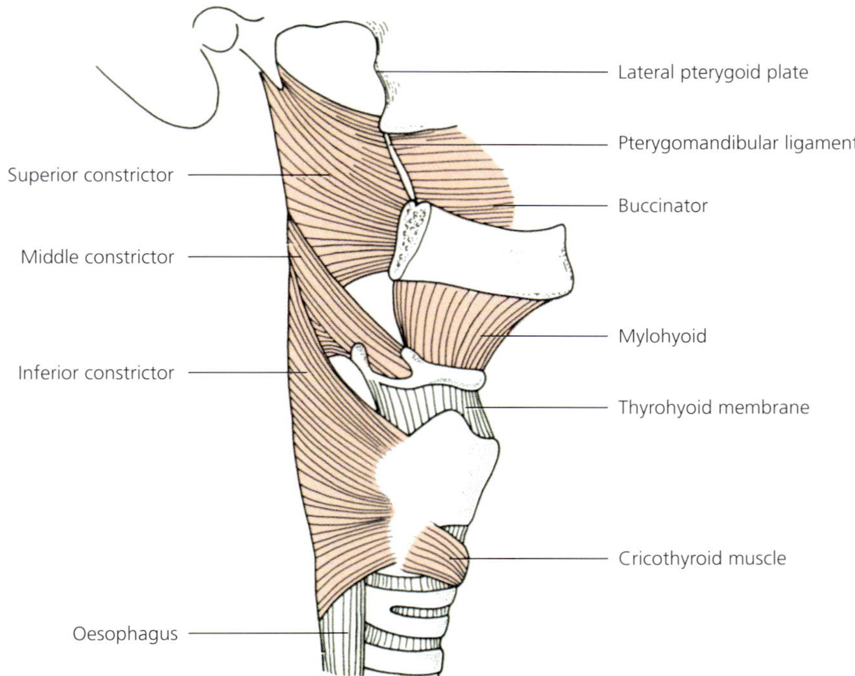

Figure 5.19 The constrictor muscles of the pharynx.

and bacteria from the respiratory passages. Moreover, during deglutition, the Eustachian auditory tube is opened, thus equalizing the pressure on either side of the ear drum.

Deglutition is a complex, orderly series of reflexes. It is initiated voluntarily but is completed by involuntary reflex actions set up by stimulation of the pharynx. If the pharynx is anaesthetized then normal swallowing cannot take place. The reflexes are co-ordinated by the deglutition centre in the medulla, which lies near the vagal nucleus and the respiratory centres.

The food is first crushed by mastication and lubricated by saliva. It is a common experience that it is well-nigh impossible to swallow a pill when the throat is dry. The bolus is then pushed back through the oropharyngeal isthmus by the pressure of the tongue against the palate, assisted by the muscles of the mouth floor.

During swallowing, the oral, nasal and laryngeal openings must be closed off to prevent regurgitation of food or fluid through them; each of these openings is guarded by a highly effective sphincter mechanism.

The nasopharynx is closed by elevation of the soft palate, which shuts against a contracted ridge of superior pharyngeal constrictor, the *ridge of Passavant*. At the same time, the tensor palati opens the ostium of the Eustachian tube. The oropharyngeal isthmus is partially blocked by contraction of palatoglossus on each side, which narrows the space between the anterior faucial pillars. The residual gap is closed by the dorsum of the tongue wedging into it.

The protection of the larynx is a complex affair, brought about not only by closure of the sphincter mechanism of the larynx but also by tucking the larynx behind the overhanging mass of the tongue and by utilizing the epiglottis to guide the bolus away from the laryngeal entrance. The central nervous component of the swallowing reflex is depressed by narcotics, anaesthesia and cerebral trauma. In these circumstances aspiration of foreign material into the pulmonary tree becomes possible, particularly if the patient is lying on his back or in a head-up position.

The laryngeal sphincters are at three levels as mentioned below:

1. The aryepiglottic folds, defining the laryngeal inlet, which are apposed by the aryepiglottic and oblique arytenoid muscles
2. The walls of the vestibule of the larynx, which are approximated by the thyroepiglottic muscles
3. The vocal cords, which are closed by the lateral cricoarytenoid and interarytenoid muscles

The larynx is elevated and pulled forwards by the action of the thyrohyoid, stylohyoid, stylopharyngeus, digastric and mylohyoid muscles so that it comes into apposition with the base of the tongue, which is projecting backwards at this phase. While the larynx is raised and its entrance closed there is reflex inhibition of respiration.

The action of the epiglottis has been the subject of much speculation. As the head of the bolus reaches the epiglottis, the latter is first tipped backwards against the pharyngeal wall and momentarily holds up the onward passage of the food. The larynx is then elevated and pulled forwards, drawing with it the epiglottis so that it now stands erect, guiding the food bolus into streams along both piriform fossae and away from the laryngeal orifice, like a rock sticking up into a waterfall. Finally, the epiglottis is seen indeed to flap backwards as a cover over the laryngeal inlet, but this occurs only after the main bolus has passed beyond it. The epiglottis acts as a laryngeal lid at this stage to prevent deposition of fragments of food debris over the inlet of the larynx during re-establishment of the airway.

The cricopharyngeus then relaxes allowing the bolus to cross the pharyngo-oesophageal junction. Fluids may shoot down the oesophagus passively under the initial impetus of the tongue action; semi-solid or solid material is carried down by peristalsis. The oesophageal transit time is about 15 seconds, relaxation of the cardia occurring just before the peristaltic wave reaches it. Gravity has little effect on the transit of the bolus, which occurs just as rapidly in the lying as in the erect position. It is, of course, quite easy to swallow fluid or solids while standing on one's head, a well-known party trick; here, oesophageal transit is inevitably an active muscular process.

Clinical Features

1 During the removal of foreign bodies from the piriform fossa, the internal laryngeal nerve may be injured if the instrument pierces the mucosa of the floor.
2 Pharyngeal pouch: The inferior constrictor muscle is made up of an upper oblique and a lower transverse part, the former arising from the side of the thyroid cartilage (the thyropharyngeus) and the latter from the cricoid (the cricopharyngeus).

Posteriorly, in the midline, there is a potential gap between these two components termed the *pharyngeal dimple* or *Killian's dehiscence*. The mucosa and submucosa of the pharynx may bulge through this weak area to form a pharyngeal pouch (Fig. 5.20), possibly as a result of muscle inco-ordination or of spasm of the cricopharyngeus. This diverticulum first protrudes posteriorly; as it enlarges, backwards extension is prevented by the prevertebral fascia and it therefore has to project to one side of the pharynx – usually to the more exposed left.

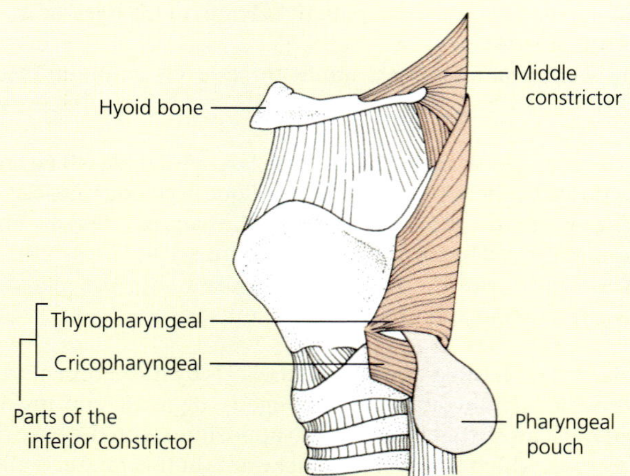

Figure 5.20 A pharyngeal pouch emerging between the two components of the inferior constrictor muscle.

With further enlargement, the pouch pushes the oesophagus aside and lies directly in line with the pharynx; most food then passes into the pouch with resulting severe dysphagia and cachexia. Spillage of the pouch contents into the larynx is very liable to cause inhalation of food material into the bronchi with respiratory infection and lung abscess as possible consequences.

Larynx

The larynx is the organ of voice. It actually has a triple function: that of an open valve in *respiration*, that of a partially closed valve whose orifice can be modulated in *phonation*, and that of a closed valve, protecting the trachea and bronchial tree during deglutition (i.e. protection of lower respiratory tract). Coughing is possible only when the larynx can be closed effectively.

Skeletal framework of larynx

The skeletal framework of the larynx is formed by nine cartilages, three unpaired (the epiglottis, thyroid cartilage, cricoid) and three paired (the arytenoids corniculate and cuneiform) (Fig. 5.21).

The larynx is slung from the U-shaped hyoid bone by the *thyrohyoid membrane* and *thyrohyoid muscle*. The hyoid bone itself is attached to the mandible and tongue by the hyoglossus, the mylohyoid, geniohyoid and digastric muscles, to the styloid process by the stylohyoid ligament and muscle and to the pharynx by the middle constrictor. Three of the four strap muscles of the neck, the omohyoid, sternohyoid and thyrohyoid, find attachment to it, only the sternothyroid failing to gain it.

The *epiglottis* is a leaf-shaped elastic cartilage lying behind the root of the tongue. It is attached anteriorly to the body of the hyoid by the hyoepiglottic ligament and below to the back of the thyroid cartilage by the thyroepiglottic ligament immediately above the vocal cords. The sides of the epiglottis are connected to the arytenoids by the aryepiglottic folds that run backwards to form the margins of the entrance, or *aditus*, of the larynx.

The upper anterior surface of the epiglottis projects above the hyoid bone; the epiglottic mucosa is reflected forwards to the base of the tongue and is raised up into a median glossoepiglottic fold and lateral pharyngoepiglottic folds. The depression on either side between these folds is termed the *vallecula*.

The *thyroid cartilage* is shield-like, being made up of two lateral plates meeting in the midline in the prominent 'V' of the 'Adam's apple', the laryngeal prominence that is easily visible in the postpubertal male.

The *cricoid* is signet-ring shaped, deepest behind. It is the only complete ring of cartilage throughout the respiratory tract. Inferiorly, it is attached to the trachea by the *cricotracheal membrane*.

The *arytenoids* sit one on each side of the posterior 'signet' of the cricoid cartilage.

In addition, there are two small nodules of cartilage at the inlet of the larynx; the *corniculate cartilage*, a nodule lying at the apex of the arytenoid, and the *cuneiform cartilage*, a flake of cartilage within the margin of the aryepiglottic fold. These

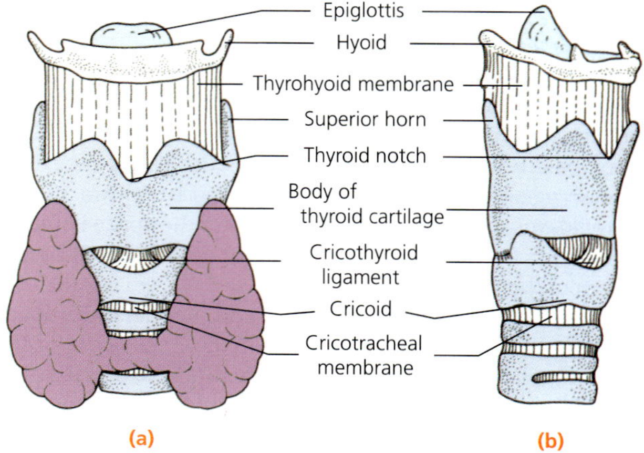

Figure 5.21 External view of the larynx. **(a)** Anterior aspect. **(b)** Anterolateral aspect.

are of no functional importance. They are, however, seen when the larynx is inspected through a laryngoscope (*see* Fig. 5.23) and, to the uninitiated, might mimic pathological nodules.

The *cricothyroid membrane* (cricovocal membrane) connects the thyroid, cricoid and arytenoid cartilages. It is composed mainly of yellow elastic tissue. Its upper edge is attached anteriorly to the posterior surface of the thyroid cartilage and behind to the vocal process of the arytenoid. Between these two structures, the upper edge of the membrane is thickened slightly to form the *vocal ligament*. Anteriorly, the membrane thickens, as the *cricothyroid ligament*; this is subcutaneous, easily felt and is used in emergency cricothyroid puncture for laryngeal obstruction.

Interior of larynx

Passing forwards from the arytenoid to the back of the thyroid cartilage, just below the epiglottic attachment, are two folds of mucosa. The upper is the *vestibular fold*, containing a small amount of fibrous tissue and forming on each side the *false vocal cord*. The lower fold (the *vocal fold* or *cord*) contains the vocal ligament (Fig. 5.22).

The mucosa is firmly adherent to the vocal ligament without there being any intervening submucosa. This accounts for the pearly white, avascular appearance of the vocal cords as seen on laryngoscopy. Oedema of the larynx cannot involve the true cords since there is no submucous tissue in which fluid can collect. The space between the vocal cords is the *rima glottidis*. These folds demarcate the larynx into the following three zones:

1. The *supraglottic compartment* (*vestibule*) above the false cords
2. The *glottic compartment* between the false and true cords
3. The *subglottic compartment* between the true cords and the 1st ring of the trachea

On either side of the larynx the pharynx forms a recess, the *piriform fossa*, in which swallowed foreign bodies tend to lodge (Fig. 5.16(b)).

The muscles of the larynx function to open the glottis in inspiration, close the vestibule and glottis in deglutition and alter the tone of the true vocal cords in phonation.

The cricothyroid (Fig. 5.19) is the only external muscle of the larynx and tenses the vocal cord (the only muscle to do so) by a slight tilting action on the cricoid. It is supplied by the external laryngeal nerve, a branch of the superior laryngeal nerve.

The remaining muscles constitute a single encircling sheet whose various attachments are denoted by the names of its separate parts: the thyroarytenoid, posterior and lateral cricoarytenoid, the aryepiglottic, thyroepiglottic and interarytenoid muscles. These are all supplied by the recurrent laryngeal nerve.

All these muscles except one have a sphincter action; the exception is the posterior cricoarytenoid on each side which, by rotating the arytenoids outwards, separates the vocal cords.

Blood supply

The larynx receives a superior and inferior laryngeal artery from the superior and inferior thyroid artery, respectively. These vessels accompany the superior and recurrent laryngeal nerves.

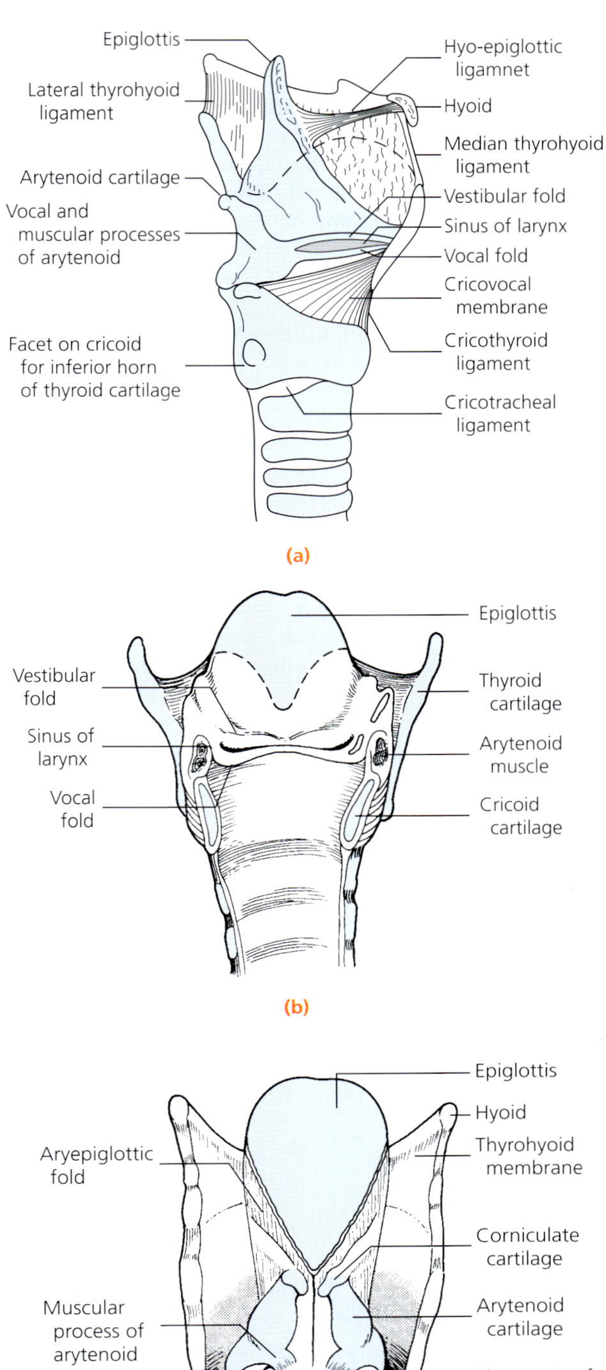

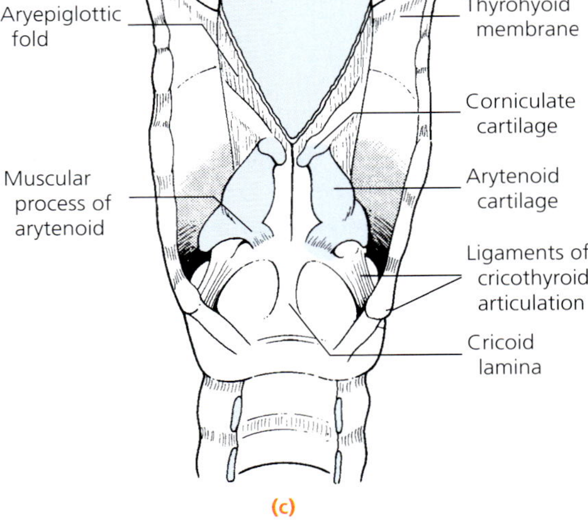

Figure 5.22 **(a)** The internal structure of the larynx – the lamina of the thyroid cartilage has been cut away. **(b)** The larynx dissected from behind, with cricoid cartilage divided, to show the true and false vocal cords with the sinus of the larynx between. **(c)** The cartilages and ligaments of the larynx seen from behind.

Lymph drainage

Above the vocal cords the larynx drains to the upper deep cervical and then to the mediastinal lymph nodes, some lymphatics passing via small nodes lying on the thyrohyoid membrane.

Below the cords, drainage is to the lower deep cervical nodes, partially via nodes on the front of the larynx and trachea.

The vocal cords themselves act as a complete barrier separating the two lymphatic areas, but posteriorly there is free communication between them; a laryngeal carcinoma may thus seed throughout the lymphatic drainage area of the larynx.

Nerve supply

The nerve supply of the larynx is of great practical importance and comprises the superior laryngeal nerve and the recurrent laryngeal nerve, both being branches of the vagus nerve (X).

The *superior laryngeal nerve* passes deep to the internal and external carotid arteries where it divides; its internal branch pierces the thyrohyoid membrane together with the superior laryngeal vessels to supply the mucosa of the larynx down to the vocal cords. The external branch passes deep to the superior thyroid artery to supply the cricothyroid muscle.

The *recurrent laryngeal nerve* has a different course on each side. The right arises from the vagus as this crosses the front of the subclavian artery, passes deep to and behind this vessel, then ascends behind the common carotid to lie in the tracheo-oesophageal groove accompanied by the inferior laryngeal vessels. The nerve then passes deep to the inferior constrictor muscle of the pharynx to enter the larynx behind the cricothyroid articulation.

The left nerve arises on the arch of the aorta, winds below it, deep to the ligamentum arteriosum, and ascends to the trachea. It then lies in the tracheo-oesophageal groove and is distributed as on the right side.

The recurrent nerves supply all the intrinsic laryngeal muscles, apart from the cricothyroid (supplied by the external branch of the superior laryngeal nerve) and the mucosa below the vocal cords.

Clinical Features

1 The laryngeal nerves bear relationships to the thyroid arteries, which are of considerable practical importance in thyroidectomy. The external branch of the superior laryngeal nerve lies immediately deep to the superior thyroid artery and may be injured in ligating this vessel.

The recurrent laryngeal nerve, lying in the tracheo-oesophageal groove, is usually behind the terminal branches of the inferior thyroid artery. Occasionally, however, the nerve lies in front of these vessels or passes between them (Fig. 5.6). Moreover, when a large thyroid is pulled forwards during thyroidectomy, the nerve is dragged forwards with it, and is therefore placed in further jeopardy. For all these reasons, meticulous care is necessary to avoid injury to the recurrent laryngeal nerve in thyroid surgery.

2 Damage to the superior nerve causes some weakness of phonation owing to the loss of the tightening effect of the cricothyroid muscle on the cord.

3 Complete division of a recurrent laryngeal nerve causes the cord on the affected side to take up the neutral (or paramedian) position between abduction and adduction. Usually the other cord is able to compensate in a remarkable way and speech is not greatly affected; if both nerves are divided, however, the voice is completely lost and breathing becomes difficult through the only partially opened glottis.

4 If the recurrent nerve is only bruised or partially damaged, the abductors (posterior cricoarytenoids) are affected more than the adductors; this is known as *Semon's law*. The affected cord adopts the midline adducted position. In bilateral incomplete paralysis, therefore, the cords come together, stridor is intense and tracheotomy may become essential.

5 The left recurrent laryngeal nerve, in its thoracic course, may become involved in a bronchial or oesophageal carcinoma, or in a mass of enlarged mediastinal nodes, or may become stretched over an aneurysm of the aortic arch. The enlarged left atrium in advanced mitral stenosis may produce a recurrent laryngeal palsy by pushing up the left pulmonary artery which compresses the nerve against the aortic arch.

Either nerve, in the neck, may be damaged by an extending thyroid carcinoma or malignant lymph nodes. For these reasons, loss of voice must always be regarded as an ominous symptom requiring careful investigation.

6 The larynx can be inspected either directly, by means of the rigid or fibre-optic laryngoscope, or indirectly through a laryngeal mirror. The base of the tongue, valleculae, epiglottis, aryepiglottic folds and piriform fossae are viewed; then the false cords, which are red and widely apart; then, between these, the pearly white true cords (Fig. 5.23).

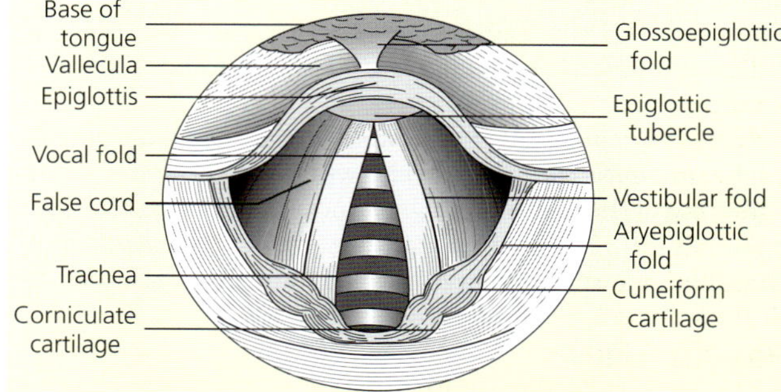

Figure 5.23 The larynx as seen at laryngoscopy.

For the passage of the rigid laryngoscope, endotracheal tube or bronchoscope it is essential to know the position which brings the axes of the mouth, oropharynx and laryngeal inlet into line; this is achieved by bringing the neck forwards and at the same time extending the head fully at the atlanto-occipital joint – it is the position in which one sniffs at the fresh air after a long day in the operating theatre.

Salivary glands

There are three pairs of large salivary gland, parotid, sabmandibular and sublingual.

Parotid gland

This is the largest of the salivary glands, lying wedged between the ramus of mandible and the mastoid process and overflowing both these bounding structures (Fig. 5.24).

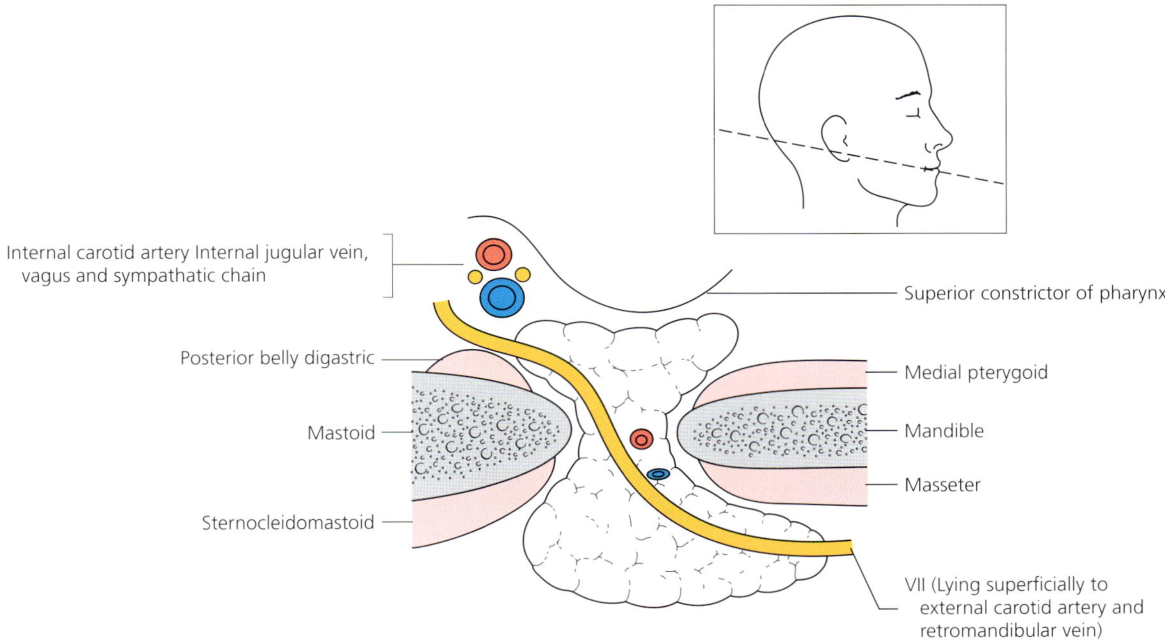

Figure 5.24 The parotid and its surrounds in a schematic horizontal section – the facial nerve is the most superficial of the structures traversing the gland. (The line of section is shown in the inset head.)

Relations

These are:

- **Above:** Lie the external auditory meatus and temporomandibular joint
- **Below:** It overlaps the posterior belly of digastric
- **Anteriorly:** It overlaps the mandibular ramus with the overlying masseter
- **Medially:** Lies the styloid process and its muscles separating the parotid from the internal jugular vein, internal carotid artery, last four cranial nerves and the lateral wall of the pharynx

Parotid fascia

The gland itself is enclosed in a split in the investing fascia, lying both on and within which are the parotid lymph nodes. Antero-inferiorly, this *parotid fascia* is thickened and is the only structure separating the parotid from the submandibular gland (the stylomandibular ligament).

Structures traversing the gland

The following structures are traversing the gland (from without in):

1. The facial nerve (*see* below)
2. The retromandibular (posterior facial) vein, formed by the junction of the superficial temporal and maxillary veins (*see* Fig. 5.33)
3. The external carotid artery, dividing at the level of the neck of the mandible into its superficial temporal and maxillary terminal branches

The *parotid duct* (*of Stensen*) is 2 in. (5 cm) long. It arises from the anterior part of the gland, runs over the masseter a finger's breadth below the zygomatic arch, dips inwards to pierce the buccinator and opens in the cheek mucosa opposite the 2nd upper molar tooth. Inspect this in the mirror in your own mouth. The duct can easily be felt by a finger rolled over the masseter if this muscle is tensed by clenching the teeth.

Relations of the facial nerve to the parotid

The facial nerve is unique in traversing the substance of a gland, a fact of considerable importance to the surgeon. This coexistence is explained embryologically; the parotid gland develops in the crotch formed by the two major branches of the facial nerve. As the gland enlarges it overlaps these nerve trunks, the superficial and deep parts fuse and the nerve comes to lie buried within the gland. The fanciful comparison between the nerve and the two parotid lobes and a sandwich-filling between two slices of bread is not valid because the two lobes of the parotid come to fuse intimately with each other both around and between the branches of the nerve.

The facial nerve emerges from the stylomastoid foramen, winds laterally to the styloid process and can then be exposed surgically in the inverted 'V' between the bony part of the external auditory meatus and the mastoid process. This has a useful surface marking, the intertragic notch of the ear, which is situated directly over the facial nerve.

Just beyond this point the nerve dives into the posterior aspect of the parotid gland and bifurcates almost immediately into its two main divisions temporofacial and cervicofacial (occasionally it divides before entering the gland). The upper temporofacial division divides into *temporal* and *zygomatic* branches; the lower cervicofacial division gives the *buccal, mandibular* and *cervical* branches (Fig. 5.25).

These two divisions may remain completely separate within the parotid, may form a plexus of intermingling connections, or, most usually, display a number of cross-communications which can be safely divided during dissection without jeopardy.

The branches of the nerve then emerge on the anterior aspect of the parotid to lie on the masseter, thence to pass to

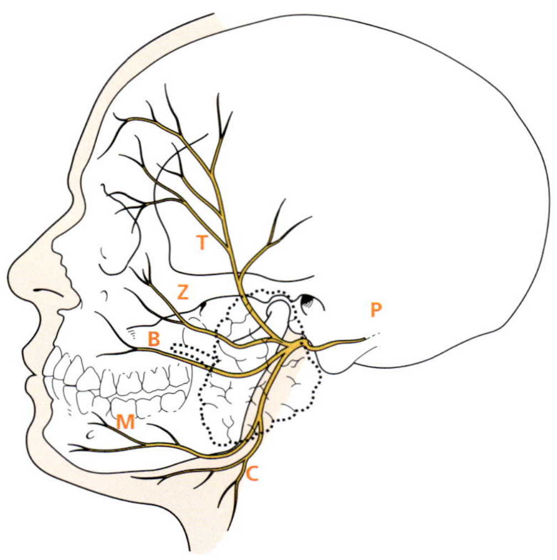

Figure 5.25 The named branches of the facial nerve which traverse the parotid gland. B, buccal; C, cervical; M, mandibular; P, posterior auricular; T, temporal; Z, zygomatic.

the muscles of the face. No branches emerge from the superficial aspect of the gland, which can therefore be completely exposed with impunity.

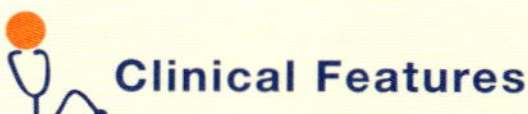

Clinical Features

1 A malignant tumour of the parotid gland, unlike benign lesions, may invade the facial nerve and produce a facial palsy.
2 In removing a benign mixed salivary tumour (pleomorphic adenoma) of the parotid, the facial nerve is exposed posteriorly in the wedge-shaped space between the bony canal of the external auditory meatus and the mastoid process. It is then traced into the gland, its main divisions defined and the tumour excised with a wide margin of normal gland, carefully preserving the exposed nerves.

   It is interesting that giant mixed tumours 'extrude' clear away from the facial nerve and can be excised with an adequate margin without even seeing the nerve.
3 The parotid duct and its ramifications can be demonstrated radiologically by injecting radio-opaque contrast through a cannula placed in the mouth of the duct (a parotid sialogram).

Submandibular gland

The submandibular gland is situated in the digastric/submandibular triangle. It is made up of a large superficial and a small deep lobe that connect with each other around the posterior border of the mylohyoid (Fig. 5.26).

The superficial lobe of the gland lies at the angle of the jaw, wedged between the mandible and the mylohyoid and overlapping the digastric muscle (Fig. 5.15). Posteriorly, it comes into contact with the parotid gland, separated only by a condensation of its fascial sheath (the stylomandibular ligament).

Superficially, the gland is covered by platysma and by its capsule of deep fascia, but it is crossed by the cervical and marginal mandibular branches of the facial nerve (VII) and by the facial vein. Its deep aspect lies against the mylohyoid for the most part, but posteriorly the gland rests against the hyoglossus muscle and here comes into contact with the lingual (V) and the hypoglossal (XII) nerves, both of which lie on hyoglossus as they pass forwards to the tongue.

The facial artery also comes into close relationship with the gland, approaching it posteriorly, then arching over its superior aspect (which it grooves), to attain the inferior border of the mandible and thence to ascend on to the face in front of the masseter.

From the medial aspect of the superficial part of the gland projects its deep prolongation along the hyoglossus deep to the mylohyoid.

The *submandibular duct* (*Wharton's duct*) arises from this deep part of the gland and runs forwards, beneath the mucosa of the floor of the mouth along the side of the tongue, to open on the sublingual papilla immediately at the side of the frenulum linguae (Fig. 5.12). Here, its orifice is readily visible and saliva can be seen trickling from it.

The sublingual gland (*see* below) lies immediately lateral to the submandibular duct.

The lingual nerve reaches the tongue by passing from the lateral side of the duct below and then medial to it – thus 'double-crossing' it.

The *submandibular lymph nodes* lie partly embedded within the gland and partly between it and the mandible.

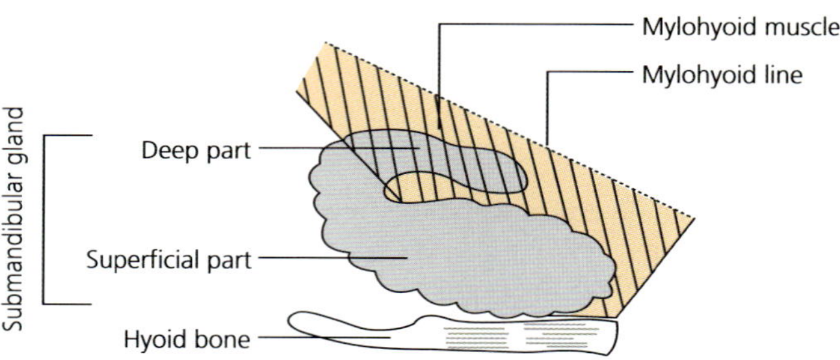

Figure 5.26 The continuity of superficial and deep parts of submandibular gland around the posterior margin of the mylohyoid muscle.

Clinical Features

1 The rather complex relations of this gland have been given at some length because excision of the gland for calculus or tumour is not uncommon. This operation is carried out through a skin crease incision below the angle of the jaw.

   The mandibular branch of VII (marginal mandibular nerve) passes behind the angle of the jaw rather less than 1 in. (2.5 cm) from it before arching upwards over the body of the mandible to supply the depressor of the lip. The incision must therefore be placed rather more than 1 in. (2.5 cm) below the angle of the jaw in order to preserve this nerve.
2 The presence of small lymph nodes actually within the substance of the gland makes removal of the gland an imperative part of block dissection of the neck.
3 In differentiating between an enlarged submandibular gland and a mass of submandibular lymph nodes, one remembers that the gland not only lies below the mandible but also extends into the floor of the mouth; it can therefore be palpated bimanually between a finger in the mouth and a finger below the angle of

(Continued ...)

(... *continued*)

the jaw. Try this on yourself. Enlarged lymph nodes are felt only at the latter site.

4 A stone in Wharton's duct can be felt bimanually in the floor of the mouth and can be seen if sufficiently large.

Sublingual gland

This is an almond-shaped salivary gland lying immediately below the mucosa of the floor of the mouth and immediately in front of the deep part of the submandibular gland. Laterally, it rests against the sublingual groove of the mandible while medially it is separated from the base of the tongue by the submandibular duct and its close companion, the lingual nerve (Fig. 5.12).

The gland opens by a series of ducts into the floor of the mouth and also in the submandibular duct.

The sublingual gland produces a mucous secretion; the parotid a serous secretion; and the submandibular gland a mixture of the two.

As well as these main salivary glands, small accessory glands are found scattered over the palate, lips, cheek, tonsil and tongue. These glands are occasional sites for development of a mixed salivary tumour.

Major arteries of the head and neck

The major arteries of the head and neck region are common carotid, external carotid, internal carotid and subclavian.

Common carotid arteries

The *left common carotid artery* arises from the aortic arch in front and to the right of the origin of the left subclavian artery. It passes behind the left sternoclavicular joint, lying in its thoracic course at first in front and then to the left side of the trachea, with the left lung and pleura, the vagus and the phrenic nerve as its lateral relations.

The *right common carotid artery* begins behind the right sternoclavicular joint at the bifurcation of the brachiocephalic artery.

In the neck, both common carotids have essentially similar courses and relationships; they ascend in the carotid fascial sheath, which contains also the internal jugular vein laterally and the vagus nerve between and rather behind the artery and vein. The cervical sympathetic chain ascends immediately posterior to the carotid sheath. These structures form a quartet which should always be considered in this inseparable manner; the relations of any one are those of the other three (Figs 5.3 and 5.27).

In the neck, each common carotid artery lies on the cervical transverse processes, separated from them by the prevertebral muscles. Medially are the larynx and trachea, with the recurrent laryngeal nerve, pharynx and oesophagus, together with the thyroid gland, which overlaps on to the anterior aspect of the carotid. Superficially, the artery is covered by the sternocleidomastoid and, in its lower part, by the strap muscles and is crossed by the intermediate tendon of omohyoid.

The common carotid artery usually gives off no side branches but terminates at the level of the upper border of the thyroid cartilage (at the vertebral level C4) into the external and internal carotids, which are more or less equal in size.

External carotid artery

This artery lies first deep to the anterior border of the sternocleidomastoid and then quite superficially in the anterior triangle of the neck, where its pulsations are usually visible as well as palpable. At first it is slightly deep to the internal carotid, then passes anterior and lateral to it. The internal jugular vein is first lateral to the external carotid then posterior

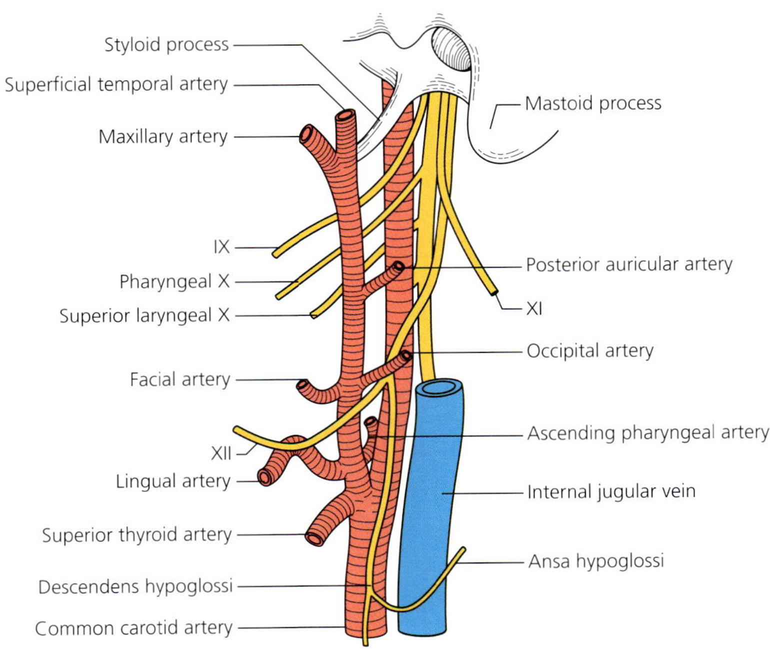

Figure 5.27 The carotid arteries, their branches and their related nerves.

to it, coming into lateral relationship to the internal carotid. The pharynx lies medially.

The external carotid artery ascends beneath the XII nerve and the posterior belly of the digastric to enter the parotid gland, within which it lies deep to the facial nerve and the retromandibular vein (Figs 5.13, 5.24 and 5.27).

The artery ends within the parotid gland at the level of the neck of the mandible by dividing into the superficial temporal and internal maxillary arteries.

Branches (Fig. 5.27)

1. The *superior thyroid artery,* giving off the superior laryngeal artery.
2. The *lingual artery*, passing deep to the hyoglossus to supply the tongue.
3. The *facial artery*, which gives off its important branch to the palatine tonsil, loops over the submandibular gland, hooks round the mandible (against which it can be felt pulsating) and ascends on to the face.
4. The *occipital artery*, running along the inferior border of the digastric muscle's posterior belly, grooving the inferior aspect of the temporal bone, to the back of the scalp, where its pulse is often palpable.
5. The *posterior auricular artery*, which supplies the skin of the back of the ear and behind the ear.
6. The *ascending pharyngeal artery*, the smallest branch, ascends between the internal carotid and the pharynx, which it helps supply.
7. The *superficial temporal artery* is the smaller terminal branch, which is given off with substance of the parotid gland. It is palpable on the zygomatic process.
8. The *maxillary artery is* the longer terminal branch, which supplies the upper and lower jaws, nasal cavity and the muscles of mastication, accompanying the various branches of the maxillary division of the trigeminal nerve, and also gives off the middle meningeal artery. This small vessel ascends through the foramen spinosum to enter the cranial cavity, where it helps to supply the meninges. Its importance in surgical practice lies in the fact that it may be torn in a skull fracture, resulting in the formation of an extradural haematoma.

Internal carotid artery

This artery commences at the bifurcation of the common carotid and ascends in the carotid sheath to reach the base of the skull. At its origin, it is dilated into the *carotid sinus*. This area receives a rich nerve supply from the glossopharyngeal nerve (IX) and acts as a baroreceptor; through this mechanism a rise of blood pressure brings about reflex slowing of the heart and peripheral vasodilatation. Tucked deep to the bifurcation is the small, yellowish *carotid body*, which is also supplied by IX. This is a chemoreceptor that produces a reflex increase in respiration in response to any rise in carbon dioxide tension or fall in the oxygen tension of the blood.

The internal carotid lies first lateral to the external carotid but rapidly passes medial and posterior to it, to ascend along the side-wall of the pharynx. It does so with the internal jugular vein, vagus and cervical sympathetic chain in the same relationship to it that they bear to the common carotid artery. At first the artery is covered superficially only by the sternocleidomastoid, the hypoglossal nerve (XII) and the common facial vein; it then passes under the posterior belly of the digastric muscle and parotid gland to the base of the skull. It is separated from the external carotid artery not only by the parotid but also by the styloid process and the muscles arising from it, by IX and by the pharyngeal branches of the vagus nerve (X) (Figs 5.24 and 5.27).

At the base of the skull, the internal carotid artery enters the carotid canal in the petrous temporal bone. Only at the skull base does the internal jugular vein lose its close lateral relation to the internal carotid, passing posterior to the artery into the jugular foramen. At this point the two vessels are separated by the emerging last four cranial nerves.

The artery gives off no branches in the neck.

The internal carotid, on entering the skull, commences an extraordinary twisted course. It passes forwards through the temporal bone, upwards into the cavernous sinus, forwards in this, upwards through the roof of the sinus to lie medial to the anterior clinoid process, turns back on itself above the cavernous sinus, then passes up once more, lateral to the optic chiasma, to end by dividing into the *anterior* and *middle cerebral arteries*. There are thus six bends in the intracranial course of this artery (readily appreciated by studying a lateral carotid arteriogram) which are believed to lessen the pulsating force of the arterial systolic blood pressure on the delicate cerebral tissues.

The *ophthalmic artery* originates from the internal carotid immediately after its emergence from the cavernous sinus, enters the orbit through the optic foramen below and lateral to the optic nerve and supplies the orbital contents and the skin above the eyebrow (via the supratrochlear and supraorbital branches). Its most important branch, however, is the *central artery of the retina*, which is the sole blood supply to this structure.

The two terminal branches of the internal carotid are distributed as follows (Fig. 5.28).

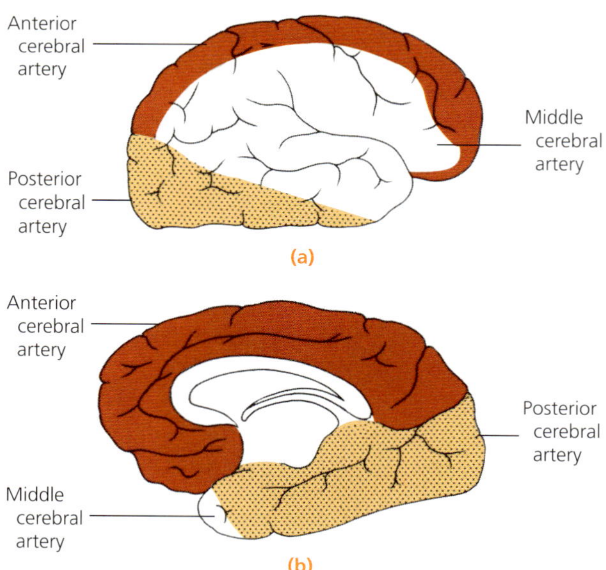

Figure 5.28 The arterial supply of the cerebral cortex. **(a)** Lateral aspect. **(b)** Medial aspect.

The *anterior cerebral artery* winds round the genu of the corpus callosum to supply the medial and superolateral aspect of the cerebral hemisphere.

The *middle cerebral artery* enters the lateral cerebral sulcus, gives off central branches to supply the internal capsule ('the *artery of cerebral haemorrhage*') and feeds most of the lateral aspect of the cerebral cortex.

The *arterial circle of Willis* (Fig. 5.29) is completed in front by the *anterior communicating artery*, which links the two anterior cerebral arteries, and behind by a *posterior communicating artery* on each side, passing backwards from the internal carotid to anastomose with the posterior cerebral, a branch of the *basilar artery*, the latter being formed by the junction of the two *vertebral arteries*.

Clinical Features

The common carotid artery can be exposed through a transverse incision over the origin of the sternocleidomastoid immediately above the sternoclavicular joint. The carotid sheath lies immediately deep to the junction between the sternal and clavicular heads of the sternocleidomastoid and is revealed either by retracting this muscle laterally or by splitting between its heads. Opening the sheath then reveals the artery lying medial to the internal jugular vein.

Ligation of the common carotid artery may be performed for intracranial aneurysm arising on the internal carotid. This operation is effective because it lowers the blood flow through the aneurysm, allowing thrombosis to occur. Adequate blood supply to the brain on the affected side is provided by free communication between the branches of the external carotid arteries on each side. Within the cranium, cross-circulation occurs through the circle of Willis.

The internal and external carotids, as well as the terminal part of the common carotid artery, can be exposed through an incision along the anterior border of the sternocleidomastoid passing downwards from the angle of the jaw. The sternocleidomastoid is retracted, the common facial vein divided, but the hypoglossal nerve, crossing the external and internal carotids just below the posterior belly of the digastric, is carefully preserved.

It may be surprisingly difficult to differentiate between the external and internal carotids at operation; the former is the anterior and rather deeper placed vessel at origin and, moreover, is the only carotid in the neck which gives off branches.

Subclavian arteries (Fig. 5.30)

The *left subclavian artery* arises from the arch of the aorta, immediately behind the commencement of the left common carotid artery. It ascends against the mediastinal surface of the left lung and pleura laterally and the trachea and oesophagus medially to lie behind the sternoclavicular joint.

The *right subclavian artery* is formed behind the right sternoclavicular joint by the bifurcation of the brachiocephalic artery; beyond this point, the course of the two arteries is much the same.

The cervical course of the subclavian arteries is conveniently divided by the scalenus anterior muscle into three parts.

The first part arches over the dome of the pleura and lies deeply placed beneath the sternocleidomastoid and the strap muscles. It is crossed at its origin by the carotid sheath and, more laterally, by the phrenic and vagus nerves. At this site, on the right side, the vagus gives off its recurrent laryngeal branch, which hooks behind the artery.

On the left side, the thoracic duct crosses the first part of the artery to open into the commencement of the left branchiocephalic vein.

The second part of the artery lies behind scalenus anterior, which separates it from the subclavian vein. Behind lie scalenus medius and also the middle and upper trunks of the brachial plexus.

The *third* part extends to the lateral border of the 1st rib, against which it can be compressed and its pulse easily felt since here it is just below the deep fascia. Immediately behind the artery is the lower trunk of the brachial plexus, which is, in fact, responsible for the 'subclavian groove' on the 1st rib.

Its branches are as follows:

- **1st Part:**
  1. The vertebral artery
  2. The thyrocervical trunk:
     a. Inferior thyroid artery
     b. Transverse cervical artery
     c. Suprascapular artery
  3. The internal thoracic artery (internal mammary artery)
- **2nd Part:** The costocervical trunk (supplying deep structures of the neck via its deep cervical branch, and the superior intercostal artery, which gives off the 1st and 2nd

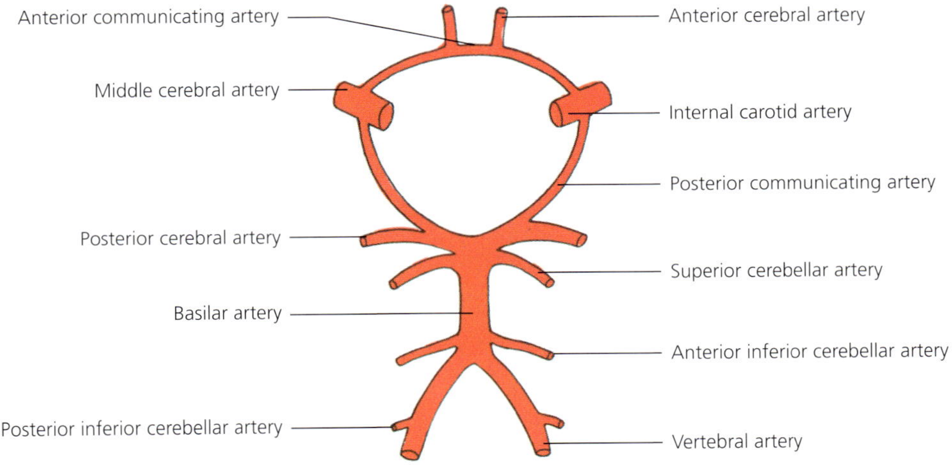

Figure 5.29 The circle of Willis.

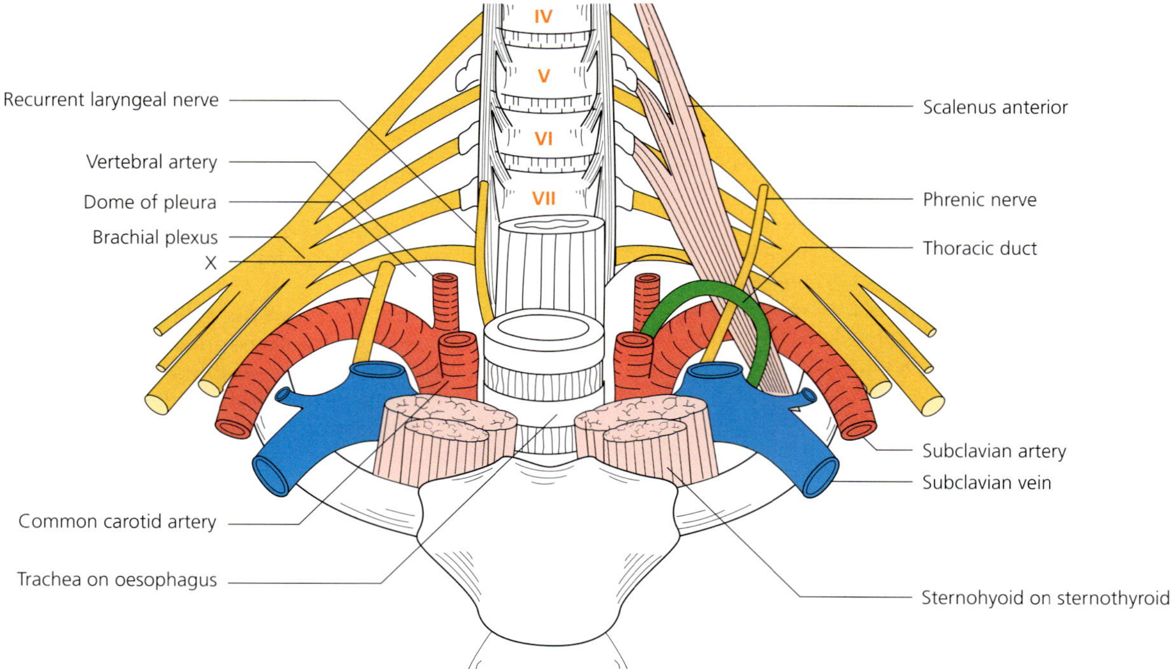

Figure 5.30 The root of the neck. For clarity, only the vagus nerve is shown on the right and only the phrenic nerve on the left, as this lies on scalenus anterior.

posterior intercostal arteries). On the left side costocervical trunk often arises from the 1st part of the subclavian artery.

- **3rd Part:** Gives no constant branch but in some cases it gives origin to the dorsal scapular artery which takes the place of a deep branch of the transverse cervical artery

Vertebral artery

This is the most important of the branches of the subclavian artery. It crosses the dome of the pleura, traverses the transverse foramina of the upper six cervical vertebrae, then turns posteriorly and medially over the posterior arch of the atlas to enter the cranial cavity at the foramen magnum by piercing the dura mater. It then runs on the anterolateral aspect of the medulla to join its fellow in front of the pons to form the *basilar artery* (Fig. 5.29).

The following are the important branches of the vertebral artery:

1. Anterior and posterior spinal arteries
2. Posterior inferior cerebellar artery

   From the basilar
3. Anterior inferior cerebellar artery
4. Superior cerebellar artery
5. Posterior cerebral artery (supplying the occipital lobe and medial aspect of the temporal lobe; Fig. 5.28)

In addition, in the neck, the vertebral artery gives off spinal branches to the cervical spinal cord and vertebrae and muscular branches. Within the foramina transversaria it is accompanied by vertebral veins and a sympathetic plexus which, together with the carotid plexus, provides sympathetic fibres to the cranial contents.

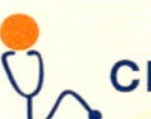

Clinical Features

1 The right subclavian artery is grafted end-to-side into the right pulmonary artery to short-circuit the pulmonary stenosis of the tetralogy of Fallot (Blalock's operation) (Fig. 1.39). It is important to note, therefore, that variations occur in the origins of the right subclavian artery, which may arise directly from the aortic arch either as its first or as its last branch. In the latter case, the right subclavian artery passes behind the trachea and oesophagus in the course to the neck; this vessel may then compress the oesophagus and produce difficulty in swallowing (*dysphagia lusoria*). Occasionally, the left subclavian artery has a common origin with the left carotid from the aortic arch.

2 An aneurysm of the subclavian artery is not rare; it never involves the thoracic part of the subclavian and its site of election is the third part of the artery. The close relation of the subclavian artery to the brachial plexus accounts for the pain, weakness and numbness in the arm which accompany this lesion. Oedema of the arm may result in compression of the subclavian vein.

3 A cervical rib may elevate the subclavian artery and render it unduly palpable; under these circumstances it may closely simulate an aneurysm and, in fact, there may be aneurysmal dilation of the artery distal to the edge of the cervical rib. Vascular changes in the arm associated with a cervical rib are probably due to peripheral emboli thrown off from thrombi forming on the walls of the compressed subclavian artery.

Veins of the head and neck

The veins of the head and neck comprise veins of the brain, venous sinuses of the dura, internal jugular vein, superficial veins and subclavian vein.

Veins of the brain

The pathways of the venous drainage of the brain are:

1. The superficial structures, e.g. the cerebral and cerebellar cortices, drain to the nearest available dural sinus (*see* the following section) by thin-walled veins
2. The deep structures drain through the *internal cerebral vein* on each side, which is formed at the interventricular foramen by the junction of the *choroid vein* (draining the choroid plexus of the lateral ventricle) with the *thalamostriate vein* (draining the basal ganglia)

The two internal cerebral veins unite to form the *great cerebral vein* (*the vein of Galen*), which emerges from under the splenium of the corpus callosum to join the inferior sagittal sinus in the formation of the straight sinus.

Venous sinuses of the dura (Fig. 5.31)

The venous sinuses lie between the layers of the dura. They receive the venous drainage of the brain and of the skull (the *diploic veins*) and disgorge ultimately into the internal jugular vein. They also communicate with the veins of the scalp, face and neck via *emissary veins* that pass through a number of the foramina in the skull.

The *superior sagittal sinus* lies along the attached edge of the falx cerebri and ends posteriorly (usually) in the right transverse sinus. Connecting with it are a number of venous lakes (*lacunae laterales*) into which project the *Pacchionian bodies* of arachnoid, filtering cerebrospinal fluid (CSF) back into the blood.

The *inferior sagittal sinus* lies in the free margin of the falx cerebri and opens into the straight sinus.

The *straight sinus* lies in the tentorium cerebelli along the attachment of the falx cerebri. It is formed by the junction of the great cerebral vein of Galen with the inferior sagittal sinus and runs backwards to open (usually) into the left transverse sinus.

The *transverse sinuses* commence at the internal occipital protuberance and run in the tentorium cerebelli on either side along its attached margin. On reaching the mastoid part of the temporal bone each passes downwards, forwards and medially as the *sigmoid sinus* to emerge through the jugular foramen as the *internal jugular vein*.

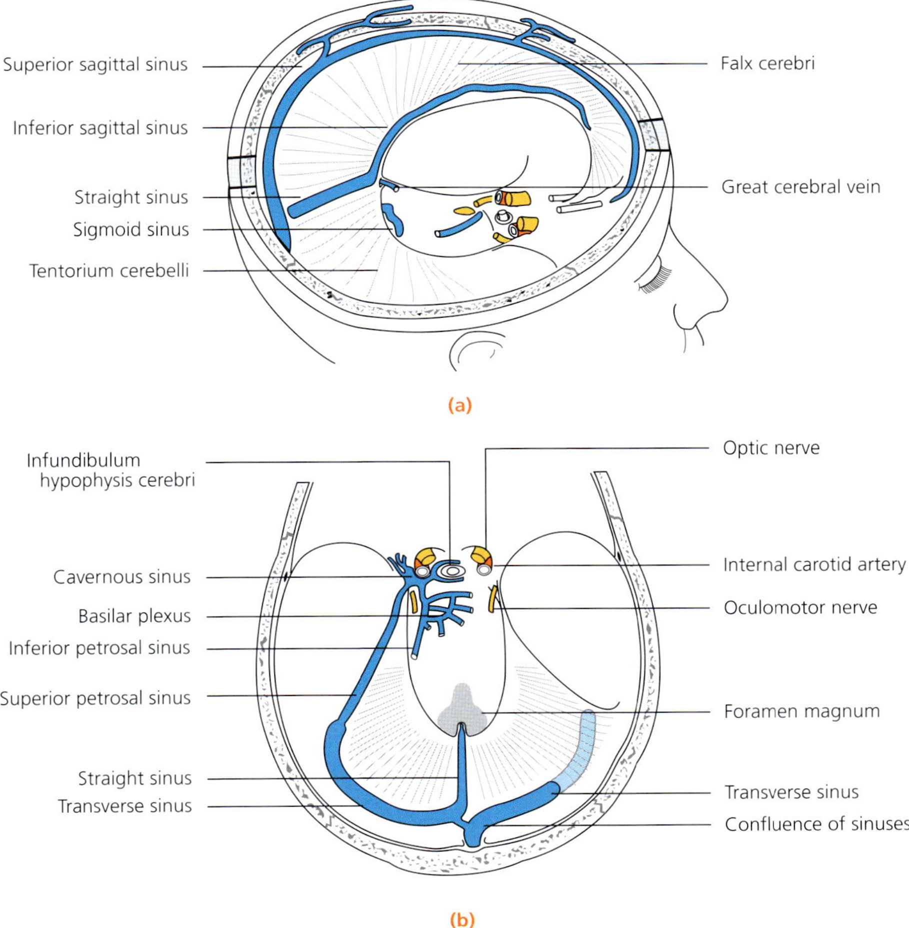

Figure 5.31 The venous dural sinuses. **(a)** Lateral view. **(b)** Superior view.

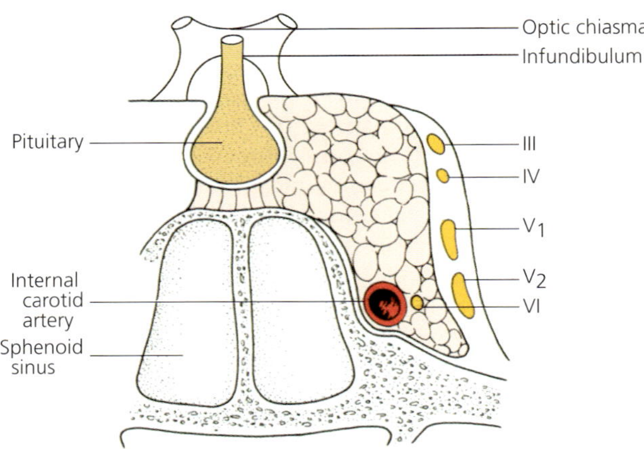

Figure 5.32 The cavernous sinus – shown in coronal section.

The *cavernous sinuses* (Fig. 5.32) lie one on either side of the body of the sphenoid against the fibrous wall of the pituitary fossa and rest inferiorly on the greater sphenoid wing. They communicate freely with each other via the *intercavernous sinuses*.

Traversing the cavernous sinus are the internal carotid artery and the cranial nerves III, IV, V (ophthalmic and maxillary divisions) and VI. The cranial nerves III, IV, V1 and V2 lies in the lateral wall of the cavernous sinus. Lying above the cavernous sinus are three important structures – the optic tract, the uncus of the temporal lobe of the cerebrum and the internal carotid artery, which first pierces the roof of the sinus then doubles back to lie against it.

The *ophthalmic veins* drain into the anterior aspect of the cavernous sinus, which also links up, through these veins, with the pterygoid venous plexus and the anterior facial vein. The cavernous sinus also receives venous drainage from the brain (the *superficial middle cerebral vein*) and from the dura (the *sphenoparietal sinus*).

Posteriorly, the *superior* and *inferior petrosal sinuses* drain the cavernous sinus into the sigmoid sinus and into the commencement of the internal jugular vein, respectively.

Clinical Features

1 The cavernous sinus is liable to sepsis and thrombosis as a result of spread of superficial infection from the lips and face via the anterior facial and ophthalmic veins, or from deep infections of the face via the pterygoid venous plexus around the pterygoid muscles, or from suppuration in the orbit or accessory nasal sinuses along the ophthalmic vein and its tributaries. A characteristic picture results – blockage of the venous drainage of the orbit causes oedema of the conjunctiva and eyelids and marked exophthalmos, which demonstrates transmitted pulsations from the internal carotid artery. Pressure on the contained cranial nerves results in ophthalmoplegia. Examination of the fundus shows papilloedema, venous engorgement and retinal haemorrhages, all resulting from the acutely obstructed venous drainage.

2 Fractures of the skull or penetrating injuries of the skull base may rupture the internal carotid artery within the cavernous sinus. A

(Continued ...)

(... continued)

caroticocavernous arteriovenous fistula results with pulsating exophthalmos, a loud bruit easily heard over the eye and, again, ophthalmoplegia and marked orbital and conjunctival oedema due to the venous pressure within the sinus being raised to arterial level.

3 The sigmoid and transverse sinuses are often together termed *the lateral sinus* by clinicians. Close relationship to the mastoid and middle ear renders these sinuses liable to infective thrombosis secondary to otitis media.

Spread of infection or thrombosis from the lateral sinus to the sagittal sinus may cause impaired CSF drainage into the latter and therefore the development of a hydrocephalus – this syndrome of raised CSF pressure associated with sinus thrombosis following ear infection is termed *otitic hydrocephalus*.

It is also possible for sagittal sinus thrombosis to follow infections of the skull, nose, face or scalp because of its diploic and emissary vein connections; if there were no emissary veins, infections of the face and scalp would never have achieved their sinister reputation.

Internal jugular vein

The internal jugular vein runs from its origin at the jugular foramen (as the continuation of the sigmoid sinus) to its termination behind the sternal extremity of the clavicle, where it joins the subclavian vein to form the brachiocephalic vein.

It lies lateral first to the internal and then to the common carotid artery within the carotid sheath and its relations are therefore identical with these vessels (Fig. 5.27). The deep cervical chain of lymph nodes lies close against the vein and, if involved by malignant or inflammatory disease, may become densely adherent to the vein. Tearing of the jugular vein for this reason is far from rare in dissections of tuberculous cervical lymph nodes.

Its tributaries are as follows:

1. The pharyngeal venous plexus
2. The common facial vein
3. The lingual vein
4. The superior and middle thyroid veins

Superficial veins

The arrangement of the superficial veins of the head and neck are somewhat variable, but the usual plan is as follows (Fig. 5.33).

The *superficial temporal* and *maxillary veins* join to form the *retromandibular vein*. This branches while traversing the parotid gland. Its posterior division, together with the *posterior auricular vein*, forms the external jugular vein, whereas the anterior division joins the *facial vein* to form the *common facial vein* which opens into the internal jugular vein.

The *external jugular vein* crosses the sternocleidomastoid in the superficial fascia, traverses the roof of the posterior triangle then plunges through the deep fascia 1 in. (2.5 cm) above the clavicle to enter the subclavian vein. You can see it in your own neck in the mirror when you perform a Valsalva manoeuvre. At times it is double.

The *anterior jugular vein* runs down one on either side of the midline of the neck, crossing the thyroid isthmus. Just above

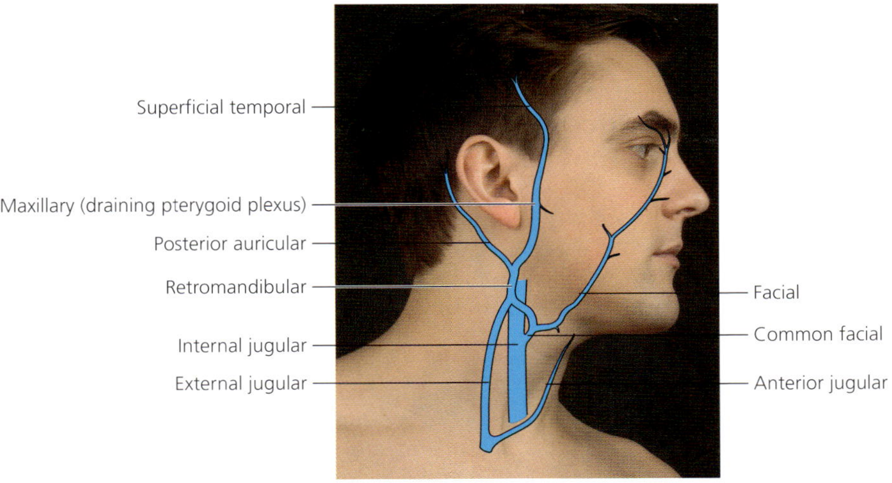

Figure 5.33 The usual arrangement of the veins in the neck.

the sternum it communicates with its fellow then passes outwards, deep to the sternocleidomastoid, to enter the external jugular vein.

Subclavian vein

This is the continuation of the axillary vein and extends from its commencement at the outer border of the 1st rib to the medial border of scalenus anterior, where it joins the internal jugular vein to form the brachiocephalic vein. During its short course it crosses, and lightly grooves, the superior surface of the 1st rib. It arches upwards and then passes medially, downwards and slightly forwards to its termination behind the sternoclavicular joint. On the left side it receives the termination of the thoracic duct. Its only tributary is the external jugular vein. Anteriorly the vein is related to the clavicle and subclavius muscle (Fig. 5.34).

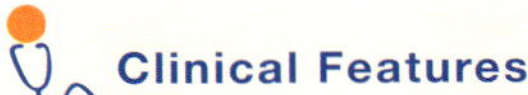

Clinical Features

Techniques of central venous catheterization are now of great clinical importance both to measure central venous pressure, for practical purposes the pressure within the right atrium, and to allow rapid blood replacement and long-term intravenous parenteral nutrition. The internal jugular vein can be cannulated by direct puncture in the triangular gap between the sternal and clavicular heads of the sternocleidomastoid immediately above the clavicle. Feel this landmark on yourself. The needle is inserted near the apex of this triangle at an angle of 30°–40° to the skin surface and is advanced caudally towards the inner border of the anterior end of the 1st rib behind the clavicle. A reflux of blood confirms venepuncture.

(Continued ...)

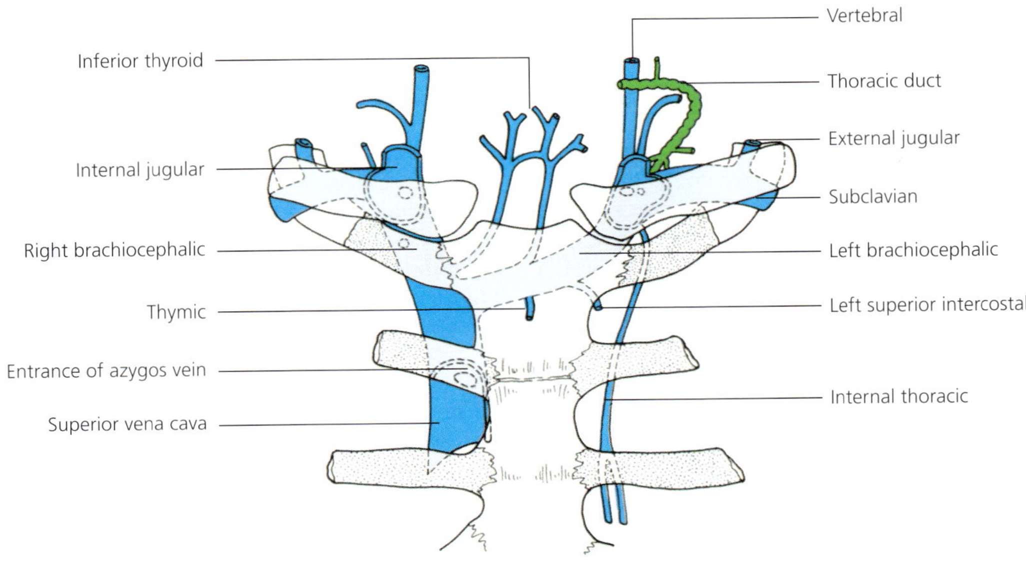

Figure 5.34 The great veins of the neck and their tributaries.

(... continued)

Subclavian venepuncture can be carried out most effectively by the infraclavicular approach (Fig. 5.35). The needle is inserted below the clavicle of the junction of its medial and middle thirds. The needle is advanced medially and upwards behind the clavicle in the direction of the sternoclavicular joint to puncture the subclavian vein at its junction with the internal jugular. When a free flow of blood is obtained by syringe aspiration, a radio-opaque plastic catheter is threaded through the needle to pass into the brachiocephalic vein.

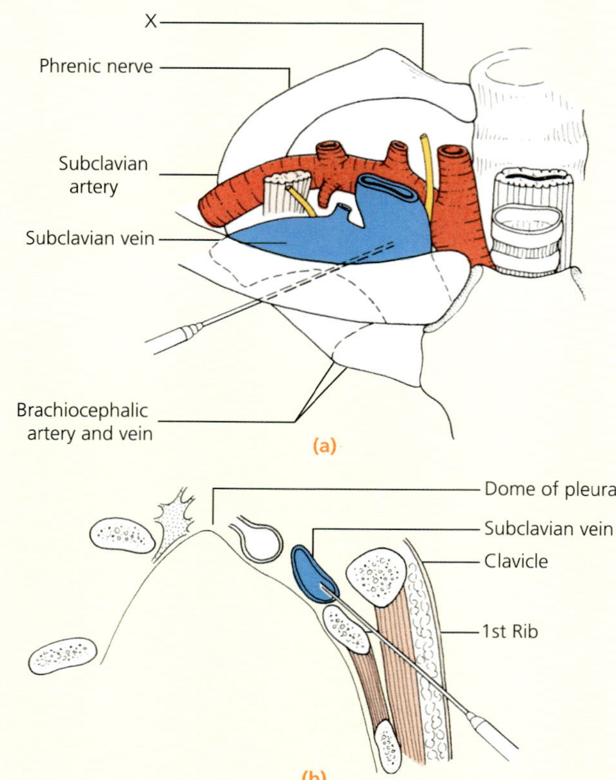

Figure 5.35 The anatomy of the infraclavicular approach to the subclavian vein. **(a)** Anterior view. **(b)** In sagittal section.

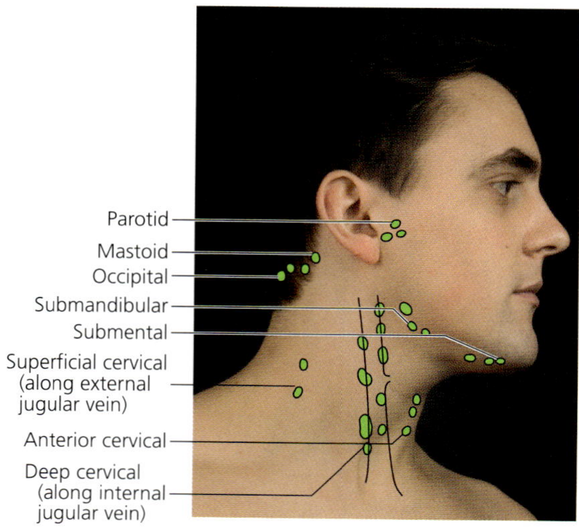

Figure 5.36 Scheme of the lymph nodes of the head and neck.

Lymph nodes of the neck

Although the lymph drainage of particular viscera is dealt with under appropriate headings (tongue, larynx, etc.), it is convenient to summarize here the arrangements of the lymph nodes of the head and neck as a whole (Fig. 5.36). There are about 800 lymph nodes in the body out of which about 300 are located in the neck only. These can be grouped into horizontally and vertically disposed aggregates.

The *horizontal nodes* form a number of groups which encircle the junction of the head with the neck and which are named, according to their position, the *submental, submandibular, superficial parotid* (or *preauricular*), *mastoid* and *suboccipital* nodes. These nodes drain the superficial tissues of the head and efferents then pass to the deep cervical nodes (although some lymph vessels pass direct to the cervical nodes, bypassing the horizontal nodes).

The *vertical nodes* drain the deep structures of the head and neck. The most important is the *deep cervical group*, which extends along the internal jugular vein from the base of the skull to the root of the neck (Fig. 5.13). The lymph then passes via the jugular trunk to the thoracic duct or the right lymphatic duct.

The *superficial cervical nodes* lie along the external jugular vein, serve the parotid and lower part of the ear and drain into the deep cervical group.

Along the front of the neck lies another group of vertically disposed nodes, the *infrahyoid* (on the thyrohyoid membrane), the *prelaryngeal* and the *pre-* and *paratracheal nodes*. These drain the thyroid, larynx, trachea and part of the pharynx and empty into the deep cervical group.

The *retropharyngeal nodes*, lying vertically behind the pharynx, drain the back of the nose, pharynx and Eustachian tube; their efferents pass to the upper deep cervical nodes.

Thus all structures in the head and neck drain through the deep cervical nodes either directly or indirectly.

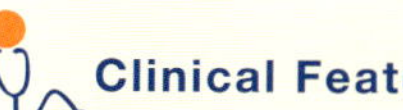

Clinical Features

1 A constant lymph node lies at the junction of the internal jugular and common facial veins – the **jugulodigastric** or **tonsillar node**. This becomes enlarged in tonsillitis and is, therefore, the commonest swelling to be encountered in the neck.

2 *Block dissection of the neck* for malignant disease is the removal of the lymph nodes of the anterior and posterior triangles of the neck and their associated lymph channels, together with those structures which must be excised in order to make this lymphatic ablation possible. It is sometimes combined with en bloc removal of the primary tumour.

The usual incision is Y-shaped, its centre being at the level of the upper border of the thyroid cartilage, its lower limb running downwards to the midpoint of the clavicle, its anterior limb extending to the symphysis menti and its posterior limb to the mastoid process. The block of tissue removed extends from the mandible above to the clavicle below and from the midline anteriorly to the anterior border of the trapezius behind. It consists of all the structures between the platysma and pretracheal fas-

(Continued ...)

(... continued)

cia enclosed by these boundaries, preserving only the carotid arteries, the vagus trunk, the cervical sympathetic chain and the lingual and hypoglossal nerves. The sternocleidomastoid, omohyoid and digastric muscles are removed in the dissection. Excision also includes the external and internal jugular veins, around each of which lymph nodes are intimately related, and the submandibular gland and the lower pole of the parotid gland, since these both contain potentially involved lymph nodes.

The accessory nerve, passing across the posterior triangle, is usually sacrificed.

3 Tuberculous disease of the neck usually involves the upper part of the deep cervical chain (from tonsillar infection). These infected nodes may adhere very firmly to the internal jugular vein, which may be wounded in the course of their excision.

Cervical sympathetic trunk

The sympathetic chain continues upwards from the thorax by crossing the neck of the 1st rib, then ascends embedded in the posterior wall of the carotid sheath to the base of the skull (Fig. 5.37). It bears the following three ganglia:

1. The *superior cervical ganglion* (the largest) lies opposite the C2 and C3 vertebrae and sends grey rami communicantes to the C1–C4 spinal nerves
2. The *middle ganglion* lies level with the C6 vertebra and sends grey rami to the C5 and C6 nerves
3. The *inferior ganglion* lies level with C7 and is tucked behind the vertebral artery. Frequently, it fuses with the 1st thoracic ganglion to form the *stellate ganglion* at the neck of the 1st rib. Grey rami pass from it to the C7 and C8 nerves

Note that these ganglia receive no white rami from the cervical nerves; their preganglionic fibres originate from the upper thoracic white rami and then ascend in the sympathetic chain.

As well as *somatic branches* transmitted with the cervical nerves, the cervical chain gives off *cardiac branches* from each of its ganglia and also *vascular plexuses* along the carotid, subclavian and vertebral vessels. The sympathetic fibres to the dilator pupillae muscle travel in this plexus along the internal carotid artery. Grey rami pass from the superior ganglion to cranial nerves VII, IX, X and XII.

Clinical Features

1 'Cervical sympathectomy' is a misnomer; it is an upper thoracic sympathectomy carried out through a cervical incision. The sympathetic chain is divided below the 3rd thoracic ganglion and the grey and white rami to the 2nd and 3rd ganglia are also cut. In this way the sudomotor and vasoconstrictor

(Continued ...)

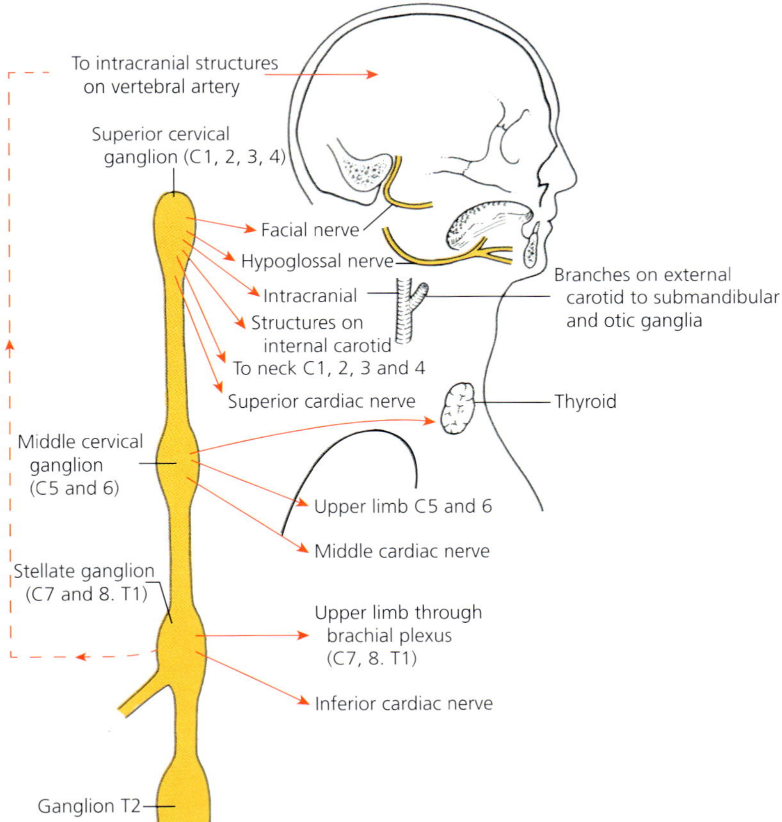

Figure 5.37 The cervical sympathetic chain.

(... continued)

pathways to the head and upper limb (from segments T2, T3 and T4) are divided, preserving the T1 connection and the stellate ganglion, which are the sympathetic connections to the eyelid and pupil. The upper thoracic chain can also be removed via a transthoracic transpleural approach through the 2nd intercostal space, or by fibre-optic endoscopy. The lung is allowed to collapse and the chain identified as it lies on the heads of the upper ribs. Resection of the T2–T4 segment results in a warm, dry hand.

2 *Horner's syndrome* results from interruption of the sympathetic fibres to the eyelids and pupil. The pupil is constricted (miosis, due to unopposed parasympathetic innervation via the oculomotor nerve), there is partial ptosis (paralysis of smooth muscle component of the levator palpebrae) and the face on the affected side is dry and flushed (sudomotor and vasoconstrictor denervation). Enophthalmos is said to occur, but this is not confirmed by exophthalmometry. The syndrome may follow spinal cord lesions at the T1 segment (tumour or syringomyelia), closed, penetrating or operative injuries to the stellate ganglion or the cervical sympathetic chain, or pressure on the chain or stellate ganglion produced by enlarged cervical lymph nodes, an upper mediastinal tumour, a carotid aneurysm or a malignant mass in the neck.

Branchial system and its derivatives

Six visceral arches form in the lateral wall of the pharyngeal wall of the foetal head between the stomodeum and the pericardial bulge. These arches are separated from each other, on the outside, by ectodermal branchial clefts and, on the inside, by five endodermal pharyngeal pouches (Fig. 5.9). In the human embryo the 5th and 6th arches do not appear externally and are represented only by a mesodermal core.

Each arch has its own nerve supply, cartilage, muscle and artery, although considerable absorption and migration of these derivatives occur in development. The 5th arch disappears entirely.

The embryological significance of many of the branchial derivatives has already been discussed under appropriate headings (the development of the face, tongue, thyroid, parathyroid and aortic arch) but Table 5.1 (*see* page 165) serves conveniently to bring these various facts together.

Branchial cyst and fistula

The 2nd branchial arch grows downwards to cover the remaining arches, leaving temporarily a space lined with squamous epithelium. This usually disappears but may persist and distend with cholesterol-containing fluid to form a *branchial cyst*. Another theory is that these cysts arise from squamous clefts in cervical lymph nodes.

If fusion fails to occur distally, a sinus persists at the anterior border of the origin of the sternocleidomastoid; this *branchial fistula* can be traced upwards between the internal and external carotids and may even open into the tonsillar fossa, demonstrating its association with the 2nd branchial arch.

Surface anatomy and surface markings of the head

Many of the important landmarks of the skull are readily felt (*see* Figs 5.39 and 5.40). Revise on your own skull the position of: the *external occipital protuberance* (the apex of this is termed the *inion*), the *nasion*, which is the depression between the two *supra-orbital margins*, and the *glabella*, which is the ridge above the nasion. Feel the sharp edge of the lateral margin of the orbit that is formed by the frontal process of the zygomatic bone; behind the zygomatic bone is the *zygomatic arch* with the *superficial temporal artery* crossing its posterior extremity and forming a convenient pulse which the anaesthetist can reach. Rather less easily felt is the *jugal point*, the junction between the zygomatic bone and the zygomatic process of the frontal bone; it is the mass of bone encountered by the finger running forwards along the upper border of the zygomatic arch, and it is a surface marking for the middle meningeal artery (*see* below). The anterior edge of the *mastoid* is easily palpable but its posterior aspect and its tip are rather obscured by the insertion of the sternocleidomastoid.

The whole of the superficial surface of the *mandible* is palpable apart from its coronoid process. The *condyloid process* can be felt by a finger placed immediately in front of, or within, the external auditory meatus while the mouth is opened and closed.

When the teeth are clenched, *masseter* and the *temporalis* can be felt contracting, respectively, over the ramus of the mandible and above the zygomatic arch. The *parotid duct* can be rolled over the tensed masseter and its orifice seen within the mouth at the level of the 2nd upper molar tooth.

The pulsation of the *facial artery* can be felt as it crosses the lower margin of the body of the mandible immediately in front of the masseter and again opposite the angle of the mouth. In the latter situation, if the cheek is gripped lightly with the finger placed within the mouth and the thumb placed on the skin surface, the pulse will be felt a little more than 0.5 in. (1.25 cm) from the angle of the mouth.

A line drawn vertically between the 1st and 2nd premolar teeth passes through the mental foramen, the infra-orbital foramen and the supra-orbital notch. Through these three orifices, lying in plumb-line, pass branches from each of the divisions of the trigeminal nerve; respectively, the mental branch of the inferior alveolar nerve (V‴), the infra-orbital nerve (V″) and the supra-orbital nerve (V′).

The *middle meningeal artery* can be represented by a line drawn upwards and somewhat forwards from a point along the zygomatic arch, two fingers' breadth behind the jugal point. The posterior branch of this artery passes backwards a thumb's breadth above, and roughly parallel to, the zygomatic arch.

The *central sulcus* of the cerebrum corresponds to a line drawn downwards and forwards from a point 0.5 in. (1.25 cm) behind the midpoint between the nasion and the inion.

Scalp

The scalp is the soft tissue covering the cranial vault. The soft tissues of the scalp are arranged in five layers (Fig. 5.38), which may be remembered by the following:

S: Skin
C: Connective tissue
A: Aponeurosis
L: Loose connective tissue
P: Periosteum

Each of these layers has features of practical importance.

The *skin* of the scalp is richly supplied with sebaceous glands and is the commonest site in the body for sebaceous cysts.

The *subcutaneous connective tissue* consists of lobules of fat bound in tough fibrous septa, very much like the connective tissue of the palm and the sole. This dense encapsulation of fat makes it unsurprising that lipomata are extremely rare at these three sites, and also that excess fat does not collect in any of these places even in the grossly obese.

The blood vessels of the scalp lie in this layer. When the head is lacerated, the divided vessels retract between the fibrous septa and cannot be picked up individually by artery forceps in the usual way. Haemorrhage is arrested by pressing with the fingers firmly down onto the skull on either side of the wound (thus compressing the vessels), by placing a series of artery forceps on the divided aponeurotic layer so that their weight again compresses these vessels and, finally, by suturing the laceration firmly in two layers (aponeurotic and cutaneous).

The haemorrhage from a scalp laceration or operation is profuse; this area has, in fact, the richest cutaneous blood supply of the body. For this reason, extensive avulsions of the scalp are usually viable providing even a narrow pedicle remains attached to the surrounding tissues.

The veins of the scalp connect with the intracranial venous sinuses via numerous *emissary veins* that pierce the skull and that also link these two venous systems with the *diploic veins* between the tables of the skull vault. A superficial infection of the scalp may spread via this system, producing an osteitis of the skull, meningitis and venous sinus thrombosis.

The *aponeurotic layer* is the occipitofrontalis, which is fibrous over the dome of the skull but muscular in the occipital and frontal regions. This muscle arises from the superior nuchal line of the occipital bone, gains a fascial insertion into the zygomatic arch, and inserts anteriorly into the subcutaneous tissues of the eyebrows and nose.

The layer of *loose connective tissue* beneath the aponeurosis accounts for the mobility of the scalp on the underlying bone; it is in this plane that the surgeon mobilizes scalp flaps, that machinery which has caught onto the hair avulses the scalp and that the Red Indians of bygone days scalped their victims.

Blood or pus collecting in this loose tissue tracks freely under the scalp but cannot pass into either the occipital or subtemporal regions because of the attachments of occipitofrontalis. Fluid can, however, track forwards into the orbits and this accounts for the orbital haematoma that may form a few hours after a severe head injury or cranial operation.

The aponeurotic layer is under tension because of its muscular component and retracts on the underlying loose layer when divided; a gaping scalp wound must, therefore, have extended at least through the aponeurosis.

The *periosteum* adheres to the suture lines of the skull; collections of pus or blood beneath this layer, therefore, outline the affected bone. This is particularly well seen in birth injuries involving the skull (*cephalohaematoma*).

Skull (Figs 5.39–5.41)

The important regional anatomy of the skull is dealt with under the appropriate headings (ear, nose, accessory sinuses, etc.). Collected together in this section are some general facts of clinical relevance followed by a general description of the floor of the cranial cavity.

The bony vault of the skull is relatively elastic in consistency (particularly in infancy and adolescence); thus a blow may injure the underlying brain without fracturing bone. Where the cranium is protected by thick muscle (the lower part of the occipital bone and the squamous temporal), the skull is correspondingly thin; if held up to the light it can be seen to be translucent at these sites.

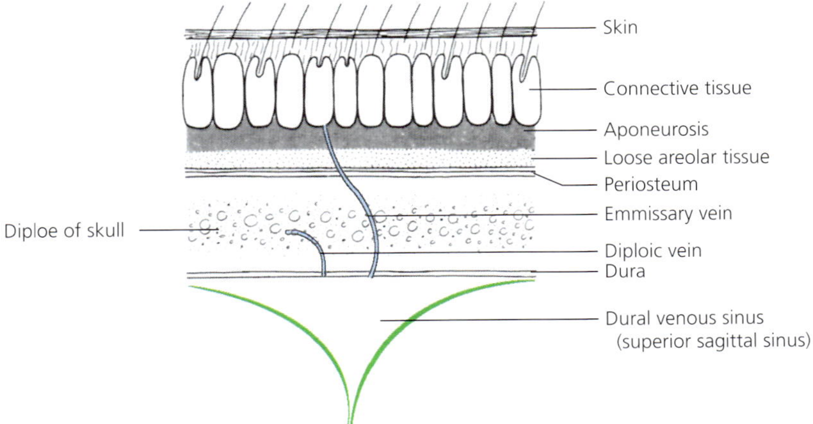

Figure 5.38 The layers of the scalp.

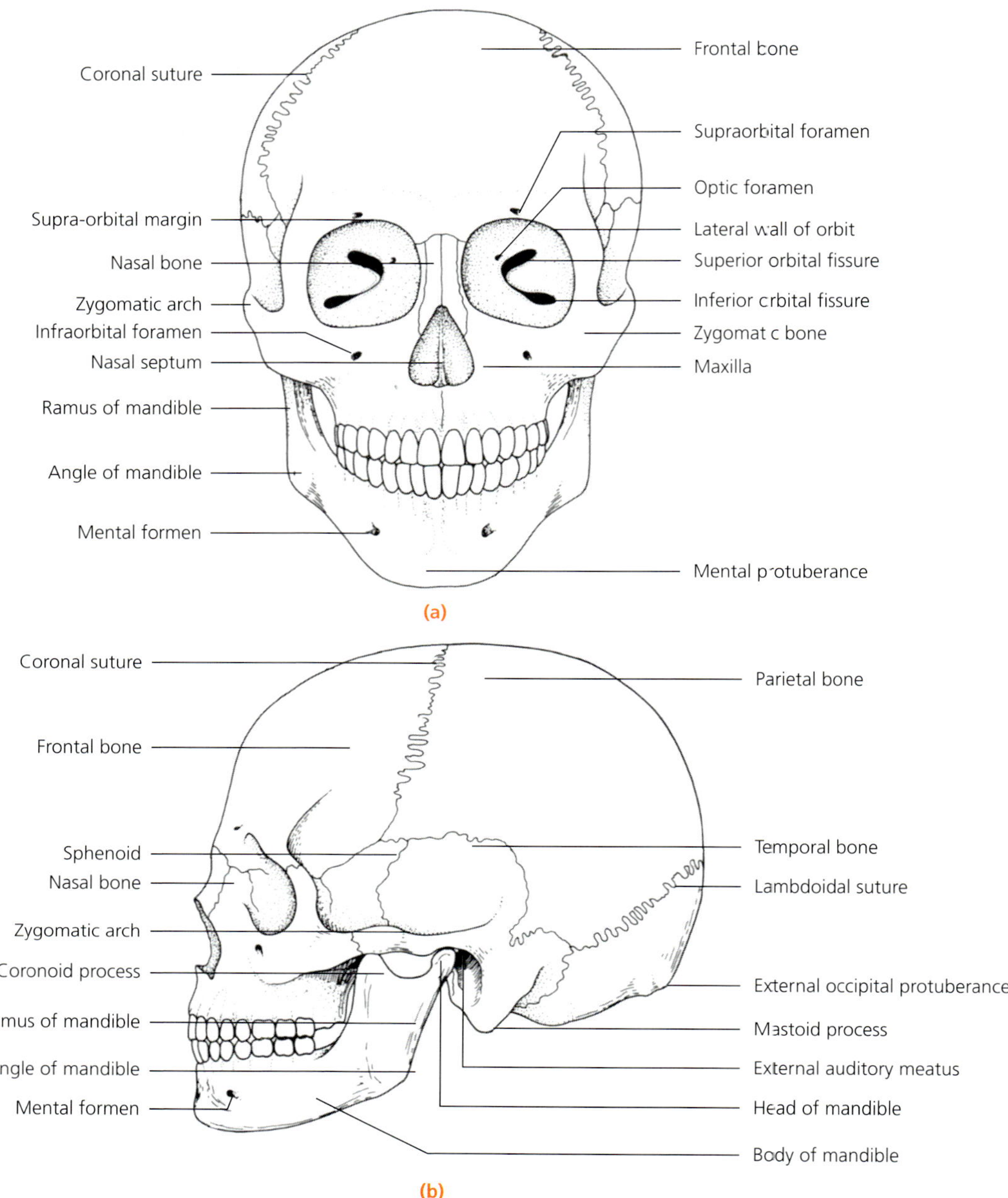

Figure 5.39 The skull. **(a)** Anterior aspect. **(b)** Lateral aspect.

The palpable landmarks of the skull are enumerated in the section on the surface anatomy of the head (*see* page 188). Radiologically, the *sutures* between the vault bones are important because they, as well as the vascular markings of the meningeal and diploic vessels, may be confused with fracture lines; however, unlike the usually straight lines of a fracture, suture lines are extremely tortuous. The *coronal* suture divides the frontal from the parietal bones, the *sagittal* suture separates the parietal bones in the midline, the *lambdoid* suture marks off the occipital from the parietal and temporal bones and the *squamosal suture* separates the squamous temporal bone from the parietal bone and greater wing of sphenoid.

In about 8% of cases the *metopic suture* persists in the midline between the two frontal bones; in the rest, this suture fuses at about the 5th year.

Occasionally, small separate areas of ossification develop between the parietal and occipital bones termed *Wormian bones*, which, again, may cause radiological confusion.

During development and infancy, the bones of cranium are separated by fibrous sutures. There are also six large membranous areas of the skull called *fontanelles* (**soft spots**). They permit the skull to undergo changes of shape (*moulding*) during child birth. The fontanelles are located one each at lambda, bregma, pterion and asterion.

The *lambda* is the point of junction of the lambdoid and sagittal sutures (the *posterior fontanelle* of infancy).

The *bregma* is the junction of the sagittal and coronal sutures (the infant's *anterior fontanelle*).

The *diploë*, between the inner and outer tables of the skull vault, is one of the sites of persistent red marrow in the adult

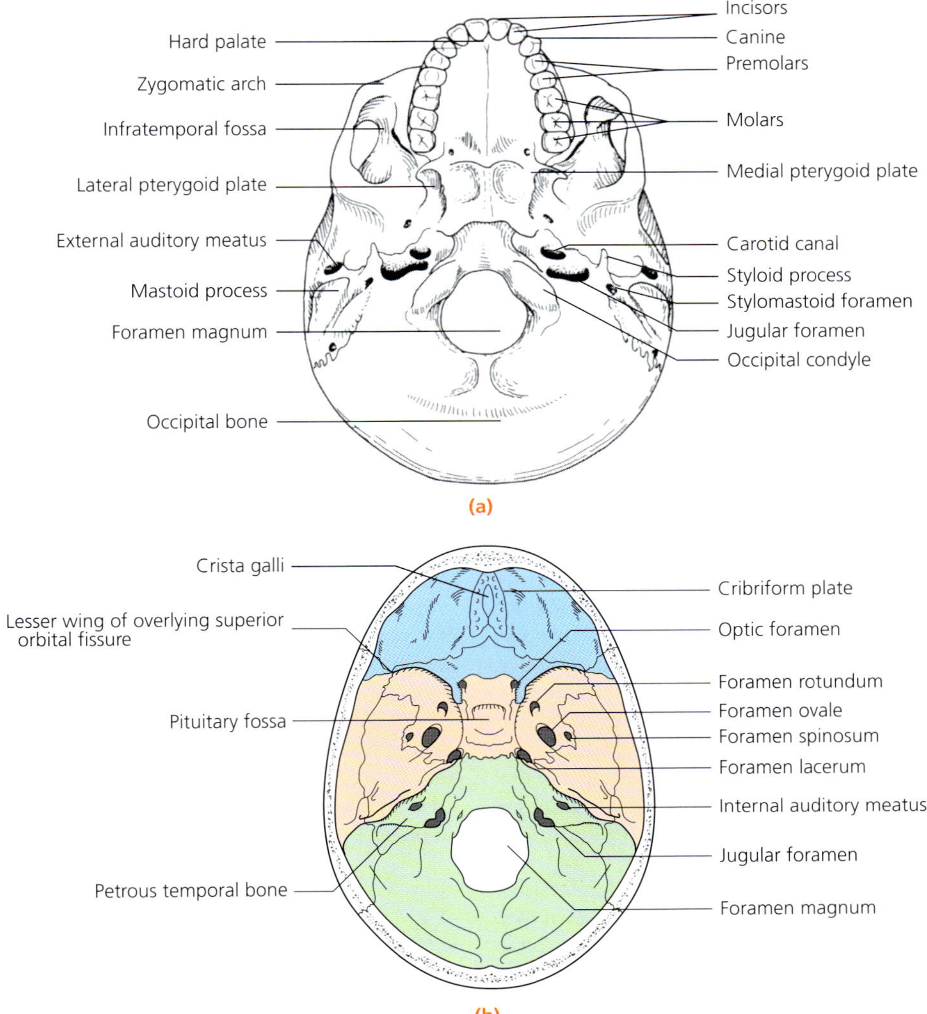

Figure 5.40 Thskull. **(a)** Inferior aspect. **(b)** Floor of the cranial cavity: the anterior, middle and posterior cranial fossae are colour coded.

skeleton. This distinction it shares with the pelvis, vertebrae, ribs, sternum, upper end of the humerus and upper end of the femur – a doubtful honour since to these sites are almost confined secondary deposits of carcinoma in bone and multiple myelomata.

Floor of the cranial cavity (Fig. 5.40(b))

The floor of the cranial cavity is the upper surface of the base of skull. In a dry skeleton it is revealed by removing the cranial vault. The cranial vault is made up of the following bones: right

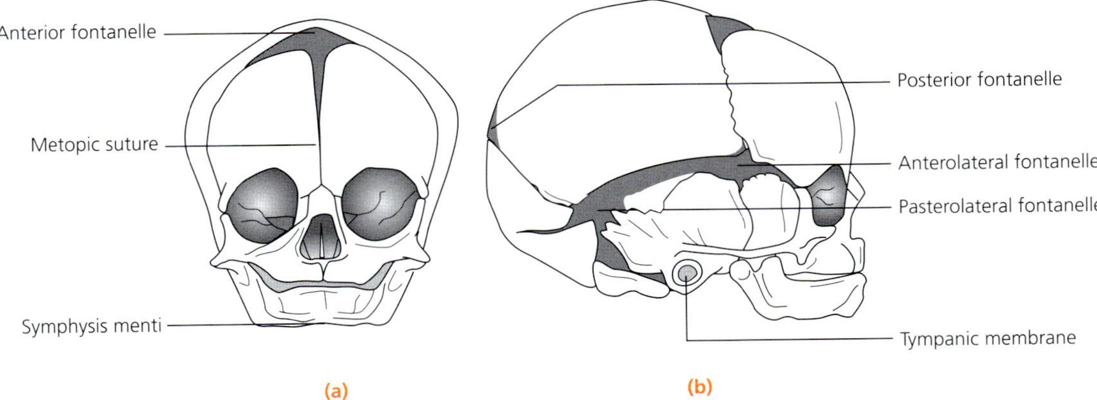

Figure 5.41 The foetal skull. **(a)** Anterior aspect. **(b)** Lateral aspect (*see* the sites of fontanelles).

and left frontal bones, right and left parietal bones, the squamous part of the right and left temporal bones and the squamous part of the occipital bone.

The floor of the cranial cavity presents a terraced arrangement of three regions (areas): anterior cranial fossa, middle cranial fossa and posterior cranial fossa. The anterior fossa is the shallowest and the smallest, whereas the posterior fossa is the deepest and largest of the three areas.

The central part of the floor of the anterior cranial fossa is a thin, somewhat depressed and perforated plate of bone, the cribriform plate of ethmoid. This forms the highest part of the roof of the nasal cavity, and is traversed on either side of the midline by the corresponding olfactory nerve filaments, and corresponding anterior ethmoidal artery. On either side of the cribriform plate, the floor of the anterior cranial fossa is raised and undulant, and constitutes the roof of the orbit of that side.

The anterior cranial fossa houses, in addition to the right and left olfactory pathways, the frontal lobes of the cerebral hemispheres and the anterior cerebral arteries as the latter course beneath the frontal lobes.

The middle cranial fossa floor shows a platform-like elevation in the centre. This is the body of the sphenoid bone; its upper surface being slightly concave and constituting the pituitary fossa. Situated above and projecting into the pituitary fossa is the pituitary gland suspended from the hypothalamus by the pituitary stalk. On either side of the central elevation, the floor is depressed and accommodates the corresponding temporal lobe of the cerebral hemisphere. Posterolateral to the pituitary fossa on either side lies the corresponding trigeminal ganglion, whereas lateral to the pituitary fossa on either side is the cavernous sinus (mentioned earlier).

Anteriorly, on either side of the midline, the middle cranial fossa communicates with the ipsilateral orbit by means of two openings: the larger and wider one being the superior orbital fissure and the smaller opening being the optic foramen (*see* Fig. 256). The latter transmits the optic nerve (ensheathed in the three meningeal layers) and ophthalmic artery, while the superior orbital fissure transmits the oculomotor (III), trochlear (IV) and abducent (VI) nerves, the ophthalmic nerve and the ophthalmic veins. On each side, the floor of the middle cranial fossa shows three significant foramina. From front to back these are the foramen rotundum, foramen ovale and foramen spinosum, which transmit, respectively, the maxillary nerve, mandibular nerve and the middle meningeal artery.

The posterior cranial fossa is the deepest and largest of the three fossae. It houses the entire cerebellum. Anterior to the cerebellum lies the brainstem comprising, from above downwards, the midbrain, pons and medulla oblongata. The medulla oblongata leaves the posterior cranial fossa through a large opening in the floor, the foramen magnum, to become the spinal cord. The 'slope' of bone which forms the anterior wall of the posterior cranial fossa, and lies in front of the brainstem, is called the *clivus*. The cerebellum is roofed by a large, thick, double-layered sheet of dura mater termed the *tentorium cerebelli*. Above the tentorium cerebelli (and therefore outside the posterior cranial fossa) lie the occipital lobes of the cerebral hemispheres.

Three significant openings, on each side, lead away from the posterior cranial fossa. These are the internal acoustic (auditory) meatus, the jugular foramen and the hypoglossal canal. The first of these transmits the VIIth (facial) and VIIIth (vestibulocochlear) cranial nerves. The jugular foramen transmits the IXth (glossopharyngeal), Xth (vagus) and XIth (accessory) cranial nerves, and also the sigmoid and inferior petrosal venous sinuses. The hypoglossal canal transmits the XIIth (hypoglossal) cranial nerve.

Development

The skull vault develops in membrane, the skull base in cartilage.

At birth (Fig. 5.41), the square anterior fontanelle and triangular posterior fontanelle are widely open. The posterior fuses at about 3 months, the anterior at about 18 months. Until then, blood can be obtained by puncturing the sagittal sinus immediately below the anterior fontanelle in the midline, and CSF aspirated by passing a needle obliquely into the lateral ventricle.

The face at birth is considerably smaller proportionally to the skull than in the adult; this is due to the teeth being nonerupted and rudimentary and the nasal accessory sinuses being undeveloped; the sinuses are evident at about 8 years but fully developed only in the late teens.

The mastoid and its air cells develop at the end of the 2nd year; until then the facial nerve is relatively superficial near its origin from the skull and may be damaged by quite trivial injuries.

With advancing age, the relative vertical measurement of the face again diminishes as a result of loss of teeth and subsequent absorption of the alveolar margins.

Development of the mandible and the teeth are considered on pages 196 and 197, respectively.

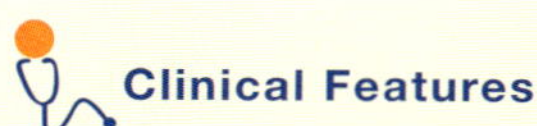

Clinical Features

Fractures of the skull

Imagine the skull as a rather elastic sphere completely filled by semifluid material; a violent blow on such a structure will produce a splitting effect commencing at the site of the blow and tending to travel along the lines of least resistance. The base of the skull is more fragile than the vault, and is thus commonly involved by such fractures. The petrous part of the temporal bone, however, forms a firm and rarely involved buttress of the skull base, the fracture line passing through less resistant areas, particularly the middle cranial fossa, the pituitary fossa and the various basal foramina.

A localized severe injury, in the adult, may produce a depressed comminuted fracture; the infant's skull is much more elastic and a similar injury here will result in a 'pond' depressed fracture, rather like the dimple produced by squeezing on a ping-pong ball.

Localizing signs in cranial fractures

Fractures of the anterior cranial fossa may involve the frontal, ethmoidal and sphenoidal sinuses and be accompanied by bleeding into the nose or mouth. In such cases CSF leakage from the nose implies coexisting tearing of the meninges; the subarachnoid space is thus put in communication with the exterior via the nasal cavity with consequent risk of meningitis.

Fractures involving the roof of the orbit are frequently associated with blood tracking forwards beneath the conjunctiva (subconjunctival haemorrhage); this must be differentiated from a small flame-shaped haemorrhage of the conjunctiva caused by direct injury to it.

A 'black eye' is not necessarily indicative of an anterior fossa fracture; it may be produced also by direct contusion of the soft tissues or by blood tracking down deep to the aponeurotic layer of the scalp (*see* 'Scalp', page 189).

Anterior basal fractures may involve the cribriform plate (with anosmia – loss of smell – due to rupture of fibres of the olfactory bulb) or the optic foramen (with primary optic atrophy and blindness).

Fractures of the middle fossa may produce bleeding into the mouth (sphenoid involvement), bleeding or CSF leakage from the ear, and facial and auditory nerve injury. Aural bleeding may, of course, be produced by direct injury to the ear – for example, rupture of the drum – without necessarily implying a skull fracture. Because of its long course, the abducent (VI) nerve may be damaged with diplopia and paralysis of the lateral rectus muscle.

Posterior fossa fractures are occasionally accompanied by cranial nerve involvement. These fractures are suggested clinically by bruising over the mastoid region extending downwards over the sternocleidomastoid.

Paranasal air sinuses

The paranasal sinuses are air-containing sacs in some bones surrounding the nasal cavity. They are lined by ciliated epithelium and communicating with the nasal cavity through narrow, and therefore easily occluded, openings (termed ostia) (Fig. 5.42). The maxillary sinus (maxillary antrum) and sphenoidal sinuses are present in a rudimentary state at birth; the rest become evident at about the 8th year. All become fully formed only in adolescence.

Frontal sinuses

The frontal sinuses are contained in the frontal bone. They vary greatly in size and one or both are occasionally absent. In section each is roughly triangular, its anterior wall forming the prominence of the forehead, its posterosuperior wall lying adjacent to the frontal lobe of the brain, and its floor abutting against the ethmoid cells, the roof of the nasal fossa and the orbit.

The frontal sinuses are separated from each other by a median bony septum, and each in turn is further broken up by a number of incomplete septa. Each sinus drains into the anterior part of the middle nasal meatus via the infundibulum into the hiatus semilunaris.

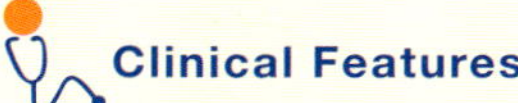

1 The close relation of the frontal sinus to the frontal lobe of the brain explains how infection of this sinus may result in the development of a frontal lobe abscess.
2 A fracture involving the sinus, severe enough to tear the dura and pia-arachnoid, will place the subarachnoid space in communication with the nasal cavity and CSF may then be detected trickling through the nostril, usually on the affected side (CSF rhinorrhoea), although, as these sinuses may communicate, a contralateral leak sometimes occurs.
3 The neurosurgeon must take into account the considerable variations in size and extent of the frontal sinus when proposing to turn down a frontal skull flap; obviously, he will want to avoid opening the sinus because of the risk of infection. He therefore consults the radiographs of the patient's skull preoperatively, which will clearly show the configuration of the sinuses.

Maxillary sinus (antrum of Highmore)

(Fig. 5.43)

This is the largest paranasal sinus. It is a pyramidal-shaped sinus occupying the cavity of the maxilla. It has anterior wall, roof, floor, medial wall and posterior wall. Its base (medial wall) is directed towards the lateral wall of the nasal cavity and apex is directed laterally towards the zygomatic bone. The medial wall of sinus forms part of the lateral wall of the nasal cavity and bears on it the inferior concha. Above this concha is the opening, or *ostium*, of the maxillary sinus into the middle meatus in the hiatus semilunaris (Fig. 5.42). This opening, unfortunately, is inefficiently placed as an adequate drainage point.

The infra-orbital nerve lies in a groove that bulges down into the roof of the sinus, while its floor bears the impressions of the upper premolar and molar roots. These roots are separated only by a thin layer of bone which may, in fact, be deficient so that uncovered dental roots project into the sinus. Note that

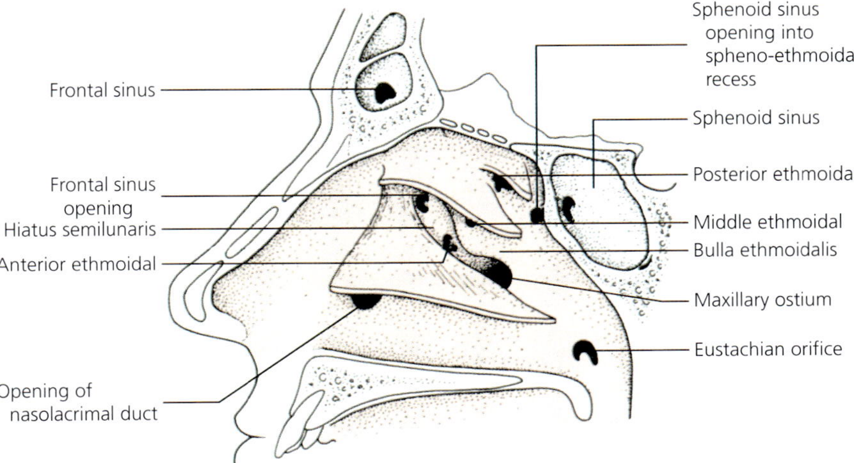

Figure 5.42 The lateral wall of the right nasal cavity; the conchae have been partially removed to show structures that drain into the nose.

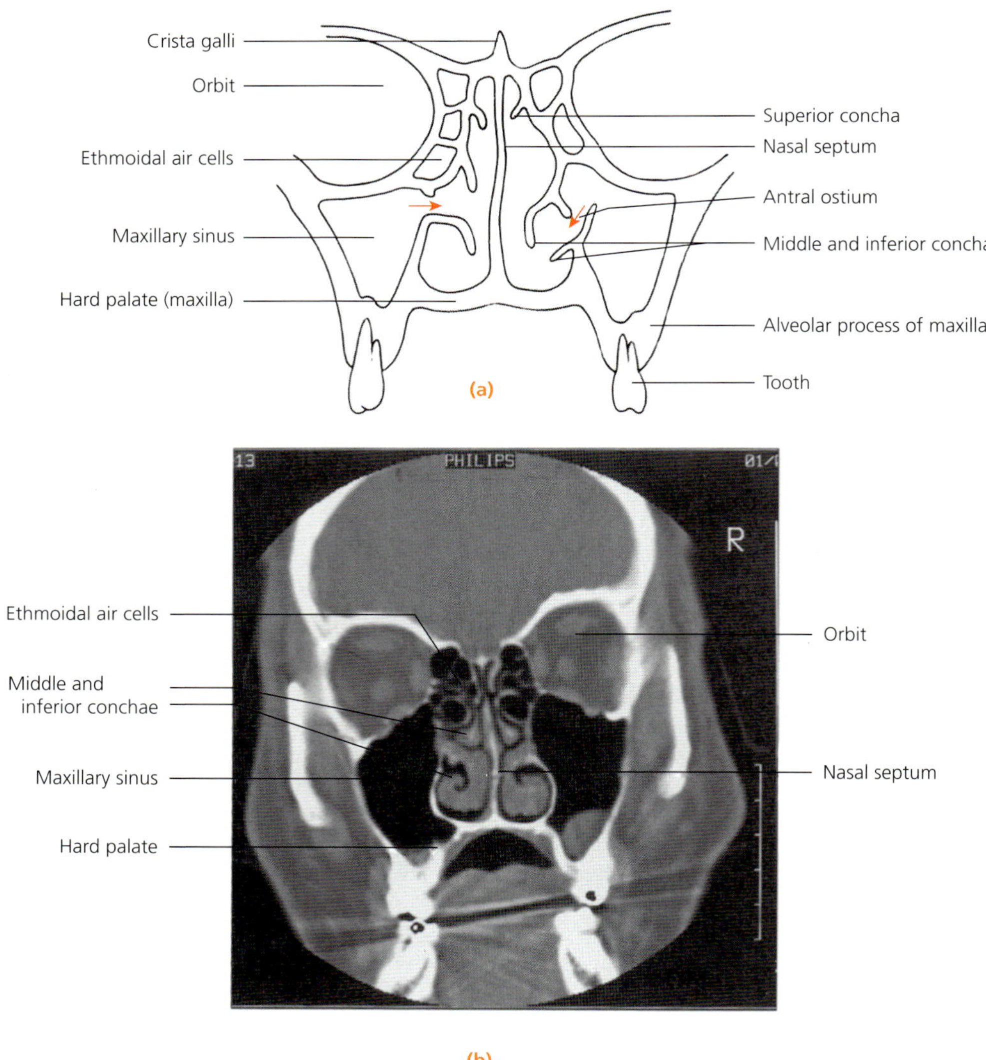

Figure 5.43 (a) The maxillary antrum in coronal section. (Note the inefficient drainage of this antrum and its close inferior relationship to the teeth.) **(b)** The corresponding computed tomography (CT) scan.

the floor of the sinus, therefore, corresponds to the level of the alveolus and not to the floor of the nasal cavity – it actually extends about 0.5 in. (1.25 cm) lower than the latter.

Clinical Features

1 The maxillary sinus, or antrum, may become infected either from the nasal cavity or from caries of the upper molar teeth.

Antral puncture can be carried out using a trocar and cannula passed through the nasal cavity in an outwards and backwards direction below the inferior concha.

More adequate drainage may require removing a portion of the medial wall of the sinus below the inferior concha or fenestrating the antrum in the gingivolabial fold (**Caldwell–Luc operation**). The old operation of draining the antrum via an extracted upper molar tooth is now seldom, if ever, performed.

(Continued ...)

(... continued)

2 The numerous symptoms and signs which may be produced by a carcinoma of the maxillary sinus are easily remembered anatomically.

- **a** Medial invasion encroaches on the nasal cavity, producing obstruction of the nares and epistaxis. Blockage of the nasolacrimal duct in this wall may cause epiphora (leakage of tears down the face).
- **b** Invasion of the orbit displaces the globe and causes diplopia. If the infra-orbital nerve becomes involved, there will be facial pain and then anaesthesia of the skin over the maxilla.
- **c** Invasion of the sinus floor may produce a visible bulge or even ulceration in the palatal roof.
- **d** Lateral spread may produce a swelling of the face or a palpable mass in the gingivolabial fold.
- **e** Posterior spread may involve the palatine nerves and produce severe pain referred to the teeth of the upper jaw.

Ethmoid sinuses

The ethmoid sinuses are made up of a group of 8–10 air cells within the lateral mass of the ethmoid and lie between the side-walls of the upper nasal cavity and the orbits (Fig. 5.43). Superiorly, they lie on each side of the cribriform plate and are related above to the frontal lobes of the brain. These cells drain into the superior and middle meatus (Fig. 5.42).

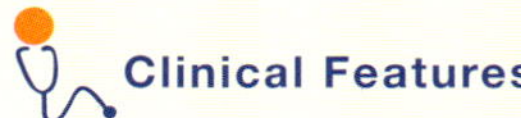

As with the frontal sinus, infection (ethmoiditis) may result in a frontal cerebral abscess and an ethmoidal fracture may cause a CSF leakage into the nasal cavity.

Sphenoidal sinuses

These lie one on either side of the midline, within the body of the sphenoid (Fig. 5.42). They vary a good deal in size and may extend laterally into the greater wing of the sphenoid or backwards into the basal part of the occipital bone.

Each sinus drains into the nasal cavity above the superior concha in the sphenoethmoidal recess.

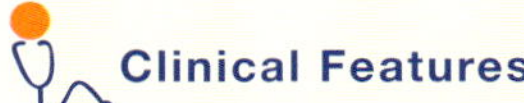

In patients with a pituitary tumour the pituitary gland may be approached endoscopically via a transnasal, trans-sphenoidal route and the tumour excised.

Mandible (Fig. 5.44)

The lower jaw comprises a horizontal *body* on each side which fuses at the *symphysis menti* (fusion occurring at the 2nd year). From the posterior part of the body projects the vertical *ramus* which, at its upper end, bears an anterior *coronoid* and a posterior *condylar* process; the latter being made up of the *head* and *neck*. Between the coronoid and condylar processes is the *mandibular notch*.

On the medial aspect of the ramus is the *mandibular foramen* for the inferior alveolar nerve, a branch of the mandibular division of the trigeminal nerve, which traverses the body within the *mandibular canal*, then emerges as the mental nerve through the *mental foramen* on the lateral surface of the body below and between the two premolars. The nerve supply to the incisors and canine runs forwards within the mandible beyond this point in the *incisive canal*.

The upper border of the body bears the *alveolar border* with 16 dental sockets or *alveoli*. The muscle attachments on mandible are shown in Fig. 5.45.

Development

The mandible develops as membrane bone in the fibrous sheath of Meckel's cartilage (the cartilage of the 1st branchial arch, which also gives rise to the malleus and incus). The cartilage itself is completely absorbed. Bony union of the two halves of the mandible occurs in the 2nd year.

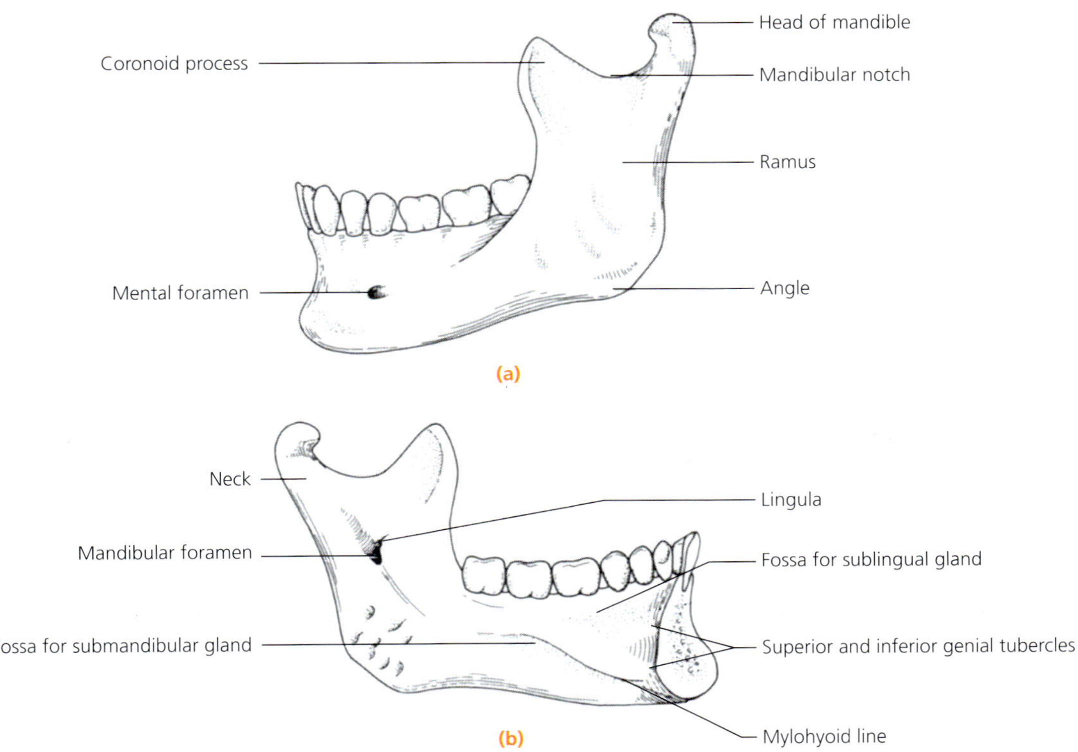

Figure 5.44 Muscle attachments on the mandible. **(a)** Lateral aspect. **(b)** Medial aspect.

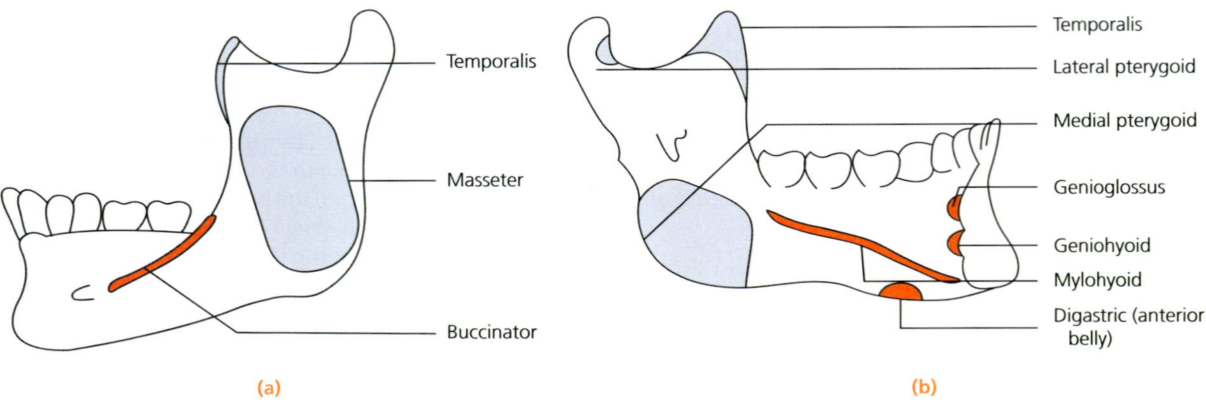

Figure 5.45 Muscle attachments on the mandible. **(a)** Lateral aspect. **(b)** Medial aspect.

Temporomandibular joint

This joint lies between the condylar process of the mandible and the articular fossa and articular eminence of the temporal bone. The articular surfaces are covered with fibrocartilage and there is also a fibrocartilaginous *articular disc* dividing the joint cavity into upper and lower compartments (Fig. 5.46).

The capsular ligament surrounding the joint is reinforced by a lateral *temporomandibular ligament* and by the *sphenomandibular ligament* which passes from the spine of the sphenoid to the *lingular process/lingula of mandible* immediately in front of the mandibular foramen; this ligament represents part of the primitive 1st arch, or Meckel's cartilage.

The lower jaw can be depressed, elevated, protruded, retracted and moved from side to side (Fig. 5.47).

The muscles effecting these movements are as follows:

- **Elevation:** Temporalis, masseter, medial pterygoid
- **Depression:** Lateral pterygoid, together with digastric, mylohyoid and geniohyoid (assisted by gravity – your jaw drops open when you fall asleep in a lecture)
- **Retraction:** Posterior fibres of temporalis
- **Protraction:** Lateral and medial pterygoids together
- **Side to side:** Lateral and medial pterygoids together, acting alternately on each side

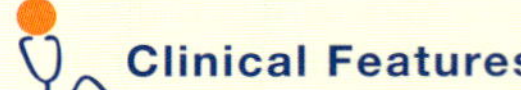

Clinical Features

Dislocation of the jaw, when uncomplicated, occurs only in a forwards direction. When the mouth is widely open, the condylar process of the mandible slides forwards onto the articular eminence; thence, a blow, or even a yawn, may cause forward dislocation into the infratemporal fossa on one or both sides. Upward dislocation can occur only in association with extensive comminution of the skull base, and backward dislocation with smashing of the bony external auditory canal and tympanic cavity that lie immediately behind the joint.

Reduction is effected by pressing down on the molar teeth with the thumbs placed in the mouth, at the same time pulling up the chin; the former stretches the masseter and temporalis muscles which are in spasm, the latter levers the mandibular head back into place.

Teeth

There are 20 deciduous or 'milk' teeth replaced by 32 permanent teeth made up, in each half jaw, as under:

- **Deciduous:** Two incisors, one canine, two molars
- **Permanent:** Two incisors, one canine, two premolars, three molars

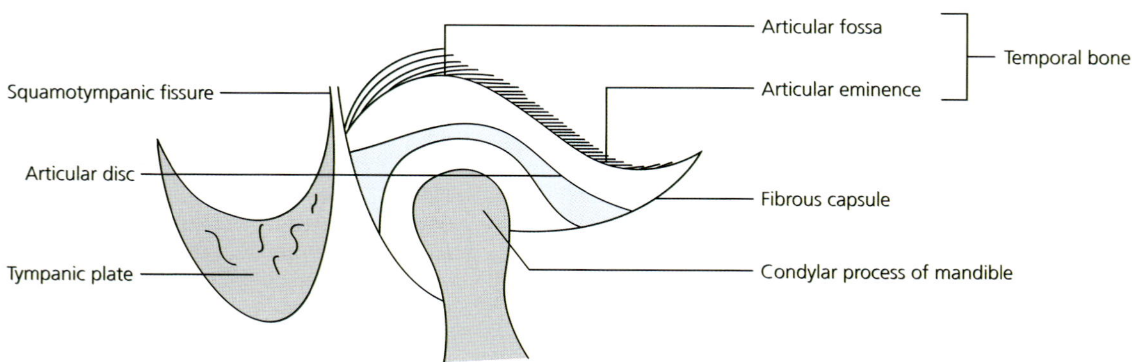

Figure 5.46 The articular surfaces of the temporomandibular joint.

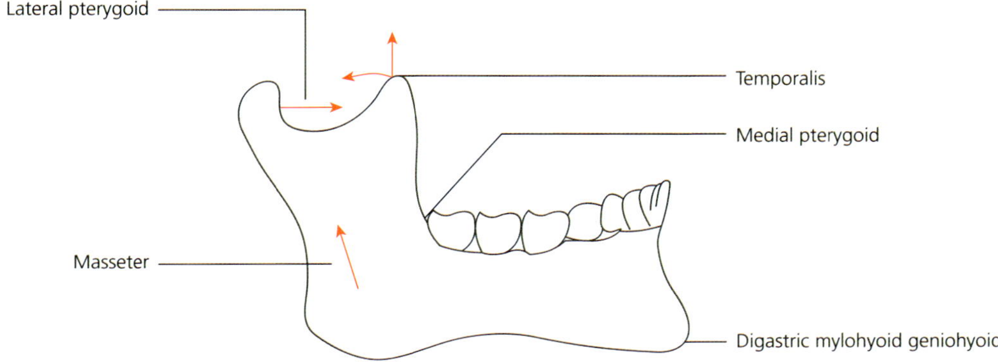

Figure 5.47 Movements of temporomandibular joints (arrow).

The times of eruption of the teeth are clinically useful milestones in a child's development as well as being of forensic interest.

As a rough guide, these times can be thought of in multiples of 6, thus:

- The 1st lower incisor deciduous tooth appears at — 6 months
- All the deciduous teeth have appeared by — 24 months
- The permanent 1st molar appear at — 6 years
- The permanent 1st incisor
- The 2nd permanent molar appears at — 12 years (approx.)
- The 3rd permanent molar appears at — 18–24 years

The lower teeth appear somewhat before their corresponding upper neighbours.

Each tooth is fixed in its socket by the *periodontal membrane*, which is, in fact, periosteum. This layer is radiotranslucent and is the dark line seen around the root of each tooth on radiography.

Development

The enamel crown of the tooth develops from a downgrowth of the alveolar epithelium (i.e. ectoderm) and represents the toughest tissue in the human body. The rest of the tooth (pulp, dentine and cement) differentiates from the underlying mesodermal connective tissue.

Inferior alveolar nerve block

This is a useful procedure for the dental surgeon because it produces complete anaesthesia of all the lower teeth on one side of the mandible. The needle is passed deep to the last molar tooth on to the inner aspect of the ramus of the mandible. Anaesthesia is produced in the lower teeth, the skin and mucosa of the lower lip (via the mental branch of the inferior alveolar nerve) and often, because of spread of the anaesthetic solution, there is loss of sensation of the side of the tongue owing to involvement of the lingual nerve, which lies immediately in front of the inferior alveolar nerve (*see* Fig. 6.21).

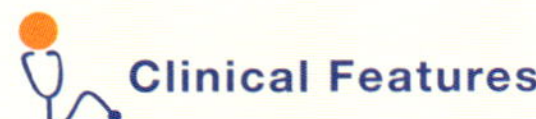

Osteomyelitis of the jaw following dental extractions is confined to the lower jaw and occurs only with the permanent dentition. The explanation of this is an anatomical one.

The lower jaw is supplied *only* by the inferior dental artery, which runs with the nerve in the mandibular canal; damage to this artery at extraction, or its thrombosis in subsequent infection, therefore, produces bone necrosis. The upper jaw, on the other hand, receives segmental vertical branches from the superior dental vessels and ischaemia does not follow injury to an individual artery. The deciduous teeth of the lower jaw are placed well clear of the mandibular canal which is, in any case, protected by the unerupted permanent teeth; damage to the artery cannot therefore occur during their removal.

Vertebral column

The vertebral column is made up of 33 vertebrae, of which 24 are discrete vertebrae and nine are fused in the sacrum and coccyx.

In the embryo the spine is curved into a gentle C shape (convex dorsally) but, with the extension of the head and lower limbs that occurs when the child first holds up its head, then sits and then stands, secondary forward curvatures appear in the cervical and lumbar region, which produce the sinuous curves of the fully developed spinal column.

The basic vertebral pattern (Fig. 5.48) is that of a *vertebral body anteriorly* and of a *neural arch* surrounding the *vertebral canal*.

The neural arch is made up of a *pedicle* on either side, each supporting a *lamina* that meets its opposite posteriorly in the midline. The pedicle bears a notch above and below which, with its neighbour, forms the *intervertebral foramen*. The arch bears a posterior *spine*, lateral *transverse processes* and upper and lower *articular facets*.

The intervertebral foramina transmit the segmental spinal nerves as follows: C1–C7 pass over the superior aspect of

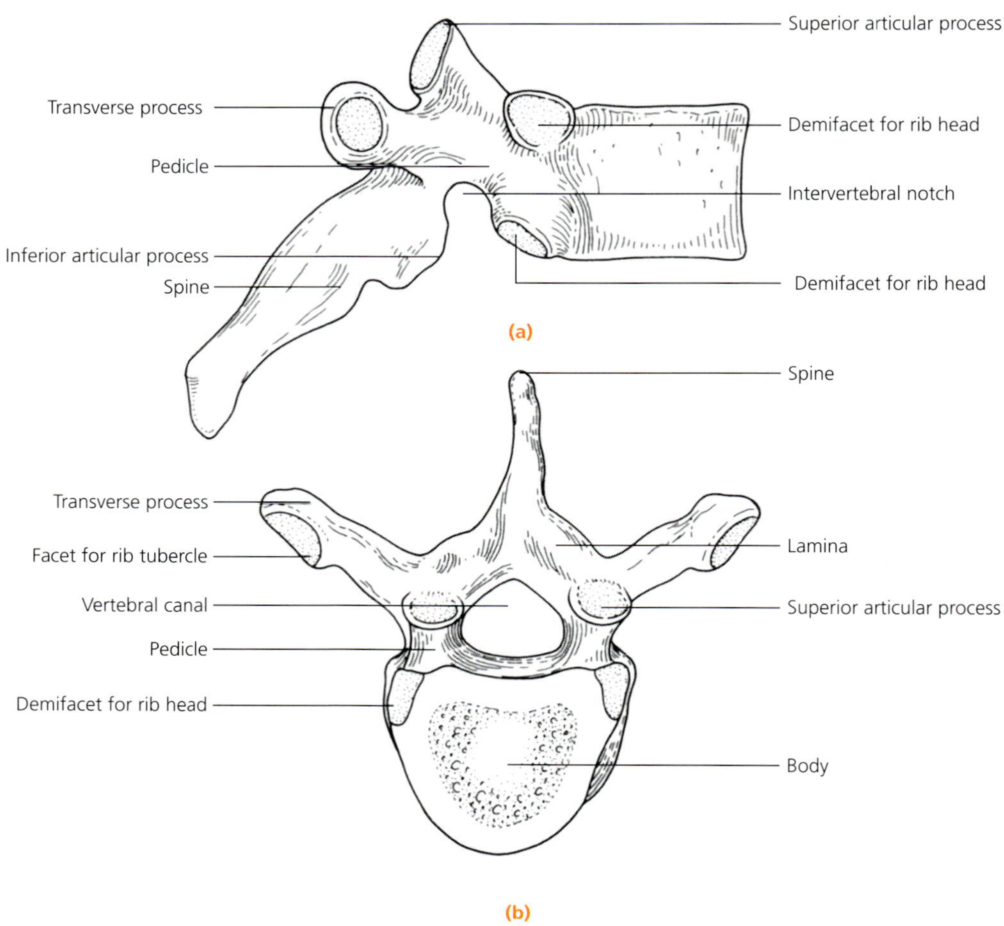

Figure 5.48 A 'typical' thoracic vertebra. **(a)** Lateral aspect. **(b)** Superior aspect.

their corresponding cervical vertebrae, C8 passes through the foramen between C7 and T1, and all subsequent nerves pass between the vertebra of their own number and the one below.

Now to consider the individual vertebrae in turn.

Cervical vertebrae (*n* = 7)

These are readily identified by the *foramen transversarium* perforating the transverse processes. These foramina transmit the vertebral artery (except that of C7), the vertebral veins and sympathetic fibres. The spines are small and bifid (except C1 and C7, which are single) and the articular facets are relatively horizontal (Fig. 5.49).

The *atlas* (C1) (Fig. 5.50) has no body. Its upper surface bears a superior articular facet on a thick lateral mass on each side that articulates with the occipital condyles of the skull.

Just posteriorly to this facet, the upper aspect of the posterior arch of the atlas is grooved by the vertebral artery as it passes medially and upwards to enter the foramen magnum.

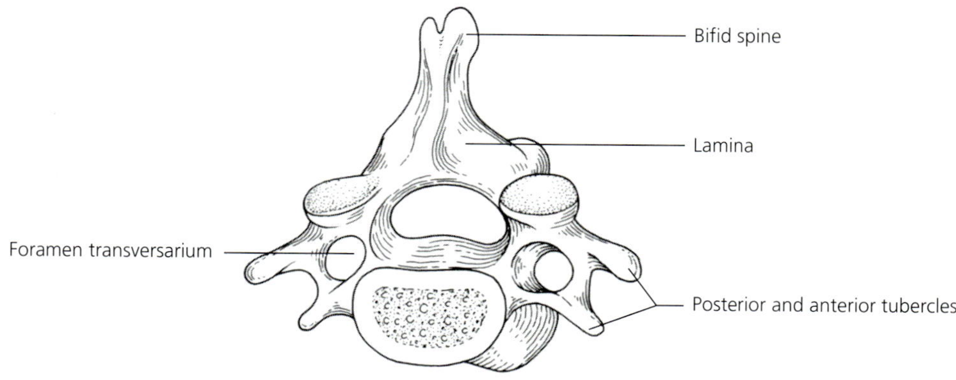

Figure 5.49 A 'typical' cervical vertebra.

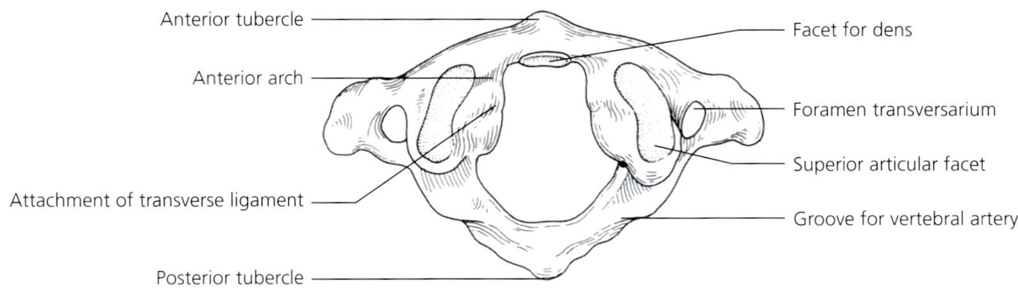

Figure 5.50 The atlas in superior view.

The *axis* (C2) (Fig. 5.51) bears the *dens* (*odontoid process*) on the superior aspect of its body, representing the detached centrum of C1.

Nodding and lateral flexion movements occur at the atlanto-occipital joint, whereas rotation of the skull occurs at the atlanto-axial joint around the dens, which acts as a pivot.

C7 is the *vertebra prominens*, so called because of its relatively long and easily felt non-bifid spine; it is the first clearly palpable spine on running one's fingers downwards along the vertebral crests, although the spine of T1 immediately below it is, in fact, the most prominent one.

The vertebral artery enters its vertebral course nearly always at the foramen transversarium of C6; it is not surprising, therefore, that the foramen of C7, which transmits only the vein, is small or even sometimes absent.

Thoracic vertebrae (*n* = 12)

These vertebrae (Fig. 5.48) are characterized by demifacets on the sides of their bodies for articulation with the heads of the ribs and by facets on their transverse processes (apart from those of the lower two or three vertebrae) for the rib tubercles. The spines are long and downward sloping and the articular facets are also relatively vertical. The lowest couple are rather 'lumbar' in appearance, have a single facet on the side of the body and no facet on the transverse process.

The bodies of T5 and T8 are worth noting; they come into relationship with the descending aorta and are a little flattened by it on their left flank. If the descending aorta becomes aneurysmally dilated, these four vertebral bodies become eroded by its pressure, although their avascular intervertebral discs remain intact. You can make this diagnosis confidently when shown a specimen of four partly worn-away vertebrae with normal intervening discs.

Lumbar vertebrae (*n* = 5)

These are of great size with strong, square, horizontal spines and with articular facets that lie in the sagittal plane (Fig. 5.52).

L5 is distinguished by its massive transverse process that connects with the whole lateral aspect of its pedicle and encroaches on its body; the transverse processes of the other lumbar vertebrae attach solely to the junction of the pedicle with the lamina.

Sacrum (comprising five fused vertebrae)

The sacrum is a triangular bone whose upper surface articulates with the body of L5 and whose lower end articulates with the coccyx. Laterally, the sacrum articulates with the corresponding hip bone.

Coccyx (comprising three, four or five fused vertebrae)

These are considered with the bony pelvis (*see* page 73).

Development

Each vertebra ossifies from three primary centres, one for each side of the arch and one for the body. The body occasionally develops from two centres and failure of one of these to form results in formation of a hemivertebra with a consequent congenital scoliosis. Failure of the two arch centres to fuse posteriorly results in the condition of spina bifida, which occurs particularly in the lumbar region. Usually this is not associated with any neurological abnormality (spina bifida occulta), although in such cases there is often an overlying dimple, lipoma or tuft of hair to warn the observant of a bony abnormality beneath. More rarely, there is a gross defect of one or several arches with protrusion of the meninges, with or without elements of the cauda equina or spinal cord; this anomaly may be associated with hydrocephalus.

L5 may occasionally fuse wholly or in part with the sacrum (sacralization of the 5th lumbar vertebra) or, more rarely, the 1st segment of the sacrum may differentiate as a separate vertebra (lumbarization of S1).

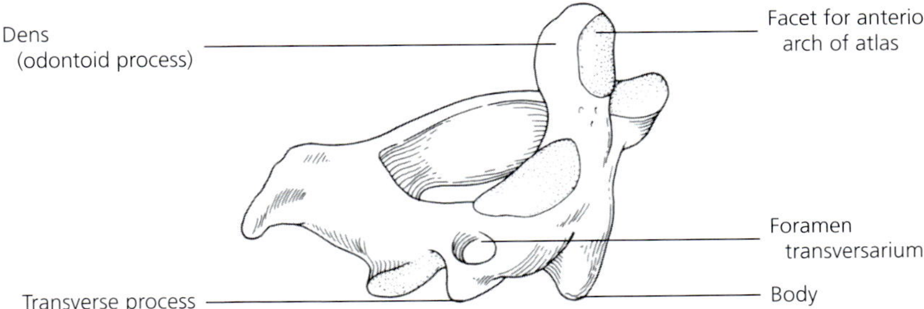

Figure 5.51 The axis in oblique lateral view.

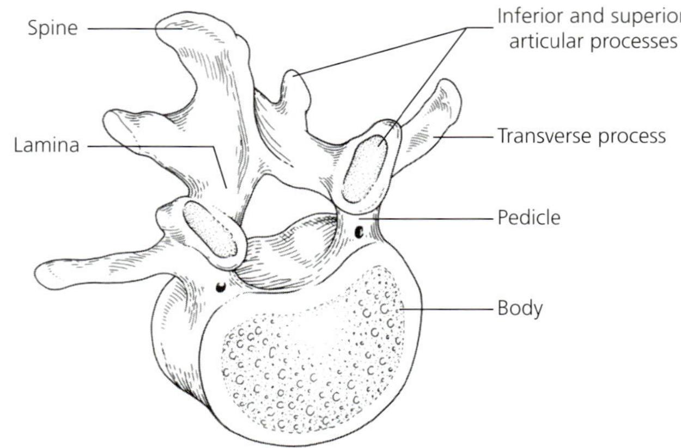

Figure 5.52 A lumbar vertebra (superior aspect).

Intervertebral joints

The spinal column is made up of individual vertebrae that articulate body to body and their articular facets. Although movement between adjacent vertebrae is slight, the additive effect is considerable. Movement particularly occurs at the cervicodorsal and dorsolumbar junctions; these are the two common sites of vertebral injury.

The vertebral laminae are linked by the *ligamentum flavum* of elastic tissue, the spines by the tough *supraspinous* and relatively weak *interspinous ligaments*, and the articular facets by *articular ligaments* around their small synovial joints. All these ligaments serve to support the spinal column when it is in the fully flexed position.

Running the whole length of the vertebral bodies, along their anterior and posterior aspects respectively, are the tough *anterior* and *posterior longitudinal ligaments*.

The vertebral bodies are also joined by the extremely strong *intervertebral discs* (Fig. 5.53). Each intervertebral disc consists of a peripheral *annulus fibrosus*, which adheres to the thin cartilage plate on the vertebral body above and below, and which surrounds a gelatinous semifluid *nucleus pulposus*. The intervertebral discs constitute approximately a quarter of the length of the spine as well as accounting for its secondary curvatures.

In old age, the discs atrophy, with resulting shrinkage in height and return of the curvature of the spine to the C shape of the newborn.

Clinical Features

1 Fractures of the spine most commonly involve T12, L1 and L2. The cause is usually a flexion–compression type of injury (for example, a fall from a height landing on the feet or buttocks, or a heavy weight falling on the shoulders), with resultant wedging of the involved vertebrae. If, in addition to compression, there is forceful forward movement, one vertebra may displace forwards on its neighbour below, with either dislocation or fracture of the articular facets between the two (fracture dislocation) and with rupture of the interspinous ligaments.

(*Continued ...*)

(*... continued*)

The cervical vertebrae (particularly C7) may be fractured or, more commonly, dislocated by a fall on the head with acute flexion of the neck, as might happen on diving into shallow water. Dislocation may even result from the sudden forward jerk that may occur when a motor car or aeroplane crashes. Note that the relatively horizontal intervertebral facets of the cervical vertebrae allow dislocation to take place without their being fractured, whereas the relatively vertical thoracic and lumbar intervertebral facets nearly always fracture in forward dislocation of the dorsolumbar region.

2 The comparatively thin posterior part of the annulus fibrosus may rupture, either because of trauma or because of degenerative changes, allowing the nucleus pulposus to protrude posteriorly into the vertebral canal – the so-called 'prolapsed intervertebral disc' (Fig. 5.53). This may sometimes occur at the lower cervical intervertebral discs (C5/6 and C6/7), very occasionally in the thoracic and upper lumbar region or, by far the most commonly, at the L4/5 or L5/S1 disc. The diagnosis of this and other spinal conditions has been greatly facilitated by the introduction of magnetic resonance imaging (MRI), which gives excellent anatomical details of this region (Fig. 5.53(b)).

A prolapsed L4/5 disc, protruding posterolaterally, to one or other side of the tough posterior longitudinal ligament, will produce pressure effects on the root of the corresponding 5th lumbar nerve. There may be consequent weakness of ankle dorsiflexion and numbness over the lower and lateral part of the leg and dorsum of the foot (L5). L5 involvement may also cause noticeable weakness of extension of the great toe (extensor hallucis longus).

A similar prolapse of the L5/S1 disc will press on the 1st sacral nerve. In the latter case, pain is referred to the back of the leg and foot along the distribution of the sciatic nerve. Hip flexion with the leg extended ('straight leg raising') is painful and limited because of the traction that this movement puts upon the already irritated and stretched nerve root. The ankle jerk may be diminished or absent and there may be weakness of plantarflexion.

Occasionally, the disc prolapses directly backwards, and, if this is extensive, may compress the whole cauda equina, producing paraplegia.

3 Lumbar puncture – *see* page 220.

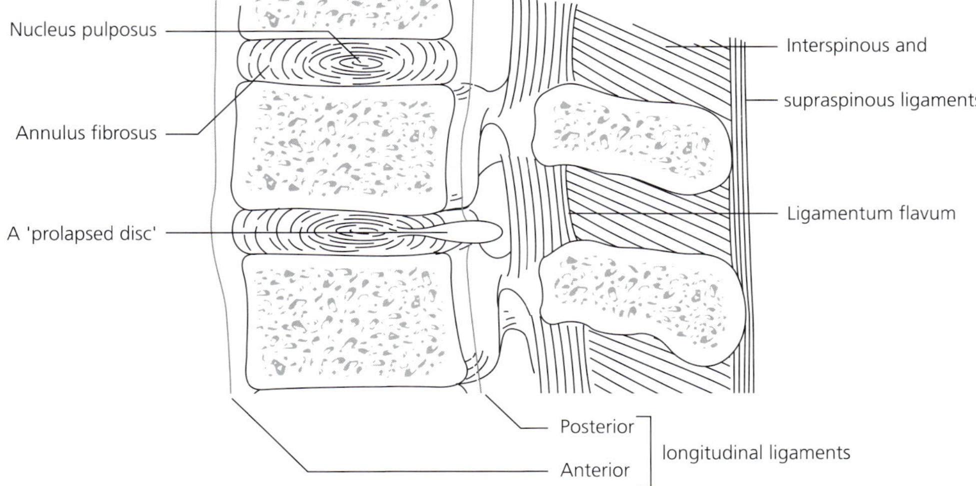

(a)

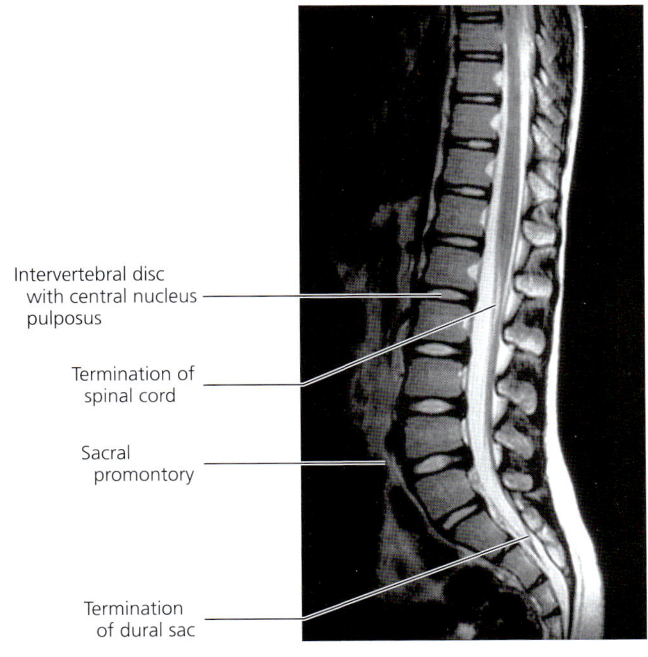

(b)

Figure 5.53 **(a)** Longitudinal section through the lumbar vertebrae showing a normal and a prolapsed intervertebral disc. **(b)** Magnetic resonance imaging (MRI) through a normal lumbar spine and sacrum. Note the excellent anatomical details.

Part VI

The nervous system

Introduction

For descriptive purposes, the nervous system can be divided, topographically, into two parts: the central nervous system and the peripheral nervous system.

The *central nervous system* comprises the brain and spinal cord, which are located, respectively, in the cranial cavity and the vertebral (spinal) canal, and are continuous with each other at the foramen magnum (where the medulla oblongata of the brain stem adjoins the spinal cord).

The *peripheral nervous system* comprises the 12 pairs of cranial nerves, 31 pairs of spinal nerves, the ganglia associated with the cranial and spinal nerves, and the right and left ganglionated sympathetic chains.

This division into central and peripheral systems is somewhat arbitrary, as the two 'systems' are physically connected and normally function in an integrated and co-ordinated manner.

Brain

The brain is a part of the central nervous system located in the cranial cavity (also called cranial cargo).

On a functional basis, the brain may be pictured as being made up of the following four major divisions:

1. Brainstem (comprising, from below upwards, the medulla oblongata, pons and midbrain)
2. Cerebellum
3. Diencephalon (comprising, mainly, the thalamus and hypothalamus)
4. Cerebrum (comprising two cerebral hemispheres)

By another convention, based on embryological development, the brain may be divided into the forebrain (comprising the cerebral hemispheres and diencephalon), midbrain and hindbrain (made up of the pons, medulla oblongata and cerebellum).

Brainstem

Extending from just above the tentorial hiatus to just below the foramen magnum, the brainstem is a stalk-like structure that is continuous superiorly with the diencephalon, and inferiorly with the spinal cord. As has been stated previously, the brainstem and the cerebellum are situated in the posterior cranial fossa.

The brainstem serves the following three major functions:

1. Housing the nuclei of all but two of the 12 pairs of cranial nerves (the exceptions being the cranial nerve pairs I and II which may both be regarded as peripheral extensions of the forebrain)
2. Acting as a 'thoroughfare' for the various ascending and descending nerve tracts running to and from the cerebral cortex, and for other tracts that project to the cerebellum
3. Containing the reticular formation (a fine and diffuse network of nerve cells and nerve fibres) and the reticular activating system. The reticular formation spans the entire length of the brainstem and harbours the '*vital centres*' – important reflex centres that regulate respiratory and cardiovascular function. The reticular formation and reticular activating system regulate the individual's level of awareness and wakefulness. Damage to the reticular formation in the upper part of the brainstem may cause the patient to be in a state of prolonged coma

Medulla oblongata

The medulla oblongata is 1 in. (2.5 cm) in length and about 0.75 in. (1.8 cm) in diameter. It is continuous below, through the foramen magnum, with the spinal cord and above with the pons; posteriorly, it is connected with the cerebellum by way of the right and left inferior cerebellar peduncles.

External features (Fig. 6.1)

The anterior surface of the medulla is grooved by an anteromedian fissure, on either side of which are longitudinal prominences termed *pyramids* which contain the pyramidal tracts. These *pyramids*, in turn, are separated from the *olivary eminences* by the anterolateral sulcus along which the rootlets of the XIIth cranial nerve emerge. Emerging from the posterolateral aspect of the olivary eminences are the rootlets of cranial nerves IX, X and XI. The posterior median sulcus of the cord is continued halfway up the medulla, where it widens out to form the inferior limits of the diamond-shaped outline of the 4th ventricle. On either side of the sulcus, the posterior columns of the spinal cord expand to form two distinct tubercles, corresponding to the gracile and cuneate nuclei.

The *blood supply* of the medulla is derived from the vertebral arteries directly and from their posterior inferior cerebellar branches.

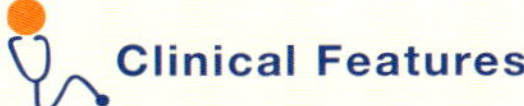

The medulla contains the respiratory, cardiac and vasomotor centres – the 'vital centres'. The respiratory centre is particularly vulnerable to compression, injury or poliomyelitis with consequent respiratory failure.

Pons

The pons lies between the medulla and the midbrain and is connected to the right and left cerebellar hemispheres by the right and left middle cerebellar peduncles, respectively. It is 1 in. (2.5 cm) in length and 1.5 in. (3.8 cm) in width.

External features (Fig. 6.1)

The ventral surface of pons presents a shallow, vertical median groove and numerous transverse ridges, which are continuous laterally on either side with the corresponding middle cerebellar peduncle. The dorsal surface of the pons forms part of the floor of the 4th ventricle. Ventrally, its junction with the medulla is marked close to the midline by the emergence of the VIth cranial nerves and, in the angle between the pons and the cerebellum, by the VIIth and VIIIth cranial nerves. Both the motor and sensory roots of the Vth cranial nerve leave the lateral part of the pons near its upper border.

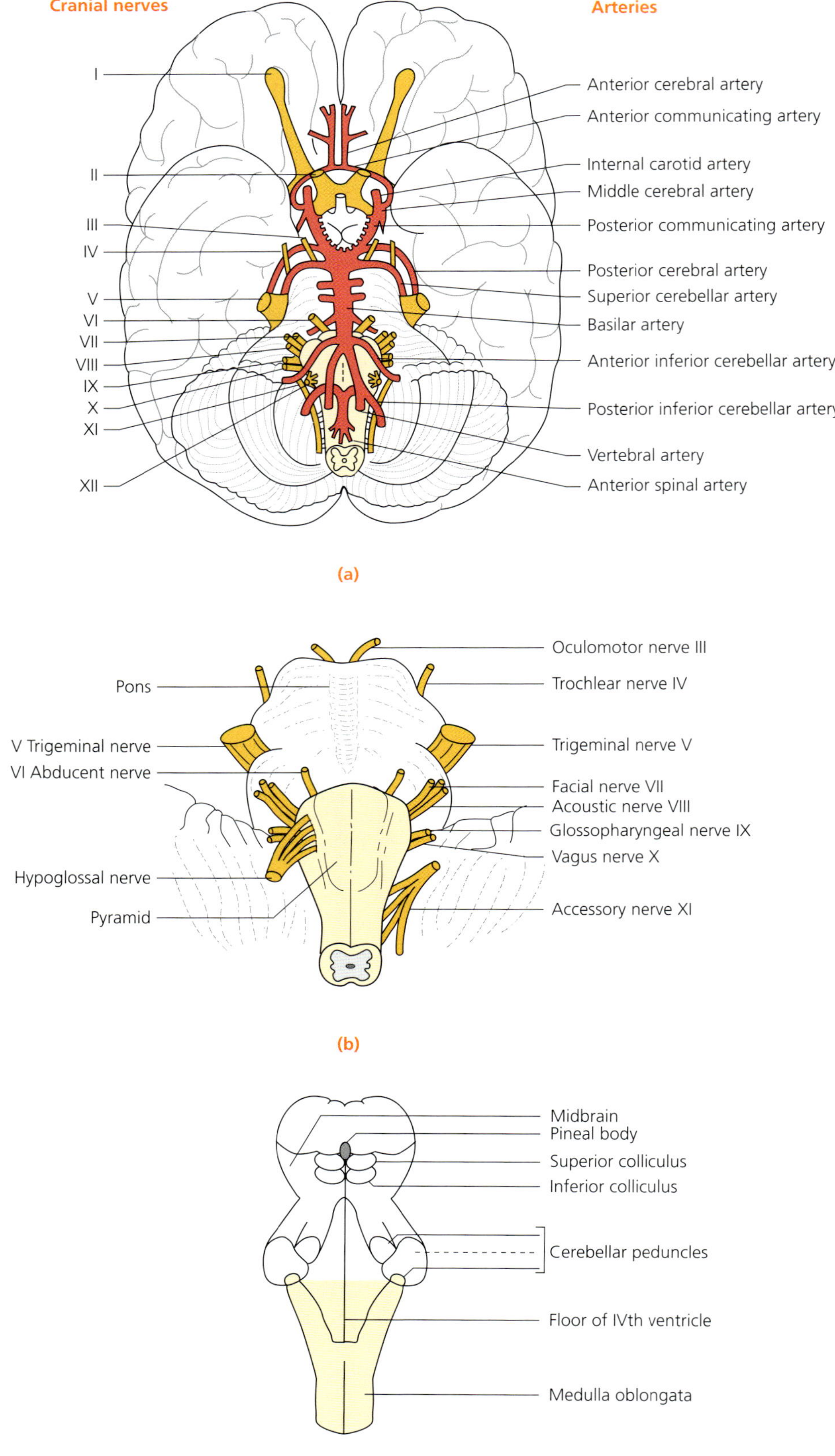

Figure 6.1 **(a)** The base of the brain showing the cranial nerve roots and their relationships to the circle of Willis. **(b)** Anterior aspect of the brainstem. **(c)** Posterior aspect of the brainstem.

The *blood supply* of the pons is derived from multiple small pontine branches of the basilar artery (Fig. 6.1), which in turn is formed by the confluence of two vertebral arteries.

Midbrain

The midbrain is the shortest part of the brainstem; it is just under 1 in. (2.5 cm) long and connects the pons and cerebellum to the diencephalon. It lies within the tentorial hiatus (the gap in the tentorium cerebelli) and is largely hidden by the surrounding structures.

External features (Fig. 6.1)

The only parts of the midbrain visible from the ventral aspect of the brain are the two *cerebral peduncles*, which emerge from the substance of the cerebral hemisphere and pass downwards and medially, connecting the internal capsule to the pons. The right and left oculomotor nerves (cranial nerve III) emerge between the two cerebral peduncles in the *interpeduncular fossa*. Viewed from the lateral aspect, the midbrain is seen to consist of three distinct portions: the basis pedunculi ventrally, the midbrain *tegmentum* centrally and the *tectum* dorsally. The trochlear nerve (IV), the optic tract and the posterior cerebral artery wind around this aspect of the midbrain. The dorsal aspect of the midbrain (Fig. 6.1(c)) presents the four *colliculi* (or *corpora quadrigemini*) and the superior *medullary velum* between the two superior cerebellar peduncles. The *pineal body* is a midline structure. It rests between the two superior colliculi and is attached by a stalk to the posterior part of the thalamus. The pineal secretes melatonin and has an important role in setting the circadian rhythm. When calcified, the pineal gland is easily identified on skull radiographs. It may then give the important radiological sign of lateral displacement by a space-occupying lesion of the cerebral hemisphere.

Cerebellum

The cerebellum is the largest part of the hindbrain and occupies most of the posterior cranial fossa.

External features (Fig. 6.1; *see* Fig. 6.3)

The cerebellum is made up of the right and left *cerebellar hemispheres* and a median *vermis*. Inferiorly, the vermis is clearly separated from the two hemispheres and lies at the bottom of a deep cleft, the *vallecula*; superiorly, it is marked off from the hemispheres only as a low median elevation. A small ventral portion of each cerebellar hemisphere lies on the middle cerebellar peduncle of its side, and is almost completely separated from the rest of the cerebellum. It is termed the *flocculus*. The surface of the cerebellum is divided into numerous narrow *folia* and, by a few deep fissures, into a number of lobules. The effect of this fissuring is to give the cerebellum in section the appearance of a many-branched tree (the *arbor vitae*) (*see* Fig. 6.10).

Internal structure

The structure of the cerebellum is remarkably uniform. It consists of a *cortex* of grey matter (in which all the afferent fibres terminate) covering a mass of white matter, in which deep nuclei of grey matter are buried.

The cerebellum is connected to the brainstem by way of three pairs of *cerebellar peduncles*. The *inferior peduncles* connect it to the dorsolateral aspect of the medulla; the *middle cerebellar peduncles* to the pons; and the *superior peduncles* to the caudal midbrain. Ventrally, the cerebellum is related to the 4th ventricle and to the medulla and pons; laterally, to the sigmoid venous sinus and the mastoid antrum and air cells; and posterosuperiorly, it is separated from the cerebral hemispheres by the *tentorium cerebelli*.

The *blood supply* of the cerebellum is derived from three pairs of arteries (Fig. 5.29); the *posterior inferior cerebellar* branches of the vertebral arteries supply the posterior aspect of the vermis and hemispheres, and the *anterior inferior* and *superior cerebellar branches of the basilar artery* supply the anterolateral part of the undersurface and the superior aspect of the cerebellum, respectively.

Functions of the cerebellum

The principal function of the cerebellum is to regulate and maintain balance, and to co-ordinate timing and precision of body movements. The cerebellum has multiple connections with the cerebral cortex, reticular formation in the brainstem, thalamus and vestibular nuclei. Through these intricate connections, the cerebellum constantly monitors proprioceptive sensory input from joints, muscles and tendons, and accordingly refines and co-ordinates the contractions of skeletal muscles.

However, unlike the cerebral cortex of the primary motor area, the cerebellum is incapable of initiating movement, nor is the cerebellum involved in the conscious perception of somatic or visceral sensations.

Clinical Features

1 As the cerebellum is principally concerned with balance and the regulation of posture, muscle tone and muscular co-ordination, it is not surprising that cerebellar lesions result in disturbance of one or more of these motor functions, manifesting as any one or more of the following: unsteady gait, ataxia, hypotonia, tremor, nystagmus, dysarthria and dysdiadokokinesia (the inability to perform alternating movements rapidly, e.g. supination/pronation).

Lesions of the cerebellum give rise to symptoms and signs on the *same side of the body*.

Destruction of the dentate nucleus (a large collection of cells within the cerebellar white matter) or the superior cerebellar peduncle results in a disability almost as severe as ablation of the entire cerebellar hemisphere.

2 Thrombosis of the posterior inferior cerebellar artery (PICA) gives rise to a characteristic syndrome (*PICA syndrome*) marked by ataxia and hypotonia of the ipsilateral limbs owing to involvement of the inferior cerebellar peduncle and cerebellar cortex, signs of cranial nerve involvement (V to X) and contralateral loss of pain and thermal sensibility (spinothalamic tract involvement).

Diencephalon

The diencephalon comprises principally the thalamus and hypothalamus, which are continuous with each other.

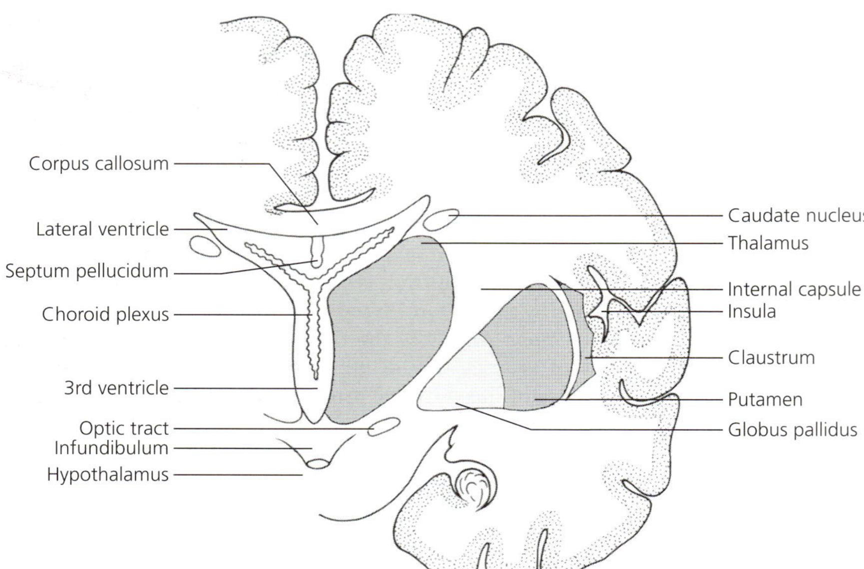

Figure 6.2 The thalamus and 3rd ventricle in coronal section.

A vertically disposed, median, cleft-like space is present between the right and left halves of the diencephalon, and is called the 3rd ventricle (Fig. 6.2). In addition to the thalamus and hypothalamus, the diencephalon includes two small but functionally important regions: the epithalamus and ventral thalamus. The epithalamus is the dorsal portion of the diencephalon and contains the pineal body. The ventral thalamus (also known as the subthalamus) contains the subthalamic nucleus, which is one of the basal ganglia. It is believed to be the main regulator and modulator of the other basal ganglia, and thus is a significant influence on motor activity.

Thalamus (Fig. 6.2; *see* Fig. 6.4)

The thalamus is an oval mass of grey matter that forms the upper part of the lateral wall of the 3rd ventricle; it extends from the interventricular foramen rostrally to the midbrain caudally. Laterally, it is related to the internal capsule (and through it to the basal ganglia), and dorsally to the floor of the lateral ventricle. Medially, it is frequently connected with its fellow of the opposite side through the *massa intermedia* (interthalamic connexus). Posteriorly, it presents three distinct eminences, the *pulvinar*, and the *medial* and *lateral geniculate bodies*, the last two are the thalamic relay nuclei of hearing and vision, respectively.

The thalamus is the principal sensory relay nucleus that projects impulses from the main sensory pathways onto the cerebral cortex. It does this via a number of thalamic radiations in the internal capsule.

The blood supply of the thalamus is derived principally from the posterior cerebral artery through its thalamostriate branches, which pierce the posterior perforated substance to supply also the posterior part of the internal capsule. Thalamic damage, by occlusion of this blood supply, results in contralateral sensory loss of the face and body.

Hypothalamus (Figs 6.1(a) and 6.2)

The hypothalamus forms the floor of the 3rd ventricle, and also the lower part of its lateral wall. Viewed from below, the hypothalamus is seen to include, from before backwards, the *optic chiasma*, the *tuber cinereum*, the *infundibular stalk* (leading down to the posterior lobe of the pituitary), the *mamillary bodies* and the posterior *perforated substance*. In each of these there is a number of cell masses or nuclei and a fibre pathway – the medial forebrain bundle – which runs throughout the length of the hypothalamus and serves to link it with the midbrain postero-inferiorly and the basal forebrain areas anterosuperiorly.

Sherrington described the hypothalamus as the head ganglion of the autonomic system. It is largely concerned with autonomic activity and can be divided into a posteromedial sympathetic area and an anterolateral area concerned with parasympathetic activity.

The hypothalamus plays an important role in endocrine control by the formation of releasing factors or release-inhibiting factors. These substances, following their secretion into the hypophyseal portal vessels, influence the production by the cells of the anterior pituitary of adrenocorticotrophin, follicle-stimulating hormone, luteinizing hormone, prolactin, somatotrophin, thyrotrophin and melanocyte-stimulating hormone.

The hormones oxytocin and vasopressin (antidiuretic hormone) are produced by two distinct aggregations of neurones (the paraventricular and supra-optic nuclei, respectively) in the hypothalamus and released at their axon terminals in the posterior pituitary. Oxytocin and antidiuretic hormone are thus neurosecretions.

In addition to its major influence on the autonomic nervous system and on pituitary function, the hypothalamus also plays a significant role in temperature regulation, water and electrolyte balance, regulation of appetite and sleep–wake patterns.

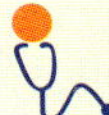

Clinical Features

1 Given its manifold functions, lesions of the hypothalamus may present to the clinician as a variety of autonomic and non-autonomic disturbances, e.g. somnolence, disturbances of temperature regulation and obesity, as well as a variety of endocrine abnormalities, e.g. hypogonadism and hypothyroidism.

(Continued ...)

(... *continued*)

2 Damage to the supra-optic nucleus or the infundibular stalk leads to diabetes insipidus, through loss of production of antidiuretic hormone.

Pituitary gland (hypophysis cerebri)

This is an example of a *'two-in-one' organ*, of which nature appears so keen; compare the two glandular components of the suprarenal cortex and medulla, and the exocrine and endocrine parts of the pancreas, testis and ovary. The pituitary comprises a *larger anterior* and *smaller posterior* lobe, the latter connected by the hollow infundibulum (pituitary stalk) to the tuber cinereum in the floor of the 3rd ventricle. The two lobes of the pituitary are connected by a narrow zone termed the pars intermedia.

The pituitary lies in the cavity of the pituitary fossa covered over by the diaphragma sellae, which is a fold of dura mater. This fold has a central aperture through which passes the infundibulum. Below the pituitary is the body of the sphenoid, laterally on either side lies the corresponding cavernous sinus and its contents separated by dura mater (*see* Fig. 5.32), with intercavernous sinuses running in front, behind and below the pituitary. The optic chiasma lies above, immediately in front of the infundibulum.

Structure

The anterior lobe is extremely cellular and consists of chromophobe, eosinophilic and basophilic cells. The pars intermedia contains large colloid vesicles reminiscent of the thyroid. The posterior lobe is made up of nerve fibres whose cell bodies lie in the hypothalamus.

Clinical Features

Tumours of the pituitary, as well as forming intracranial space-occupying lesions, may have two special features: their endocrine disturbances and their relationship to the opticchiasma.

The *chromophobe adenoma* is the commonest pituitary tumour. As it enlarges, it expands the pituitary fossa (sella turcica) and this may be demonstrated radiologically. Compression of the optic chiasma produces the very rapid typical bitemporal hemianopia (*see* 'Optic nerve (II) and the visual pathway', page 221, and Fig. 6.18). The tumour itself is non-secretory and gradually destroys the normally functioning gland. The patient develops hypopituitarism with loss of sex characteristics, hypothyroidism and hypoadrenalism. In childhood there is an arrest of growth. As the tumour extends there may be involvement of the hypothalamus with diabetes insipidus and obesity.

The *eosinophil adenoma* secretes the pituitary growth hormones. If it occurs before puberty, which is unusual, it produces gigantism; after puberty, it results in acromegaly.

The *basophil adenoma* is small, produces no pressure effects and may be associated with Cushing's syndrome, although this more often results from hyperplasia or tumour of the suprarenal cortex.

The close relationship of the pituitary to the sphenoid sinus makes it possible to insert fibre-optic instruments into the pituitary gland by a transnasal, trans-sphenoidal approach. This is now the preferred approach to surgery of pituitary tumours, rather than through a frontal bone flap.

Development

The posterior lobe is derived from a diverticulum of the diencephalon. The anterior lobe and the pars intermedia develop from Rathke's pouch in the roof of the embryonic buccal cavity. Occasionally, a tumour grows from remnants of the epithelium of this pouch (craniopharyngioma). These tumours are often cystic and calcified.

Owing to their strikingly different histological appearances and different embryological origins, the anterior and posterior lobes of the pituitary are also referred to as the *adenohypophysis* and *neurohypophysis*, respectively.

Cerebrum

The cerebrum is the largest part of the brain. It comprises right and left cerebral hemispheres which are mostly separated from each other by a median cleft, occupied by fold of dura mater, the *falx cerebri*.

The cerebral hemispheres which, in man, have developed out of all proportion to the rest of the brain, comprise the cerebral cortex, the basal ganglia, and their afferent and efferent connections. The lateral ventricles, containing cerebrospinal fluid (CSF), are at their centre.

Cerebral cortex

The cortex of the cerebral hemispheres is divided on topographical and functional grounds into four lobes – frontal, parietal, temporal and occipital (Fig. 6.3).

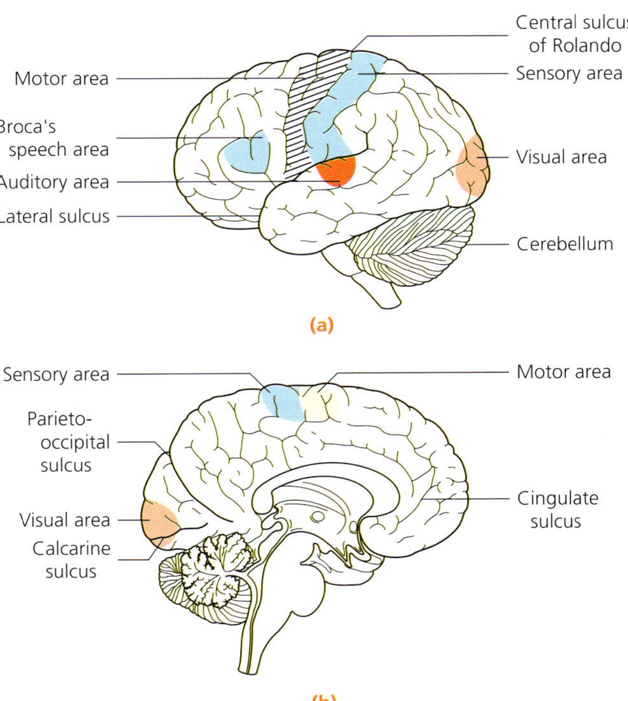

Figure 6.3 Localization of function in the cerebral cortex. **(a)** Lateral aspect. **(b)** Medial aspect.

Frontal lobe

This includes all the cortex anterior to the *central sulcus of Rolando*. Its important cortical areas are as follows:

1. **The motor cortex:** The primary motor area occupies a large part of the precentral gyrus. It receives afferents from the premotor cortex, thalamus and cerebellum and is concerned with voluntary movements. Stimulation of this area results in discrete muscle movements. Details of localization of function in the motor cortex are considered on page 213.
2. **The premotor cortex:** This lies anterior to the precentral gyrus and the adjoining lower part of the frontal gyri. It, too, is concerned with voluntary movement, but its stimulation results in movements of groups of muscles with a common function, and thus lacks the precise definition of muscle movement that is a feature of stimulation of the precentral gyrus.
3. **Eye motor field:** This lies in the middle frontal area anterior to the premotor cortex. Lesions of this area result in impaired eye movement with deviation of gaze to the side of the lesion.
4. **Broca's speech area:** Lesions of the area around the posterior part of the inferior frontal gyrus of the dominant hemisphere (the left hemisphere in 98% of individuals) were shown by Broca to affect the motor element in speech.
5. **Frontal association cortex (clinically called the prefrontal cortex):** This comprises a considerable part of the frontal lobe and is one of the remarkable, evolutionary advances seen in the human brain. Its afferents are derived from the thalamus, limbic area and also from other cortical areas; it probably sends efferents to the thalamus and hypothalamus. From a functional point of view, the lateral aspect of the frontal lobe appears to be related to 'intellectual activity' (i.e. cognitive functions – analysis, judgement and planning), the medial and orbital surfaces to affective (or emotional) behaviour and the control of autonomic activity.

Parietal lobe

The parietal lobe is bounded anteriorly by the central sulcus and behind by a line drawn from the parieto-occipital sulcus to the preoccipital sulcus and below by a line extending from posterior end of the lateral (Sylvian) sulcus to the first line. The important cortical areas of the parietal lobe are as follows.

1. The *primary somatosensory cortex*. The postcentral gyrus receives afferent fibres from the thalamus and is concerned with all forms of somatic sensation. Details of localization along the sensory cortex are considered on pages 212 and 213.
2. The *parietal association cortex*, comprising the remainder of the parietal lobe, is concerned largely with the recognition of somatic sensory stimulation and its integration with other forms of sensory information. It also receives afferents from the thalamus and, when damaged, gives rise to more complex defects than simple loss of sensation. An example of this is the inability to recognize somatic stimuli, which is called *astereognosis*; put a pen or a coin in the patient's hand – he is aware of the object but is unable to recognize what it is. The lower part of the parietal lobe in the subject's dominant hemisphere interacts with the somatosensory visual and auditory associations and has a key role in language.

Temporal lobe

This is arbitrarily separated from the occipital lobe by a line drawn vertically downwards from the preoccipital sulcus to preoccipital notch and from parietal lobe by the posterior ramus of the lateral sulcus.

The important cortical areas of the temporal lobe are the following:

1. **The auditory cortex:** This lies in the superior temporal gyrus on the lateral and superior surfaces of the hemisphere. Its afferent fibres are from the medial geniculate body and it is concerned with the perception of auditory stimuli.
2. **The temporal association cortex:** The area surrounding the auditory cortex is responsible for the recognition of auditory stimuli and for their integration with other sensory modalities. Lesions of this area result in auditory agnosia, i.e. the inability to recognize or to understand the significance of meaningful sounds. The cortical region just above and behind this area on the dominant hemisphere (*Wernicke's area*) is of considerable importance in the sensory aspects of language comprehension. This visual area of the occipital lobe connects with the temporal lobe and is concerned with visual recognition. The antero-inferior aspect of the frontal lobe connects with the medial aspect of the temporal lobe and is concerned with behaviour.

Parahippocampal gyrus

The cortex of the most medial part of the undersurface of the temporal lobe is known as the parahippocampal gyrus, much of which is referred to as the *entorhinal cortex*. It receives widespread association cortical afferents and is a significant source of inputs to the hippocampus. Anteriorly, it is related to the olfactory cortex of the uncus. Medially, it is in direct continuity with the layer of in-rolled cortex which is the *hippocampus* and which is one of the most important sources of afferents to this structure. The hippocampus occupies the whole length of the floor of the inferior horn of the lateral ventricle and extends to the amygdala. It sends its efferents into the overlying layer of white matter known as the *alveus*. The fibres of the alveus collect on the medial margin of the hippocampus to form a compact bundle, the *fimbria*, which, as it arches under the corpus callosum, becomes known as the *fornix*. The fornix passes forwards and then downwards in front of the interventricular foramen and finally backwards into the hypothalamus to terminate in the *mamillary body*. It also gives fibres to the thalamus and the hypothalamus.

Projection of the hippocampus to the hypothalamus is part of the *limbic system*. This is an important substrate for emotions, behaviour and memory. The circuit is completed by projections of the hypothalamus to the thalamus, from the thalamus to the cingulate gyrus and from thence back to the hippocampus. Bilateral hippocampal damage results in inability to form new long-term memories.

Amygdaloid nuclear complex

The amygdaloid nuclear complex is also a prominent temporal lobe structure, situated immediately rostral to the hippocampus. It is conveniently divided into three groups of nuclei: corticomedial, central and basolateral, which receive largely olfactory, gustatory and association cortical afferents, respectively. These divisions also have more or less separable projections to the hypothalamus and septum, brainstem autonomic centres and ventral striatum. The amygdala is involved in the control of emotional behaviour and conditioned reflexes. Its neuroanatomical connections are clearly appropriate for such a role, since it is in a position to affect emotional responses in endocrine, autonomic and motor domains. Destruction of the amygdala is particularly associated with reduced aggressive behaviour, whereas the very high density of benzodiazepine receptors here has suggested amygdaloid involvement in anxiety and stress and their treatments.

Occipital lobe

The occipital lobe lies behind the parietal and temporal lobes. On its medial aspect it presents the Y-shaped *calcarine* and *postcalcarine sulci* (Fig. 6.3). The following cortical areas are noteworthy:

1. The *visual cortex* surrounds the calcarine and postcalcarine sulci and receives its afferent fibres from the lateral geniculate body of the thalamus of the same side; it is concerned with vision of the opposite (contralateral) half field of sight (Fig. 6.4).
2. The *occipital association cortex* lies anterior to the visual cortex. This area is particularly concerned with the recognition and integration of visual stimuli.

Insula (Figs 6.2 and 6.4)

If the lips of the lateral sulcus are separated, it is seen that there is a considerable area of cortex buried in the floor of this sulcus. This area is known as the *insula of Reil*. It is divided into a number of small gyri and is crossed by the middle cerebral artery. Apart from its upper part, which abuts on the sensory cortex and probably represents the taste area of the cerebral cortex, the function of the insula is unknown. Its stimulation excites visceral effects such as belching, increased salivation, gastric movements and vomiting.

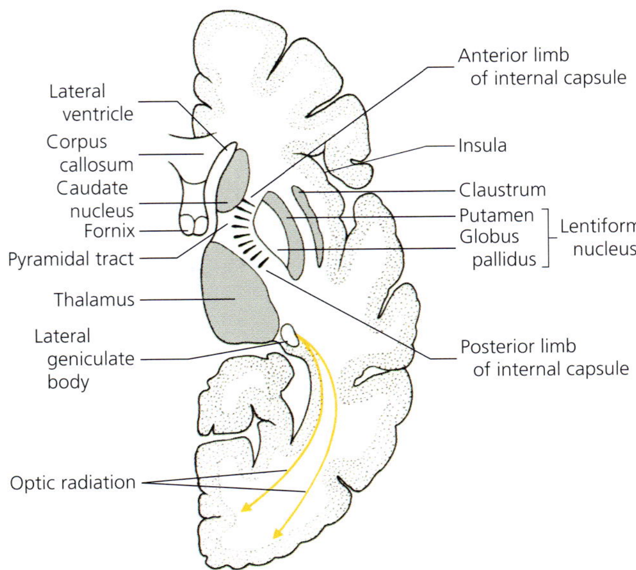

Figure 6.4 The basal ganglia and internal capsule shown in horizontal section through the cerebrum.

Connections of the cerebral cortex

As has been indicated, most areas of the cerebral cortex receive their main afferent input from the thalamus, but, in addition to this, there are well-established *commissural connections* with the corresponding area of the opposite hemisphere by way of the *corpus callosum*. *Intracortical association fibres* also link neighbouring cortical areas on the same side and, in some cases, connect distant cortical areas; thus, the frontal, occipital and temporal lobes within the same hemisphere are directly connected by long association pathways.

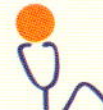

Clinical Features

It is convenient to summarize here the clinical effects of lesions affecting the principal cortical areas.

1. *Frontal cortex* – Impairment of higher mental functions and emotions.
2. *Precentral (motor) cortex* – Weakness of the opposite side of the body; lesions low down the cortex affecting the face and arm, high lesions affecting the leg. Midline lesions (meningioma, sagittal sinus thrombosis or a gunshot wound) may produce paraplegia by involving both leg areas.
3. *Sensory cortex* – Contralateral hemianaesthesia (distributed in the same pattern as the motor cortex) affecting especially the higher sensory modalities such as stereognosis and two-point position sense.
   (For area localizations along the motor and sensory cortex, *see* page 213.)
4. *Occipital cortex* – Contralateral homonymous hemianopia.
5. Lesions adjacent to the *lateral sulcus* in the frontal, parietal or temporal lobes of the dominant hemisphere result in aphasia.

Basal ganglia (Figs 6.2 and 6.4)

These compact masses of grey matter are situated deep in the substance of the cerebral hemisphere and comprise the *corpus striatum* (composed of the caudate nucleus, the putamen and the globus pallidus) and the *claustrum*. Together with the cerebellum, they are involved in co-ordination and control of movement.

Corpus striatum

The *caudate nucleus* is a large homogeneous mass of grey matter consisting of a *head*, anterior to the interventricular foramen and forming the lateral wall of the anterior horn of the lateral ventricle; a *body*, forming the lateral wall of the body of the ventricle; and an elongated *tail*, which forms the roof of the inferior (temporal) horn of the ventricle. It is largely separated from the putamen by the *internal capsule*, but the two structures are connected anteriorly. The *putamen* is a roughly ovoid mass closely applied to the lateral aspect of the *globus pallidus*; together, they are called the *lentiform nucleus*. The corpus striatum receives afferent connections from the cerebral cortex and sends efferents to the globus pallidus. From there, fibres project to the thalamus and, thence, back to the premotor cortex. Dopaminergic fibres project from the substantia nigra to the corpus striatum and efferent fibres also pass to the thalamus, hypothalamus, red nucleus, substantia nigra and the inferior olivary nucleus.

Neural pathways

The neural pathways are of two types: ascending and descending. The following text deals with the long ascending (afferent) and descending (motor) pathways:

Somatic afferent pathways (Fig. 6.5)

The somatic afferent pathways carry two types of sensory modalities: (a) proprioceptive and tactile modalities and (b) pain and temperature modalities.

1. Proprioceptive and tactile impulses pass uninterruptedly through the posterior root ganglia, through the ipsilateral *posterior columns* of the spinal cord to the *gracile* and *cuneate nuclei* in the lower part of the medulla. In the posterior columns there is a fairly precise organization of the afferent fibres; those from sacral and lumbar segments are situated medially in the tracts whereas fibres from thoracic and cervical levels are successively added to their lateral aspect. This arrangement according to body segments is maintained in the gracile and cuneate nuclei and in the efferents from these nuclei to the contralateral thalamus. The fibres arising from the gracile and cuneate nuclei immediately cross over to the opposite side in the *sensory decussation* of the medulla and continue up to the thalamus as a compact contralateral bundle – the *medial lemniscus*.
2. Dorsal root fibres subserving pain and temperature, together with some tactile afferents, end ipsilaterally in the *substantia gelatinosa* of the posterior horn. They then synapse and cross

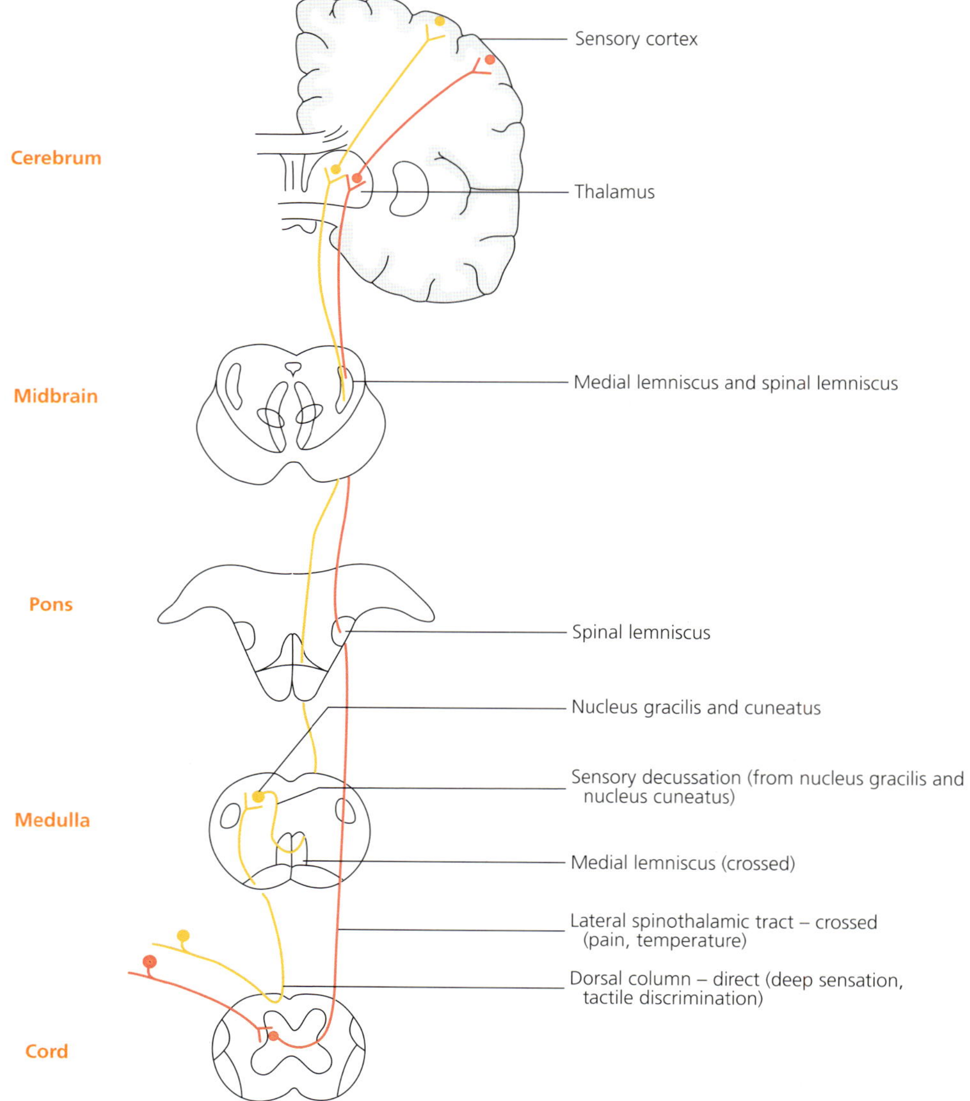

Figure 6.5 The long ascending pathways of the dorsal columns (yellow lines) and spinothalamic tracts (red lines).

to the contralateral anterior lateral columns of the cord and are relayed to the contralateral thalamus. The fibre crossing occurs in the anterior white commissure of the spinal cord. In the brainstem these fibres come to lie immediately lateral to the medial lemniscus and are sometimes known as the *spinal lemniscus* (Fig. 6.5). They terminate in the thalamus.

These somatic afferents are relayed from the thalamus, through the posterior limb of the internal capsule (Fig. 6.4) to the somatic sensory cortex of the *postcentral gyrus*. In the internal capsule the fibres are arranged in the sequence 'face, arm, trunk and leg' from before backwards, and this segregation persists in the sensory cortex, where the leg is represented on the dorsal and medial part of the cortex, the trunk and arm in its middle portion and the face most inferiorly. Since the size of the area of cortical representation reflects the density of the peripheral innervation and hence complexity of the function being performed rather than the area of the receptive field, there is a good deal of distortion of the body image in the cortex, the cortical representation of the face and hand being much greater than that of the limbs and trunk.

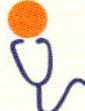

Clinical Features

1 Lesions of the sensory pathway most commonly occur in the internal capsule following some form of cerebrovascular accident. If complete, these result in a total hemianaesthesia of the opposite side of the body. In partial lesions the area of sensory loss will be determined by the site of the injury/ischaemia in the internal capsule and, from a knowledge of the sensory (and motor) loss, it is usually possible to determine with some degree of accuracy the site of a lesion in the capsule.

2 Since there is modality segregation below the decussation of the medial lemniscus, lesions of the sensory pathways at cord level result in dissociation of sensation, with an area of analgesia contralaterally together with impairment of tactile sensibility ipsilaterally (for further details, *see* pages 217–218).

The auditory, visual and olfactory pathways are dealt with later under the appropriate cranial nerves.

Motor pathways (Fig. 6.6)

It is customary to divide the motor pathways of the brain and spinal cord into pyramidal and extrapyramidal systems. Although the latter is an imprecise term, it nevertheless provides a useful collective term for the many motor structures not confined to the pyramidal tracts in the medulla.

Pyramidal tract

The pyramidal system is the main 'voluntary' motor pathway and derives its name from the fact that projections to the motor neurones in the spinal cord are grouped together in the medullary pyramids. The fibres in this pathway arise from a wide area of the cerebral cortex. About two-thirds derive from the motor and premotor cortex of the frontal lobes; however, about one-third arise from the primary somatosensory cortex. In both the motor and premotor cortex there is an organization comparable to that seen in the sensory area. Again, the body is inverted so that the 'leg area' is situated in the dorsomedial part of the precentral gyrus encroaching on the medial surface of the hemisphere, supplied by the anterior cerebral artery. The 'face area' is near the lateral sulcus, while the 'arm area' occupies a central position, both supplied by the middle cerebral artery. Again, the body image is greatly distorted; the areas representing the hand, lips, eyes and foot are exaggerated out of proportion to the rest of the body and in accordance with the complexity of the tasks they perform.

From the cortex, the motor fibres pass through the posterior limb of the *internal capsule* (Fig. 6.4) where they are again organized in the sequence of 'face, arm, leg', anteroposteriorly. From the internal capsule the fibres form a compact bundle that occupies the central third of the cerebral peduncle. From there they pass through the ventral pons, where they are broken up into a number of small bundles between the cells of the *pontine nuclei* and the transversely disposed *pontocerebellar fibres*. Near the lower end of the pons they again collect to form a single bundle, which comes to lie on the ventral surface of the medulla and forms the elevation known as the 'pyramid'. As it passes through the brainstem, the pyramidal system gives off, at regular intervals, contributions to the somatic and branchial arch efferent nuclei of the cranial nerves. Most of these *corticobulbar fibres* cross over in the brainstem, but many of the cranial nerve nuclei are bilaterally innervated.

Near the lower end of the medulla the great majority of the pyramidal tract fibres cross over to the opposite side and come to occupy a central position in the lateral white column of the spinal cord. This is the so-called '*crossed pyramidal tract*' shown in Fig. 6.12. A small proportion of the fibres of the medullary pyramid, however, remain uncrossed until they reach the segmental level at which they finally terminate. This is the *direct* or *uncrossed pyramidal tract*, which runs downwards close to the anteromedian fissure of the cord, with fibres passing from it at each segment to the opposite side.

In view of the frequent involvement of the pyramidal tract in cerebrovascular accidents, its blood supply is listed here in some detail:

- **Motor cortex:** Leg area: anterior cerebral artery; face and arm areas: middle cerebral artery
- **Internal capsule:** Branches of the middle cerebral artery
- **Cerebral peduncle:** Posterior cerebral artery
- **Pons:** Pontine branches of basilar artery
- **Medulla:** Anterior spinal branches of vertebral artery
- **Spinal cord:** Segmental branches of anterior and posterior spinal arteries.

Extrapyramidal motor system

This should, by definition, include all those motor projections that do not pass physically through the medullary pyramids. It was once thought to control movement in parallel with and, to a large extent, independently of the pyramidal motor system and the pyramidal/extrapyramidal division was used clinically to distinguish between two motor syndromes: one characterized by spasticity and paralysis whereas the other involved involuntary movements, or immobility without paralysis. It is now clear that many 'extrapyramidal' structures, particularly the *basal ganglia*, actually control movement by altering activity in the premotor cortex and, thus, the pyramidal motor projections. This clearly emphasizes the blur between the two systems.

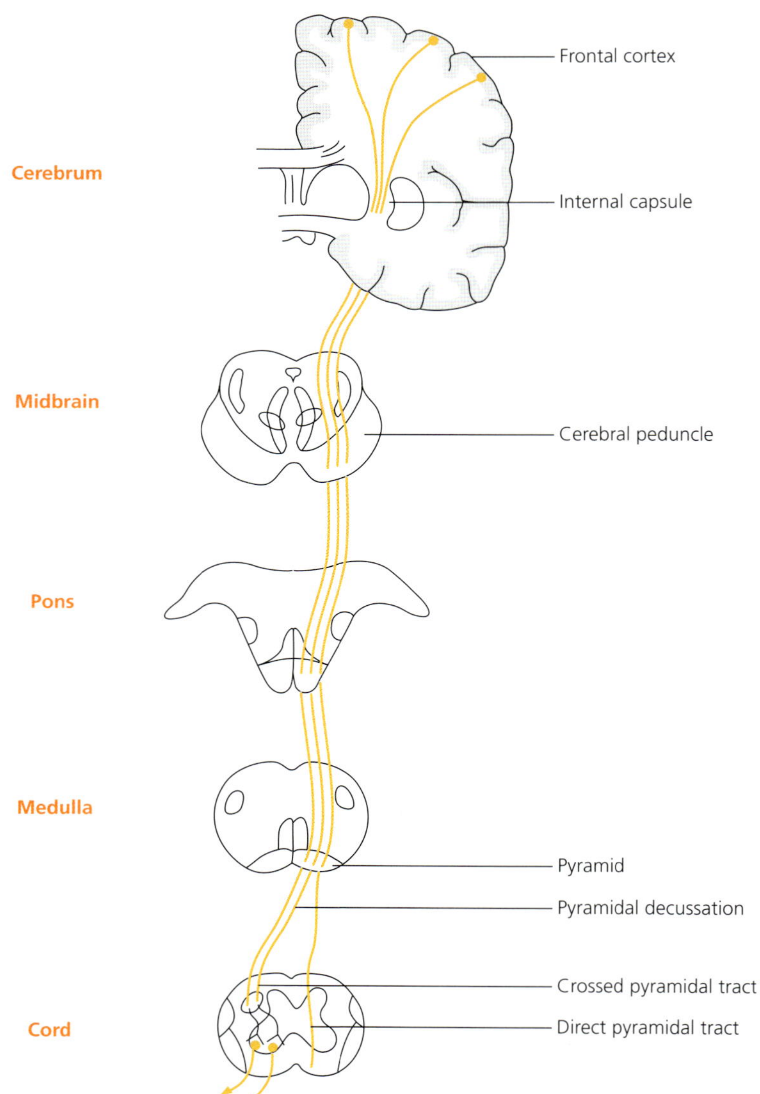

Figure 6.6 The long descending pathway of the pyramidal tract.

Components of the extrapyramidal system include the red nuclei, vestibular nuclei, superior colliculus and reticular formation in the brainstem, all of which project via discrete pathways to influence spinal cord motor neurones. Cerebellar projections (*see* page 207) are also included since they influence not only these brainstem motor pathways but also the motor cortex itself via the dentatothalamic projection.

Perhaps the most important structures to retain an extrapyramidal definition are the basal ganglia (*see* pages 211 and 212). The neostriatum (caudate and putamen) receives widespread cortical afferents, including those from high-order sensory association and motor areas, and projects mainly to the globus pallidus. The latter nucleus is the major outflow for the basal ganglia and, via the ventral anterior thalamus, exerts its major influence on premotor and hence the motor cortices. This pattern of connections suggests that the basal ganglia are involved in complex aspects of motor control, including motor planning and the initiation of movement.

A variety of motor disorders are associated with basal ganglia pathology and, in some instances, neuroanatomically discrete deficits in specific neurotransmitters. For example, Parkinson's disease involves the degeneration of dopaminergic neurones in the substantia nigra in the midbrain. This pigmented nucleus provides the neostriatum with a dense dopaminergic innervation which may be completely lost in severe cases of Parkinsonism. Knowledge of this selective chemical neuropathology has resulted in the development of a treatment of the disease which involves the oral administration of the dopamine precursor l-dopa.

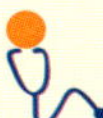

Clinical Features

1 It is important to remember that, in the motor cortex, movements are represented rather than individual muscles; lesions of this pathway result in paralysis of voluntary movement on the opposite side of the body, although the muscles themselves are not paralysed and may cause involuntary movements. This

(Continued ...)

(... *continued*)

is the essential difference between an 'upper motor neurone' lesion (i.e. a lesion of the central motor pathway) and a 'lower motor neurone' lesion (i.e. a lesion affecting the cranial nerve nuclei, or the anterior horn cells or their axons). In both types of lesion muscular paralysis results; in the latter, reflex activity is abolished and flaccidity and muscular atrophy follow, whereas, in pyramidal lesions, there is spasticity, increased tendon reflexes and an extensor plantar response.

2 Experimental lesions strictly confined to the pyramidal tract are not followed by increased muscular tone in the affected part (spasticity), but clinically this is a feature of upper motor neurone lesions; it is attributable to concomitant involvement of the extrapyramidal system, hence demonstrating the oversimplification of the pyramidal and extrapyramidal concept.

3 The pyramidal tract is most frequently involved in cerebrovascular accidents where it passes through the internal capsule. Indeed, the artery supplying this area – the largest of the perforating branches of the middle cerebral artery – has been termed the *artery of cerebral haemorrhage*.

4 A list of the more important related signs is given here for involvement of the pyramidal tract at each level.

  a *Cortex* – Isolated lesions may occur here, resulting in loss of voluntary movement in, say, only one contralateral limb, but often the sensory cortex is also involved. Aphasia in dominant hemisphere lesions (usually left), involving Broca's and Wernicke's areas and the cortex between them, is not uncommon.

  b *Internal capsule* – Usually all parts of the tract are involved, giving a complete contralateral hemiplegia with associated sensory loss. The lesion may extend back to involve the visual radiation, giving a contralateral homonymous field defect (hemianopia).

  c *Cerebral peduncle and midbrain* – The fibres from the IIIrd nerve are often concomitantly involved so that there are the associated signs of a IIIrd nerve palsy.

  d *Pons* – Here the VIth nerve is often involved, alone or together with the VIIth cranial nerve. There may then be a hemiplegia affecting the arm and leg of the opposite side, an ipsilateral facial palsy of the lower motor neurone type and failure to abduct the ipsilateral eyeball.

  e *Medulla* – Because of the proximity of the pyramids to one another, medullary lesions often affect both sides of the body. Paralysis of the tongue on the side of the lesion is due to involvement of the XIIth nerve or its nucleus. The respiratory, vasomotor and swallowing centres may also be affected.

  f *Spinal cord* – The paralysis following lesions of the spinal cord is ipsilateral and accurately depends on the level at which the pyramidal tract is involved. Lower motor neurone lesion signs can be detected at the level of the spinal trauma (direct injury) and upper motor neurone lesion signs below. The proximity of the pyramidal tracts to the ascending sensory pathways accounts for the concomitant sensory changes which are usually found.

Membranes of the brain and spinal cord (the meninges)

Three concentrically arranged membranes, known as meningeal layers or meninges, surround the brain and spinal cord. From outside in, these three layers are the dura mater, arachnoid mater and pia mater.

The *dura* is a dense membrane which, within the cranium, is often described as being made up of two layers. This description requires some qualification. The so-called outer layer of the dura is intimately adherent to the inner surface of the skull; the inner layer, which is the true dural layer, is for the most part fused with the outer layer except where the two layers are separated by the *intracranial dural venous sinuses* and where the inner layer projects inwards to form four, prominent, reduplicated sheets (Fig. 5.31):

- The falx cerebri
- The falx cerebelli
- The tentorium cerebelli
- The diaphragma sellae

These dural reduplications serve to compartmentalize the cranial cavity and act as partitions between different parts of the brain, thereby performing the hugely important function of minimizing the considerable torsional stresses to which the brain is normally subjected.

The *arachnoid* is a delicate membrane applied, throughout, to the inner surface of the dura, and separated from the dura by the potential *subdural space*.

The *pia* is closely moulded to the surface of the brain and spinal cord. It dips down into all the cerebral sulci. The interval between the pia mater and the overlying arachnoid is termed the *subarachnoid space*. This space contains cerebrospinal fluid and is traversed by trabeculae of fine fibrous strands that run from the arachnoid to the pia.

Ventricular system and the cerebrospinal fluid circulation

The ventricles of the brain comprise two lateral ventricles, one in each cerebral hemisphere, 3rd ventricle in diencephalon and 4th ventricle in hindbrain. The ventricles are connected to each other and to the central canal of the spinal cord.

The CSF is formed by the secretory activity of the epithelium covering the choroid plexuses in the lateral, 3rd and 4th ventricles; it circulates through the ventricular system of the brain and drains into the subarachnoid space from the roof of the 4th ventricle before being reabsorbed into the dural venous system.

The general appearance of the ventricular system is indicated in Fig. 6.7. The two *lateral ventricles*, which are by far the largest components of the system, occupy a considerable part of the cerebral hemispheres. Each has an *anterior horn* (in front of the interventricular foramen), a *body*, above and medial to the body of the caudate nucleus, a *posterior horn* in the occipital lobe and an *inferior horn* reaching down into the temporal lobe. The choroid plexuses of the lateral ventricles, which are responsible for the production of most of the CSF, extend from the inferior horn, through the body, to the interventricular foramen where they become continuous with the plexus of the 3rd ventricle (Fig. 6.2).

The *3rd ventricle* is a narrow midline slit-like cavity between the two halves of the diencephalon. Thus the upper part of the 3rd ventricle lies between the two halves of the thalamus, while the lower part of the ventricle is between the two halves of the hypothalamus. The floor of the 3rd ventricle is formed, from front to back, by the optic chiasma, tuber cinereum, infundibulum and mamillary bodies. The hypothalamus

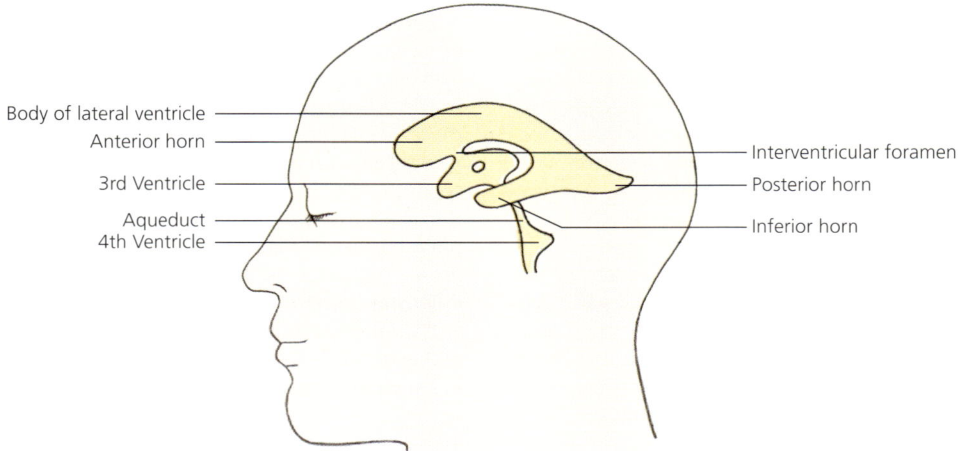

Figure 6.7 The ventricular system.

thus contributes to both the lateral wall and floor of the 3rd ventricle. From the 3rd ventricle the CSF passes through the narrow *cerebral aqueduct* (*of Sylvius*) in the midbrain to reach the 4th ventricle.

The *4th ventricle* is diamond-shaped when viewed from above and tent-shaped as seen from the side. Its floor is formed caudally by the medulla and rostrally by the pons. Its roof is formed by the cerebellum and the superior and inferior medullary vela. The CSF escapes from the 4th ventricle into the subarachnoid space by way of the *median* and *lateral apertures* (of *Magendie* and *Luschka*, respectively) and then flows over the surface of the brain and spinal cord.

In certain areas the subarachnoid space is considerably enlarged to form distinct *cisterns*. The most important of these are the *cisterna magna* between the cerebellum and the dorsum of the medulla; the *cisterna pontis* over the ventral surface of the pons; the *interpeduncular cistern* between the two cerebral peduncles; the *cisterna ambiens* between the splenium of the corpus callosum and the superior surface of the cerebellum (containing the great cerebral vein and the pineal gland); and the *chiasmatic cistern* around the optic chiasma. Re-absorption of CSF is principally by way of the superior sagittal sinus and to a lesser extent by the other dural venous sinuses, the modified arachnoid of the *arachnoid granulations* piercing the dura and bringing the CSF into direct contact with the sinus mesothelium. Along the superior sagittal sinus, these granulations (or *arachnoid villi*) clump together to form the *Pacchionian bodies*, which produce the pitted erosions readily seen along the median line of the inner aspect of the skull cap.

About one-fifth of the CSF is absorbed along similar spinal villi or escapes along the nerve sheaths into the lymphatics.

Clinical Features

1 Computed tomography (CT scanning) has quite revolutionized the investigation of intracranial space-occupying lesions (post-traumatic haematoma, abscesses and neoplasms), both by delineating the lesion itself and by demonstrating displacement of the ventricular system. Figures 6.8 and 6.9 are representative

(Continued ...)

(... continued)

transverse cuts through the skull to illustrate normal anatomical features; note that the details of the anatomy of the ventricles are clearly visualized.

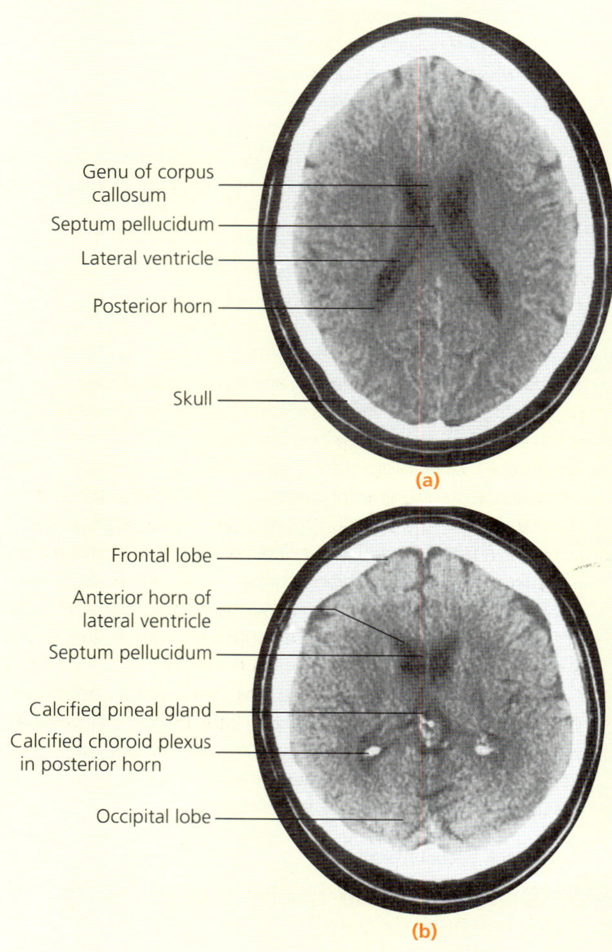

Figure 6.8 (a) Computed tomography (CT) scan of the skull through the level of the bodies of the lateral ventricles. **(b)** CT scan cut through the level of the anterior horns of the lateral ventricles.

(Continued ...)

(... *continued*)

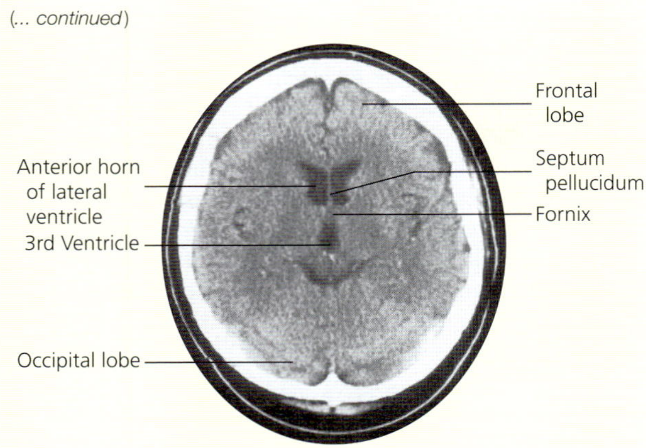

Figure 6.9 Computed tomography (CT) scan cut through the level of the 3rd ventricle.

2 Magnetic resonance imaging (MRI) is particularly valuable in producing high-quality images of the central nervous system (Fig. 6.10).

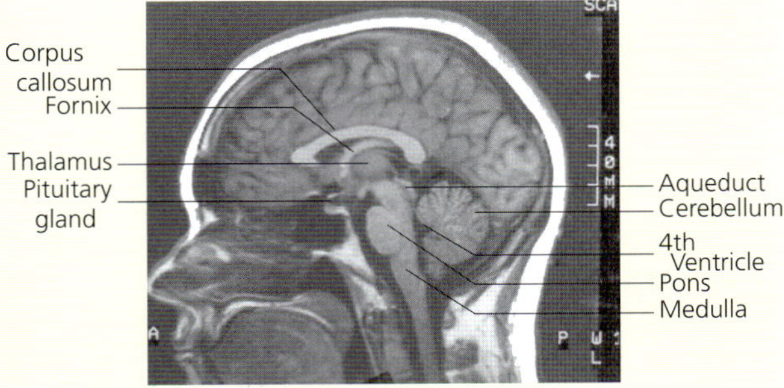

Figure 6.10 Magnetic resonance imaging (MRI) sagittal section of the head. Note the fine details of brain structure which can be visualized by this technique.

3 The CSF serves several purposes, including the provision of a protective water-jacket and a regulating mechanism of intracranial pressure with changing cerebral blood flow.

4 The total capacity of the CSF in the adult is about 150 mL, of which some 25 mL is contained within the spinal theca; it is normally under a pressure of about 100 mm of water (with a range of 80–180) in the lateral horizontal position. The dural theca acts as a simple hydrostatic system, so that, when the patient sits up, the CSF pressure in the lumbar theca rises to between 350 and 550 mm, whereas the ventricular fluid pressure falls to below atmospheric.

5 Certain parts of the CSF pathway are narrow and easily obstructed. These sites are the interventricular foramina, the 3rd ventricle, the aqueduct, the exit foramina of the 4th ventricle and the subarachnoid space around the midbrain in the tentorial notch. Obstruction to the system causes increased intracranial pressure and ventricular dilatation (*hydrocephalus*).

6 The meningeal coverings, together with the subarachnoid space, are prolonged along the optic nerve. Raised CSF pressure is transmitted along this space and may compress the venous drainage of the eye, thus producing *papilloedema*. This swelling of the optic disc can be detected by ophthalmoscopic examination of the fundus.

7 Lumbar puncture – *see* page 220.

This absorption of CSF is passive, depending on its hydrostatic pressure being higher than that of the venous blood.

Spinal cord

The spinal cord is a long cylindrical part of the central nervous system located in the vertebral canal. It is 18 in. (45 cm) long. It is continuous above with the medulla oblongata at the level of the foramen magnum and ends below at the level of the lower border of the 1st lumbar vertebra. Inferiorly, it tapers into the *conus medullaris*, from which a prolongation of pia mater, the *filum terminale*, descends to be attached to the back of the coccyx.

The cord is somewhat flattened pasteroanteriorly, making it oval in cross section. It bears a deep longitudinal *anterior fissure*, a narrower *posterior septum* and, on either side, a *posterolateral sulcus* along which the *posterior (sensory) nerve roots* are serially arranged (Fig. 6.11).

These posterior roots each bear a *ganglion*, which constitutes the first cell-station of the sensory nerves (*see* Fig. 6.37).

The *anterior (motor) nerve roots* emerge serially along the anterolateral aspect of the cord on either side. Both the anterior and posterior nerves arise by a series of rootlets from the cord.

At each intervertebral foramen the anterior and posterior nerve roots unite to form a *spinal nerve* that immediately divides into its *anterior* and *posterior primary rami*, each transmitting both motor and sensory fibres.

The length of the roots increases progressively from above downwards owing to the disparity between the length of the cord and the vertebral column; the lumbar and sacral roots below the termination of the cord at vertebral level L2 continue as a leash of nerve roots termed the *cauda equina*.

Structure (Fig. 6.11)

In transverse section of the cord is seen the *central canal* around which is the 'H'-shaped *grey matter*, surrounded in turn by the *white matter*, which contains the long ascending and descending tracts.

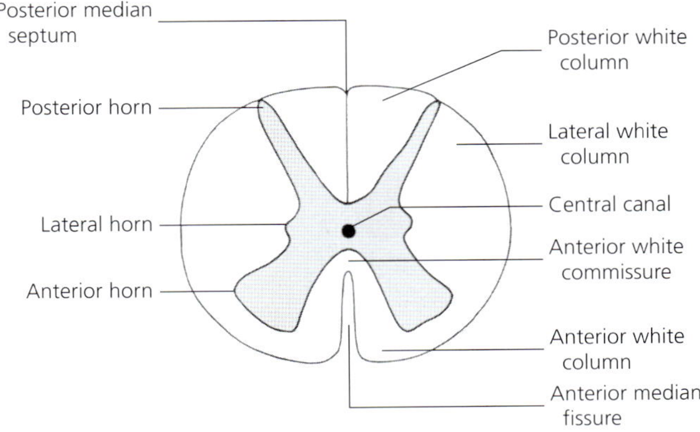

Figure 6.11 The spinal cord – transverse section through a thoracic segment.

Within the *posterior horns* of the grey matter, capped by the *substantia gelatinosa*, terminate many of the sensory fibres entering from the posterior nerve roots. In the large *anterior horns* lie the motor cells that give rise to the fibres of the anterior roots.

In the thoracic and upper lumbar cord are found the *lateral horns* on each side, containing the cells of origin of the sympathetic system.

The more important long tracts in the white matter will now be dealt with.

Descending tracts (Fig. 6.12)

The two major descending tracts are pyramidal and direct pyramidal.

1. *The pyramidal (lateral cerebrospinal* or *crossed motor) tract.* The motor pathway commences at the pyramidal cells of the motor cortex, decussates in the medulla, then descends in the pyramidal tract on the contralateral side of the cord. At each spinal segment, fibres enter the anterior horn and connect up with the motor cells there – the tract therefore becomes progressively smaller as it descends.
2. *The direct pyramidal (anterior cerebrospinal* or *uncrossed motor) tract* is a small tract descending without medullary decussation. At each segment, however, fibres pass from it to the ventral horn (anterior) motor cells of the opposite side.

Ascending tracts (Fig. 6.12)

The two major ascending tracts comprise posterior and anterior spinocerebellar tracts, lateral and anterior spinothalamic tracts and posterior spinal columns.

1. The *posterior* and *anterior spinocerebellar tracts* ascend on the same side of the cord and enter the cerebellum through the inferior and superior cerebellar peduncles, respectively.
2. The *lateral* and *anterior spinothalamic tracts.* Pain and temperature fibres enter the posterior roots, ascend a few segments, relay in the substantia gelatinosa, then cross to the opposite side to ascend in these tracts to the thalamus, where they are relayed to the sensory cortex.
3. The *posterior columns* comprise a medial and lateral tract, termed, respectively, the *fasciculus gracilis* (*of Goll*) and *fasciculus cuneatus* (*of Burdach*). They convey 1st order sensory fibres subserving fine touch, vibration sense and proprioception (position sense), mostly uncrossed, to the gracile and cuneate nuclei in the medulla where, after synapse, the 2nd order fibres decussate, pass to the thalamus and, after further synapse, 3rd order fibres are relayed to the sensory cortex. Some fibres pass from the medulla to the cerebellum along the inferior cerebellar peduncle.

Blood supply

The *anterior* and *posterior spinal arteries* descend in the subarachnoid space from the intracranial part of the vertebral artery. They are reinforced serially by spinal branches from the ascending cervical, the cervical part of the vertebral, the posterior intercostal arteries and the lumbar arteries.

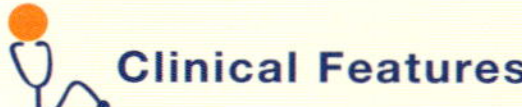

1 Complete transection of the cord is followed by total loss of sensation in the regions supplied by the cord segments below the level of injury together with flaccid muscle paralysis. As the cord distal to the section recovers from a period of spinal shock, the paralysis becomes spastic, with exaggerated reflexes. Voluntary sphincter control is lost but reflex emptying of bladder and rectum subsequently return, provided that the cord centres situated in the sacral zone of the cord are not destroyed.

2 Destruction of the centre of the cord, as occurs in *syringomyelia* and in some intramedullary tumours, first involves the decussating spinothalamic fibres so that initially there is bilateral loss of pain and temperature sense below the lesion; proprioception and fine touch are preserved until late in the uncrossed posterior columns.

3 Hemisection of the cord is followed by the *Brown-Séquard syndrome*; there is paralysis on the affected side below the lesion (pyramidal tract) and also loss of proprioception and fine discrimination (dorsal columns). Pain and temperature senses are lost on the *opposite* side below the lesion, because the affected spinothalamic tract carries fibres which have decussated below the level of cord hemisection.

(*Continued ...*)

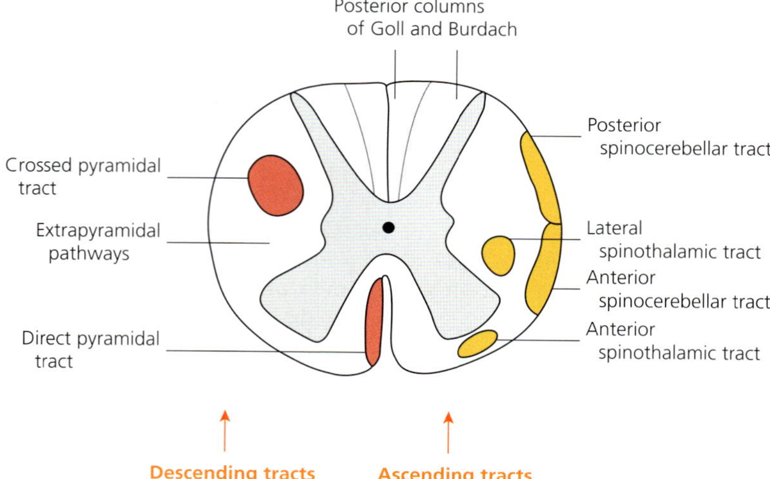

Figure 6.12 The location of the important spinal tracts. (The descending tracts are shown on the left and the ascending tracts on the right.)

(... *continued*)

4 *Tabes dorsalis*, which is a syphilitic degenerative lesion of the posterior columns and posterior nerve roots, is characterized by loss of proprioception; the patient becomes ataxic, particularly if he closes his eyes, because he has lost his position sense for which he can partially compensate by visual knowledge of his spatial relationship (Romberg's sign).
5 Intractable pain can be treated in selected cases by cutting the appropriate posterior nerve roots (*posterior rhizotomy*) or by division of the spinothalamic tract on the side opposite the pain (cordotomy). A knife passed 0.125 in. (3 mm) into the cord anterior to the denticulate ligament and then swept anteriorly from this point will sever the spinothalamic tract but preserve the pyramidal tract lying immediately posterior to it.
6 *Cauda equina syndrome* is the term for a condition in which there is extrinsic compression of the nerve roots which make up the cauda equina. The cause is usually a prolapsed intervertebral disc (at L4–L5 level or L5–S1 level). The condition may also be caused by tumours or trauma. Less common causes include arteriovenous malformations in the spinal canal, abscesses and haematomas. The clinical presentation of the condition includes urinary and/or recto-anal dysfunction, saddle anaesthesia, lower limb motor weakness and low back pain.

Age differences

Up to the 3rd month of foetal life the spinal cord occupies the full extent of the vertebral canal. The vertebrae then outpace the cord in the rapidity of their growth so that, at birth, the cord reaches the level of only the 3rd lumbar vertebra (Fig. 6.13).

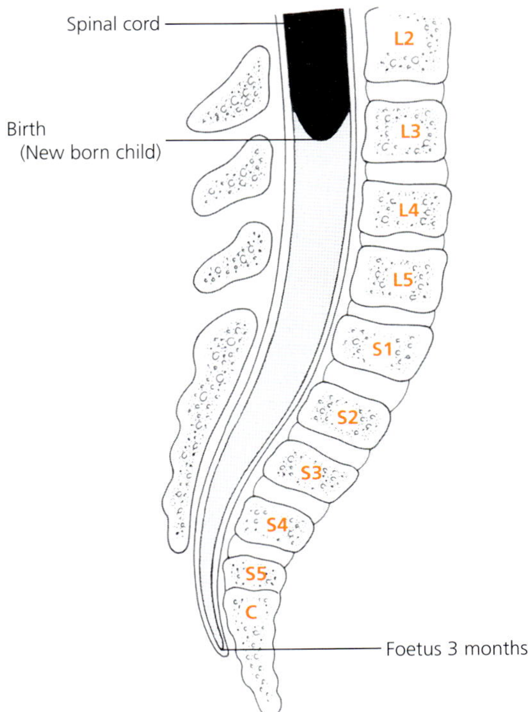

Figure 6.13 The relationship between the spinal cord and the vertebrae in the 3-month foetus and in the newborn child.

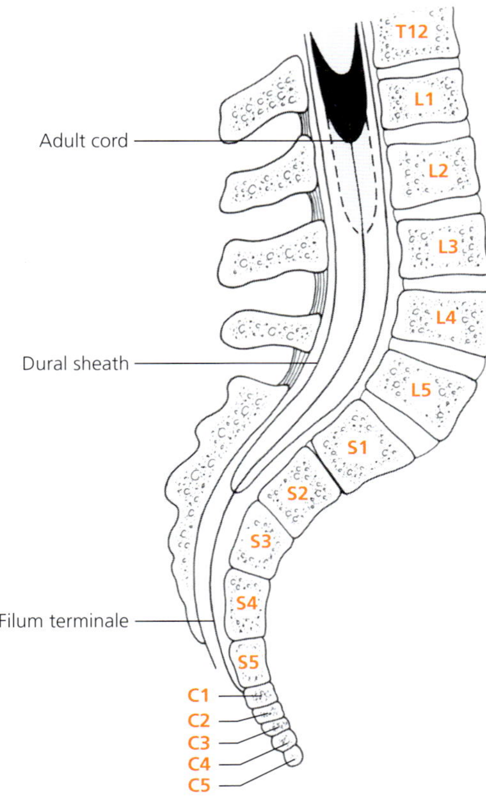

Figure 6.14 The range of variation in the termination of the spinal cord in the adult.

Further differential growth up to the time of adolescence brings the cord to its definitive position at the approximate level of the disc between the 1st and 2nd lumbar vertebrae (Fig. 6.14).

Membranes of the cord (the meninges)

(Fig. 6.15)

The spinal cord, like the brain, is closely ensheathed by the *pia mater*. This is thickened on either side between the nerve roots to form the *denticulate ligament*, which passes laterally to adhere to the dura. Inferiorly, the pia continues as the *filum terminale*, which pierces the distal extremity of the dural sac and becomes attached to the coccyx.

The *arachnoid mater* lines the *dura mater*, leaving an extensive *subarachnoid space*, containing CSF, between it and the pia. Both pia and arachnoid are continued along the spinal nerve roots.

The dura itself forms a tough sheath to the cord. It ends distally at the level of the 2nd sacral vertebra. It also continues along each nerve root and blends with the sheaths of the peripheral nerves.

The *extradural* (or *epidural*) *space* is the compartment between the dural sheath and the spinal canal. It extends downwards from the foramen magnum (above which the dura becomes two-layered) to the sacral hiatus. It is filled with semiliquid fat and contains lymphatics (although there are no lymphatics within the nervous system deep to the dura), together with arteries and large, thin-walled veins. These can be considered equivalent to the cerebral venous sinuses which lie between the two layers of cerebral dura.

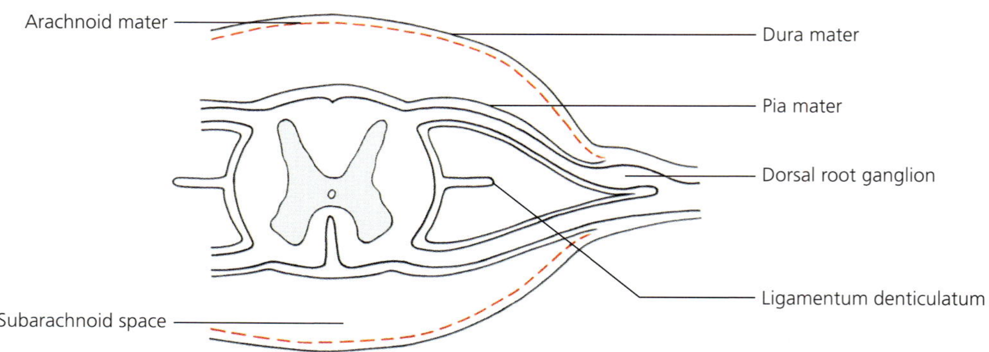

Figure 6.15 The membranes of the spinal cord.

Whereas the arteries of this space are relatively insignificant, the extradural veins form a rich network of intercommunicating vessels termed the internal vertebral venous plexus. This plexus receives the *basivertebral veins*, which emerge from the posterior aspect of each vertebral body. In addition, the internal vertebral venous plexus links up with both the pelvic veins below and the cerebral veins above – thereby allowing a pathway for the spread of both bacteria and tumour cells. This accounts, for example, for the ready spread of prostatic cancer to the sacrum and vertebrae (*Batson's 'valveless vertebral venous plexus'*), the spread of aggressive carcinomas of the breast to the thoracic vertebrae and the spread of follicular cancers of the thyroid to the cervical vertebrae.

Clinical Features

Lumbar puncture to withdraw CSF from the spinal subarachnoid space must be performed well clear of the termination of the cord. A line joining the summits of the iliac crests corresponds to the level of the 4th lumbar vertebra (Fig. 2.1) and therefore the intervertebral spaces immediately above or below this landmark can be used with safety. The spine must be fully flexed (with the patient either seated or lying in the left or right lateral position) so that the vertebral interspinous spaces are opened to their maximal extent (Fig. 6.16). The needle is passed inwards and somewhat cranially exactly in the midline and at right angles to the spine; the supraspinous and interspinous ligaments are traversed and then the dura is penetrated, the latter with a distinct 'give'. Occasionally, root pain is experienced if a root of the cauda equina is impinged upon, but usually these float clear of the needle.

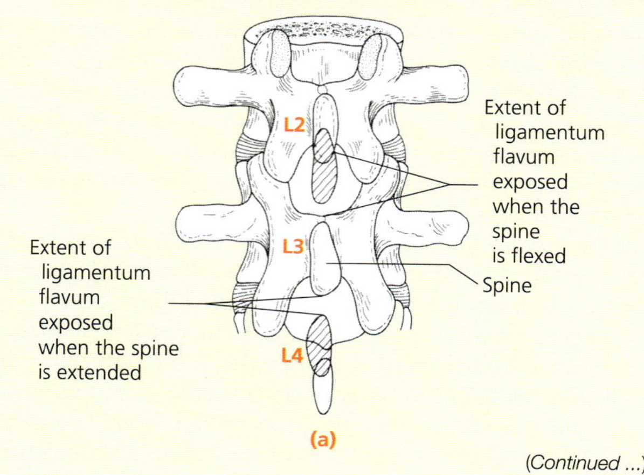

(Continued ...)

(... continued)

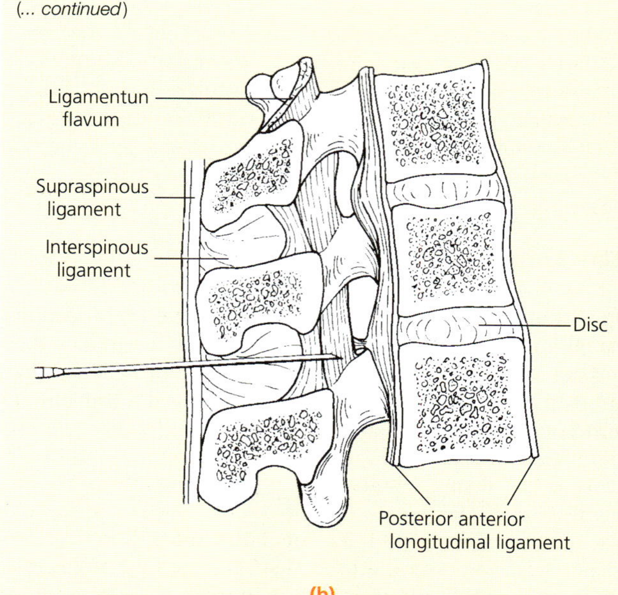

Figure 6.16 (a) The lumbar interlaminar gap when the spine is flexed; this anatomical fact makes lumbar puncture possible. The locations of the spines of L2 and L4 in. the extended position are shown cross-hatched. **(b)** The anatomy of lumbar puncture.

At spinal puncture CSF can be obtained for examination; antibiotics, radio-opaque contrast medium or anaesthetics may be injected into the subarachnoid space, and the CSF pressure can be estimated (normal, when lying on the side, 80–180 mm CSF). A block in the subarachnoid space above the point of puncture, produced, for example, by a spinal tumour, can be revealed by *Queckenstedt's test* as follows.

Pressure is applied to the neck in order to compress the internal jugular veins; this reduces venous outflow from the cranium and raises the intracranial pressure. Consequently, CSF is displaced into the spinal sac and the CSF pressure, as determined by lumbar puncture and manometry, rises briskly by at least 40 mm. This rise in pressure is not seen if a block is present in the subarachnoid space.

Extradural block. The extradural space can be entered by a needle passed either between the spinal laminae or via the sacral hiatus (caudal or sacral anaesthesia, *see* page 78).

Cranial nerves

Just as the 31 pairs of spinal nerves are regarded as the peripheral nerves of the spinal cord, so may the 12 pairs of cranial nerves be considered the peripheral nerves of the brain. The name of each cranial nerve suggests either the main function of the nerve or some characteristic anatomical feature of the nerve. It is also conventional to refer to the 12 cranial nerves by Roman numerals. Thus, cranial nerve I (olfactory nerve) is the uppermost one to emerge from the brain, and cranial nerve XII (hypoglossal nerve) the lowermost. Cranial nerves I and II are generally regarded as extensions of the forebrain, while the remaining cranial nerves (III–XII) originate in, and emerge from, the brainstem.

Clinically it is helpful to categorize the cranial nerves into one or other of the following three groups (as this classification determines the approach to the clinical testing of the cranial nerve): (1) exclusively sensory (cranial nerves I, II, VIII); (2) exclusively motor (cranial nerves III, IV, VI, XI, XII) and (3) mixed motor and sensory (V, VII, IX, X).

Olfactory nerve (I)

The fibres of the olfactory nerve, unlike other afferent fibres, are unique in being the central processes of the olfactory cells and not the peripheral processes of a central group of ganglion cells.

The central processes of the olfactory receptors pass upwards from the olfactory mucosa in the upper part of the superior nasal concha and septum, through the cribriform plate of the ethmoid bone to end by synapsing with the dendrites of mitral cells in the olfactory bulb. The mitral cells in turn send their axons back in the olfactory tract to terminate in the cortex of the uncus, the adjacent inferomedial temporal cortex and the region of the anterior perforated space. The further course of the olfactory pathway is uncertain in man, but it is now clear that the hippocampus–fornix system is not directly concerned with olfaction.

Optic nerve (II) and the visual pathway

(For a description of the eye itself, *see* the section on special senses, page 234.)

Clinical Features

1 The sense of smell is not highly developed in man and is easily disturbed by conditions affecting the nasal mucosa generally (e.g. the common cold). However, *unilateral anosmia* may be an important sign in the diagnosis of frontal lobe tumours. Tumours in the region of the uncus may give rise to the so-called 'uncinate' type of fit, characterized by olfactory hallucinations associated with impairment of consciousness and involuntary chewing movements.

2 *Bilateral anosmia* due to interruption of the olfactory nerve may occur after head injuries, particularly in association with anterior cranial fossa fractures, when leakage of CSF through the cribriform plate may present as rhinorrhoea.

The optic nerve is the nerve of vision. It is not a true cranial nerve but should be thought of as a brain tract that has become drawn out from the cerebrum. Embryologically, it is developed, together with the retina, as a lateral diverticulum of the forebrain. Devoid of neurilemmal sheaths, its fibres, like other brain tissues, are incapable of regeneration after division.

From a *functional* point of view, the retina can be regarded as consisting of three cellular layers: a layer of receptor cells – the *rods* and *cones*; an intermediate layer of *bipolar cells*; and a layer of *ganglion cells*, whose axons form the optic nerve (Fig. 6.17). From all parts of the retina these axons converge on the *optic disc*, whence they pierce the sclera to form the optic nerve.

The optic nerve passes backwards and medially to the optic foramen, through which it reaches the optic groove on the dorsum of the body of the sphenoid. Here, all the fibres from the medial half of the retina (i.e. those concerned with the temporal visual field) cross over in the *optic chiasma* to the optic tract of the opposite side, while the fibres from the lateral half of the retina (nasal visual field) pass back in the optic tract of the same side. The great majority of the fibres in the optic tract end in the *lateral geniculate body* of the thalamus. From the lateral geniculate body the fibres of the optic radiation sweep laterally to the temporal lobe before passing backwards to the occipital visual cortex (the striate area surrounding the calcarine fissure) where they terminate in such a way that the upper and lower halves of the retina are represented on the upper and lower lips of the fissure, respectively (Figs 6.3 and 6.18).

However, a small proportion of fibres in the optic tract, subserving pupillary, ocular and head and neck reflexes, bypass the geniculate body to reach the superior colliculus and pretectal nucleus of the midbrain. From the pretectal nucleus, fibres connect with the Edinger–Westphal nucleus of both sides. This pathway explains the direct and consensual pupillary response.

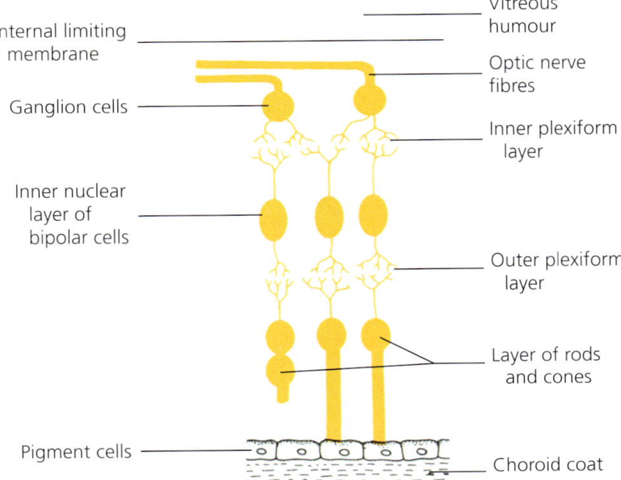

Figure 6.17 The layers of the retina.

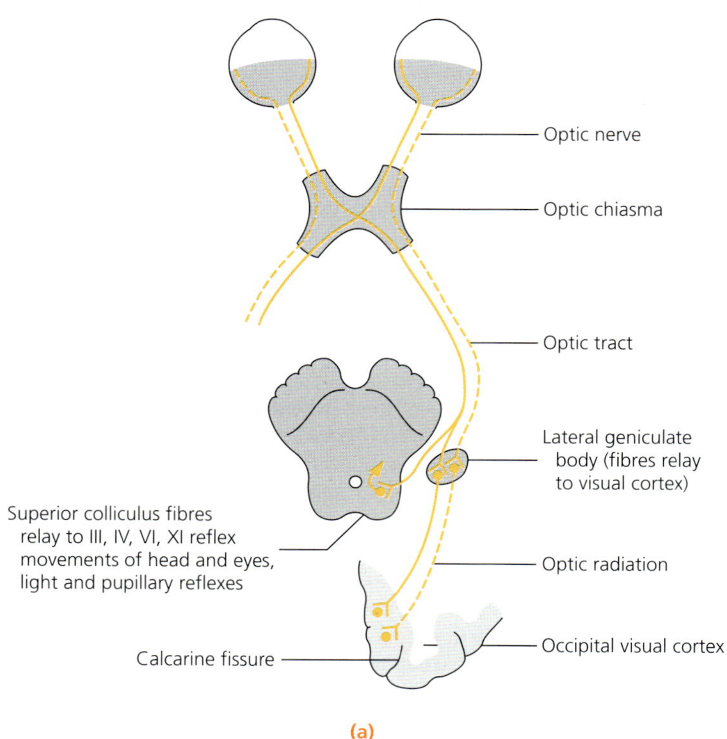

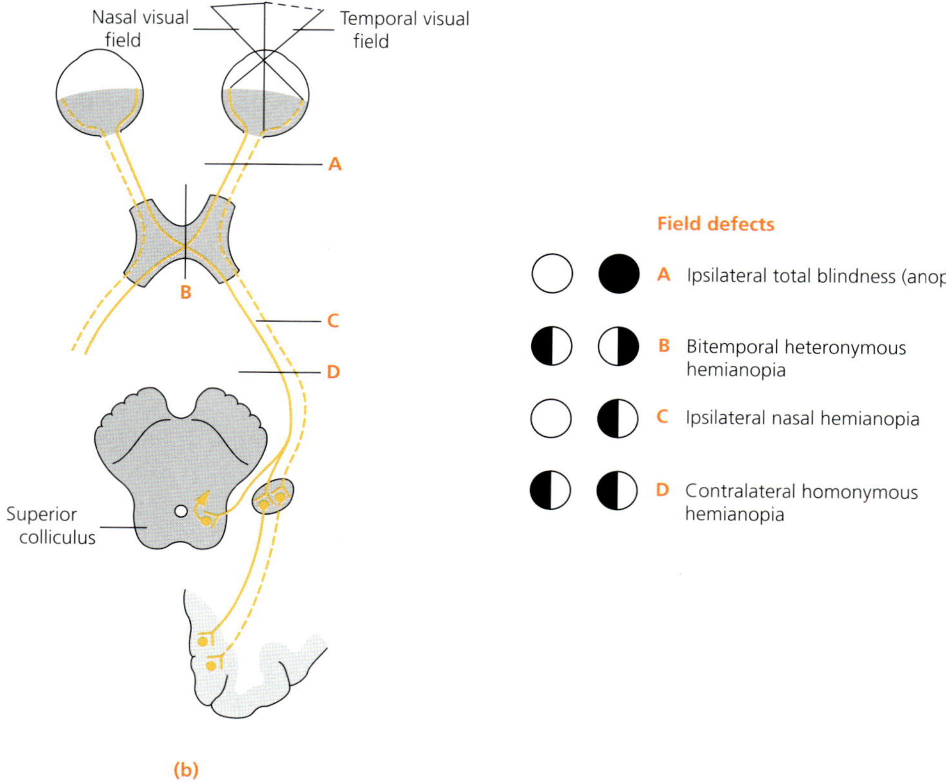

Figure 6.18 **(a)** The optic pathway. **(b)** Scheme of field defects. **A–D** denote sites of interruption of the visual pathway.

Clinical Features

1 Lesions of the retina or optic nerve result in *ipsilateral blindness* in the affected segment, but lesions of the optic tract and central parts of the visual pathway result in contralateral *homonymous defects*. Similarly, lesions of the optic chiasma (e.g. from an expanding pituitary tumour) will give rise to a *bitemporal hemianopia* (*tunnel vision*), i.e. there will be a loss of vision in both temporal eye-fields.

2 The lesion responsible for the *Argyll Robertson pupil* is thought to be in the vicinity of the pretectal area. The pupil is constricted, does not respond to light but responds to accommodation; there is no satisfactory explanation why the pupillary reaction to light should be abolished while the convergence–accommodation reflex is preserved. It is classically seen in syphilis affecting the CNS.

Oculomotor nerve (III)

In addition to supplying most of the extrinsic eye muscles, the oculomotor nerve conveys the preganglionic parasympathetic fibres for the sphincter of the pupil via the ciliary ganglion. Its nucleus of origin lies in the midbrain and consists essentially of two components: the *somatic efferent nucleus*, which supplies the extrinsic ocular muscles, and the *Edinger–Westphal nucleus*, from which the preganglionic parasympathetic fibres are derived. The former is referred to as the *main oculomotor nucleus*, and the latter is termed the *accessory oculomotor nucleus*.

From these nuclei, fibres pass vertically through the midbrain tegmentum to emerge just medial to the cerebral peduncle. Passing forwards between the superior cerebellar and posterior cerebral arteries, the nerve pierces the dura mater to run in the lateral wall of the cavernous sinus (Fig. 6.19) as far as the superior orbital fissure. Before entering the fissure it divides into a superior and inferior branch; both branches enter the orbit through the tendinous ring from which the recti arise (*see* Fig. 6.23). The superior branch passes lateral to the optic nerve to supply the superior rectus muscle and levator palpebrae superioris; the inferior branch supplies three muscles, the medial rectus, the inferior rectus and the inferior oblique, the nerve to the last conveying the parasympathetic fibres to the ciliary ganglion.

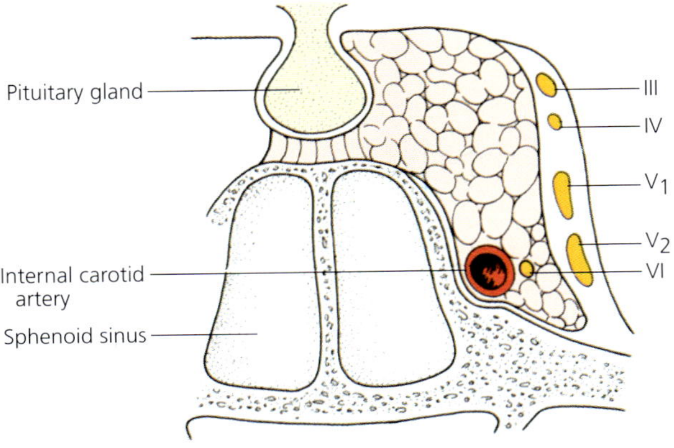

Figure 6.19 The cavernous sinus – showing the relations of the IIIrd, IVth, Vth and VIth cranial nerves.

Ciliary ganglion

This small but important ganglion lies near the apex of the orbit just lateral to the optic nerve. It receives, in addition to the preganglionic parasympathetic fibres from the Edinger–Westphal nucleus, a sympathetic (postganglionic) root ultimately from the plexus on the internal carotid artery, and a sensory root from the nasociliary nerve (a branch of the ophthalmic division of the trigeminal nerve). Of these fibres, only the *parasympathetic* synapse in the ganglion, the others pass directly through it. The postganglionic efferent fibres from the ganglion pass to the ciliary muscle and the muscles of the iris by way of about 10 *short ciliary nerves*. Stimulation results in pupillary constriction and in accommodation of the lens. The sympathetic and sensory fibres are, respectively, vasoconstrictor and pupillodilator, and sensory to the globe of the eye.

(Note that the majority of sympathetic dilator pupillae nerve fibres are transmitted to the eye in the long ciliary branches of the nasociliary nerve.)

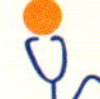

Clinical Features

Complete division of the IIIrd nerve results in a characteristic group of signs:

- *Ptosis* – Due to paralysis of the levator palpebrae superioris
- A *divergent squint* – Due to the unopposed action of the superior oblique and lateral rectus muscles, rotating the eyeball laterally
- *Dilatation of the pupil* – The dilator action of the sympathetic fibres being unopposed
- *Loss of the accommodation–convergence* and *light reflexes* – Due to constrictor pupillae paralysis
- Diplopia (*double vision*)

Trochlear nerve (IV)

The trochlear nerve is the most slender of the cranial nerves and supplies only one eye muscle, the *superior oblique*.

Emerging on the dorsum of the pons (being the only cranial nerve to arise from the dorsal aspect of the brainstem), the nerve winds round the cerebral peduncle and then passes forwards between the superior cerebellar and posterior cerebral arteries to pierce the dura. It then runs forwards in the lateral wall of the cavernous sinus (Fig. 6.19) between the oculomotor and ophthalmic nerves to enter the orbit through the superior orbital fissure, lateral to the tendinous ring from which the recti take origin. It then passes medially over the optic nerve to enter the superior oblique muscle.

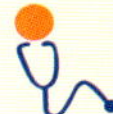

Clinical Features

A lesion of the trochlear nerve results in paralysis of the superior oblique muscle, resulting in diplopia that occurs when the patient attempts to look downwards and laterally. This can be remembered as 'the *tramp's nerve*' – it makes the eye go 'down and out'!

Trigeminal nerve (V) (Figs 6.20 and 6.21)

The trigeminal nerve is the largest cranial nerve. As the name suggests, this nerve consists of three divisions. Together they supply sensory fibres to the greater part of the skin of the head and face, the mucous membranes of the mouth, nose and paranasal air sinuses and, by way of a small motor root, the muscles of mastication. In addition it is associated with four autonomic ganglia, the ciliary, pterygopalatine, otic and submandibular.

Trigeminal ganglion

This ganglion, which is also termed the *semilunar ganglion*, is equivalent to the dorsal sensory ganglion of a spinal nerve. It is crescent-shaped and is situated within an invaginated pocket of dura in the middle cranial fossa. It lies near the apex of the petrous temporal bone, which is somewhat hollowed for it. The motor root of the trigeminal nerve and the greater superficial petrosal nerve both pass deep to the ganglion. Above lies the hippocampal gyrus of the temporal lobe of the cerebrum; medially lies the internal carotid artery and the posterior part of the cavernous sinus. The trigeminal ganglion represents the first cell-station for all sensory fibres of the trigeminal nerve except those subserving proprioception.

V_1: Ophthalmic division (Fig. 6.21)

This is the smallest division of the trigeminal nerve; it is wholly sensory and is responsible for the innervation of the skin of the forehead, the upper eyelid, cornea and most of the nose. Passing forwards from the trigeminal ganglion, it immediately enters the lateral wall of the cavernous sinus where it lies beneath the trochlear nerve (Fig. 6.19). Just before entering the orbit it divides into three branches, frontal, lacrimal and nasociliary.

The *frontal nerve* runs forwards just beneath the roof of the orbit for a short distance before dividing into its two terminal branches, the *supratrochlear* and *supra-orbital nerves*, which supply the upper eyelid and the scalp as far back as the lambdoid suture.

The *lacrimal nerve* supplies the lacrimal gland (with post-ganglionic parasympathetic fibres from the pterygopalatine ganglion which reach it by way of the maxillary nerve) and the lateral part of the conjunctiva and upper lid.

The *nasociliary nerve* gives branches to the ciliary ganglion, the eyeball, cornea and conjunctiva, the medial half of the upper eyelid, the dura of the anterior cranial fossa, and to the mucosa and skin of the nose.

V_2: Maxillary nerve (Fig. 6.21)

The maxillary nerve is also purely sensory. Passing forwards from the central part of the trigeminal ganglion, close to the cavernous sinus, it leaves the skull by way of the *foramen rotundum* and emerges into the upper part of the pterygopalatine fossa. Here, it gives off a number of branches before continuing through the inferior orbital fissure and the infra-orbital canal as the *infra-orbital* nerve, which supplies the skin of the cheek and lower eyelid.

The maxillary nerve has the following named branches:

1. The *zygomatic nerve*, whose zygomaticotemporal and zygomaticofacial branches supply the skin of the temple and cheek, respectively
2. *Superior alveolar (dental) branches* to the teeth of the upper jaw
3. The *branches from the pterygopalatine ganglion*, which run a descending course and are distributed as follows: the *greater* and *lesser palatine nerves*, which pass through the

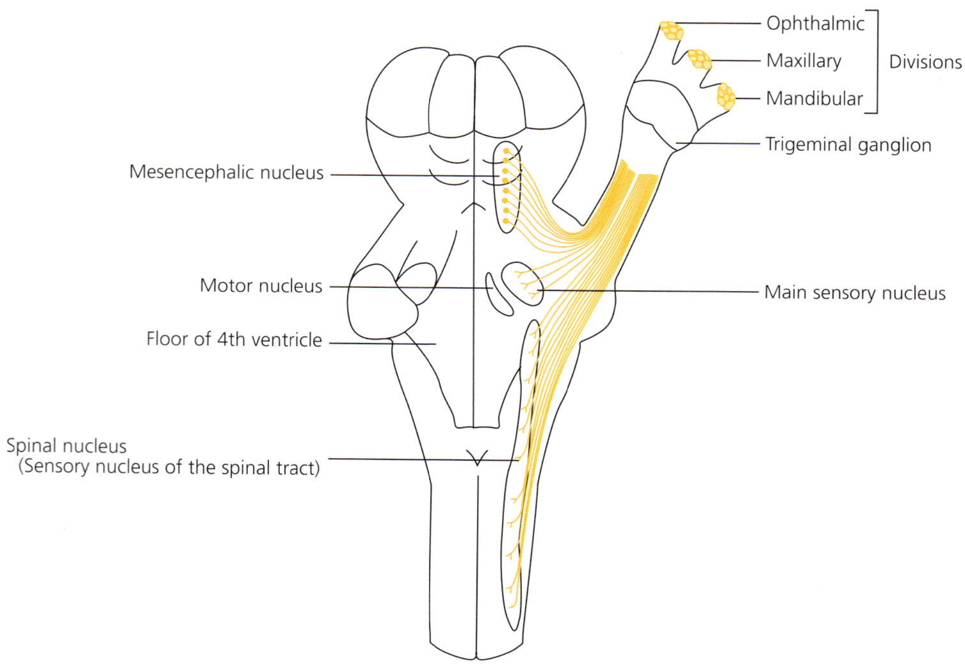

Figure 6.20 Plan of the trigeminal nerve and its nuclei in dorsal view.

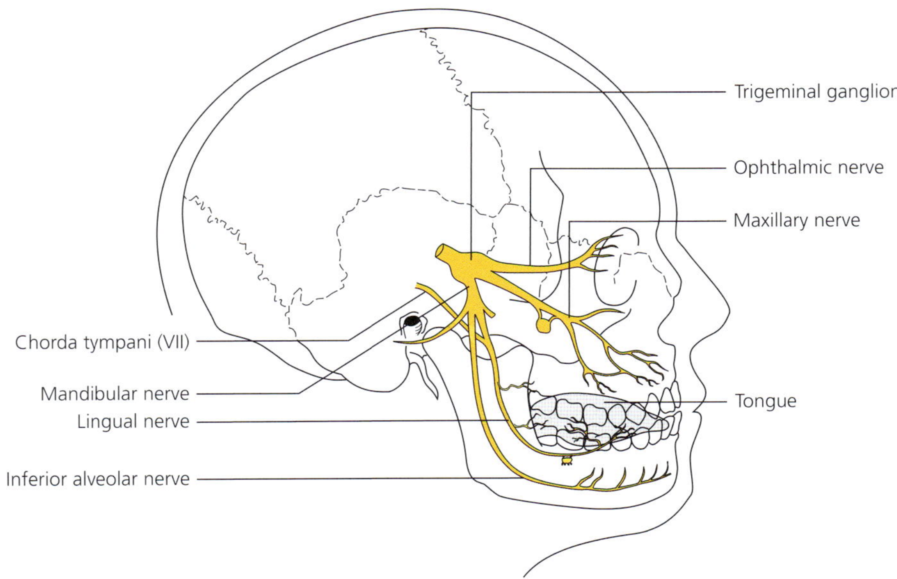

Figure 6.21 Distribution of the trigeminal nerve.

corresponding palatine foramina to supply the mucous membrane of the hard and soft palates, the uvula and the tonsils, and the mucous membrane of the nose, and a *pharyngeal branch* supplying the mucosa of the nasopharynx. The *nasopalatine nerve* (long sphenopalatine) supplies the nasal septum then emerges through the incisive canal of the hard palate to supply the gum behind the incisor teeth. The *posterior superior lateral nasal nerves* (short sphenopalatine) supply the posterosuperior lateral wall of the nose

Pterygopalatine ganglion

Associated with the maxillary division of V as it lies in the pterygopalatine fossa is the relatively large pterygopalatine ganglion. This receives its parasympathetic or secretomotor root from the greater superficial petrosal branch of VII, its *sensory* component from two pterygopalatine branches of the maxillary nerve and its *sympathetic* root from the internal carotid plexus. Its parasympathetic efferents pass to the lacrimal gland through a communicating branch to the lacrimal nerve. Parasympathetic efferents from the pterygopalatine ganglion are also distributed to the mucous and serous glands of the nose, palate and paranasal sinuses. Sensory and sympathetic (vasoconstrictor) fibres are distributed to nose, nasopharynx, palate and orbit.

V_3: Mandibular nerve (Fig. 6.21)

This is the largest of the three divisions of the trigeminal nerve and the only one to convey motor fibres. In addition to supplying the skin of the temporal region, part of the auricle and the lower face, the mucous membrane of the anterior two-thirds of the tongue and the floor of the mouth, it also conveys the motor root to the muscles of mastication and secretomotor fibres to the salivary glands.

Passing forwards from the trigeminal ganglion, it almost immediately enters the foramen ovale through which it reaches the infratemporal fossa. Here, it divides into a small anterior and a larger posterior trunk, but before doing so it gives off the *nervus spinosus* to supply the dura mater and the *nerve to the medial pterygoid muscle* from which the *otic ganglion* is suspended and through which motor fibres are transmitted to tensor palati and tensor tympani.

The *anterior trunk* gives off the following:

1. A sensory branch, the *buccal nerve*, which supplies part of the skin of the cheek and the mucous membrane on its inner aspect.
2. Motor branches to the masseter, temporalis and lateral pterygoid muscles.

The *posterior trunk*, which is principally sensory, divides into the following three branches:

1. The *auriculotemporal nerve*, which conveys sensory fibres to the skin of the temple and auricle and secretomotor fibres from the otic ganglion to the parotid gland.
2. The *lingual nerve*, which passes downwards under cover of the ramus of the mandible to the side of the tongue (Fig. 5.12), where it supplies the mucous membrane of the floor of the mouth, the anterior two-thirds of the tongue (including the taste buds by way of fibres which join it from the chorda tympani), and the sublingual and submandibular salivary glands.
3. The *inferior alveolar* (*dental*) *nerve*, which passes down into the mandibular canal and supplies branches to the teeth of the lower jaw. A side branch, *the mental nerve*, emerges from the mental foramen to supply the outer gingiva of the lower jaw, skin of the chin and lower lip. The inferior alveolar nerve is the only branch of the posterior trunk that carries motor fibres. These motor fibres are conveyed in the nerve to mylohyoid, a branch of the inferior alveolar nerve given off before the latter enters the mandibular foramen. The *nerve to the mylohyoid* supplies the muscle of that name and the anterior belly of the digastric.

Otic ganglion

The otic ganglion is unique among the four ganglia associated with the trigeminal nerve in having a motor as well as parasympathetic, sympathetic and sensory components. It lies immediately below the foramen ovale medial to the trunk of the mandibular nerve.

Its *parasympathetic* fibres reach the ganglion by the lesser superficial petrosal branch of the glossopharyngeal nerve; these relay in the ganglion and pass via the auriculotemporal nerve to the parotid gland, and are its secretomotor supply. The *sympathetic* fibres are derived from the superior cervical ganglion along the plexus which surrounds the middle meningeal artery, while the *sensory* fibres arrive from the auriculotemporal nerve; they are, respectively, vasoconstrictor and sensory to the parotid gland.

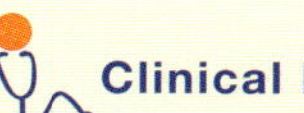

Clinical Features

1 Section of the whole trigeminal nerve results in ipsilateral anaesthesia of the face and anterior part of the scalp, the auricle and the mucous membranes of the nose, mouth and anterior two-thirds of the tongue, together with paralysis and wasting of the ipsilateral muscles of mastication. Lesions of individual divisions of the trigeminal nerve give rise to corresponding sensory deficits in the area of distribution of the affected nerve. Injury to the mandibular division will result in sensory and motor deficits.

2 *Trigeminal neuralgia* may affect any one or more of the three divisions, giving rise to the characteristic acute, lancinating, episodic pain over the appropriate area (Fig. 6.22).

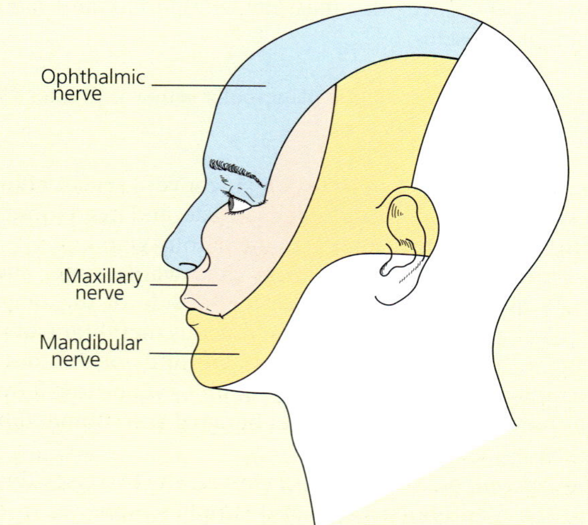

Figure 6.22 Areas of the face and scalp supplied by the three divisions of the trigeminal nerve.

3 Pain is frequently referred from one segment to another. Thus, a patient with a carcinoma of the tongue (lingual nerve) frequently complains bitterly of earache (auriculotemporal nerve). The classical description of such a case is an old gentleman sitting in the outpatients department spitting blood and with a piece of cotton wool in his ear.

Motor fibres pass through the ganglion from the nerve to the medial pterygoid (a branch of the mandibular nerve) and supply the tensor tympani and tensor palati muscles.

Submandibular ganglion

This is suspended from the lower aspect of the lingual nerve. Its *parasympathetic* supply is derived from the chorda tympani branch of the facial nerve (*see* Fig. 6.24) by which it is conveyed to the lingual nerve. It carries the secretomotor supply to the submandibular and sublingual salivary glands.

Sympathetic fibres are transmitted from the superior cervical ganglion via the plexus on the facial artery and supply vasoconstrictor fibres to these same two salivary glands. The *sensory* component is contributed by the lingual nerve itself, which provides sensory fibres to these salivary glands and also to the mucous membrane of the floor of the mouth.

Central connections of the trigeminal nerve

The central processes of the trigeminal ganglion cells enter the lateral aspect of the pons and divide into ascending and descending branches, which terminate in one or other component of the sensory nucleus of V (Fig. 6.20). This nucleus consists of three parts, each of which appears to subserve different sensory modalities: a chief sensory nucleus in the pontine tegmentum concerned with touch; a descending, or spinal, nucleus subserving pain and temperature; and a mesencephalic nucleus receiving proprioceptive afferents. The *motor root of the trigeminal nerve* lies just medial to the sensory nucleus in the upper part of the pons; its efferents pass out with the sensory fibres and are distributed by way of the mandibular division of the nerve.

Abducent nerve (VI)

The abducent nerve has the longest intracranial course. Like the trochlear nerve, the abducent nerve supplies only one extrinsic ocular muscle, the *lateral rectus*. Its nucleus lies in the pons and from there its fibres emerge on the base of the brain at the junction of the pons and medulla. The nerve then passes forwards to enter the cavernous sinus (Fig. 6.19). Here, it lies lateral to the internal carotid artery and medial to the IIIrd, IVth and Vth nerves. Passing through the tendinous ring just below the IIIrd nerve, it enters the orbit to pierce the deep surface of the lateral rectus (Fig. 6.23).

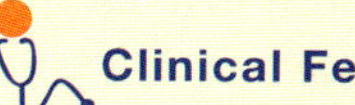

Clinical Features

On account of its long intracranial course, the VIth nerve is frequently involved in injuries to the base of the skull. When damaged, it gives rise to diplopia and a convergent squint. The patient is unable to deviate the affected eye laterally.

Facial nerve (VII)

In addition to supplying the muscles of facial expression, the facial nerve conveys secretomotor fibres to the sublingual and submandibular salivary glands and the lacrimal gland as well as to the nasal mucosa; it also carries taste fibres from the anterior two-thirds of the tongue.

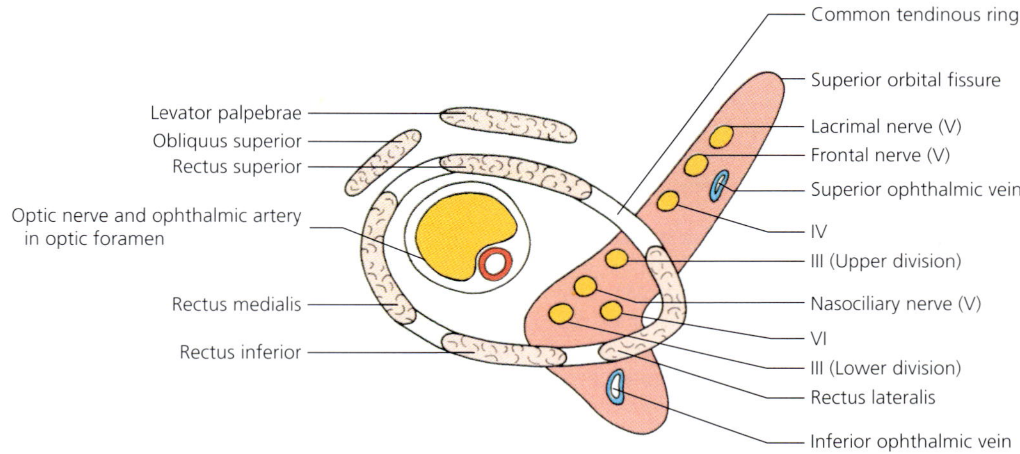

Figure 6.23 The superior orbital fissure and tendinous ring of origin of the extrinsic orbital muscles, showing the relations of the cranial nerves as they enter the orbit (schematic; left orbit viewed from the front).

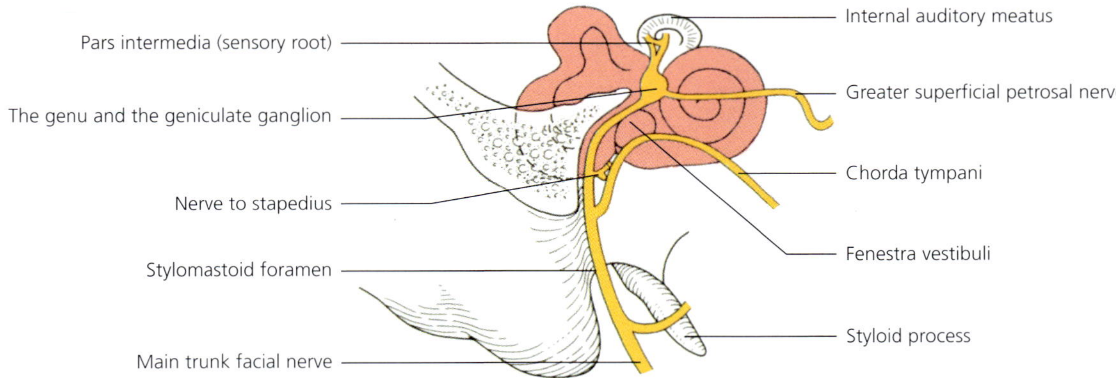

Figure 6.24 Distribution of the facial nerve within the temporal bone.

The fibres innervating the facial muscles have their nucleus of origin in the ventral part of the caudal pons; the secretomotor fibres for the salivary glands are derived from the superior salivary nucleus. The sensory fibres associated with the nerve have their cells of origin in the facial (geniculate) ganglion.

Originating in the motor nucleus, the motor fibres of the facial nerve run a tortuous course within the pons before emerging from the lateral aspect of the pons together with cranial nerve VIII in the cerebellopontine angle.

The sensory and motor fibres of the facial nerve pass together into the internal auditory meatus, at the bottom of which they leave the VIIIth nerve and enter the facial canal. Here, they run laterally over the vestibule before bending sharply backwards over the promontory of the middle ear. This bend, or *genu of the facial nerve*, as it is called, marks the site of the facial ganglion and the point at which the secretomotor fibres for the lacrimal gland leave to form the greater superficial petrosal nerve. The facial nerve then passes downwards, medial to the middle ear, to reach the stylomastoid foramen (Fig. 6.24).

Just before entering this foramen it gives off the branch, known as the *chorda tympani*, which runs back through the middle ear between the incus and malleus, exits via the fissure between the tympanic and petrous parts of the temporal bone (*petrotympanic fissure*) to enter the infratemporal fossa where it joins the lingual nerve. Hence its taste fibres reach the anterior two-thirds of the tongue and its secretomotor fibres are conveyed to the submandibular ganglion, thence to the submandibular and sublingual salivary glands.

On emerging from the stylomastoid foramen, the nerve supplies the stylohyoid and the posterior belly of digastric muscle. It then enters the parotid gland, where it divides into five divisions for the supply of the muscles of facial expression (*mimetic muscles*): the temporal, zygomatic, buccal, mandibular and cervical branches (Figs 5.24 and 6.25).

Clinical Features

1 It is important to distinguish between '*nuclear*' and '*infranuclear*' *facial palsies* on the one hand and '*supranuclear*' *palsies* on the other. Both nuclear and infranuclear palsies result in a facial

(*Continued ...*)

(... *continued*)

paralysis that is complete and that affects *all* the muscles on one side of the face. In supranuclear palsies there is no involvement of the muscles above the palpebral fissure since the portion of the facial nucleus supplying these muscles receives fibres from both cerebral hemispheres. Furthermore, in such cases the patient may involuntarily use the facial muscles but will be unable to do so on request.

2 *Supranuclear facial palsies* most frequently result from vascular involvement of the corticobulbar pathways, e.g. in cerebral haemorrhage. Nuclear palsies may occur in poliomyelitis or other forms of bulbar paralysis, while infranuclear palsies may result from a variety of causes including compression in the cerebellopontine angle (as by an acoustic neuroma), fractures of the temporal bone and invasion by a malignant parotid tumour. However, by far the commonest cause of infranuclear facial paralysis is *Bell's palsy*, which is generally described as a condition of unknown aetiology. Nevertheless, there is, in many cases, a fairly strong association between Bell's palsy and viral infections (particularly herpes simplex infections and influenza).

When the intracranial part of the nerve is affected or when it is involved in fractures of the base of the skull there is usually loss of taste over the anterior two-thirds of the tongue and an associated loss of hearing (VIIIth nerve damage).

Auditory (vestibulocochlear) nerve (VIII)

The VIIIth nerve consists of two sets of fibres: cochlear and vestibular. The *cochlear fibres* (concerned with hearing) represent the central processes of the bipolar spiral ganglion cells of the cochlea which traverse the internal auditory meatus to reach the lateral aspect of the medulla, at the cerebellopontine angle (together with VII), where they terminate in the *dorsal* and *ventral cochlear nuclei*. The majority of the projection fibres from these nuclei cross to the opposite side, and ascend to reach the *inferior colliculus* and the *medial geniculate body*; from the former, fibres reach the motor nuclei of the cranial nerves and form the pathway of auditory reflexes; from the latter, fibres sweep laterally in the *auditory radiation to the auditory cortex* in the superior temporal gyrus (Fig. 6.3).

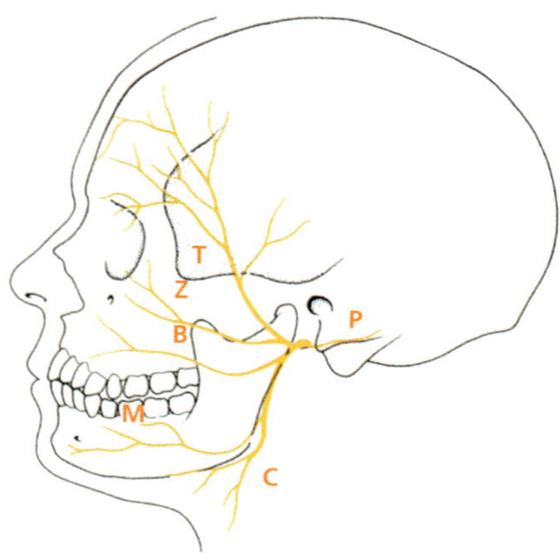

Figure 6.25 Distribution of the facial nerve: B, buccal; C, cervical; M, mandibular; P, posterior auricular branch; T, temporal; Z, zygomatic.

The *vestibular fibres* (concerned with equilibrium) enter the medulla just medial to the cochlear division and terminate in the *vestibular nuclei*. Many of the fibres from these nuclei pass to the cerebellum in the inferior cerebellar peduncle together with fibres bypassing the vestibular nuclei and passing directly to the cerebellum.

Other vestibular connections are to the nuclei of III, IV, VI and XI and to the upper cervical cord (via the vestibulospinal tract). These connections bring the eye and neck muscles under reflex vestibular control.

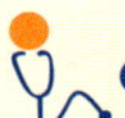

Clinical Features

1 *Lesions of the cochlear division* result in deafness which may, or may not, be accompanied by tinnitus.

The differential diagnosis between middle ear deafness and cochlear (inner ear) or auditory nerve lesions can be made clinically by the use of a tuning fork. Air conduction (the fork being held beside the ear) is normally louder than bone conduction (the fork being held against the mastoid process). If the middle ear is damaged, the reverse will hold true.

2 Apart from injury to the cochlear nerve itself, unilateral lesions of the auditory pathway do not greatly affect auditory acuity because of the bilaterality of the auditory projections.

3 Temporal lobe tumours may give rise to auditory hallucinations if they encroach upon the auditory (superior temporal) gyrus.

4 *Lesions of the vestibular division* of the labyrinth or of the vestibulocerebellar pathway result in vertigo, a subjective feeling of rotation, together with nausea, ataxia and nystagmus.

Glossopharyngeal nerve (IX) (Fig. 5.26)

The glossopharyngeal nerve contains sensory fibres for the pharynx and the posterior one-third of the tongue (including the taste buds), motor fibres for the stylopharyngeus muscle and secretomotor fibres for the parotid gland. It also supplies the carotid sinus (baroreceptor) and carotid body (chemoreceptor). It is attached to the upper part of the medulla by four or five rootlets along the groove between the olive and the inferior cerebellar peduncle (Fig. 6.1(b)) and leaves the skull by way of the jugular foramen in which it gives off its tympanic branch.

Below the jugular foramen, the nerve courses downwards and forwards between the internal carotid artery and the internal jugular vein to reach the styloid process. From here it passes along the stylopharyngeus muscle to enter the pharnyx between the superior and middle constrictors. Here, it breaks up into its terminal branches, which supply the posterior one-third of the tongue and the mucous membrane of the pharynx (including the tonsil).

The *tympanic branch*, which is continued as the *lesser superficial petrosal nerve*, conveys the preganglionic parasympathetic fibres to the otic ganglion (parotid secretomotor fibres).

The only other branch of significance is the *carotid nerve*, which arises just below the skull and runs down on the internal carotid artery to supply both the carotid body and carotid sinus. This small twig serves as the afferent limb of the baroreceptor and chemoreceptor reflexes from the carotid sinus and body, respectively (Fig. 6.26).

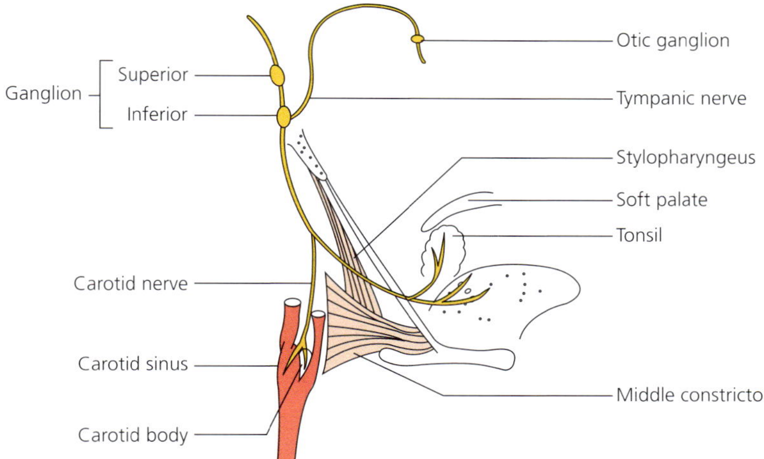

Figure 6.26 The extracranial course of glossopharyngeal nerve.

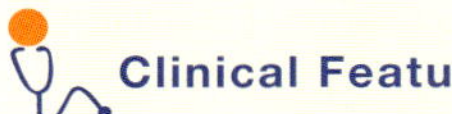

Clinical Features

Complete section of the glossopharyngeal nerve results in sensory loss in the pharynx, loss of taste and common sensation over the posterior one-third of the tongue, some pharyngeal weakness and loss of salivation from the parotid gland. However, such lesions are frequently difficult to detect and rarely occur as isolated phenomena since there is so often associated involvement of the vagus or its nuclei.

Vagus nerve (X)

The vagus is a longest cranial nerve. It has the most extensive distribution of all the cranial nerves, innervating the heart and the major part of the respiratory and alimentary tracts.

Central connections

The *dorsal nucleus* of the vagus in the medulla is a mixed visceral afferent and efferent nucleus. It receives sensory fibres from the heart, the lower respiratory tract and the alimentary tract as far as the distal transverse colon; in addition, it gives rise to preganglionic parasympathetic motor fibres to the heart and to the smooth muscles of the bronchi and gut.

From the *nucleus ambiguus* efferent fibres pass to the striped muscles of the pharynx and larynx.

Distribution

The nerve is connected to the side of the medulla by about 10 filaments that lie in series with the glossopharyngeal nerve along the groove between the olive and the inferior cerebellar peduncle (Fig. 6.1(b)). These filaments unite to form a single bundle that passes beneath the cerebellum to the jugular foramen. Two sensory ganglia are associated with this part of the nerve: a superior, within the jugular foramen, and an inferior, immediately beneath the skull.

The vagus then passes vertically downwards to the root of the neck, lying in the posterior part of the carotid sheath between the internal jugular vein and the internal and then common carotid arteries (Fig. 5.30). There are a number of important branches in the neck: *pharyngeal* to the pharyngeal and palatal musculature by way of the pharyngeal plexus; *superior laryngeal*, supplying the interior of the larynx above the vocal folds and the cricothyroid and inferior constrictor muscles; and the superior and inferior *cardiac branches* which are inhibitory to the heart.

Below the level of the subclavian arteries, the course and relations of the nerve on the two sides differ.

On the *right side*, the *recurrent laryngeal branch* is given off as the vagus crosses the subclavian artery; beyond this, the vagus descends through the superior mediastinum in close association with the great veins. Behind the root of the lung it takes part in the formation of the *pulmonary plexus* and then passes on to the oesophagus to form, with its fellow, the *oesophageal plexus*.

The *left vagus* enters the thorax in close association with the great arteries, lying at first lateral to the common carotid and then crossing the arch of the aorta (Fig. 1.44). The *left recurrent laryngeal branch*, which is given off as the vagus crosses the aortic arch, passes below the ligamentum arteriosum, behind the arch and then ascends in the groove between the trachea and the oesophagus (Fig. 1.40(a)). The vagus then passes behind the root of the lung, enters into the formation of the pulmonary plexus and passes on to the oesophagus to form a plexus from which emerge two trunks, named anterior and posterior vagal trunks, each comprising fibres from both the left and right vagus.

The two vagi then enter the abdomen through the oesophageal opening in the diaphragm, the anterior vagus passing on to the anterior surface and the posterior passing to the posterior aspect of the stomach (Fig. 2.15). Beyond this it is difficult to trace the course of the nerves, but branches are given to the *coeliac*, *hepatic* and *renal plexuses* and, by way of these plexuses, are distributed to the fore- and midgut and to the kidneys.

Clinical Features

1 Isolated lesions of the vagus nerve are uncommon, but it may be involved in injuries or disease of related structures.
2 A simple test for the integrity of the vagus relies on its innervation of the muscles of the palate. In unilateral paralysis, the uvula deviates to the normal side when the patient says 'Ah'.
3 Vagotomy (*See* page 45).
4 Injuries to the recurrent laryngeal nerve (*See* page 176).

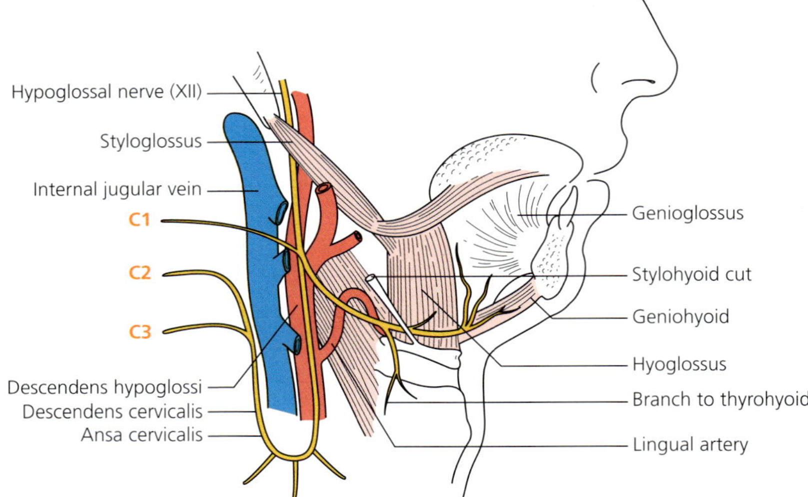

Figure 6.27 The distal course of the hypoglossal nerve.

Accessory nerve (XI) (Figs 5.27 and 6.1(b))

The accessory nerve is conventionally described as having a cranial and a spinal root. According to standard descriptions, the cranial root is formed by a series of rootlets that emerge from the medulla between the olive and the inferior cerebellar peduncle. These rootlets are considered to join the spinal root, travel with it briefly, then separate within the jugular foramen and are distributed with the vagus nerve to supply the musculature of the palate, pharynx and larynx.

A recent, detailed dissection study has demonstrated that all the medullary rootlets that do not join to form the glossopharyngeal nerve (IX) join the vagus nerve at the jugular foramen. All the rootlets that form the accessory nerve arise caudal to the olive and no connections can be demonstrated between the accessory nerve and the vagus in the jugular foramen. Thus, according to this study the accessory nerve has no cranial component and consists only of the structure hitherto referred to as the spinal root of the accessory nerve.

This spinal root is formed by the union of fibres from an elongated nucleus in the anterior horn of the upper five cervical segments, which leave the cord midway between the anterior and posterior roots, join, then pass upwards through the foramen magnum. The accessory nerve and the converging rootlets of the vagus nerve then enter the jugular foramen in a shared sheath of dura. The glossopharyngeal nerve enters the jugular foramen anterior to the vagus through a separate dural sheath.

The accessory nerve passes backwards over the internal jugular vein to the sternocleidomastoid muscle, which it pierces (and supplies), and then crosses the posterior triangle of the neck to enter and supply the deep surface of the trapezius.

Surface marking of the spinal accessory nerve

The extracranial course of the spinal accessory nerve can be marked out by a line which runs from the tragus of the ear to a point at the junction of the middle and lower thirds of the anterior border of the trapezius. This line will be seen to cross the palpable transverse process of the atlas (which lies immediately inferior to the mastoid process) and also the junction of the upper and middle thirds of the posterior border of the sternocleidomastoid muscle. There is, however, a good deal of variation in the precise position of the nerve as it crosses the posterior triangle of the neck.

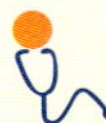

Clinical Features

Division of the accessory nerve results in paresis of the sternocleidomastoid and trapezius muscles. This follows, for example, most block dissections of the lymph nodes of the neck, the nerve being sacrificed in clearing the posterior triangle. The accessory nerve may also be damaged inadvertently during a supraclavicular lymph node biopsy. Great care must be exercised to avoid this complication.

Division of the accessory nerve results in paralysis of sternocleidomastoid and trapezius. Sternocleidomastoid is tested clinically by asking the patient to turn his/her face to the opposite side against the resistance of the examining clinician's hand, while trapezius is tested by asking the patient to elevate his/her shoulder against the resistance applied by the clinician's hand. (A paralysed trapezius results in flattening and drooping of the ipsilateral shoulder.)

Injury to the accessory nerve in the posterior triangle will result in paralysis of trapezius with the sternocleidomastoid being spared.

Hypoglossal nerve (XII)

The hypoglossal nerve is entirely motor and supplies all the intrinsic and extrinsic muscles of the tongue (with the exception of the palatoglossus). From its nucleus, which lies in the floor of the 4th ventricle, a series of about a dozen rootlets leave the side of the medulla in the groove between the pyramid and the olive (Fig. 6.1(b)). These rootlets unite to leave the skull by way of the hypoglossal canal (also known as the anterior condylar canal) in the floor of the posterior cranial fossa just above the lateral margin of the foramen magnum. Lying at first deep to the internal carotid artery and the jugular vein, the nerve passes downwards between these two vessels to just above the level of the angle of the mandible. Here, it passes forwards over the internal and external carotid arteries, and gives off its descending and thyrohyoid branches. It then crosses the hyoglossus and genioglossus muscles to enter the tongue (Fig. 6.27). Its descending branch (*descendens hypoglossi*) actually derives from a twig of the 1st cervical nerve and therefore transmits C1 fibres. It passes more or less vertically downwards upon the internal carotid artery to join the descending cervical nerve (C2 and C3) to form a loop known as the *ansa cervicalis* (or *ansa hypoglossi*) just above the omohyoid muscle. From this loop branches are given to three infrahyoid muscles – sternothyroid, sternohyoid and omohyoid.

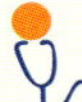

Clinical Features

1 Division of the hypoglossal nerve, or lesions involving its nucleus, result in an ipsilateral paralysis and wasting of the muscles of the tongue. This is detected clinically by deviation of the protruded tongue to the affected side.
2 Supranuclear paralysis (due to an upper motor neurone lesion involving the corticobulbar pathways) leads to paresis but not atrophy of the muscles of the contralateral side.

Special senses

The special senses comprise smell, hearing and balance, sight and taste. They are located in complex receptor organs such as nose, ear, eye and tongue, respectively.

Nose (*See also* 'The paranasal sinuses (accessory nasal sinuses)', page 193)

The *external nose* consists of a bony and cartilaginous framework closely overlaid by skin and fibrofatty tissues. The bones are the two nasal bones and the frontal processes of the maxilla. The *ala* (*the lateral margin*) is composed solely of fatty tissue at its lower free edge.

The *nasal cavity* is divided into right and left halves by a median *nasal septum* formed by the *perpendicular plate* of the *ethmoid bone*, the *septal cartilage* and the *vomer* (Fig. 6.28). Each cavity extends from the nostril (or anterior nares) in front to the posterior nasal aperture behind, communicating through the latter with the nasopharynx. The *lateral wall* is very irregular, owing to the projection of the three *conchae* (superior, middle and inferior) and the underlying meatuses (superior, middle and inferior) (Figs 5.42 and 5.43).

The superior meatus receives the opening of the posterior ethmoidal air cells. Opening into the middle meatus are (from before backwards) the frontal and maxillary sinuses and the anterior and middle ethmoidal air cells. Only the nasolacrimal duct opens, in splendid isolation, into the inferior meatus. The roof of the cavity is horizontal in its central portion, where it is formed by the cribriform plate of the ethmoid, but slopes downwards both anteriorly (the frontal and nasal bones) and posteriorly (the sphenoid). The *floor* corresponds to the roof of the mouth; it comprises the palatine process of the maxilla and the horizontal process of the palatine bone.

Mucous membrane

The *olfactory portion*, which is confined to the superior concha and the adjacent upper part of the septum, is thin and dull yellow in colour; it contains the olfactory receptors and supporting cells. The remaining *respiratory portion* is thick, vascular and moist with secretions of mucous glands; its epithelium is ciliated.

The upper part of the nasal cavity receives its arterial supply from the ethmoidal branches of the ophthalmic artery, a branch of the internal carotid. The sphenopalatine branch of the maxillary artery, a terminal of the external carotid, supplies the lower part of the cavity. Just within the vestibule of the nose, on the antero-inferior part of the septum, it links with a septal branch of the facial artery and it is from this zone, *Little's area*, that 90% of nosebleeds occur. The veins drain downwards into the facial vein and upwards to the ethmoidal tributaries of the ophthalmic veins.

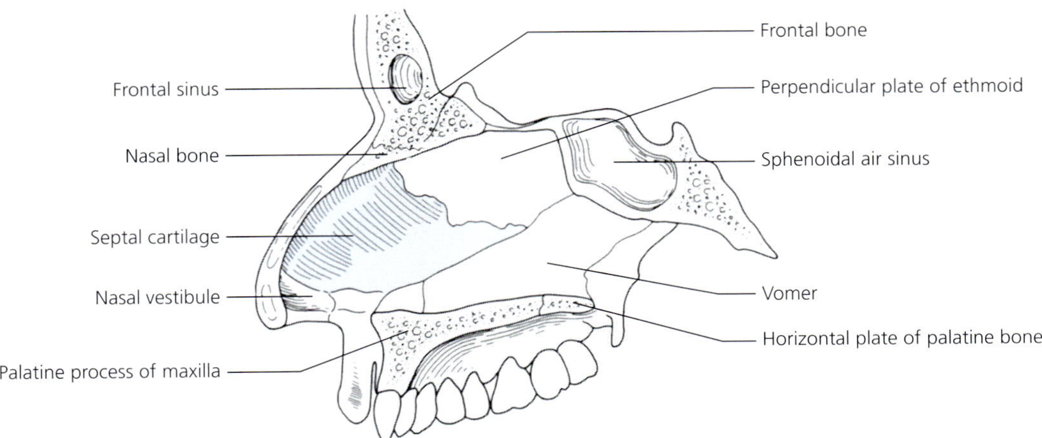

Figure 6.28 The septum of the nose.

Clinical Features

1 The skin of the external nose contains many sebaceous glands and hair follicles that may become blocked and infected. The significance of this fact is that the facial veins, which may become secondarily infected, communicate directly with the ophthalmic veins and hence with the cavernous sinus. For this reason, this zone is often known as the 'danger area of the face'.
2 The extensive relations of the nasal cavity are important in the spread of infection. Observe that it is in direct continuity with (1) the anterior cranial fossa (via the cribriform plate of the ethmoid bone); (2) the nasopharynx and, through the pharyngotympanic tube, the middle ear; (3) the paranasal air sinuses; and (4) the lacrimal apparatus and conjunctiva.
3 The septum is frequently deviated to one or other side, interfering both with inspiration and with drainage of the nose and accessory sinuses.

Ear

The ear is the organ of hearing and balance (equilibrium). It consists of three parts: the external ear, the middle ear and the inner ear.

External ear (Fig. 6.29)

The external ear comprises the auricle and external auditory meatus. The *auricle* (also called pinna) for the most part, consists of a cartilaginous framework to which the skin is closely applied. The intrinsic and extrinsic muscles described for the ear are of no significance in man.

The *external auditory meatus* extends inwards to the tympanic membrane. It is about 1.5 in. (3.7 cm) long, and has a peculiar 'S'-shaped course, being directed first medially upwards and forwards, then medially and backwards and, finally, medially forwards and downwards. The outer third of the canal is cartilaginous and somewhat wider than the medial osseous portion. The whole canal is lined by skin, which is closely adherent to the

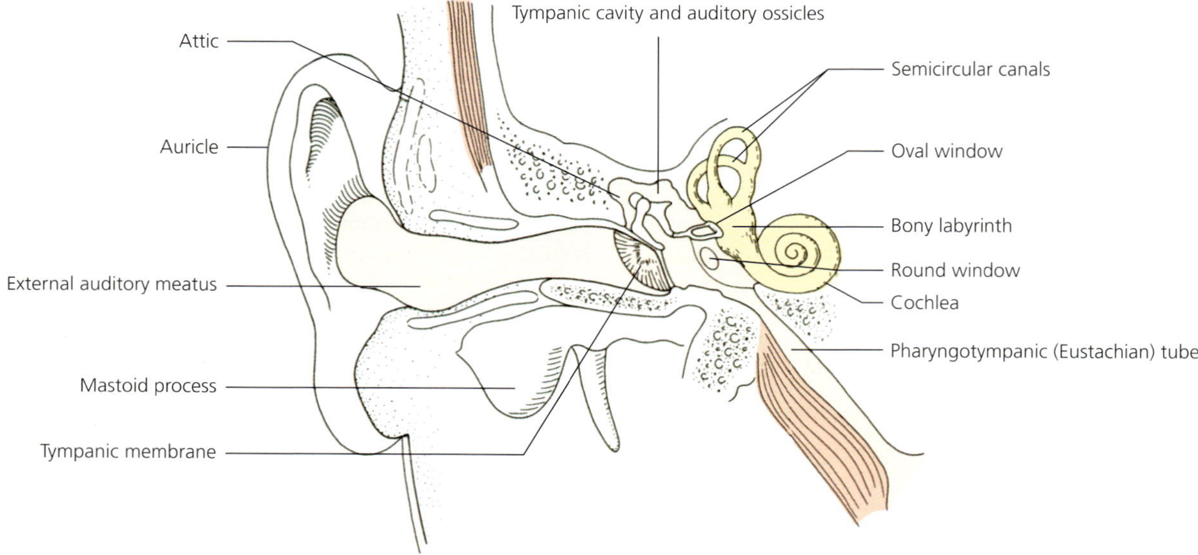

Figure 6.29 General view of the ear.

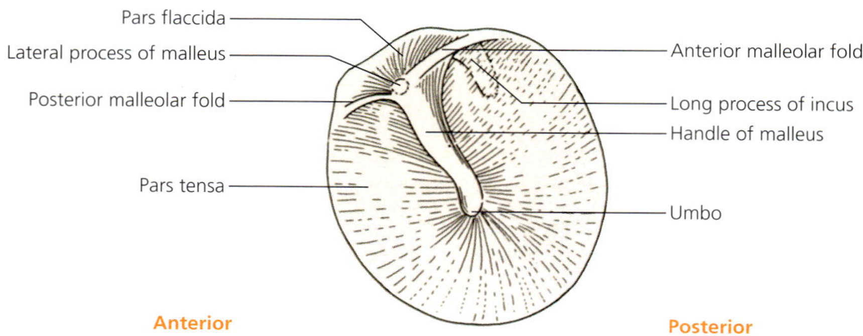

Figure 6.30 The tympanic membrane as seen through an otoscope.

osseous portion but is separated from the cartilaginous part by the ceruminous glands in the subcutaneous tissue.

The *tympanic membrane*, or *ear drum* (Figs 6.29 and 6.30), separates the middle ear from the external auditory meatus. It is made up of an outer cutaneous layer, continuous with the skin of the external auditory meatus, a middle fibrous layer and an inner mucous layer continuous with the mucoperiosteum of the rest of the tympanic cavity. It is oval in outline, a little less than 0.5 in. (1.25 cm) in its greatest (vertical) diameter, and faces laterally, downwards and forwards; it is slightly concave outwards. Since it is translucent (except at its margin where it is attached to the medial aspect of the external auditory meatus), it is possible on examination to see the underlying malleus and part of the incus. The greater part of the membrane is taut and is known as the *pars tensa*, but above the lateral process of the malleus there is a small triangular area where the membrane is thin and lax – the *pars flaccida*. This area is bounded by two distinct malleolar folds that reach down to the lateral process of the malleus. The point of greatest concavity of the membrane is known as the *umbo*; this marks the attachment of the handle of the malleus to the membrane.

Middle ear

The *middle ear*, or *tympanic cavity*, is the narrow slit-like cavity in the petrous part of the temporal bone containing the three auditory ossicles: malleus (the hammer), incus (the anvil) and stapes (the stirrup) (Fig. 6.29).

The walls of the cavity and its important relations are as follows.

The *lateral wall* is formed mainly by the tympanic membrane, which separates the tympanic cavity from the external auditory meatus, and above this by the squamous part of the temporal bone; the part of the cavity above the tympanic membrane is known as the *epitympanic recess* or *attic*; this part of the cavity contains the incus and the head of the malleus.

The *medial wall*, which separates the cavity from the internal ear, presents the *fenestra cochleae* (round window), closed by the secondary tympanic membrane; the *fenestra vestibuli* (oval window), occupied by the base (foot-piece) of the stapes; the *promontory*, formed by the first turn of the cochlea; and the *prominence* caused by the underlying canal for the facial nerve (Fig. 6.24).

The *floor* is a thin plate of bone separating the cavity from the bulb of the jugular vein.

The *roof* is formed by the thin sheet of bone known as the *tegmen tympani*, which separates it from the middle cranial fossa and the temporal lobe of the brain.

Anteriorly, the cavity communicates with the pharynx by way of the pharyngotympanic or Eustachian tube.

Posteriorly, it communicates with the mastoid or tympanic antrum and the mastoid air cells.

The *mastoid antrum* is a small cavity in the posterior part of the petrous temporal bone connected to the epitympanic recess of the middle ear by way of the narrow *aditus*. Its importance is twofold: it is in communication with the *mastoid air cells* (hence the portal through which infection may spread to these spaces from the middle ear) and it is intimately related posteriorly to the sigmoid sinus and the cerebellum, both of which may be involved from a middle ear infection.

The *mastoid air cells* arise postnatally as diverticula from the tympanic antrum, becoming obvious first at 2 years. They may invade not only the mastoid process but also the squamous part of the temporal bone. They are lined by a mucoperiosteum continuous anteriorly with that of the tympanic cavity.

The *pharyngotympanic* (*Eustachian*) *tube* reaches downwards, forwards and medially from the anterior part of the tympanic cavity to the lateral walls of the nasopharynx. In all it is about 1.5 in. (3.7 cm) long, the first 0.5 in. (1.25 cm) being bony while the rest is cartilaginous. It is lined by a ciliated columnar epithelium. The mucous membrane is thin in its bony part but the cartilaginous segment contains numerous mucous glands and, near its pharyngeal orifice, a considerable collection of lymphoid tissue termed the *tubal tonsil*. This may become swollen in infection, producing blockage of the tube. The tube is widest at its pharyngeal end and narrowest at the junction of the bony and cartilaginous portions.

Conduction of sound through the middle ear is by way of the malleus, incus and stapes. The *malleus* is the largest of the three and is described as having a handle, attached to the tympanic membrane, a rounded head, which articulates with the incus, and a lateral process, which can be seen through the tympanic membrane and from which the malleolar folds radiate. The *incus* comprises a body, which articulates with the malleus, and two processes, a short process attached to the posterior wall of the middle ear and a long process for articulation with the stapes. The shadow of the long process can often be seen through an auroscope running downwards behind the handle of the malleus. The *stapes* has a head for articulation with the incus, a neck and a base, which is firmly fixed in the fenestra vestibuli (the oval window).

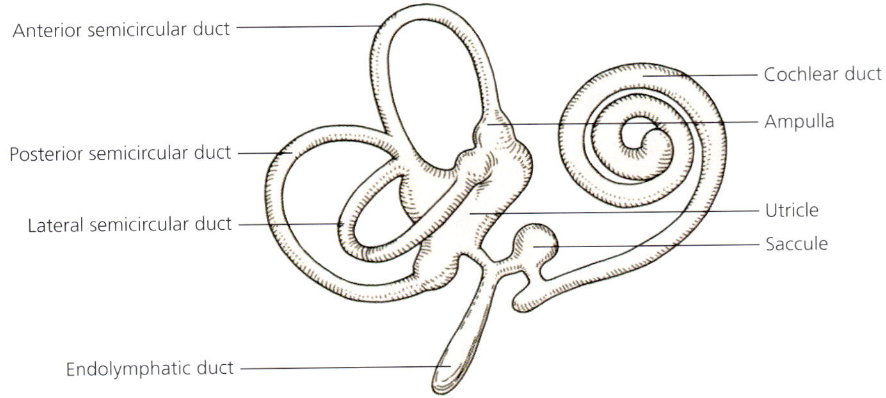

Figure 6.31 Detail of the membranous labyrinth.

Two small muscles are associated with these ossicles: the *stapedius*, which is attached to the neck of the stapes and is supplied by the facial nerve, and the *tensor tympani*, which is inserted into the handle of the malleus and is supplied by the mandibular division of V. Both serve to damp high-frequency vibrations.

Internal ear (Fig. 6.31)

The internal ear consists essentially of a complicated bony labyrinth made up of a central *vestibule*, which communicates posteriorly with three semicircular ducts and anteriorly with the spiral cochlea. This cavity contains a fluid known as *perilymph* and encloses the *membranous labyrinth*, comprising the *utricle* and *saccule*, which communicate, respectively, with the semicircular ducts and the cochlear duct. The duct system is filled with *endolymph*.

In each component of the membranous labyrinth there are specialized sensory receptor areas known as the *maculae* of the utricle and saccule, the *ampullary crests* of the semicircular canals and the *spiral organ of Corti* in the cochlea.

The disposition of the semicircular canals in three planes at right angles to each other renders this part of the labyrinth particularly well suited to signal changes in position of the head. The organ of Corti is adapted to record the sound vibrations transmitted by the stapes at the oval window.

Eye and associated structures (for optic nerve and visual pathway, *see* page 221)

The eye and associated structures comprise eyeball, orbital muscles , eyelids and conjunctiva.

Eyeball (Fig. 6.32)

The eyeball, which is just under 1 in. (2.5 cm) in all diameters, is formed by segments of two spheres of different size: a prominent anterior segment, which is transparent and forms about one-sixth of the eyeball, and a larger posterior segment, which is opaque and constitutes five-sixths of a sphere. The optic nerve enters the eye about 0.125 in. (3 mm) to the nasal (medial) side of the posterior pole.

The eyeball is made up of three coats: a fibrous outer coat, a vascular middle coat and an inner neural coat – the retina.

Fibrous coat

The fibrous coat comprises a transparent anterior part, the cornea, and an opaque posterior portion, the sclera. Peripherally, the *cornea* is continuous with the sclera at the *sclerocorneal junction*. The *sclera* is a tough, fibrous membrane which is responsible for the maintenance of the shape of the eyeball and which receives the insertion of the extra-ocular

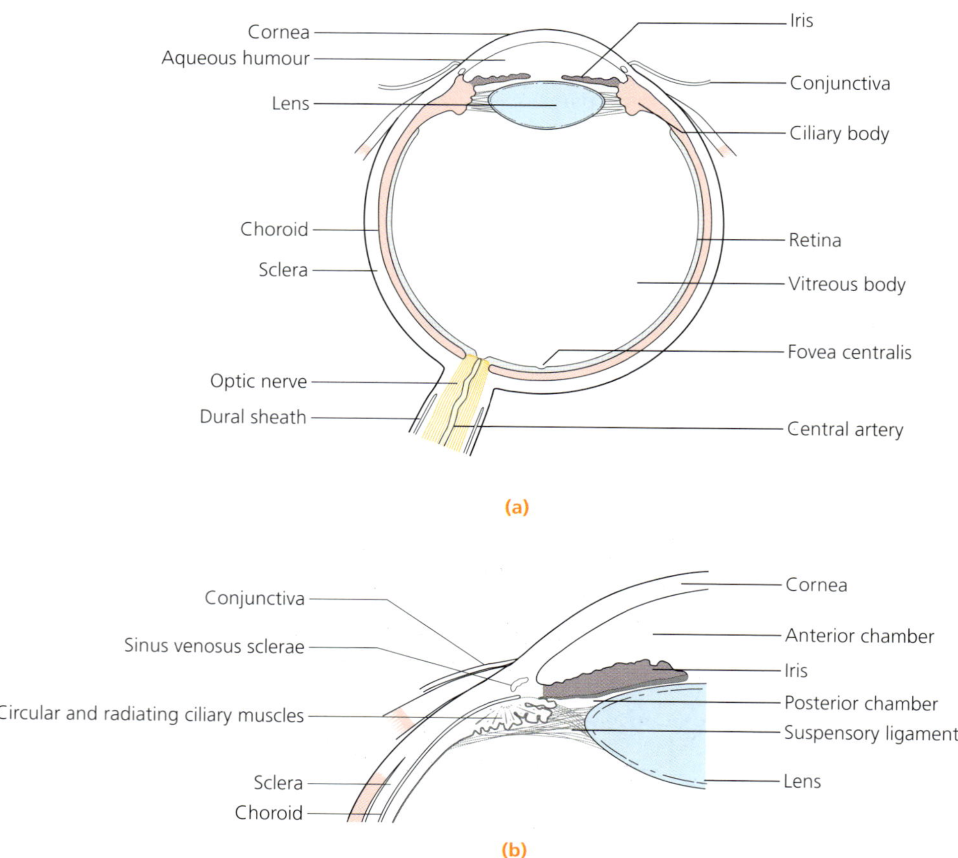

Figure 6.32 **(a)** The eyeball in section. **(b)** Detail of the ciliary region.

muscles. Posteriorly, it is pierced by the optic nerve, with whose dural sheath it is continuous.

Vascular coat

This is made up of the choroid, the ciliary body and the iris. These three components together form the *uveal tract*.

The *choroid* is a thin but highly vascular membrane lining the inner surface of the sclera. Posteriorly it is pierced by the optic nerve and anteriorly it is connected to the iris by the ciliary body.

The *ciliary body* includes the *ciliary ring*, a fibrous ring continuous with the choroid, the *ciliary processes*, a group of 60–80 folds arranged radially between the ciliary ring and the iris and connected posteriorly to the suspensory ligament of the lens, and the *ciliary muscles*, an outer radial and inner circular layer of smooth muscle responsible for the changes in convexity of the lens in accommodation and supplied by parasympathetic fibres transmitted in the oculomotor nerve (III).

The *iris* is the contractile disc surrounding the pupil. It consists of the following four layers:

1. An anterior mesothelial lining
2. A connective tissue stroma containing pigment cells
3. A group of radially arranged smooth muscle fibres – the dilator of the pupil (supplied by the sympathetic system) and a circular group, the pupillary sphincter (supplied by the parasympathetic fibres in the oculomotor nerve)
4. A posterior layer of pigmented cells which is continuous with the ciliary part of the retina

Neural coat

The neural coat or *retina* is formed by an outer pigmented and an inner nervous layer, and is interposed between the choroid and the hyaloid membrane of the vitreous. Anteriorly, it presents an irregular edge, the *ora serrata*, while posteriorly the nerve fibres on its surface collect to form the optic nerve. Its appearance as seen through an ophthalmoscope is shown in Fig. 6.33. Near its posterior pole there is a pale yellowish area, the *macula lutea*, the site of central vision, and just medial to this is the pale *optic disc* formed by the passage of nerve fibres through the retina, corresponding to the 'blind spot'. The *central artery of the retina* emerges from the disc and then divides into upper and lower branches; each of these in turn divides into a nasal and temporal branch. Histologically, the retina consists of a number of layers but from a functional point of view only three need be considered: an inner receptor cell layer – the layer of rods and cones; an intermediate layer of bipolar neurones; and the layer of ganglion cells, whose axons form the superficial layer of optic nerve fibres (Fig. 6.17).

Contents of the eyeball

Within the eyeball are found the *lens*, the *aqueous humour* and the *vitreous body*. The *lens* is biconvex and is placed between the vitreous and the aqueous humour, just behind the iris. The *aqueous humour* is a filtrate of plasma secreted by the vessels of the iris and ciliary body into the *posterior chamber* of the eye (i.e. the space between the lens and the iris). From here it passes through the pupillary aperture into the *anterior chamber* (between the cornea and the iris) and is re-absorbed into the ciliary veins by way of the *sinus venosus sclerae* (or *canal of Schlemm*). The *vitreous body*, which occupies the posterior four-fifths of the eyeball, is a thin transparent gel contained within a delicate membrane – the *hyaloid membrane* – and pierced by the lymph-filled *hyaloid canal*. The anterior part of the hyaloid membrane is thickened, receives attachments from the ciliary processes and gives rise to the *suspensory ligament of the lens*. This ligament is attached to the capsule of the lens in front of its equator and serves to retain it in position. It is relaxed by contraction of the radial fibres of the ciliary muscle and so allows the lens to assume a more convex form in accommodation (close reading).

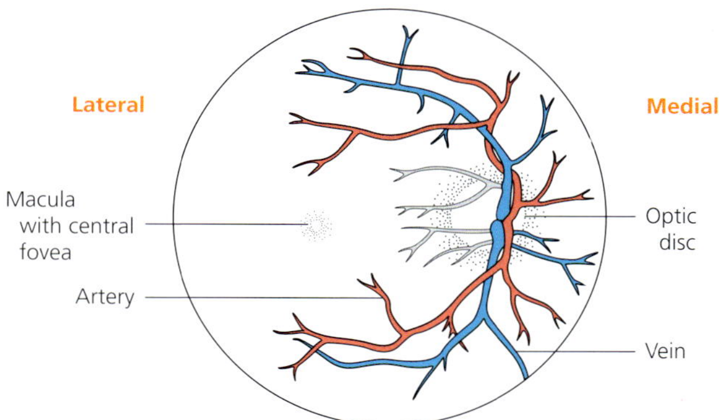

Figure 6.33 The right fundus oculi as seen through an ophthalmoscope.

Orbital muscles (Fig. 6.23; *see* Fig. 6.35)

These are the levator palpebrae superioris and the extra-ocular muscles; the medial, lateral, superior and inferior recti and the superior and inferior obliques. The four *recti* arise from a tendinous ring around the optic foramen and the medial part of the superior orbital fissure and are inserted into the sclera anterior to the equator of the eyeball. The lateral rectus is supplied by the VIth nerve, the others by the IIIrd. The *superior oblique* arises just above the tendinous ring and is inserted by means of a long tendon that loops around a fibrous pulley on the medial part of the roof of the orbit into the sclera just lateral to the insertion of the superior rectus. It is supplied by the IVth nerve. The *inferior oblique* passes like a sling from its origin on the medial side of the orbit around the undersurface of the eye to insert into the sclera between the superior and lateral recti; it is supplied by III.

Both the oblique muscles insert behind the equator of the eyeball.

The eyeball is capable of elevation, depression, adduction, abduction and rotation. The medial and lateral recti move the eyeball in one axis only.

The other following four muscles move it on all three axes:

- Rectus superior: Elevation, adduction and medial rotation
- Rectus inferior: Depression, adduction and lateral rotation
- Superior oblique: Depression, abduction and medial rotation
- Inferior oblique: Elevation, abduction and lateral rotation

Pure elevation and depression of the eyeball are produced by one rectus acting with its opposite oblique – rectus superior with inferior oblique producing pure elevation and rectus inferior with the superior oblique producing pure depression.

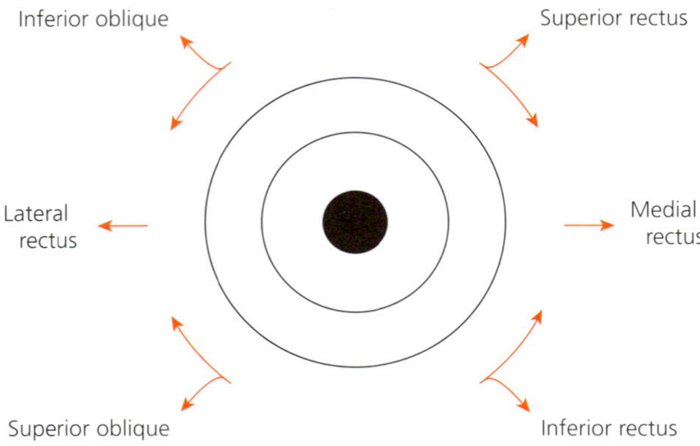

Figure 6.34 The direction of action of the muscles acting on the eyeball from the primary position (i.e. looking directly forwards).

A useful mnemonic is that the superior oblique is 'the *tramp's muscle*' – it moves the eye 'down and out'!

The actions of these muscles are shown in Fig. 6.34.

The *fascial sheath of the eye* (*Tenon's capsule*) is the membrane enclosing the eyeball from the optic nerve behind to the sclerocorneal junction in front. It is pierced by the vessels and nerves of the eye and by the tendons of the extraocular muscles. It is thickened inferiorly, where it forms the suspensory ligament.

Eyelids and conjunctiva (Fig. 6.35)

Of the two eyelids, the upper is the larger and more mobile, but, apart from the presence of the levator palpebrae superioris in this lid, the structure of the eyelids is essentially the same. Each consists of the following layers, from without inwards: skin, loose connective tissue, fibres of the orbicularis oculi muscle, the tarsal plates, of very dense fibrous tissue, tarsal glands and conjunctiva. The eyelashes arise along the mucocutaneous junction and immediately behind the lashes there are the openings of the *tarsal* (*Meibomian*) *glands*. These are large sebaceous glands whose secretion helps to seal the palpebral fissure when the eyelids are closed and forms a thin layer over the exposed surface of the open eye; if blocked, they distend into Meibomian cysts.

The *conjunctiva* is the delicate mucous membrane lining the inner surface of the lids from which it is reflected over the anterior part of the sclera to the cornea. Over the lids it is thick and highly vascular, but over the sclera it is much thinner and over the cornea it is reduced to a single layer of epithelium. The line of reflection from the lid to the sclera is known as the conjunctival fornix; the superior fornix receives the openings of the lacrimal glands.

Movements of the eyelids are brought about by the contraction of the orbicularis oculi and levator palpebrae superioris muscles. The width of the palpebral fissure at any one time depends on the tone of these muscles and the degree of protrusion of the eyeball.

Lacrimal apparatus (Fig. 6.36)

The *lacrimal gland* is situated in the upper, lateral part of the orbit in what is known as the lacrimal fossa. The main part of the gland is about the size and shape of an almond, but it is connected to a small terminal process that extends into the posterolateral part of the upper lid. The gland is drained by a series of 8–12 small ducts that open into the lateral part of the superior conjunctival fornix whence its secretion is spread over the surface of the eye by the action of the lids.

The tears are drained by way of the *lacrimal canaliculi*, whose openings, the *lacrimal puncta*, can be seen on the small elevation near the medial margin of each eyelid known as the *lacrimal papilla*. The two canaliculi, superior and inferior, open into the *lacrimal sac*, which is situated in a small depression on the medial surface of the orbit. This in turn drains through the nasolacrimal duct into the anterior part of the inferior meatus of the nose. The nasolacrimal duct, which not uncommonly becomes obstructed, is about 0.75 in. (2 cm) in length and lies in its own bony canal that leads from the fossa for the lacrimal sac along the lateral wall of the nasal cavity.

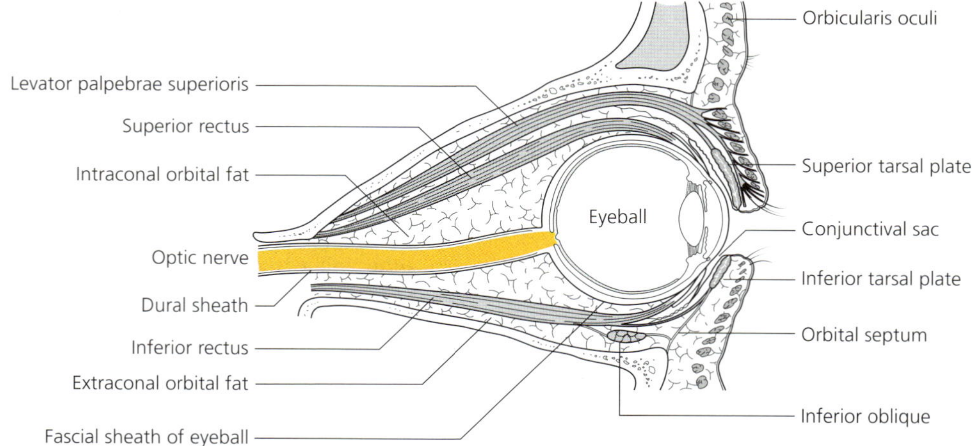

Figure 6.35 Compartments of the orbit.

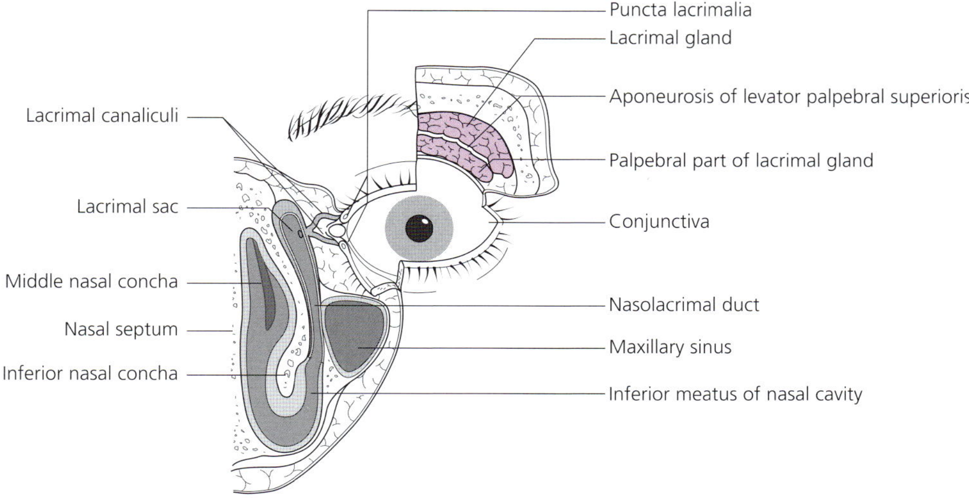

Figure 6.36 The lacrimal gland and its drainage system.

Autonomic nervous system

The nervous system is divided into two great subgroups: the *cerebrospinal system*, made up of the brain, spinal cord and the peripheral cranial and spinal nerves, and the *autonomic system* (also termed the *vegetative, visceral* or *involuntary system*), comprising the autonomic ganglia and nerves. Broadly speaking, the cerebrospinal system is concerned with the responses of the body to the external environment. In contrast, the autonomic system is concerned with the control of the internal environment, exercised through the innervation of the non-skeletal muscle of the heart, blood vessels, bronchial tree, gut and the pupils and the secretomotor supply of many glands, including those of the alimentary tract and its outgrowths, the sweat glands and, as a rather special example, the suprarenal medulla.

The two systems should not be regarded as being independent of each other, for they are linked anatomically and functionally. Anatomically, autonomic nerve fibres are transmitted in all of the peripheral and some of the cranial nerves; moreover, the higher connections of the autonomic system are situated within the spinal cord and brain. Functionally, the two systems are closely linked within the brain and spinal cord.

The characteristic feature of the autonomic system is that its efferent nerves emerge as medullated fibres from the brain and spinal cord, are interrupted in their course by a synapse in a peripheral ganglion and are then relayed for distribution as fine non-medullated fibres. In this respect they differ from the somatic efferent nerves, which pass without interruption to their terminations (Fig. 6.37).

The autonomic system is subdivided into the sympathetic and parasympathetic systems on anatomical, functional and, to a considerable extent, pharmacological grounds.

Anatomically, the *sympathetic nervous system* has its motor cell-stations in the lateral grey column of the thoracic and upper two lumbar segments of the spinal cord. The parasympathetic system is less neatly defined anatomically since it is divided into a *cranial outflow*, which passes along the cranial

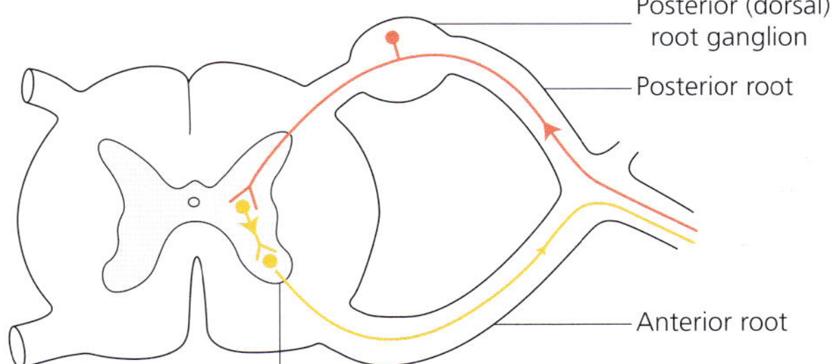

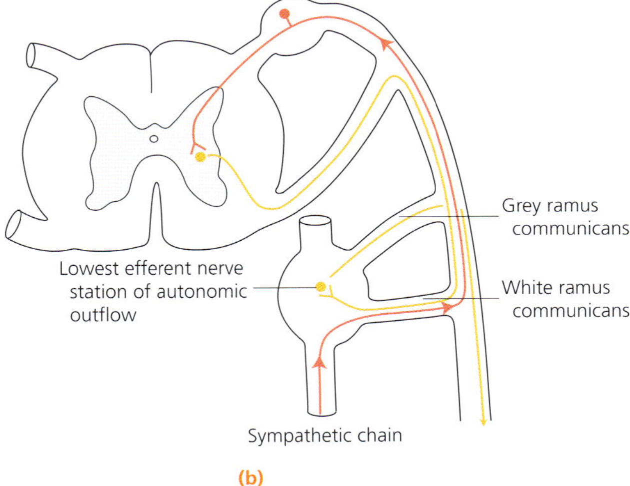

Figure 6.37 The essential difference between the cerebrospinal and autonomic outflows: **(a)** the cerebrospinal system has its lowest efferent nerve cell-stations within the central nervous system; **(b)** the autonomic system has its lowest efferent cell-stations in a peripheral ganglion (here illustrated by a typical sympathetic nerve ganglion). Red, afferent pathway; yellow, efferent pathway.

nerves III, VII, IX and X, and a *sacral outflow*, with cell-stations in the 2nd, 3rd and sometimes 4th sacral segments of the cord.

Functionally, the sympathetic system is concerned principally with stress reactions of the body. When this system is stimulated, the pupils dilate, peripheral blood vessels constrict, the force, rate and oxygen consumption of the heart increase, the bronchial tree dilates, visceral activity is diminished by inhibition of peristalsis and increase of sphincter tone, glycogenolysis takes place in the liver, the suprarenal medulla is stimulated to secrete, and there is cutaneous sweating and pilo-erection. The sympathetic pelvic nerves inhibit bladder contraction and are motor to the internal vesical sphincter.

Coronary blood flow is increased, partly by a direct sympathetic effect and partly produced by indirect factors, which include more vigorous cardiac contraction, reduced systole, relatively increased diastole and an increased concentration of vasodilator metabolites.

The *parasympathetic system* tends to be antagonistic to the sympathetic system (Table 6.1). Its stimulation results in constriction of the pupils, diminution in the rate, conduction and excitability of the heart, an increase in gut peristalsis with sphincter relaxation and enhanced alimentary glandular secretion. In addition, the pelvic parasympathetic nerves inhibit the vesical internal sphincter and are motor to the detrusor muscle of the bladder.

The sympathetic system tends to have a 'mass action' effect; stimulation of any part of it results in a widespread response. In contrast, parasympathetic activity is usually discrete and localized. This difference can be explained, at least in part, by differences in anatomical peripheral connections of the two systems, as will be shown below.

It is useful to think of the two systems as acting synergistically. For example, reflex slowing of the heart is effected partly from increased vagal and partly from decreased sympathetic stimulation. In addition, some organs receive their autonomic innervation from one system only; for example, the suprarenal medulla and the cutaneous arterioles receive only sympathetic fibres, whereas neurogenic gastric secretion is entirely under parasympathetic control via the vagus nerve.

Pharmacologically, the sympathetic postganglionic terminals release adrenaline (epinephrine) and noradrenaline (norepinephrine), with the single exception of the terminals to the sweat glands which, in common with all the parasympathetic postganglionic terminations, release acetylcholine.

Sympathetic system

The efferent fibres of the sympathetic system arise in the lateral grey column of the spinal cord (Figs 6.37 and 6.38) from segments T1–L2. From each of these segments small medullated axons emerge into the corresponding anterior primary ramus and pass via a white ramus communicans into the sympathetic trunk.

The spinal segments responsible for the sympathetic innervation of the various parts of the body are approximately as follows:

- Head and neck, T1–T2
- Upper limb, T2–T5
- Thoracic viscera, T1–T5
- Abdominal viscera, T4–L2
- Pelvic viscera, T10–L2
- Lower limb, T11–L2

Stimulation of a single white ramus communicans would thus obviously have widespread effects – the anatomical basis of the 'mass action' response of sympathetic stimulation.

Sympathetic trunk

The sympathetic trunk on each side is a ganglionated nerve chain that extends from the base of the skull to the coccyx in close relationship to the vertebral column, maintaining

Table 6.1 Summary of effects of sympathetic and parasympathetic stimulation

	Sympathetic stimulation	Parasympathetic stimulation
Eye	Pupil dilates	Pupil constricts; accommodation of lens
Lacrimal gland	Vasoconstrictor	Secretomotor
Heart	Increase in force, rate, conduction and excitability	Decrease in force, rate, conduction and excitability
Lung	Bronchi dilate	Bronchi constrict; secretomotor to mucous glands
Skin	Vasoconstrictor	
	Pilo-erection	
	Secretomotor to sweat glands	
Salivary glands	Vasoconstrictor	Secretomotor
Musculature of alimentary canal	Peristalsis inhibited	Peristalsis activated; sphincters relax
Acid secretion of stomach	–	Secretomotor
Pancreas	–	Secretomotor
Liver	Glycogenolysis	–
Suprarenal	Secretomotor	–
Bladder	Detrusor inhibited	Detrusor stimulated
	Sphincter stimulated	Sphincter inhibited
Uterus	Uterine contraction	Vasodilatation
	Vasoconstriction	

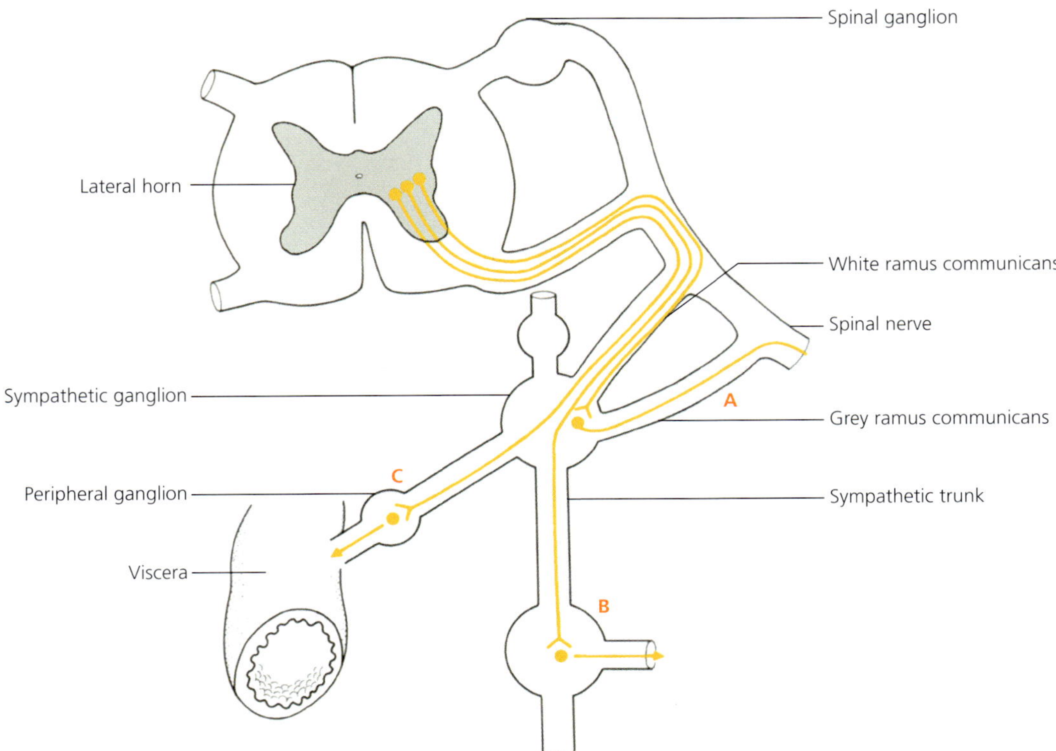

Figure 6.38 The three fates of sympathetic white rami. These may **(a)** relay in their corresponding ganglion and pass to their corresponding spinal nerve for distribution, **(b)** ascend or descend in the sympathetic chain and relay in higher or lower ganglia, or **(c)** pass without synapse to a peripheral ganglion for relay.

a distance of about 1 in. (2.5 cm) from the midline throughout its course. Commencing in the superior cervical ganglion beneath the skull base, the chain descends closely behind the posterior wall of the carotid sheath, enters the thorax anterior to the neck of the 1st rib, descends over the heads of the upper ribs and then on the sides of the bodies of the last three or four thoracic vertebrae. The chain then passes into the abdomen behind the medial arcuate ligament of the diaphragm and descends in a groove between psoas major and the sides of the lumbar vertebral bodies, overlapped by the abdominal aorta on the left and the inferior vena cava on the right. The chain then passes behind the common iliac vessels to enter the pelvis anterior to the ala of the sacrum and then descends medial to the anterior sacral foramina. The sympathetic trunks end below by meeting each other at the *ganglion impar* on the anterior face of the coccyx.

The details of the cervical, thoracic and lumbar portions of the trunk are given on pages 187, 29 and 90, respectively.

The sympathetic trunk bears a series of ganglia along its course that contain motor cells with which preganglionic medullated fibres enter into synapse and from which non-medullated postganglionic axons originate. Developmentally, there was originally one ganglion for each peripheral nerve, but by a process of fusion these have been reduced in man to three cervical, 12 or fewer thoracic, two to four lumbar and four sacral ganglia. Only the ganglia of T1–L2 receive white rami directly; the higher and lower ganglia must receive their preganglionic supply from medullated nerves that travel through their corresponding ganglia without relay and that then ascend or descend in the sympathetic chain. Still other preganglionic fibres pass intact through the ganglia to peripheral visceral ganglia for relay.

There are thus the following three fates which may befall white rami (Fig. 6.38):

1. To enter into synapse from the corresponding sympathetic ganglion (this applies only to the T1–L2 segments)
2. To ascend or descend in the sympathetic chain with relay in higher or lower ganglia
3. To traverse the ganglia intact and relay in peripheral ganglia

Pharmacologically, the sympathetic postganglionic terminals release adrenaline (epinephrine) and noradrenaline (norepinephrine), with a single exception of the sweat glands, which, in common with all the parasympathetic postganglionic terminations, release acetylcholine.

Distribution

The branches of the sympathetic ganglionic chain have somatic and visceral distribution.

Somatic distribution

Each spinal nerve receives one or more grey rami from a sympathetic ganglion that distributes postganglionic non-medullated sympathetic fibres to the segmental skin area supplied by the spinal nerve. These fibres are vasoconstrictor to the skin arterioles, sudomotor to sweat glands and pilomotor to the cutaneous hairs.

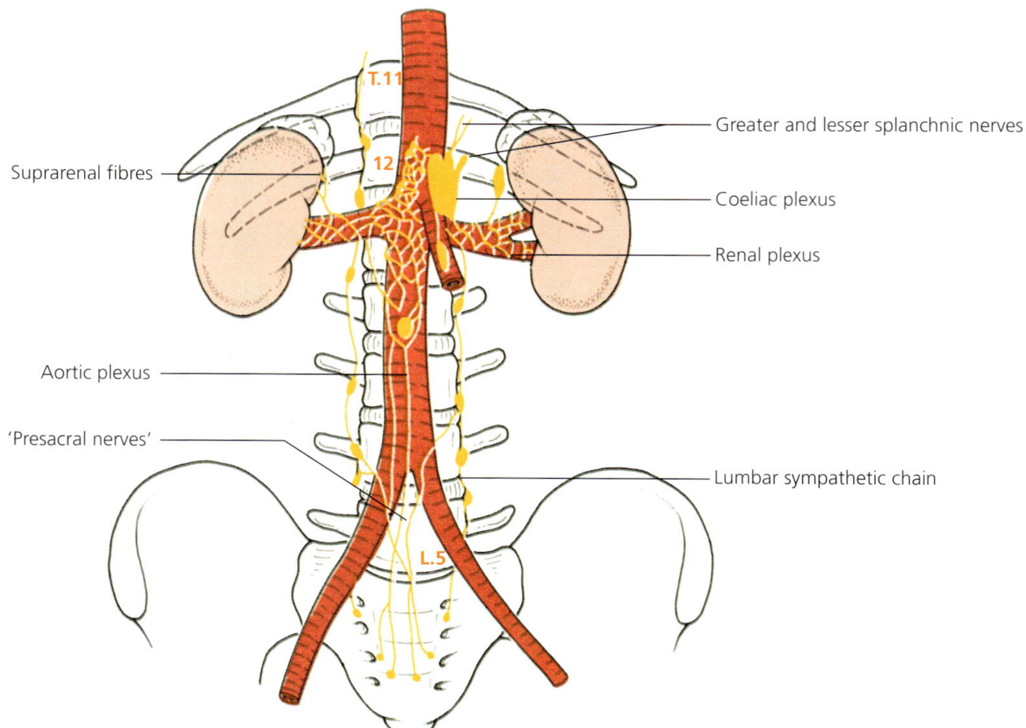

Figure 6.39 The abdominal sympathetic plexuses.

Visceral distribution

Postganglionic fibres to the head and neck and to the thoracic viscera arise from the ganglion cells of the sympathetic chain. Those to the head ascend along the internal carotid and vertebral arteries, whereas those to the thoracic organs are distributed by the cardiac, pulmonary and oesophageal plexuses.

The abdominal and pelvic viscera, however, are supplied by postganglionic fibres that have their cell-stations in more peripherally placed prevertebral ganglia – the coeliac, hypogastric and pelvic plexuses – which receive their preganglionic fibres from the splanchnic nerves (Fig. 6.39). These nerves are detailed on page 31, and shown in Fig. 6.38(a) and (b).

The suprarenal medulla has a unique nerve supply comprising a rich plexus of preganglionic fibres that pass without relay from the coeliac ganglion to the gland. These fibres end in direct contact with the chromaffin medullary cells and liberate acetylcholine (as in all autonomic ganglia), which stimulates the secretion of adrenaline (epinephrine) and noradrenaline (norepinephrine) by the suprarenal medulla.

The chromaffin cells of the suprarenal medulla may thus be regarded as sympathetic cells that have not developed postganglionic fibres; indeed, embryologically both the medulla and the sympathetic nerves have a common origin from the neural crest.

Afferent sympathetic fibres

As well as the efferent sympathetic system, there are also important *afferent sympathetic fibres.* These arise from the thoracic, abdominal and pelvic viscera and are concerned with the afferent arc of the autonomic reflexes and also – of great importance from the clinical point of view – with the conduction of visceral pain sensation to the higher centres. The afferent sympathetic fibres pass from receptors in the walls of the viscera, and ascend in the autonomic sympathetic plexuses. The afferent course from any viscus is therefore along the same pathway as the efferent autonomic fibres which supply that organ. They have their cell-stations in the dorsal root ganglia of the spinal nerves (Fig. 6.37).

(Note that, although afferent fibres are conveyed in both sympathetic and parasympathetic nerves, they are independent – they do not relay in the autonomic ganglia and terminate, just like somatic sensory fibres, in the dorsal ganglia of the spinal and cranial nerves. They merely use the autonomic nerves as a convenient anatomical conveyor system from the periphery to the brain.)

The afferent sympathetic fibres ascend centrally to the hypothalamus and thence to parts of the cerebral cortex and the limbic system along as yet undefined pathways.

Normally we are unaware of the afferent impulses from our viscera. Indeed, the thoracic, abdominal and pelvic organs are insensitive to cutting or burning. Thus, haemorrhoids can be injected, polyps in the stomach or colon biopsied and oesophageal varices or bleeding peptic ulcers injected without the patient being aware of this. Visceral pain may be provoked by distension, traction, excessive involuntary muscle contraction, inflammation or ischaemia; hence, the pain of coronary artery occlusion, intestinal obstruction, biliary or ureteric colic and the uterine contractions in childbirth.

In contrast to somatic pain, which is usually sharp and well localized, visceral pain is poorly localized and dull, and difficult to describe. Of considerable diagnostic importance, however, is referral of pain to the cutaneous areas that correspond to the segments of visceral nerves involved.

Referred pain can be from the following:

- **Heart (T1–T5):** To the front of the left chest, epigastrium, or medial side of the left arm
- **Stomach, adnexae, foregut, midgut (T5–T12):** To the epigastrium and upper and mid-abdomen (the gall bladder typically gives referred pain to the lower pole of the scapula, T7)
- **Kidney and ureter (T10–T12, L1):** Lumbar region, flank, groin and, in the male, the testis
- **Gonads (T10–T11):** To the iliac fossa and loin
- **Pelvic viscera (S2–S4):** Sacral area, the buttocks and posterior aspects of the thighs

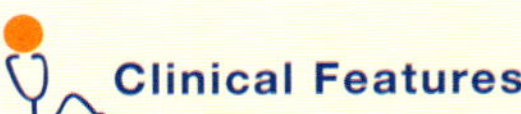

Clinical Features

- *Coeliac plexus block* may be used to treat the intractable pain of chronic pancreatitis or upper gastrointestinal malignancy.
- *Presacral nerve block* may similarly be used in the management of pain from pelvic malignant disease.
- *Cervical sympathectomy* (*See* page 187).

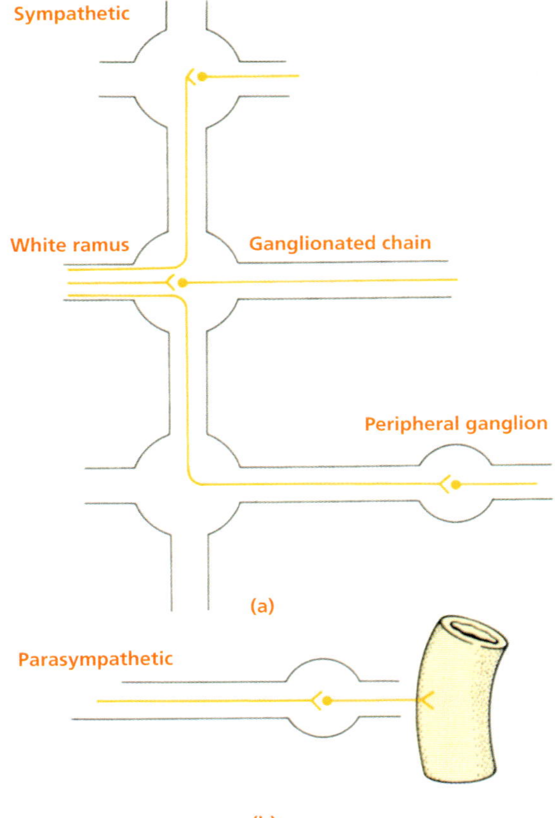

Figure 6.40 The anatomical basis of widespread sympathetic and local parasympathetic response. **(a)** The widespread distribution of postganglionic fibres from a single sympathetic white ramus. **(b)** The localized distribution of postganglionic parasympathetic fibres.

Parasympathetic system

As already stated, this system has a cranial and a sacral component. Its medullated preganglionic fibres synapse with ganglion cells that lie close to, or actually in the walls of, the viscera supplied. Postganglionic fibres therefore have only a short and direct course to their effector cells, and there is thus the anatomical pathway of a local discrete response to parasympathetic stimulation (Fig. 6.40).

Cranial outflow

The cranial component of the parasympathetic system is conveyed in cranial nerves III, VII, IX and X, of which X (the vagus) is the most important and the most widely distributed. The functions of this group of nerves can be summarized as follows:

1. **Pupils:** Constrictor to pupil, motor to ciliary muscle (accommodation)
2. **Salivary glands:** Secretomotor
3. **Lacrimal glands:** Secretomotor
4. **Heart:** Inhibitor of cardiac conduction, contraction, excitability and impulse formation (with consequent slowing of the heart and diminution of its contraction force)
5. **Lungs:** Bronchoconstrictor, secretomotor to mucous glands
6. **Alimentary canal:** Motor to gut muscles as far as the region of the ascending colon; inhibitor to the pyloric sphincter; secretomotor to the glands and adnexae of the stomach and intestine

The parasympathetic distribution of III, VII and IX is carried out via four ganglia from which postganglionic fibres relay. These ganglia also transmit (without synapse and therefore without functional connection) sympathetic and sensory fibres which have similar peripheral distribution. These ganglia are the ciliary (*see* page 223), pterygopalatine (*see* page 224), submandibular (*see* page 226) and otic (*see* page 226).

The Xth (vagal) distribution conveys by far the most important and largest contributions of the parasympathetic system. It is responsible for all the functions of the parasympathetic cranial outflow enumerated above, apart from the innervation of the eye and the secretomotor supply to the salivary and lacrimal glands. The efferent fibres are derived from the dorsal nucleus of X and are distributed widely in the cardiac, pulmonary and alimentary plexuses. Postganglionic fibres are relayed from tiny ganglia that lie in the walls of the viscera concerned; in the gut, these constitute the submucosal *plexus of Meissner* and the myenteric *plexus of Auerbach*.

Sacral outflow

The anterior primary rami of S2, S3 and occasionally S4 give off nerve fibres termed the *pelvic splanchnic nerves* or *nervi erigentes*, which join the sympathetic pelvic plexus for distribution to the pelvic organs. Tiny ganglia in the walls of the viscera then relay postganglionic fibres.

The sacral parasympathetic system has been termed by Cannon 'the mechanism for emptying'. It supplies visceromotor fibres to the muscles of the rectum and inhibitor fibres to the internal anal sphincter, motor fibres to the bladder wall and inhibitor fibres to the internal vesical sphincter. In addition, vasodilator fibres supply the erectile cavernous sinuses of the penis and the clitoris.

Afferent parasympathetic fibres

Parasympathetic afferent fibres are conveyed in the glossopharyngeal nerve (IX), transmitting baroreceptor fibres from the carotid sinus and chemoreceptor fibres from the carotid body, afferent fibres of the vagus nerve (X) from the heart, lungs and alimentary tract, and along the pelvic splanchnic nerves (S2, S3 and S4) from the pelvic viscera.

Like the afferent fibres conveyed in the sympathetic system (*see* page 240), these do not relay in the autonomic ganglia and have their cell-stations, just like somatic sensory fibres, in the dorsal ganglia of the spinal and cranial nerves. They simply use the autonomic nerves as a convenient anatomical pathway from the viscera to the brain.

Autonomic control of micturition, defecation and sexual function

The detrusor muscle in the urinary bladder is innervated by the parasympathetic fibres. These originate in the 2nd, 3rd and possibly 4th sacral segments of the spinal cord and reach the bladder via the pelvic splanchnic nerves and inferior hypogastric plexuses. Thus, detrusor contractility is exclusively under parasympathetic control. The smooth muscle in the bladder neck and the superficial trigonal muscle are, however, innervated by sympathetic fibres. Normal bladder emptying is the result of pelvic parasympathetic stimulation and reciprocal sympathetic inhibition. Damage to the pelvic parasympathetic fibres will therefore result in an atonic bladder with neither voluntary nor reflex control.

The autonomic control of sexual function in the male is as follows: penile erection is mediated by pelvic parasympathetic fibres (an alternative name for the pelvic parasympathetics is *nervi erigentes*, the nerves of erection; of course, the parasympathetics mediate a great deal more than just penile erection!). The penile branches of the pelvic parasympathetics, upon stimulation, produce vasodilatation of the arteries in the penile erectile tissue, i.e. corpora cavernosa and corpus spongiosum. Ejaculation is, by contrast, essentially mediated by sympathetic nerves. These nerves, when stimulated, result in contraction of the bladder neck muscle (thereby preventing retrograde ejaculation) and simultaneous contraction of seminal vesicles, prostatic muscle and the muscle in the walls of the vas deferens and epididymis.

The initiation of defecation is brought on by stimulation of receptors in the rectal wall. This provokes a parasympathetic reflex response resulting in peristalsis. The urge to defecate can, up to a point, be overridden by higher (cortical) centres. The anal sphincter complex has the following two components:

1. An internal anal sphincter, which is a smooth muscle sphincter and is under sympathetic control (L1–L2 segments); the internal anal sphincter normally accounts for 40–50% of the resting anal tone;
2. An external anal sphincter, which is the larger of the two sphincters. It is a striated muscle sphincter and thus under voluntary control. It is innervated by a somatic nerve – the inferior rectal branch of the pudendal nerve.

Glossary of eponyms

In spite of their being 'unscientific', eponymous terms are still commonly used – more so among clinicians, it is true, than among professional anatomists. This glossary gives brief biographical details of the names mentioned in the text. Entries appear alphabetically according to the person whose name is used adjectivally in the term: *valves of Ball* under Ball, *column of Burdach* under Burdach, and so on.

transpyloric plane of Addison A transverse (horizontal) plane half-way between the sternal notch and the upper edge of the pubic symphysis. It corresponds to the level of the lower border of the 1st lumbar vertebra.
Christopher Addison (1869–1951), Professor of Anatomy, University of Sheffield. He subsequently took up a full-time career in politics, becoming a member of parliament in 1910. Shortly after the end of the First World War, he became Britain's first ever Minister of Health.

Alcock's canal Fascial tunnel on the lateral wall of the ischiorectal fossa that conveys the pudendal vessels and nerve.
Benjamin Alcock (1801–?), Professor of Anatomy, first in Dublin and then Cork. He emigrated to America and disappeared from the scene.

Argyll Robertson pupil The pupil does not respond to light but reacts to accommodation. It is classically seen in neurosyphilis.
Douglas Argyll Robertson (1837–1909), ophthalmic surgeon at the Royal Infirmary, Edinburgh.

Auerbach's plexus Nerve plexus between the circular and longitudinal muscle coats of the intestine.
Leopold Auerbach (1828–1897), Professor of Pathology, Breslau.

valves of Ball Valve-like folds that connect the distal extremities of the columns of Morgagni (q.v.) in the upper half of the anal canal.
Sir Charles Ball (1851–1916), Regius Professor of Surgery, Dublin, and an early pioneer of rectal surgery.

Bartholin's gland The greater vestibular gland. Mucus-secreting gland in the posterior labium majus.
Caspar Bartholin (1655–1738), Professor of Anatomy, Copenhagen.

Batson's venous plexus The 'valveless vertebral veins' communicate with the prostatic plexus of veins and explain the readiness with which carcinoma of the prostate spreads to the pelvis and lumbar vertebrae.
Oscar Bătson (1894–1979), Professor of Anatomy, University of Pennsylvania.

Bell's palsy Viral infection of the facial (VII) nerve.
Sir Charles Bell (1774–1842), surgeon at the Middlesex Hospital, London.

Bennett's fracture Fracture dislocation of the base of the metacarpal of the thumb.
Edward Hallaran Bennett (1837–1907), Professor of Surgery at Trinity College, Dublin. He described this fracture in 1882.

Bigelow's Y-shaped ligament The tough iliofemoral ligament of the hip joint.
Henry James Bigelow (1818–1890), surgeon at Harvard Medical School, Boston, MA.

Blalock's operation The right subclavian artery is anastomosed end-to-side into the right pulmonary artery in order to overcome the pulmonary stenosis of the tetralogy of Fallot (q.v.).
Alfred Blalock (1899–1964), Professor of Surgery, Johns Hopkins Hospital, Baltimore, MD.

Bochdalek's foramen The pleuroperitoneal canal of the developing diaphragm.
Vincent Bochdalek (1801–1883), anatomist in Prague.

Broca's area The anterior portion of the inferior frontal gyrus; on the dominant side it is the motor area for speech.
Pierre Broca (1824–1880), Professor of Clinical Surgery, Paris.

Brown-Séquard syndrome Produced by hemisection of the spinal cord.
Charles Edouard Brown-Séquard (1817–1894), born in Mauritius, practised as a neurologist in Paris, at Harvard and at the National Hospital, Queen's Square, London.

Brunner's glands The characteristic submucosal acinar glands of the duodenum.
Johann Brunner (1653–1727), Swiss anatomist who became Professor of Anatomy at Heidelberg and later at Strasbourg. It is said that his father-in-law, J. J. Wepfer, actually discovered these glands!

Bryant's triangle Used in measurement of the hip.
Thomas Bryant (1828–1914), surgeon at Guy's Hospital, London; President of the Royal College of Surgeons of England.

column of Burdach The lateral tract (fasciculus cuneatus) of the posterior column of the spinal cord.
Charles Burdach (1776–1847), Professor of Anatomy and Medicine, Konigsberg.

Caldwell–Luc operation For drainage of the maxillary sinus.
George Walter Caldwell (1866–1946), ENT surgeon in New York.
Henri Luc (1855–1925), ENT surgeon in Paris.

Calot's triangle Triangle formed by the liver, common hepatic duct and cystic duct.
Jean François Calot (1861–1941), surgeon at the Rothschild Hospital, Paris, where he specialized in the treatment of surgical tuberculosis in children.

Camper's fascia The superficial fatty layer of the superficial fascia of the lower abdominal wall.
Peter Camper (1722–1789), Professor of Medicine, Amsterdam, and then Professor of Medicine, Surgery, Anatomy and Botany, Groningen.

Cannon's description of the sacral parasympathetic system as the 'mechanism for emptying'.
William Bradford Cannon (1871–1945), George Higginson Professor of Physiology, Harvard University, Boston, MA.

Cloquet's gland Lymph node situated in the femoral canal.
Jules Cloquet (1790–1883), Professor of Anatomy and Surgery, Paris.

Colles' fascia The perineal fascia.

Colles' fracture Fracture of the lower end of the radius with dorsal displacement.
Abraham Colles (1773–1843), Professor of Anatomy and Surgery, Royal College of Surgeons in Ireland, Dublin.

ligament of Cooper The iliopectineal fascia.

ligaments of Cooper Fibrous septa in the breast.
Sir Astley Paston Cooper (1768–1841), surgeon at Guy's Hospital, London; President of the Royal College of Surgeons.

organ of Corti The sound receptor organ in the cochlea.
Alfonso Corti (1822–1888), Italian histologist who worked mainly on the retina and the ear.

Cowper's glands Two glands situated in the deep perineal pouch which drain into the bulbous urethra.
William Cowper (1666–1698), surgeon in London.

Cushing's syndrome Endocrine abnormality associated with hyperplasia or tumour of the adrenal cortex or of a basophil adenoma of the anterior pituitary.
Harvey Cushing (1869–1939), pioneer neurosurgeon at the Peter Bent Brigham Hospital, Boston, MA.

fascia of Denonvilliers Fascia which separates the prostate from the rectum.
Charles Pierre Denonvilliers (1808–1872), Professor of Anatomy, Paris.

Dormia basket A device consisting of fine, interlinked wires that can be manipulated through an endoscope into a body cavity or tube to retrieve a calculus or similar object.
Enrico Dormia (1928–2009), Professor of Urology, University of Milan, Italy. Acknowledged to be the first practitioner of minimally invasive surgery in Italy.

arcuate line of Douglas The lower margin of the posterior rectus sheath.

pouch of Douglas The recto-uterine peritoneal pouch.
James Douglas (1675–1742), anatomist and obstetrician in London.

Dupuytren's contracture Contraction and fibrosis of the palmar (and occasional plantar) fascia.
Baron Guillaume Dupuytren (1777–1835), surgeon at the Hôtel Dieu, Paris.

Edinger–Westphal nucleus Supplies the parasympathetic fibres of the oculomotor nerve.
Ludwig Edinger (1855–1918), German anatomist and neurologist.
Karl Westphal (1833–1890), neurologist in Berlin. Described the nucleus in the adult 2 years after this had been demonstrated in the fetus by Edinger.

Erb–Duchenne paralysis Results from injury to the C5 and C6 roots of the brachial plexus.
Wilhelm Erb (1840–1921), Professor of Neurology, Heidelberg.
G. B. A. Duchenne (1806–1875), neurologist in Paris; also described Duchenne's muscular dystrophy.

Eustachian tube The pharyngotympanic tube.
Bartolomeo Eustachi (1524–1574), Professor of Anatomy, Rome.

Fallopian tube The uterine tube.
Gabrielle Fallopio (1523–1562), Professor of Anatomy, Padua, and a pupil of Vesalius.

Fallot's tetralogy Congenital heart disease comprising pulmonary stenosis, right ventricular hypertrophy, ventricular septal defect and overriding of the aorta.
Etienne Fallot (1850–1911), Professor of Medicine, Marseilles.

Galen's vein The great cerebral vein.
Claudius Galen (130–200 ad), physician to the emperor Marcus Aurelius. Taught anatomy in Rome and prolific author of text books.

duct of Gartner Mesonephric duct remnant in the female.
Hermann Gartner (1785–1827), Danish surgeon.

Gimbernat's ligament The lacunar portion of the inguinal ligament.
Manuel Gimbernat (1734–1816), Professor of Anatomy, Barcelona.

column of Goll The medial tract of the posterior column of the spinal cord (fasciculus gracilis).
Friedrich Goll (1829–1903), both a neurologist and anatomist; Professor of Anatomy, Zurich.

Graafian follicle Maturing ovarian follicle.
Regnier de Graaf (1641–1673), physician and anatomist in Delft.

Hartmann's pouch Dilatation of the gall bladder proximal to its neck.
Henri Hartmann (1860–1952), Professor of Surgery, Faculty of Medicine, Paris.

Henry's method A method of locating the posterior interosseous branch of the radial nerve in the forearm.
Arnold Henry (1886–1962), Professor of Surgery, Cairo University, and, subsequently, Professor of Anatomy, the Royal College of Surgeons in Ireland, Dublin.

antrum of Highmore The maxillary sinus.
Nathaniel Highmore (1613–1685), physician in Sherborne, Dorset. His claim to fame is tenuous since the maxillary sinus was well known to previous anatomists and was illustrated by Leonardo da Vinci.

Hilton's law Nerves crossing a joint supply the muscles acting on the joint and the joint itself.
John Hilton (1805–1878), surgeon at Guy's Hospital, London.

Hippocratic method For reduction of dislocation of the shoulder.
Hippocrates (*c.* 460–375 bc), lived in the Greek island of Cos. He is generally acknowledged as the *Father of Medicine*.

bundle of His Atrioventricular conduction fibres in the heart.
Wilhelm His, Jr (1863–1934), Swiss-born anatomist and cardiologist. Professor of Medicine, University of Berlin.

Horner's syndrome Ptosis and constriction of the pupil resulting from interruption of the sympathetic innervation to the eyelids and pupil.
Johann Horner (1831–1886), Professor of Ophthalmology, Zurich.

Houston's valves The three lateral folds of the rectum.
John Houston (1802–1845), lecturer in surgery, Dublin.

Hunter's canal The subsartorial canal.
John Hunter (1728–1793), surgeon at St George's Hospital, London. He described ligation of the femoral artery in the subsartorial canal for popliteal aneurysm.

Killian's dehiscence The potential gap between the two parts of the interior constrictor muscle through which a pharyngeal pouch protrudes.
Gustav Killian (1860–1921), ENT surgeon in Berlin.

Klumpke's paralysis Injury to the lowest root of the brachial plexus.
Augusta Dejerine-Klumpke (1859–1927), neurologist in Paris. Married another famous neurologist, Joseph Dejerine.

Kocher's incision The subcostal approach to the gall bladder.

Kocher's manoeuvre Mobilization of the duodenum by incising its lateral peritoneal attachment.

Kocher's method For reduction of dislocation of the shoulder.
Theodore Kocher (1841–1917), Professor of Surgery in Berne. Winner of the Nobel Prize for Medicine or Physiology in 1909. The first surgeon ever to receive this accolade.

islets of Langerhans Clumps of insulin-secreting cells in the pancreas.
Paul Langerhans (1847–1888), Professor of Pathology, Freiburg. He described the islet cells in his doctorate studies in 1869, at the age of 22.

nerve of Latarjet The fibres of the vagus nerve that supply the gastric antrum.
André Latarjet (1876–1947), Professor of Anatomy, Lyons.

dorsal tubercle of Lister A palpable prominence on the dorsal surface of the distal radius. Immediately to its ulnar side lies the tendon of extensor pollicis longus.
Joseph (Lord) Lister (1827–1912), Professor of Surgery, successively at the Universities of Glasgow and Edinburgh, and at King's College Hospital, London.

Little's area Area of arterial anastomosis on the antero-inferior part of the nasal septum.
James Lawrence Little (1836–1885), Professor of Surgery, University of Vermont, New England.

angle of Louis The angulated articulation between the manubrium sterni and mesosternum.
Pierre Charles Louis (1787–1872), Physician to the Hôpital de la Pitié, Paris. He was, in his day, a leading authority on pulmonary tuberculosis.

Ludwig's angina Infection of the submandibular region.
Wilhelm Ludwig (1790–1865), Professor of Surgery, Tubingen.

foramina of Luschka The lateral openings of the fourth ventricle.
Hubert Lushka (1820–1875), Professor of Anatomy, Tubingen.

Mackenrodt's ligaments The transverse cervical (or cardinal) ligaments of the female pelvis.
Alwin Mackenrodt (1859–1925), Professor of Gynaecology, Berlin.

foramen of Magendie The midline opening of the fourth ventricle.
François Magendie (1783–1855), physician at the Hôtel Dieu, Paris.

vein of Mayo A constant vein that crosses the junction of the pylorus with the duodenum.
Charles Mayo (1865–1939), with his father and his brother, William, founded the Mayo Clinic, Rochester, MN. The vein of Mayo was described earlier by Latarjet (q.v.).

McBurney's point Two-thirds of the way laterally along the line from the umbilicus to the anterior superior iliac spine; the usual site of maximum tenderness in acute appendicitis and the centre of the skin incision for appendicectomy.
Charles McBurney (1845–1913), Professor of Surgery, New York. A pioneer of early surgery in acute appendicitis.

Meckel's cartilage The cartilage of the first branchial arch.

Meckel's diverticulum The remains of the embryonic vitellointestinal duct and present in approximately 2% of subjects.
Johann Meckel (1781–1833), Professor of Anatomy, Halle. His grandfather, who was Professor of Anatomy in Berlin, described the pterygopalatine ganglion and the dural space which contains the ganglion of the trigeminal nerve. Johann's father was also Professor of Anatomy in Halle.

Meibomian glands The tarsal glands of the eyelid. If blocked, they distend into Meibomian cysts.
Heinrich Meibom (1638–1700), Professor of Medicine, Helmstadt.

Meissner's plexus The nerve plexus in the submucosal layer of the intestine.
George Meissner (1829–1905), anatomist and physiologist, Professor successively in Basle, Freiburg and Gottingen. He also described Meissner's corpuscles, the cutaneous sensory end-organs.

glands of Montgomery The modified sebaceous glands of the areola of the nipple.
William Montgomery (1797–1859), practised obstetrics in Dublin.

columns of Morgagni Vertical columns of mucosa in the anal canal.

foramen of Morgagni Gap between the xiphoid and costal origins of the diaphragm.

hydatid of Morgagni The appendix epididymis, the remnant of the mesonephros.
Giovanni Morgagni (1682–1771), Professor of Anatomy, Padua – a post he held for 59 years!

Morison's pouch The right subhepatic space.
James Rutherford Morison (1853–1939), Professor of Surgery, University of Durham. He had served as a surgical dresser to Joseph Lister.

Müllerian duct The paramesonephric duct.
Johannes Müller (1801–1858), Professor of Anatomy, Berlin.

Naegele's pelvis Absence or underdevelopment of one-half of the sacrum resulting in a contracted, ovate pelvis.
Franz Karl Naegele (1778–1851), obstetrician, Dusseldorf.

Nelaton's line A line joining the anterior superior iliac spine to the ischial tuberosity. The greater trochanter normally lies distal to this line.
Auguste Nelaton (1807–1873), Professor of Surgery, Paris, and surgeon to Napoleon III.

sphincter of Oddi The sphincter around the termination of the common bile duct.
Ruggero Oddi (1845–1906), surgeon in Rome. The sphincter had already been described by Glisson in the seventeenth century!

Pacchionian bodies Clumps of arachnoid villi along the superior sagittal sinus.
Antoine Pacchioni (1665–1726), Professor of Anatomy, Rome.

Pancoast's syndrome Invasion of the brachial plexus by an apical tumour of the lung.
H. K. Pancoast (1875–1939), Professor of Radiology, University of Pennsylvania, the first such appointment in the USA.

Parkinson's disease Tremor and rigidity due to lesions of the substantia nigra.
James Parkinson (1755–1824), medical practitioner, Shoreditch, London. His small book *An Essay on the Shaking Palsy* in 1817 was based mainly on close observation of one case.

Passavant's ridge Produced by contraction of the superior pharyngeal constrictor in deglutition.
Philipp Passavant (1815–1893), surgeon in Frankfurt.

Perthes' disease Avascular necrosis of the femoral head in children.
Georg Perthes (1869–1927), Professor of Surgery, Tubingen.

Pfannenstiel incision Transverse lower abdominal incision employed usually for pelvic surgery.
Hermann Johannes Pfannenstiel (1862–1909), gynaecologist in Breslau (then part of Prussia).

Pott's disease Spinal tuberculosis.

Pott's fracture Fracture–dislocation of the ankle.
Percival Pott (1714–1789), surgeon at St Bartholomew's hospital, London.

Poupart's ligament The inguinal ligament.
Francois Poupart (1661–1708), surgeon at the Hôtel Dieu, Paris.

Pringle's manoeuvre Compression of the hepatic artery at the foramen of Winslow (q.v.) in the control of haemorrhage.
James Hogarth Pringle (1863–1941), surgeon at the Royal Infirmary, Glasgow.

Queckenstedt's test Compression of the internal jugular vein during lumbar puncture produces a rise in cerebrospinal fluid pressure.
H. H. G. Queckenstedt (1876–1918), neurologist in Rostock. He described his test in 1916 while serving in the German army during the First World War. He was killed in a road accident 2 days before the armistice.

Rathke's pouch Origin of the anterior pituitary in the root of the embryonic buccal cavity.
Martin Heinrich Rathke (1793–1860), Professor of Zoology and Anatomy, Königsberg, Prussia.

island of Reil The insula of the cerebral cortex.
Johann Reil (1759–1813), Professor of Medicine, Halle and, later, Berlin.

cave of Retzius The retropubic space.
Andreas Retzius (1797–1860), Professor of Anatomy, Karolinska Institute, Stockholm.

fissure of Rolando The central cerebral fissure.
Luigi Rolando (1773–1831), Professor of Anatomy, Turin.

Romberg's sign Ataxia when the eyes are closed because of loss of position sense. Characteristic of posterior column lesions.
Moritz Romberg (1795–1873), Director of the University Hospital in Berlin and author of the first systematic book on neurology.

duct of Santorini The accessory pancreatic duct.
Giovanni Santorini (1681–1737), Professor of Anatomy, Venice.

Sappey's plexus The plexus of lymphatics below the nipple.
Marie Sappey (1810–1896), Professor of Anatomy, Paris.

Scarpa's fascia The fibrous layer of superficial fascia of the lower abdomen.
Antonio Scarpa (1747–1832), Professor of Anatomy and Surgery, Pavia. His name is also attached to the femoral triangle.

canal of Schlemm The sinus venosus sclerae, draining the aqueous humour from the anterior chamber of the eye.
F. S. Schlemm (1795–1858), Professor of Anatomy, Berlin.

Seldinger technique A method of percutaneous puncture and catheterization of arteries and other hollow tubes (under radiological control), using a guidewire over which is passed a Seldinger catheter.
Sven-Ivar Seldinger (1921–1998), radiologist, Mora (near Uppsala).

Semon's law In partial damage of the recurrent laryngeal nerve, the abductors of the vocal cords are affected more than the adductors.
Felix Semon (1849–1921), graduated in Berlin but emigrated to England and became a laryngologist at St Thomas' Hospital, London.

Sherrington's description of the hypothalamus As the 'head ganglion of the autonomic nervous system'.
Charles Scott Sherrington (1857–1952), Waynfleet Professor of Physiology, University of Oxford.

Stensen's duct The duct of the parotid gland.
Niels Stensen (1638–1686), Professor of Anatomy, University of Copenhagen.

aqueduct of Sylvius Between the third and fourth ventricle.

fissure of Sylvius The lateral cerebral fissure.
François de la Boe Sylvius (1614–1672), Professor of Medicine, Leyden.

Tenon's capsule The fascial sheath of the eye.
Jacques Tenon (1724–1816), surgeon at the Salpetrière, Paris.

suspensory ligament of Treitz Peritoneal fold from the right crus of the diaphragm to the duodenal termination.
Wenzel Treitz (1819–1872), Professor of Pathology, Prague.

Trendelenburg's test A clinical test for hip stability.
Friedrich Trendelenburg (1844–1924), Professor of Surgery, Leipzig. He attempted a pulmonary embolectomy (unsuccessfully) in 1908.

bloodless fold of Treves The ileocaecal fold.
Sir Frederick Treves (1853–1923), surgeon at the London Hospital. Drained the appendix abscess of King Edward VII in 1902.

Valsalva manoeuvre Forcible exhalation of inhaled air against a closed airway (nose and mouth).
Antonio Mario Valsalva (1666–1723), physician and anatomist, Bologna.

ampulla of Vater The ampulla of the common bile duct.
Abraham Vater (1684–1751), Professor of Anatomy, Wittenberg.

Volkmann's contracture Produced by ischaemic fibrosis of the forearm muscles.
Richard von Volkmann (1830–1889), Professor of Surgery, Halle, and one of the pioneers of Lister's antiseptic surgical technique.

Waldeyer's ring The ring of lymphoid tissue comprising the nasopharyngeal tonsil, the palatine tonsils and the lymphoid nodules on the dorsum of the tongue.

Heinrich Waldeyer (1836–1921), Professor of Anatomy, first in Strasbourg and then Berlin. He also described the plasma cell in 1875.

Wernicke's speech area Superior area of the temporal lobe of the cerebral cortex.
Karl Wernicke (1848–1904), psychiatrist, first in Breslau then Halle.

Wharton's duct The duct of the submandibular salivary gland.
Thomas Wharton (?1616–1673), physician at St Thomas' Hospital, London. His name is also given to the mucoid substance of the umbilical cord (Wharton's jelly).

circle of Willis The arterial anastomosis at the base of the brain.
Thomas Willis (1621–1675), practised medicine in Oxford and then London. Buried in Westminster Abbey.

foramen of Winslow The opening into the lesser sac (epiploic foramen).
Jacob Winslow (1669–1760), born in Denmark and became Professor of Anatomy and Surgery, Paris.

Wirsung's duct The main pancreatic duct.
Johann Wirsung (1600–1643), Professor of Anatomy, Padua, where he was assassinated!

Wolffian body and ducts The mesonephros and its ducts.
Caspar Wolff (1733–1794), born in Berlin; Professor of Anatomy, St Petersburg. One of the pioneers of embryology.

Wormian bones Occasional accessory bones between the parietal and occipital bones.
Ole Worm (1588–1654), Professor of Anatomy, Copenhagen.

Index

A

B

C

F

I

J

K

L

M

N

O

P

Q

R

T

W

X

Y

Z